Length

INCHES TO CENTIMETERS

1 inch increments Example: To obtain centimeters equivalent to 22 inches, read "20" on top scale, "2" on side scale; equivalent is 55.9 centimeters.

Inches	0	10	20	30	40
0	0	25.4	50.8	76.2	101.6
1	2.5	27.9	53.3	78.7	104.1
2	5.1	30.5	55.9	81.3	106.7
3	7.6	33.0	58.4	83.8	109.2
4	10.2	35.6	61.0	86.4	111.8
5	12.7	38.1	63.5	88.9	114.3
6	15.2	40.6	66.0	91.4	116.8
7	17.8	43.2	68.6	94.0	119.4
8	20.3	45.7	71.1	96.5	121.9
9	22.9	48.3	73.7	99.1	124.5

One-quarter (¼) inch increments Example: To obtain centimeters equivalent to 14¾ inches, read "14" on top scale, "¾" on side scale; equivalent is 37.5 centimeters.

10–15 Inches

	10	11	12	13	14	15
0	25.4	27.9	30.5	33.0	35.6	38.1
¼	26.0	28.6	31.1	33.7	36.2	38.7
½	26.7	29.2	31.8	34.3	36.8	39.4
¾	27.3	29.8	32.4	34.9	37.5	40.0

16–21 Inches

	16	17	18	19	20	21
0	40.6	43.2	45.7	48.3	50.8	53.3
¼	41.3	43.8	46.4	48.9	51.4	54.0
½	41.9	44.5	47.0	49.5	52.1	54.6
¾	42.5	45.1	47.6	50.2	52.7	55.2

NOTE: 1 inch = 2.540 centimeters. Centimeter equivalents rounded one decimal place by adding 0.1 when second decimal place is 5 or greater, for example, 33.48 becomes 33.5.

Weight (Mass)

POUNDS AND OUNCES TO GRAMS

Example: To obtain grams equivalent to 6 pounds, 8 ounces, read "6" on top scale, "8" on side scale; equivalent is 2948 grams.

						POUNDS									
	0	1	2	3	4	5	6	7	8	9	10	11	12	13	14
0	0	454	907	1361	1814	2268	2722	3175	3629	4082	4536	4990	5443	5897	6350
1	28	482	936	1389	1843	2296	2750	3203	3657	4111	4564	5018	5471	5925	6379
2	57	510	964	1417	1871	2325	2778	3232	3685	4139	4593	5046	5500	5953	6407
3	85	539	992	1446	1899	2353	2807	3260	3714	4167	4621	5075	5528	5982	6435
4	113	567	1021	1474	1928	2381	2835	3289	3742	4196	4649	5103	5557	6010	6464
5	142	595	1049	1503	1956	2410	2863	3317	3770	4224	4678	5131	5585	6038	6492
6	170	624	1077	1531	1984	2438	2892	3345	3799	4252	4706	5160	5613	6067	6520
7	198	652	1106	1559	2013	2466	2920	3374	3827	4281	4734	5188	5642	6095	6549
8	227	680	1134	1588	2041	2495	2948	3402	3856	4309	4763	5216	5670	6123	6577
9	255	709	1162	1616	2070	2523	2977	3430	3884	4337	4791	5245	5698	6152	6605
10	283	737	1191	1644	2098	2551	3005	3459	3912	4366	4819	5273	5727	6180	6634
11	312	765	1219	1673	2126	2580	3033	3487	3941	4394	4848	5301	5755	6209	6662
12	340	794	1247	1701	2155	2608	3062	3515	3969	4423	4876	5330	5783	6237	6690
13	369	822	1276	1729	2183	2637	3090	3544	3997	4451	4904	5358	5812	6265	6719
14	397	850	1304	1758	2211	2665	3118	3572	4026	4479	4933	5386	5840	6294	6747
15	425	879	1332	1786	2240	2693	3147	3600	4054	4508	4961	5415	5868	6322	6776

(Side scale = OUNCES)

NOTE: 1 pound = 453.59237 grams; 1 ounce = 28.349523 grams; 1000 grams = 1 kilogram. Gram equivalents have been rounded to whole numbers by adding 1 when the first decimal place is 5 or greater.

Handbook of Neonatal Intensive Care

GERALD B. MERENSTEIN, M.D., F.A.A.P.

Professor of Pediatrics;
Director of Newborn Services;
Director, Lubchenco Center for Perinatal Research,
Education, Follow-up, and Epidemiology,
University of Colorado Health Sciences Center,
Denver, Colorado

SANDRA L. GARDNER, R.N., M.S., P.N.P.

Neonatal/Perinatal/Pediatric Consultant;
Director, Professional Outreach Consultation;
Formerly Assistant Professor,
University of Colorado School of Nursing,
Denver, Colorado

SECOND EDITION

with 229 illustrations

The C.V. Mosby Company

ST. LOUIS · BALTIMORE · PHILADELPHIA · TORONTO   1989

📖 Mosby

Editor: William Grayson Brottmiller
Senior developmental editor: Sally Adkisson
Project manager: Kathleen L. Teal
Manuscript editor: Judith Bange
Design: Liz Fett
Production: Ginny Douglas, Judith Bange

SECOND EDITION

The C.V. Mosby Company
11830 Westline Industrial Drive, St. Louis, Missouri 63146

Library of Congress Cataloging in Publication Data

Handbook of neonatal intensive care.

Includes bibliographies and index.
1. Neonatal intensive care—Handbooks, manuals, etc.
2. Pediatric nursing—Handbooks, manuals, etc.
I. Merenstein, Gerald B. II. Gardner, Sandra L.
[DNLM: 1. Critical Care—in infancy & childhood.
2. Infant, Newborn, Diseases—nursing. WS 420 H236]
RJ253.5.H36 1989   618.92'01   88-13712
ISBN 0-8016-3415-6

V/D/D 9 8 7 6 5

Contributors

Steven H. Abman, M.D.
Assistant Professor of Pediatrics,
University of Colorado Health Sciences Center,
Denver, Colorado

Eugene W. Adcock III, M.D.
Professor of Pediatrics and of Obstetrics, Gynecology,
   and Reproductive Sciences;
Director, Division of Neonatal-Perinatal Medicine,
University of Texas Health Science Center,
Houston, Texas

Joanne Bartram, R.N., M.S.
Perinatal Clinical Specialist,
Albuquerque, New Mexico

Patricia Beachy, R.N., M.S.
Manager of Perinatal Services,
The Children's Hospital/St. Anthony Hospital,
Denver, Colorado

Carita Bird, R.N., LTC, ANC, USA
Head Nurse, Pediatrics,
Darnall Army Hospital,
Fort Hood, Texas

W. Woods Blake, M.D.
Neonatologist,
TC Thompson Children's Hospital Medical Center,
Chattanooga, Tennessee

Coralie Bonnabel, R.N., B.S., M.B.A.
Nursing Administrator II,
University of Colorado Health Sciences Center,
Denver, Colorado

Sara Browder, R.N., M.S.N.
Assistant Nurse Manager, Pediatric Renal Unit,
University Children's Hospital at Hermann,
University of Texas Health Science Center,
Houston, Texas

Frederic W. Bruhn, M.D., Col, MC
Chief, Department of Pediatrics,
Fitzsimons Army Medical Center,
Aurora, Colorado

John Burrington, M.D.
Pediatric Surgeon,
The Children's Hospital,
Denver, Colorado

Brian Carter, M.D., Maj, MC
Fellow in Neonatal-Perinatal Medicine,
University of Colorado Health Sciences Center,
Denver, Colorado

William H. Clewell, M.D., F.A.C.O.G.
Phoenix Perinatal Associates,
Associate Director, Maternal-Fetal Medicine,
Good Samaritan Hospital,
Phoenix, Arizona

Carol Ann Consolvo, R.N., M.S.
Assistant Professor of Pediatrics,
University of Texas Health Science Center,
Houston, Texas

Audrey J. Costello, M.S.W., L.S.W. II
Social Worker, Department of Pediatrics,
University of Colorado Health Sciences Center,
Denver, Colorado

Elaine Daberkow, R.N., M.S.N.
Pediatric Cardiology, Clinical Specialist,
University of Colorado Health Sciences Center;
Senior Instructor, University of Colorado School of
   Nursing,
Denver, Colorado

Jane E. DiGiacomo, M.D.
Fellow in Neonatal-Perinatal Medicine,
University of Colorado Health Sciences Center,
Denver, Colorado

Susan M. DiStefano, R.N., M.S.N.
Nurse Manager, Turner Neonatal Intensive Care Unit,
University Children's Hospital at Hermann,
University of Texas Health Science Center,
Houston, Texas

Cheryl Ellis-Vaiani, R.N., M.S.N., Maj, ANC
Formerly Clinical Nurse Specialist, Newborn Service,
Fitzsimons Army Medical Center,
Aurora, Colorado

Loretta Forlaw, R.N., M.S.N., Maj, ANC
Clinical Nurse Specialist, Nutritional Support,
    Department of Nursing,
Walter Reed Army Medical Center,
Washington, D.C.

C. Gilbert Frank, M.D., Lt Col, MC
Chief, Newborn Service,
Fitzsimons Army Medical Center,
Aurora, Colorado

Sandra L. Gardner, R.N., M.S., P.N.P.
Neonatal/Perinatal/Pediatric Consultant;
Director, Professional Outreach Consultation;
Formerly Assistant Professor,
University of Colorado School of Nursing,
Denver, Colorado

Kelduyn R. Garland, M.S.W., L.C.S.W.
Executive Director,
The RPLG Group, Inc.,
Chapel Hill, North Carolina

Stephen M. Golden, M.D.
Director, Neonatology,
Overlook Hospital,
Summit, New Jersey;
Associate Professor of Pediatrics,
Uniformed Services University of the Health
    Sciences,
Bethesda, Maryland;
Clinical Associate Professor of Pediatrics,
Columbia University, College of Physicians and
    Surgeons,
New York, New York

Olga R. Gunnell, R.N., M.S.N., CCRN
Martin Army Community Hospital,
Fort Benning, Georgia

Mary I. Hagedorn, R.N., M.S.
Pediatric Practitioner-Teacher,
University of Colorado Health Sciences Center,
Denver, Colorado

William W. Hay, Jr., M.D.
Professor of Pediatrics;
Head, Section of Neonatology;
Director, Neonatal Clinical Research Center,
University of Colorado Health Sciences Center,
Denver, Colorado

Betty Jones, R.N., B.S.N.
Formerly Infection Control Nurse,
Letterman Army Medical Center,
Presidio of San Francisco, California

Joseph W. Kaempf, M.D.
Fellow in Neonatal-Perinatal Medicine,
University of Colorado Health Sciences Center,
Denver, Colorado

Howard W. Kilbride, M.D.
Neonatologist,
Children's Mercy Hospital;
Associate Professor, Department of Pediatrics,
University of Missouri School of Medicine,
Kansas City, Missouri

Cyndi J. Lepley, R.N., M.S., P.N.P.
Director of Maternal Child Nursing,
St. Francis Regional Medical Center,
Wichita, Kansas

Lula O. Lubchenco, M.D.
Professor Emerita,
University of Colorado Health Sciences Center,
Denver, Colorado

Gerald B. Merenstein, M.D., F.A.A.P.
Professor of Pediatrics;
Director of Newborn Services;
Director, Lubchenco Center for Perinatal Research,
    Education, Follow-up, and Epidemiology,
University of Colorado Health Sciences Center,
Denver, Colorado

Stacy L. Merenstein, O.T.R.
The Children's Hospital,
Denver, Colorado

Chester J. Minarcik, Jr., M.D.
Head, Division of Pediatric Neurology;
Director, Pediatric EEG Laboratory;
Assistant Professor of Pediatrics and Neurology,
University of Medicine and Dentistry/Robert Wood
    Johnson Medical School at Camden,
Camden, New Jersey

Claudia Moore, R.N.
Staff Nurse, University Hospital,
University of Colorado Health Sciences Center,
Denver, Colorado

Askold D. Mosijczuk, M.D., Col, MC
Chief, Pediatric Hematology-Oncology Section,
Department of Pediatrics,
Fitzsimons Army Medical Center,
Aurora, Colorado;
Clinical Associate Professor of Pediatrics,
University of Colorado Health Sciences Center,
Denver, Colorado

M. Gail Murphy, M.D., Maj, MC
Assistant Professor of Pediatrics and Pharmacology,
Uniformed Services University of the Health
    Sciences,
Bethesda, Maryland;
Clinical Pharmacologist, Walter Reed Army Institute
    Research,
Washington, D.C.

Jayne P. O'Donnell, R.N., M.S., Maj, ANC
Doctoral Student,
University of Texas at Austin,
Austin, Texas

William H. Parry, M.D., Col, MC
Commander,
Irwin Army Community Hospital,
Fort Riley, Kansas

Dolores Y. Peters, RNC, M.S.N., C.R.N.P.
Clinical Nurse Specialist, Neonatal;
Formerly Coordinator of Comprehensive Neonatal
    Care Course,
Newborn and Intensive Care Nurseries,
Naval Hospital,
Bethesda, Maryland

Gary Pettett, M.D., Col, MC, USA
Director, Section on Neonatal Medicine,
Department of Pediatrics,
Uniformed Services University of the Health
    Sciences,
Bethesda, Maryland

John R. Pierce, M.D., Col, MC
Consultant in Pediatrics to the Surgeon General
    (Army);
Washington, D.C.

Ronald Portman, M.D.
Assistant Professor of Pediatrics,
Pediatric Nephrology Division;
Pediatric Nephrologist, Pediatric Renal Unit,
University Children's Hospital at Hermann,
University of Texas Health Science Center,
Houston, Texas

Linda Powers, R.N., B.S.N.
Administrative Nursing Supervisor,
The Children's Hospital,
Denver, Colorado

Julie Sandling, M.Div.
Chaplain,
University of Colorado Health Sciences Center,
Denver, Colorado

Roberta Siegel, M.S.W.
Perinatal Social Worker,
The Children's Hospital,
Denver, Colorado

John W. Sparks, M.D.
Associate Professor of Pediatrics;
Chairman, Ethics Committee,
University Hospital,
University of Colorado Health Sciences Center,
Denver, Colorado

Barbara S. Turner, R.N., M.A., M.S., Ph.D., Maj, ANC
Director of Research Nursing,
Walter Reed Army Medical Center,
Washington, D.C.

Reginald L. Washington, M.D., F.A.A.P., F.A.C.C.
Associate Professor of Pediatrics,
University of Colorado Health Sciences Center;
Staff Cardiologist,
The Children's Hospital,
Denver, Colorado

Leonard E. Weisman, M.D., Lt Col, MC
Assistant Professor of Pediatrics,
Uniformed Services University of the Health
   Sciences,
Bethesda, Maryland

To Bonnie, Scott, Stacy, and Ray with love
for their patience and understanding
G.B.M.

In memory of Stephanie Marie Gardner,
whose three days of life did have a purpose
S.L.G.

NOTICE

Since some of the drugs mentioned in this book have not been approved by the FDA for use in neonates, caution should be exercised in their use. We have tried to ensure that the dosage schedules provided are accurate and meet current conventional standards. Changes in treatment may occur with new information from research or clinical experience. The reader should consult the package insert for changes in dosage, indications, and contraindications.

Preface

The concept of the team approach is important in neonatal intensive care. Each health professional must not only perform the duties of his or her own role, but must also understand the roles of other involved professionals. Nurses, physicians, and other health care professionals must work together in a coordinated and efficient manner to achieve optimal results when they are caring for patients in the neonatal intensive care unit (NICU).

Because this team approach is so important in the field of neonatal intensive care, we believed that it was necessary that this book contain input from both major fields of health care—medicine and nursing. Therefore it has been coedited by a physician and a registered nurse. In addition, the chapters have been contributed by both physicians and nurses.

The book is divided into five parts. Parts I through IV are the clinical sections, and this second edition contains several additions—a chapter on obstetric influences on the fetus and newborn, a chapter on neonatal kidney physiology and problems, and a chapter on pharmacology in neonatal intensive care. An easy reference guide to tables, figures, and lists of particular importance to the clinician has been added in order to make them more accessible to the reader. The combina-

tion of physiology and pathophysiology and separate emphasis on clinical application in these sections is designed for neonatal intensive care nurses, nursing students, medical students, and pediatric, surgical, and family practice housestaff. These sections are comprehensive enough for physicians and nurses, yet are basic enough to be useful to all ancillary personnel.

Part V presents the psychosocial aspects of neonatal care. The medical, psychologic, and social aspects of providing care for the ill neonate and family are discussed. This second edition contains a new chapter on the impact of the NICU enviornment on neonatal development and a chapter on ethical issues in the NICU. This section will benefit social workers and clergy who frequently deal with family members of patients in the NICU. Of course, it will also be a valuable resource for all other involved health care professionals.

In this handbook we present physiologic principles and practical applications and point out areas as yet unresolved. **All material that is clinically applicable is set in boldface type so that it will be easily identified.**

Gerald B. Merenstein
Sandra L. Gardner

Acknowledgments

I would like to thank the numerous fellows, housestaff, and nurses at Fitzsimons Army Medical Center and University Hospital, University of Colorado Health Sciences Center, who have taught me the importance of the team approach to neonatal intensive care and shared the joys and disappointments of our patients and their families over the years. William Silverman, M.D., and Lillian Blackmon, M.D., taught me the art and science of neonatology. They taught me to always question our practices and to try to improve our knowledge and understanding so that we could provide more appropriate care to our patients and ideally minimize any harm we might cause. Daniel Plunket, M.D., James Shira, M.D., and Fred Battaglia, M.D., have always provided me full support for clinical and research activities within their department. Fred Battaglia, M.D., Lula O. Lubchenco, M.D., and L. Joseph Butterfield, M.D., welcomed me into the Denver neonatal community and encouraged my professional growth. There are no words to express my deep appreciation for their support, guidance, and friendship.

G.B.M.

Many personal and professional experiences have influenced the writing of this book. Thomas A. Courtenay, M.D., stimulated my earliest interest in neonatal care, and Celia D. Blanks, R.N., M.S., challenged me to develop to my maximal potential. In an overcrowded, understaffed neonatal intensive care unit at the Children's Hospital (Louisville, Kentucky), I learned from colleagues such as Sherry Walsh, R.N., and the medical staff what "collaborative care" really means. As Perinatal Outreach Education Coordinator (National Foundation March of Dimes Grant), I had the opportunity to work with L. Joseph Butterfield, M.D., and Frederic C. Battaglia, M.D. While patiently enduring my attempts "to change the world in a week," they both encouraged my creativity, independence, teaching, and management skills. Such teaching associates as Bev Morgan, R.N., Linda Tauchen, R.N., M.S., and B.J. Snell, R.N., M.S., contributed quality and expertise to every program. Colleagues Cyndi Lepley, R.N., M.S., P.N.P., and Rosalind Losey, R.N., M.S., are always a source of strategy as well as support in perinatal community projects. A special thanks to Jimmie Lynne Avery, Executive Director, Lact-Aid International, for her special editorial assistance with the breastfeeding chapter. Kelduyn Garland, M.S.W., L.C.S.W., a perinatal social worker with whom I have taught, discussed, and mutually experienced crisis and grief, has facilitated a deeper understanding of myself and the families I serve.

S.L.G.

Contents

Important Figures, Tables, and Lists

Chapter 25   Ethics in neonatal intensive care

PART I

Support of the Neonate

CHAPTER 1

Regionalization and transport in perinatal care

GARY PETTETT · CORALIE BONNABEL · CARITA BIRD

REGIONALIZATION
History

Care of the high-risk perinatal patient has been one of the most rapidly evolving areas of pediatrics and obstetrics. From its beginning with a relatively few, small premature centers staffed by dedicated physicians and nurses, neonatology has grown into a labor- and capital-intensive, technologically sophisticated subspecialty area. The apparent success of neonatology and newborn intensive care in reducing neonatal mortality has been gratifying.[11,17,47,50] More recently obstetricians have developed techniques for identifying and managing pregnancies believed to be at a particular risk for adverse perinatal outcome.[20,26] Support for these programs rests with the concept that early assessment and planned management by the perinatal team will further reduce perinatal mortality and morbidity.

The factors responsible for this growing interest in reproductive efficiency are multiple. During the first half of this century, the approach to medical care in the United States was rather individualistic. Communities, hospitals, and professional groups attempted to provide up-to-date medical care in a singular and competitive fashion. Using this approach, infant mortality continually declined through the 1940s. Then between 1950 and 1965 neither infant, neonatal, nor perinatal mor-

□ The opinions and assertions in this chapter are those of the authors and do not necessarily represent those of the Department of the Army or the Department of Defense.

tality declined significantly.[37] Attitudes toward medical care in general and perinatal care in particular began to change. The number of live births lessened, fertility rates fell, families became smaller, and the use of contraceptives increased.

In 1966 the American Medical Association Committee on Maternal and Child Care focused attention on the problem of infant mortality.[14] The committee placed emphasis on the identification of risk factors and problems of prematurity; organization and delivery of special care services; use of manpower; further development of perinatal research; and education of obstetricians, pediatricians, and expectant parents. In addition, the Eighty-ninth Congress passed two major federal health acts that were forerunners of regionalized health care. Public Law 89-239, Regional Medical Programs (RMP), concentrated on delivery of service by disease category, and Public Law 89-749, Comprehensive Health Planning (CHP), dealt with plans for using resources. Unfortunately, neither act carried any real administrative or financial authority.

Perhaps the most important statement on perinatal care was made in 1971 by the American Medical Association (AMA).[1] The policy statement, "Centralized Community or Regionalized Perinatal Intensive Care," pressed for the development of centrally operated special care facilities. It encouraged the training of personnel, formulation of guidelines and evaluations, and development of adequate facilities. The AMA Maternal and Child Care Committee was directed to establish the necessary guidelines for regional perinatal programs.[3] In 1972, in conjunction with the National Foundation–March of Dimes, representatives of the American Academy of Pediatrics, the American College of Obstetricians and Gynecologists, the American Academy of Family Physicians, and the American Medical Association met to draft these guidelines. Operating as the Committee on Perinatal Health, their recommendations were published in 1975.[45]

By the middle of the 1970s, the road to regionalization was becoming well traveled. The Robert Wood Johnson Foundation awarded nearly $20 million to eight institutions to test the premise that regional perinatal services improve the possibilities for satisfactory pregnancy outcome. Federal expansion of Title V (Social Security Act of 1935) by Public Law 92-345 required all organized maternal and child health programs to address five separate areas:

1. Maternal and infant care
2. Family planning
3. Child and youth programs
4. Dental care
5. Intensive infant care

Each state was required to develop programs in intensive infant care that addressed the location of perinatal centers, type of care offered, type of transport systems used, and plans for regionalization. Regional centers were to serve as resources for referral while establishing education and counseling services for parents and the community.

In December of 1975 the AMA House of Delegates adopted a resolution entitled "Availability of Health Services in Rural Areas." This report included the following recommendation[2]:

That the AMA communicate with state medical associations suggesting that they, through their component societies, work with appropriate local health planning bodies to assist rural communities in a logical health services area to coordinate and share their health resources on a regional basis.

Administrative and financial authority for regionalization were given new strength with the passage of Public Law 93-641, the National Health Planning and Resource Development Act. The intent of this legislation was to standardize effective methods of delivering health care, redistribute health care facilities, and offset the increasing costs of health care. Planning was facilitated by establishing Health Systems Agencies (HSA) or State Health Planning Agencies. Regional goals were to be developed by joint efforts of health care professionals and local citizenry working within a health department or HSA subunit. By 1979 there were more than 200 recognized regional neonatal and perinatal centers in the United States.[44]

Intensive care transport is now an integral part of regional perinatal programs. Recognition of this fact has led to a willingness by third-party and state insurance carriers to pay transport costs.[33] However, recent changes in the economics of medical practice (health maintenance organizations, diagnostic related groups) present new challenges for regionalization. Today, the concept of regionalization and perinatal transport must interface with a new and intensely competitive medical practice environment.[22]

Objectives

The efficient management of limited health care resources has been one of the major reasons behind efforts to regionalize perinatal care. The capital necessary to underwrite the technology, facilities, manpower, training, and liability exposure for a perinatal/neonatal center is enormous. If every hospital providing pediatric or obstetric care were to invest in tertiary neonatal-perinatal care, the costs to the consumer and public might well price these services beyond affordability. In many metropolitan areas the duplication of services risks the underutilization of perinatal/neonatal centers. The skills of highly trained individuals would be infrequently practiced when high-risk pregnancies (10% to 20% of all deliveries) and potentially ill neonates (5% to 10% of all newborns) are spread throughout a system with redundant services. As specialized skills become rusty, the quality of care tends to drop, and the final impact on perinatal outcome may be less than anticipated.

Since the common goal for the entire program is to improve the outcome of pregnancy, development of a regional perinatal system requires optimal distribution of facilities and personnel, balancing a reliable access to care against the costs, and efficient use of limited resources. Attention must be given to coordinating efforts; communicating information; developing educational programs for health professionals and consumers; and establishing the guidelines by which the program will be monitored and evaluated.

Planning

The process of planning and decision making are the tools by which the separate elements of the regional system are drawn together in a cohesive unit. The fundamentals of regional planning can be outlined in a general fashion[37,53]:

I. Regional survey
    A. Demography
    B. Geography and climate
    C. Relation of existing medical centers to pediatric and obstetric units
II. Assessment of current facilities
    A. Number of beds
    B. Available equipment
    C. Available manpower
III. Regional and administrative organization
    A. Establish objectives
    B. Provide for general administration, planning, consultation, and surveillance
    C. Monitor outcome
    D. Evaluate cost and cost-effectiveness
IV. Organization of lines of communication
V. Organization of transportation

The methods by which a regional program accomplishes these fundamental tasks will be important to the success of regionalization.

Although political boundaries (states) may not always coincide with regional boundaries, for economic and legislative reasons it is probably most appropriate to organize professional and community support for regionalization at the state level. Participants in regional planning will vary from area to area depending on the existing health care systems. Representation should be gathered from broadly based groups reflecting the area's geographic and demographic diversity. Local groups in particular can be active in helping define regional problems and suggesting remedial activities. In many instances established local programs can be strengthened or expanded. Institutional and individual priorities must be assessed while continually seeking the understanding and support of both the local and regional constituency.

Coordination of effort at the planning stage alone can be a tremendous administrative task. It may frequently be easiest to form a perinatal regional planning committee within previously existing organizational structures (Figure 1-1). Model recommendations have been provided by the AMA Maternal and Child Care Committee through its *Action Guide for Maternal and Child Care Committees.*[3]

Implementation

The implementation of a regional perinatal program requires specific operational objectives for the network of providers[35]:

1. High-risk perinatal patients must be identified during the early prenatal period, intrapartum period, and neonatal period.
2. Hospitals must establish criteria for the transfer of mothers and infants within the region.
3. Support systems must be developed for consultation, laboratory services, education, and transport.

A conceptual model of a regional perinatal system is presented in Figure 1-2. The Committee on Perinatal Health has developed specific guidelines for the division of services within a region[45]

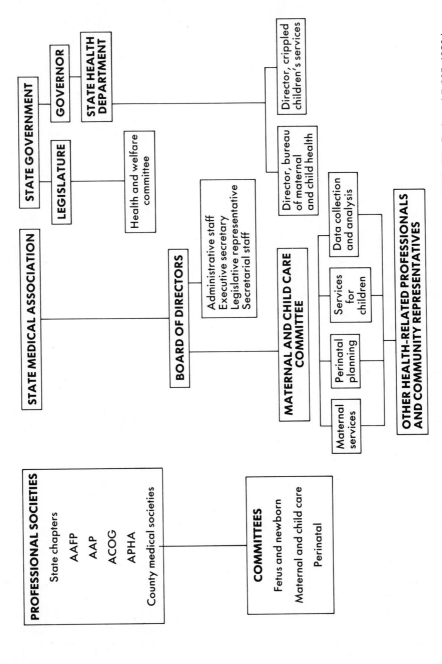

Figure 1-1. Organization of state maternal and child care committee. (From Meyer HBP: Clin Perinatol 7:205, 1980.)

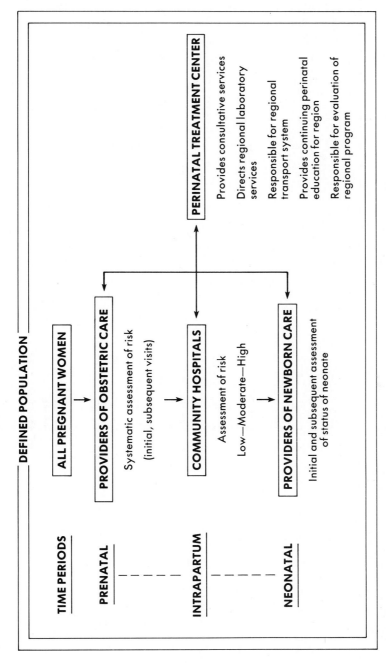

Figure 1-2. Conceptual model of regional perinatal system within defined geographic area. (From Merkatz IR and Johnson KG: Clin Perinatol 3:271, 1976.)

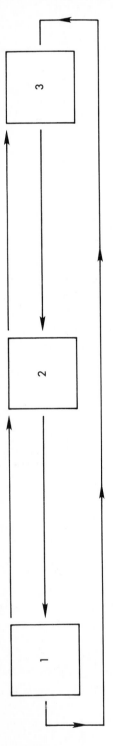

LEVEL 1 TO LEVEL 2

COMPLICATED CASES NOT
REQUIRING INTENSIVE CARE

LEVEL 1 TO LEVEL 3

COMPLICATED CASES
REQUIRING INTENSIVE CARE

LEVEL 1
(RESPONSIBILITIES)

1. Uncomplicated maternity
    and neonatal care for areas
    not served by other units

2. Emergency management of
    unexpected complications

SPECIAL SERVICES

1. Early identification of
    high-risk patients

2. Preventive and social
    services

LEVEL 2 TO LEVEL 3

COMPLICATED CASES REQUIRING
INTENSIVE CARE
1. Labor less than 34 weeks gestation
2. Severe isoimmune disease
3. Severe medical complications
4. Anticipated need for neonatal surgery

LEVEL 2
(RESPONSIBILITIES)

1. Complete maternity and neonatal
    care for uncomplicated and
    most high-risk patients

SPECIAL SERVICES

1. 15-minute start-up time for
    cesarean section
2. 24-hour in-house anesthesia
    for obstetrics
3. Short-term assisted ventilation
    of newborn
4. 24-hour clinical laboratory
    services
5. 24-hour radiology services
6. 24-hour blood bank services
7. Fetal monitoring
8. Special care nursery

**LEVEL 3 OR LEVEL 2 TO HOSPITAL OF
ORIGIN**

FOR GROWTH AND DEVELOPMENT OF
INFANTS NO LONGER REQUIRING
INTENSIVE CARE

LEVEL 3
(RESPONSIBILITIES)

1. Complete maternity and neonatal
    care plus intensive care of intrapartum
    and neonatal high-risk
    patients

SPECIAL SERVICES

1. 24-hour consultation service for
    region
2. Coordination of transport system
3. Development and coordination of
    educational program for region
4. Data analysis for region

Figure 1-3. Consultation and possible transfer patterns in regional system. (From Ryan GM: Am J Obstet Gynecol 46:375, 1975.)

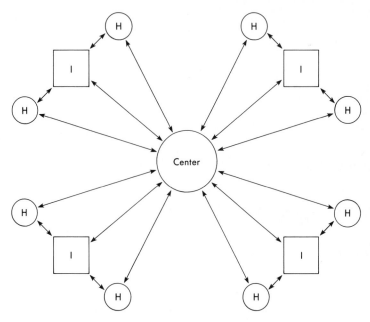

Figure 1-4. Lines of communication and referral in regional perinatal system. *H*, Community hospital; *I*, intermediate care facility. (Redrawn from Butterfield LJ: Clin Perinatol 3:281, 1976.)

(Figure 1-3). Detailed criteria for the various levels of care are contained in this committee's published report. For regionalization to work, the unique roles of the various professionals within the system must be recognized. The division of services (level I, level II, etc.) represents a consensus of community investment and does not reflect the level of local professional talent. The pregnant woman and her infant must remain the focus of attention and concern.

A perinatal/neonatal center is commonly located at a university or large community medical facility. The center provides the focal point for the entire region. Figuratively, it forms the axle in the wheel of a regional perinatal program (Figure 1-4). Among its responsibilities are services for consultation, education, communication, transportation, and data accumulation and analysis. The center's personnel must recognize the fact that some faculty members will spend large portions of their time outside the center to provide

these services. In corporate terms these individuals function as the "detail team," updating customers on recent developments and executing the public relations work crucial to the marketing of perinatal services. These tasks must be recognized within the academic environment as a part of the center's responsibilities.

Results

Areas in which regional perinatal programs have been developed are reporting improved survival rates from neonatal intensive care units.[30,43,51,52] Retrospective studies in Arizona[36] and Wisconsin[46] before the development of regional programs found that 40% to 50% of the perinatal casualties could have been prevented with techniques currently available but poorly distributed. With established intensive care programs, neonatal mortality began to drop. Perhaps some of the most demonstrative data come from the Quebec Perinatal Committee.[54] Comparative data

TABLE 1-1

Perinatal Mortality and Utilization of Neonatal Intensive Care (IC) Services, Quebec 1967-1969

	INTRAMURAL NEONATAL IC	REFERRAL NEONATAL IC	NEITHER INTRAMURAL NOR REFERRAL NEONATAL IC
Number of births	20,176	35,289	105,467
Neonatal mortality per 1000 live births			
1001-2500 g	64	74	81
Over 2500 g	2.0	2.1	3.4
Total	6.3	7.4	9.4
Stillbirth rate per 1000 total births	8.5	9.5	9.9
Perinatal mortality per 1000 total births	14.7	16.9	19.1

From Avery GB: Neonatology, ed 2, Philadelphia, 1981, JB Lippincott Co. Data obtained from obstetric services in Montreal and Quebec City delivering more than 1000 infants per year, considering births over 1000 g birth weight and deaths up to 7 days. By permission of the Quebec Perinatal Committee, 1973.

TABLE 1-2

Reduction in Perinatal Asphyxia with Perinatal Intensive Care (Royal Victoria Hospital, Montreal)

	1965-1969 (BEFORE PERINATAL UNIT)	1970-1972 (WITH PERINATAL UNIT IN OPERATION)	1970 (PROVINCE OF QUEBEC)
Number of births	14,619	5784	—
Severe birth asphyxia per 1000 births	11.7	5.9	—
Postasphytic convulsions per 1000 births	1.2	0.2	—
Postasphytic cerebral depression per 1000 births	2.8	1.7	—
Asphytic fetal deaths during labor per 1000 births	3.6	1.2	2.8

From Avery GB: Neonatology, ed 2, Philadelphia, 1981, JB Lippincott Co. Modified from Gosselin P, Roy A, Desjardins DA, and Usher R: By permission of the Quebec Perinatal Committee, 1973.

show that neonatal mortality was lower when an intensive care referral unit was used with a further reduction in neonatal mortality when the intensive care unit was actually located at the point of delivery (Table 1-1). Similar improvements in perinatal morbidity and mortality were shown in other Canadian cities with the development of neonatal centers (Tables 1-2 and 1-3).

Since 1975 several studies have attempted to show further reduction in perinatal mortality with high-risk antenatal maternal transfer.[12,24,34,40] Despite the fact that the logic seems correct and data from these studies show lower mortality and morbidity among antepartum transfers, firm proof is lacking. Comparison of maternal and neonatal transfers is probably not legitimate. Maternal referrals are generally made for *potential* problems (which may be alleviated after referral), whereas neonates are more likely referred for *actual* problems. The lower mortality among antenatal referral patients is not surprising; however, evaluation of maternal transfers will likely need more refined measures of outcome to prove any distinct advantage.[41]

TABLE 1-3

Impact of Intensive Care (IC)

	HOSPITAL	BEFORE IC	AFTER IC		
Stillbirth rate (per	St. Boniface, Winnipeg	8.8	3.5	1973	
1000 births)	St. Joseph's, London	10.4	7.3	1969	
	Women's College, Toronto	—	8.3	1978	
	Royal Victoria, Montreal	—	6.9	1970-1972	Fetal and neonatal IC
	Queen's, Halifax	20.8	12.0	1965-1968	
Neonatal mortality	St. Boniface, Winnipeg	5.0	3.5	1973	<1000 g
rate (up to 6 days,	Women's College, Toronto	10.6	6.2	1971	
per 1000 live	Women's College, Toronto	—	5.6	1978	
births)	Jewish General, Montreal	7.6	6.4	1973	
	Jewish General, Montreal	—	3.7	1974	
	Jewish General, Montreal	—	3.4	1975	
	Queen's, Halifax	17.0	9.9	1965-1968	<500 g
Perinatal mortality	St. Boniface, Winnipeg	13.9	7.0	1973	<1000 g
rate (per 1000 live	St. Joseph's, London	21.6	19.0	1969	<500 g + SB
births)	Women's College, Toronto	20.5	14.8	1971	Neonatal IC
	Women's College, Toronto	—	13.9	1978	Fetal and neonatal IC
	Royal Victoria, Montreal	19.1	15.2	1970-1972	Neonatal IC
	Royal Victoria, Montreal	—	11.6	1970-1972	Fetal and neonatal IC
	Jewish General, Montreal	20.9	14.9	1973	
	Jewish General, Montreal	—	9.0	1974	
	Queen's, Halifax	—	8.9	1975	
	Grace, Halifax	12.5	7.7		Before and after fetal IC

From Avery GB: Neonatology, ed 2, Philadelphia, 1981, JB Lippincott Co.

REGIONAL TRANSPORT

An established perinatal transport service is a key element in a regional perinatal program. In its most efficient form the transport service functions within a region of graded health care responsibilities. At the primary care level methods must exist to identify high-risk mothers and infants, project potential health care needs, and locate the appropriate support. The transport service provides the patient(s) with access to the required level of care. In addition, it should ensure that mothers and infants reach the appropriate facility without jeopardizing or interrupting their care. Neither the transport service nor the regional center can support a *triage en masse* of all high-risk mothers or infants. The system must be selective and above all based on a reasonable anticipation of the patient's needs.

Maternal referrals

Many high-risk pregnancies can be identified before the onset of labor.[20,26] Social, demographic, and medical-obstetric risk factors that correlate with fetal outcome have been identified.[27] Some of these factors can be elicited with a thorough maternal history and physical examination on the first prenatal visit. Other factors appear only during follow-up prenatal visits, and a final group may not appear until the intrapartum period. Some of the most commonly encountered risk factors include:

I. Prenatal
  A. History
    1. Sociodemographic
      a. Low socioeconomic status
      b. Ethnic minority
      c. Low educational level

d. Emotional instability
e. Substance abuse (use)
    (1) Alcohol
    (2) Drugs, medications
    (3) Cigarettes
f. Age (over 35 or under 15 years)
g. Multiparity

2. Medical-obstetric
    a. Moderate to severe renal disease
    b. Chronic hypertension
    c. Moderate to severe toxemia
    d. Organic heart disease, class 2 to 4
    e. Prior Rh sensitization, prior history of erythroblastosis fetalis
    f. Previous stillbirth
    g. Previous premature infant
    h. Previous neonatal death
    i. Previous cesarean section
    j. Habitual abortion
    k. Prior infant over 10 pounds birth weight
    l. Sickle cell disease
    m. History of tuberculosis or PPD positive
    n. History of genital herpes

B. Physical examination and prenatal follow-up
    1. Severe toxemia, hypertension
    2. Severe renal disease
    3. Severe heart disease, class 2 to 4
    4. Acute pyelonephritis
    5. Diabetes mellitus
    6. Uterine malformation
    7. Incompetent cervix
    8. Abnormal fetal position
    9. Polyhydramnios or oligohydramnios
    10. Abnormal cervical cytology
        a. Dysplasia
        b. Herpes
    11. Multiple pregnancy
    12. Rh sensitization
    13. Positive serology
    14. Vaginal bleeding

II. Intrapartum
    A. Maternal
        1. Moderate to severe toxemia
        2. Polyhydramnios or oligohydramnios
        3. Amnionitis
        4. Uterine rupture
        5. Premature rupture of membranes
        6. Premature labor
        7. Labor lasting over 20 hours
        8. Second stage of labor over 2½ hours
        9. Precipitous labor (<3 hours)
        10. Prolonged latent phase of labor
        11. Uterine tetany
    B. Placenta
        1. Placenta previa
        2. Abruptio placentae
        3. Postterm (over 42 weeks completed gestation)
        4. Meconium-stained amniotic fluid
    C. Fetal
        1. Abnormal presentation
        2. Multiple pregnancy
        3. Fetal bradycardia
        4. Prolapsed cord
        5. Fetal weight less than 2500 g
        6. Fetal acidosis, pH less than 7.25
        7. Fetal tachycardia
        8. Operative or vacuum delivery
        9. Difficult forceps delivery

Both retrospective and prospective studies have shown a strong statistical correlation between pregnancy risks and fetal morbidity and mortality.[25,49] In actual practice risk assessment provides an appropriate means for grouping populations of patients into risk groups, but it functions somewhat less optimally in determining the necessity of a referral for the individual patient. Part of this discrepancy may be accounted for by the variability with which risk factors may cluster in a given patient, part may relate to the interaction of simultaneously occurring risk factors, and part may represent the variable impact of each individual factor on the pregnancy.

Pregnancy screening represents only a general

mechanism by which the physician may categorize patients for management. Consultation and referral decisions will have to be made based on more concrete information from each individual pregnancy.

The following specific maternal conditions are examples of the types of problems that frequently lead to specialized care in a perinatal center.[10] This specialized care is especially necessary when the probability of any of the following conditions exists for delivery of an infant before 34 weeks of gestation and/or at an estimated weight of less than 2000 g:

I. Obstetric complications
   A. Premature rupture of the fetal membranes
   B. Premature onset of labor
   C. Severe preeclampsia or hypertension
   D. Multiple gestation
   E. Intrauterine growth retardation with evidence of fetal distress
   F. Third trimester bleeding
   G. Rh isoimmunization
   H. Premature cervical dilation
II. Medical complications
   A. Maternal infection that may affect the fetus or lead to premature birth
   B. Severe organic heart disease, class 3 to 4
   C. Thyrotoxicosis
   D. Renal disease with deteriorating function or hypertension
   E. Drug overdose
III. Surgical complications
   A. Trauma requiring intensive care
   B. Acute abdominal emergencies
   C. Thoracic emergencies requiring intensive care

Occasionally, high-risk pregnancies will be identified that are not covered by any of the preceding situations. The decision to transport to a perinatal care center must be based on the relationship between the patient's projected care needs and the locally available resources.

In many instances patient referral may not be nearly as essential as medical consultation. Certainly if treatment within the home community is a prime objective, consultative services provide an important support element, which will affect both the quantity and quality of perinatal transports. The practical considerations of individual patients and of the diverse medical communities will continue to require decisions unique to each regional program.

Neonatal referrals

The transport service in a regional perinatal system must be capable of responding to both maternal and neonatal problems. Despite maximal efforts to detect maternal risk, nearly 30% of all perinatal mortality will occur in women not suspected of being at risk.[29] In other instances complications may occur acutely during the intrapartum period when transport is not reasonable. For the critically ill neonate, immediate care and stabilization must occur at the point of delivery. Supportive care needs to be maintained until the infant is either out of danger or the transport team has arrived and assumed care.

Selection of appropriate infants for neonatal transport is generally somewhat easier than for maternal transport. For neonatal referrals, unlike maternal transfers, the object of major concern, the infant, is readily available for direct examination and observation.

Before the development of specialized care centers for neonates, birth weight alone was the most commonly used indicator of maturity and morbidity-mortality risk. Little was known of deviations in intrauterine growth patterns. As interest in the premature infant has increased, data have been accumulated on the physical characteristics and neurologic developments that occur with increasing gestational age.[4,39] Examination of the newborn provides the most satisfactory method for assessing or confirming gestational age. Estimates may be obtained from physical characteristics, neurologic examination, or a combination of the two.[18] The larger the number of items examined, the more accurate is the assessment. For prediction of particular problems, information on gestational age should be obtained as soon after birth as possible. Unfortunately, portions of the examination may not be valid at this time. Particularly in infants with severe intrapartum stress (asphyxia), the neurologic examination may not be reliable. For such infants a combination of physical characteristics and pregnancy milestones (heart tones, fundal heights, ultrasound studies) may be the most accurate. Several examination methods using numeric indexes and computed averages for gestational aging have been published.[6,18] The error in prediction for the majority of these examinations is approximately ±2 weeks. By combining weight and accurate gestational aging, growth patterns for both the fetus and neonate can be constructed.[31] Together these factors allow us to classify each newborn into one of nine possible birth weight (small, appropriate, and large) and gestational age (term, preterm, postterm) categories.[32] Having determined the infant's birth weight, gestational age, and intrauterine growth pattern, the physician or nurse is better able to project potential mortality, morbidity, and the most likely causes of each.[8,30]

Once the gestational age–birth weight assessment and risk analysis have been made, attention needs to be directed toward those factors accounting for potential risks. Many of these abnormalities show a particular propensity for certain intrauterine growth patterns.[30] **The following outline lists factors that need to be addressed during stabilization for each growth group:**

I. **Premature infants**
   A. **Support pulmonary transition to extrauterine life**
      1. **Maintain oxygenation and ventilation**
      2. **Watch for respiratory distress and apnea**
   B. **Support cardiovascular function**
      1. **Maintain pulmonary and tissue perfusion**
      2. **Watch for hypovolemia and shock**
   C. **Provide temperature support**
      1. **Increased heat losses**
      2. **Restricted ability to generate body heat**
   D. **Avoid central nervous system complications**
      1. **Poorly coordinated suck and swallow may delay enteral feeding**
      2. **Impaired respiratory control with apnea and bradycardia**
   E. **Appreciate renal immaturity**
      1. **Lower glomerular filtration rate**
      2. **Impaired ability to excrete or conserve a salt and water load**
   F. **Follow bilirubin**
      1. **Increased production**
      2. **Poor albumin-bilirubin binding**
      3. **Delayed conjugation and excretion**
   G. **Monitor hematologic status**
      1. **Stress may lead to disseminated intravascular coagulation**
      2. **Watch for hemorrhagic diathesis and intracranial hemorrhage**

II. **Term infants**
   A. **Provide thermal support**
      1. **Avoid cold stress**
   B. **Record and follow vital signs**
   C. **Screen for hypoglycemia, polycythemia, and hypothyroidism**
   D. **Watch for analgesic and narcotic depression**
   E. **Screen for congenital anomalies**

III. **Postterm infants**
   A. **Provide thermal support**
      1. **Relative high surface area/metabolic rate ratio**
   B. **Observe for respiratory distress and aspiration**
   C. **Screen for hypoglycemia and polycythemia**
   D. **Record vital signs and observe through transitional period**

IV. **Large-for-dates infants**
   A. **Screen for congenital anomalies and syndromes**

B. **Screen for hypoglycemia and hypocalcemia**

C. **Screen for Rh isoimmunization, and infant of a diabetic mother**

D. **Watch for respiratory distress, especially in the infant of a diabetic mother**

E. **Provide thermal support**

V. **Small-for-dates infants**

A. **Search for anomalies and syndromes**

B. **Screen for perinatal infections**

C. **Watch for withdrawal symptoms (narcotics, barbiturates)**

D. **Provide thermal support, prevent cold stress**

E. **Assess for hypoglycemia and polycythemia**

The decision to transfer a high-risk or ill neonate is similar to the decision to transfer the high-risk mother. Specific criteria will have to be developed within each region based on needs (real or projected) of the infant and local resources. Premature infants from 28 to 34 weeks gestation will generally need maximal physiologic support and should be best cared for in a well-equipped intensive care unit. Between 34 and 38 weeks gestation, premature infants can frequently be managed in a less complicated environment. Attention to considerations such as thermal support, glucose levels, fluid therapy, hematocrit, bilirubin, ventilation, and perfusion may frequently be of a lower order of magnitude than in the very small infant.

The major problems that the term infant faces are those of adaptation. Many of these transitional problems are under the direct control of the delivery room or hospital staff. The most serious problems are generally the result of intrapartum events. Asphyxia neonatorum and meconium aspiration may frequently be severe enough to warrant extensive support and prompt referral. Life-threatening congenital anomalies or those requiring surgical intervention are best dealt with at a specialized center.

Postterm infants are at greatest risk during the latter part of pregnancy. Deterioration of placental function may result in suboptimal intrauterine nutrition and depleted fetal metabolic reserves. Many of these infants are candidates for antenatal transfer for fetal monitoring. Postdates infants transferred in the neonatal period are most likely to be those suffering the consequences of intrapartum stress (asphyxia neonatorum and meconium aspiration).

Large-for-gestational-age infants are often the offspring of large parents. Mothers of growth-accelerated infants tend to be older, taller, heavier, and of greater parity.[30] Maternal height and infant birth weight have been positively correlated. Several perinatal problems common to large infants may need to be handled in the perinatal center; these include Beckwith-Wiedemann syndrome, Rh isoimmunization, and transposition of the great vessels. A macrosomic infant of the diabetic mother (usually class A) can usually be cared for at the same hospital as the mother except perhaps for infants with congenital defects.

Unlike the large-for-gestational-age infant, pathologic conditions frequently occur in infants who are small-for-gestational-age. Anatomic malformations, structural malformations, and perinatally acquired infections (viral and protozoal) most frequently require referral.

Communication and consultation

Communication systems are important factors in any regional perinatal program. Any one of a variety of devices may be used. The particular format selected will depend on the type of information to be transmitted and the population to be targeted:

1. Television and newspaper—public information, human interest stories
2. Pamphlets and brochures—periodic reports, reviews of specialized or general interest
3. Videotape and closed-circuit television—educational and informational material to health care personnel within the region
4. Radio—specialized communication systems for use during transport (ground-to-ground, ground-to-air)

Despite these alternatives, the telephone remains the most commonly used link in the perinatal network. Within the communication system, the highest priority must be placed on requests for medical consultation and/or consideration for patient referral. This service generally can be provided by a dedicated telephone line to the center. The line must be unencumbered by other requirements of the special care unit. The use of dedicated telephone lines is not new to medical or emergency units. Service of this type can frequently be made available through the telephone system serving the receiving hospital.

Direct and immediate communication with the perinatal center should be made as easy as possible. Toll free or "800" telephone numbers can be employed. Mnemonics such as "-BABY," "NEWBORN," or "-NICU" for all or parts of the center's phone number can be of assistance in remembering the appropriate number. For the most frequent users, a direct, nondial "hot line" can provide immediate access to the unit. Appropriate consultants should be available at the center on a 24-hour-a-day, 7-day-a-week basis. Although it may not be necessary to have a physician (neonatologist or perinatologist) respond to each call, one should be readily available at all times. Cost for the system should be borne by the regional program and not by the referring physician, hospital, or patient.

Information transmitted over the telephone must be relevant to the caller and the patient's particular problem. For critically ill neonates, the initial call may be crucial to the infant's survival. The referring personnel must be able to provide the center staff with the most accurate medical information possible. It is frequently helpful to have a checklist of pertinent information available (Figure 1-5). This can help guide patient assessment and suggestions for interim care while awaiting the transport team.

Based on the initial conversation with the referring facility, the individual receiving the call may have to make a number of decisions:

1. Determine the need for medical consultation with a neonatologist or perinatologist.
2. If multiple calls have been received, priorities must be assigned.
3. Determine the composition of the team.
4. Determine whether extra or accessory equipment may be needed (e.g., ventilator).
5. Alert the receiving center of potential diagnostic and therapeutic needs.

Whether the calls are received by a physician, transport team member, or professionally (medically) trained dispatcher will vary with different regional programs. Junior personnel (trainees) and staff members who are not active in newborn or maternal transport should not perform this function. These individuals generally lack experience in neonatal and maternal care. For a variety of reasons, they frequently do not interact well with referring physicians or other health professionals.

A final and perhaps most overlooked priority in communication occurs at the conclusion of a transport. Once the patient has arrived at the center, a call should be placed to the referring physician, parents, and/or spouse. The purpose of the call is to relay information regarding the patient's condition and to indicate the scope of immediate care plans. If parents do not accompany their infant(s), or a husband his wife, a number at the center should be made available for the family to maintain contact. Ideally the center unit would make frequent calls to the parents, keeping them informed on both progress and problems. At all times a line of immediate contact must be available should the patient's condition suddenly change.

Preparation for transport

The goal of every transport is to bring a sick neonate or high-risk mother to a tertiary care center in stable condition. To avoid intra-transfer complications, the infant should be as stable as possible before leaving the referring hospital. In most instances this process should

INFANT TRANSPORT	TODAY'S DATE	
(Worksheet only - NOT TO BE FILED IN MEDICAL RECORD)		

TIME CALL RECEIVED	REFERRING HOSPITAL	TIME DEPART MAMC	TIME ARRIVED DESTINATION

VEHICLE USED

☐ AMBULANCE   ☐ HELICOPTER   ☐ AIRPLANE

PHYSICIAN	NURSE	91C

✓	CHECKLIST
	1. Unit clean and ready to use.
	2. Battery pack.
	3. Oxygen pressure:
	Bottom tanks:
	4. Heart rate monitor.
	5. Temperature monitor, (skin sensor) rectal thermometer.
	6. Oxygen monitor.
	7. Holter pump, extra tubing and solution.
	8. Oxygen mask, bag, Hope/Dragger, tubing and adapter.
	9. Extra apparatus for provision of CPAP.
	10. Gavage set (feeding tube and syringe).
	11. Stethescope.
	12. Wash cloths and Septisol.
	13. Diapers, cloth and disposable.
	14. Infant blankets, silver swaddler.
	15. Suction equipment: DeLee and bulb syringe.
	16. Umbilical catheter set.
	17. Medications not kept in med box: Heparin

COMMENTS

Continued.

Figure 1-5. Infant transport form.

DATE		DATE OF DELIVERY		TIME OF DELIVERY		

INFANT'S NAME			SEX		GESTATION	

MOTHER		AGE	RACE	RELIGION

FATHER		AGE		SSN

OCCUPATION	BRANCH	RANK	UNIT		HOME PHONE

EMPLOYER	ATTENDING PHYSICIAN	PHONE

HOSPITAL OF DELIVERY	TYPE OF DELIVERY	BIRTH WEIGHT	WEIGHT AT TRANSPORT	APGAR

✓	Must-have list
	1. Copy of infant's chart
	2. List any vital information of family
	3. Laboratory flow sheet
	4. Last blood gases: pH P_{O_2} P_{CO_2} HCO_3 BE O_2 Sat %
	5. Have eyes been rinsed with $AgNO_3$?
	6. Has vitamin K been given?
	7. Feedings: NPO H_2O Glucose H_2O Formula Breast
	8. Has infant voided? Had BM?
	9. Blood type: Baby: Mother: Cord specimen: Maternal specimen:
	10. Has infant been baptized? By whom? Date:
	11. Stomach contents emptied?
	12. Instructions for future contact with family: *HAVE MOTHER TOUCH.*
	13. Last vital signs before transport: T P R B/P
	14. Respiratory effort: RA Oxygen CPAP Respirator
	15. Medications: (a) Mother during pregnancy:
	(b) Infant to include IV:

COMMENTS

Figure 1-5, cont'd. Infant transport form.

actually begin before the transport team arrives. The primary physician and hospital personnel should have a good understanding of what these processes are (see Chapters 2 through 8).

In maternal transport the most common reasons for referral include premature rupture of the membranes, premature onset of labor, and pregnancy-associated hypertension. The factors requiring most immediate attention in these instances are the likelihood of labor, status of delivery, and fetal well-being. A good physical and obstetric examination, prenatal record review, and evaluation of fetal heart rate and activity would constitute a minimum of data. After consultation with the receiving hospital, further measures may be indicated before transport, depending on the referring hospital's capabilities. These include an ultrasound examination, nonstress test, fetal scalp pH test, and an amniocentesis. If needed, magnesium sulfate, tocolytic agents, antibiotic agents, or antihypertensive agents should be administered at this time. A complete copy of the patient's records (hospital and prenatal), results of any laboratory tests, heart rate monitor strips, x-ray examination, and notation of all medications (with the times and doses given) should be ready to accompany the patient.

Although the reasons for neonatal referral may be quite diverse, the most frequent indications are respiratory distress or complications of prematurity. The following procedures should begin as soon as the infant's problems are recognized to ready the patient for transfer[19]:

1. Administer vitamin K (Aquamephyton), 0.5 to 1 mg intramuscularly (IM).
2. Administer narcotic antagonist in the face of potential narcotic depression—Narcan (Naloxone), 0.005 mg/kg intravenously (IV) or IM.
3. Record all intake and output from the time of delivery.
4. Record the time of the first urine and meconium passage.
5. Record the quantity of gastric aspirate in the delivery room.
6. Record vital signs.
7. Record the oxygen concentration given.
8. Record the temperature of the neonate (skin, axillary) and incubator.
9. Record treatment rendered in the delivery room, positive-pressure ventilation, amount of oxygen used, drugs given, fluid given, and Apgar scores.
10. Record all results of x-ray reports, laboratory tests, and any significant signs and symptoms.
11. Maintain good color; monitor blood gases if possible.
12. Maintain a clear airway.
13. Maintain thermal support.
14. Maintain adequate hydration.
15. Obtain a maternal blood sample (clotted).
16. Obtain maternal vaginal cultures for amnionitis cases or prolonged rupture of the membranes.
17. Obtain a copy of all neonatal laboratory and x-ray results and records.
18. Obtain consent forms for immediate procedures.
19. Obtain a copy of prenatal and intrapartum records.
20. Obtain the family background and historical information.

As with maternal transfers, copies of all the obtained information (just listed) should be available at the time of transfer. When possible, a properly fixed placenta should be sent for pathologic examination. The mother and/or infant should always remain at the hospital until the transport team arrives. It is never wise to send the patient ahead with plans to meet the transport en route.

Whenever possible, the transport team should make contact with the parents (in a neonatal transport) or spouse (in a maternal transport) before departing for the center. This offers the parents or spouse the opportunity to meet the interim care team, ask questions, and receive information about where and how the patient will be cared for. The transport team leader can explain how the transport will occur, approximately how long it will take, and what will be done en route. In the case of neonatal transports, the parent(s) should be encouraged to touch, look at, and talk to the baby. No matter how long or short the separation will be, this may be an important factor in the bonding of the parent(s) to the infant and how well they tolerate the impending separation.[28] This brief period of time spent with the parents may go a long way in helping parents deal with the emotional trauma they are experiencing and may well continue to face.

Information regarding the tertiary center should be left with the parents. This should include:

1. Exact location of the unit—address, map
2. Visiting hours and hospital rules
3. Telephone numbers
4. Names of individuals likely to be involved with the patient's care
5. Information on the special care unit—what it is, what it does
6. Location of parking facilities, nearby lodging, and rules regarding young children (siblings)
7. Any particular rules or regulations regarding the special care unit

Transport team

The critically ill infant or high-risk mother is best served when he or she is accompanied in transit by personnel who are adequately trained in the areas of neonatal and perinatal care.[15] If transport is not an everyday affair, team personnel can generally be drawn from the nursery or perinatal duty roster. When transports are more frequent than 1 per day (300 per year), a separate team and roster may be required to prevent chronic understaffing at the center.[19] The organizational structure of regional programs will frequently place the transport team at the perinatal center, but depending on the regional referral pattern and hospital loca-

tions, there may be instances, such as with an intermediate or community hospital, where the transport team is not located at the center.[23] In a metropolitan area or where a transport team serves more than one local center, the team members may be drawn from multiple units.[13,42]

Transport teams have been composed of a variety of different personnel.[42] This is not surprising when one remembers that a central theme in regionalization has to do with efficient use of *available* resources. There are two common principles to be met for membership on the transport team. First, the members of the transport team must have documented evidence of their ability to care for maternal and neonatal problems. Second, the transport team should reflect as closely as possible the patient's needs.

As with perinatal care in general, the central figures of the team will always be the physician and nurse. The decision to use a physician in transport must be balanced against the other, equally important responsibilities of a physician. Availability of physician coverage in the center must be weighed against the patient's potential problems in transport. For most appropriately staffed centers, coverage at the center should be an exceedingly rare problem. Some of the larger referral services may have physicians specifically assigned to transport or a diversity of resources from which to draw.[13,19] There are circumstances where a physician's presence may be specifically indicated. Still, a significant number of transports can be safely and efficiently accomplished with appropriately trained and ancillary personnel.[42] These circumstances should be predetermined for each individual transport service.[10,19]

In the last few years increasing emphasis has been placed on the expanding role of nurses in the clinical setting. Nurse clinicians now exist in a number of health care areas, including pediatrics, obstetrics, and neonatology. In obstetrics nurses have become active in following the course of pregnancy through delivery as nurse midwives. As the nurse's training and responsibilities have increased, his or her inclusion in various aspects of neonatal or perinatal care, including transport, have been logical if not necessary steps.[9] Throughout the country, regional perinatal programs have developed nurse training courses to help fill the need for perinatal personnel. Most of these programs combine both formal teaching sessions and practical on-the-job training. Their duration varies from 6 months to 1 year. At the completion of training the nurse should be able to[7,19]:

1. Identify risk factors during pregnancy and predict problems at delivery
2. Perform neonatal resuscitation
3. Identify and treat respiratory distress, asphyxia, pulmonary air leaks, and apnea in the newborn
4. Handle psychosocial problems of families and mothers
5. Obtain a complete family, social, economic, and medical history
6. Perform a neonatal examination for clinical condition and gestational age
7. Provide perinatal teaching to community and local hospital personnel
8. Collaborate effectively with other perinatal health team members
9. Participate in relevant perinatal experimental and clinical research

For personnel who are frequently involved in air transport, the following additional requirements are appropriate:

10. Have a thorough knowledge of flight physiology
11. Have knowledge of aircraft and aircraft safety

Respiratory therapists have been a third frequently mentioned member of the neonatal transport team.[19] Their presence may be particularly helpful with infants with respiratory disease who require ventilatory assistance. Members should be thoroughly familiar with neonatal respiratory needs and be drawn from a pool of therapists who would normally work within the newborn special care unit.

Ambulance drivers, attendants, and pilots have traditionally not been active in nor specifically trained for neonatal care. As their training is upgraded (emergency medical technician, paramedic), it is conceivable that their roles could increase.[21]

One of the most important aspects of the transport team is its need to function as a unit. To this end, all members from ambulance driver to physician must participate in some shared training and evaluation. Each member of the team must recognize the unique abilities and responsibility of every other member. Together they must appreciate the needs of the patient and be able to jointly plan the safest and most expedient transport. Ongoing educational sessions and transport critiques provide excellent means for this interaction to occur. Frequently overlooked but ever present is the need for the entire team to be involved in accident survival drills to prepare for the unforeseen intratransport accident.

The lines of responsibility during a transport must be clearly defined. Written job descriptions may provide useful tools for achieving this goal. When a physician is present, he or she is clearly charged with the medical responsibility. In the absence of the physician, the senior transport nurse must assume that role. Responsibility for the vehicle is generally that of the ambulance driver or pilot. CAUTION: The decision to move in inclement weather, the route to follow, and the maintenance of a safe speed are best decided by an appropriately trained driver or pilot who has been informed of the patient's condition. This information should be shared and updated during the entire transport. The lives and safety of the team and patient must take precedence over expedience. Melodrama should be confined to the television screen.

In their capacity as a transport team, members must interact with the medical personnel at the regional hospitals. Regardless of the patient's condition when the team arrives, it is best to remember that the local hospital personnel have likely performed to the limits of their capabilities and are duly concerned for the patient's welfare. A demeaning or patronizing attitude with editorial overtones on the part of team members can easily defeat months of work establishing interhospital liaison. Rather, the team should view the hospital visit as both a learning and teaching experience. Members of the transport team should become familiar with the region's hospitals, their capabilities, and the people who make them function. The objective is to establish rapport and an esprit de corps toward a common goal. During the visit the transport team may have the opportunity to demonstrate techniques of stabilization, discuss management problems, or perhaps offer advice on recent or projected equipment purchases. The best results occur where both the team and the referring personnel learn, so that both may function better for the experience.

Equipment

The biomedical equipment and pharmaceutical industries are developing products for the neonate at a rate that is virtually impossible to keep up with. One need only glance at a few current pediatric or obstetric journals to appreciate the volume of advertisements for a great variety of equipment. The scope of this section does not allow us to consider all equipment in detail. Publications dealing solely with transport have touched on these issues.[20,48] The goal in this section is to discuss equipment needs in general terms and to point out some of the key factors in equipment selection.

Maternal transports can frequently require the addition of a significant amount of equipment. If the mother is not in active labor or delivery is remote, only equipment to continue the mother's care is necessary. However, if the mother is in labor, on tocolysis, or the transport time is quite long, it may be necessary to carry equipment for maternal treatment, delivery, and resuscitation of the infant. In these instances space and weight considerations can be important factors in determining the timing and mode of transport. A list of commonly used equipment for maternal transport is given below[19]:

I. Equipment
  A. Kelly clamps (4)
  B. Cord clamps
  C. Sponges (4 by 4 inches)
  D. Sponge stocks (2)
  E. Tape
  F. Red top laboratory tubes (4)
  G. Gloves (variety of sizes)
  H. Suture (repair) set
  I. Pudendal block set
  J. IV infusion equipment
    1. IV poles
    2. One-half normal saline (two 1 L bottles)
    3. 5% dextrose in water (D_5W) (two 1 L bottles)
    4. Ringer's lactate (two 1 L bottles)
    5. Blood administration set
    6. Infusion pump
    7. 25% and 50% dextrose vials
    8. Assorted needles and syringes
    9. Angiocatheters
    10. Adult arm boards
  K. Blood pressure apparatus
  L. Tourniquet
  M. Fetal heart monitor
  N. Assorted suture material
  O. Speculum
  P. Portable light source
  Q. Buckets (2)
  R. Scissors (2)
  S. Suction bulb and ear syringe
  T. Povidone-iodine (Betadine) sticks
  U. Adult oxygen masks and nasal cannula
II. Drugs
  A. Meperidine (Demerol) ampules, 50 mg, 75 mg
  B. Hydralazine (Apresoline), 20 mg ampule (5)
  C. Naloxone (Narcan), adult, 0.4 mg ampule
  D. Magnesium sulfate, 10% IV solution, 50% IM solution
  E. Phenobarbital, 120 mg vial
  F. Promethazine (Phenergan), 25 mg/ml

G. Diazoxide (Hyperstat), 300 mg ampule
H. Furosemide (Lasix), 20 mg or 40 mg
I. Hydroxyzine (Vistaril), 50 mg/ml
J. Oxytocin (Pitocin), 10 units/ml
K. Calcium gluconate, 1 g/10 ml
L. Methergine, 0.2 mg/ml
M. Lidocaine (Xylocaine), 1%, no epinephrine
N. Isoxsuprine (Vasodilan), 10 mg/ml
O. Terbutaline (Brethine), 80 mg in 500 ml $D_5\frac{1}{4}$ normal saline
P. Ritodrine (Yutopar) solution, 150 mg/500 ml (0.3 mg/ml)

The equipment required for neonatal transport is similar to that used in the newborn intensive care unit. Essential equipment includes that for environmental control; cardiorespiratory, temperature, blood pressure, and oxygen monitoring; suction; IV therapy; and ventilatory support. When selecting equipment, consideration must be given to the geography of the region, its climate, and the modes of transport that will likely be used.

Since much of the major equipment is electronic, these units must be easily adaptable to the types of power supply used in transport. All electronic equipment used in transport should be supplied with battery-operated capability. The batteries should be able to support the equipment for the entire transport if no other power source is available. Conversion devices are often needed to allow use of 12 V and $^{24}/_{28}$ V DC and 100 V/60 Hz AC current. For aircraft transport a converter for 100 V AC current may also be useful. Adequate grounding of electrical equipment is as important during transport as it is in the special care unit. Equipment used in air transport must also meet Federal Aviation Agency's (FAA) requirements. Some of the monitoring devices on the market today may interfere with aircraft navigational equipment. Equipment of this type should not be taken on air transport, particularly where instrument flying is to be used.

In most system designs, the transport incubator is the central piece of neonatal equipment. It must be capable of controlling the infant's immediate environmental condition and of allowing sufficient access to manage a critically ill patient. In regions where extreme climates may be encountered, the unit should possess satisfactory heating and ventilation capabilities. The incubator should be mounted on or built into an easily movable stand that can be locked or fixed into position during transport. Some transport incubators are designed to include all the required monitoring devices. Since the incubator will need to be lifted on and off the transport craft, total weight becomes an important factor in selecting these units. The unit must be light enough to be easily lifted by the crew or transport team.

Since many neonates are transported for reasons of respiratory distress, oxygen and air-blended mixtures are essential. Therefore a source of oxygen and air, plus an appropriate blender and oxygen analyzer, are required. The most convenient gas form for transport is the compressed gas cylinder. The FAA has strict regulations about compressed gas cylinders in aircraft. The transport team should be familiar with these regulations and use appropriately designed cylinders.[19,48] To provide air and oxygen sources within the aircraft, compressed gas cylinders may be carried on board and carried off for use while traveling to and from the aircraft. The transport team should estimate the amount of oxygen and air required for a transport by approximating the distance, time, and infant's needs. The capacity of standard gas cylinders and expected life of the cylinder at various flow rates are listed in Table 1-4. Table 1-5 gives the flow rates of oxygen and air required to produce various oxygen concentrations (FIO_2). From this information, estimated gas consumption can be derived.

The neonatal ventilator selected for transport should be appropriate for the type of transport vehicle used, suitably sized to the entire equipment system, and familiar to the transport team. Ventilators may be time cycled, volume cycled, or pressure cycled, and pressure (gas) driven or electrically driven. Ideally the ventilator should be affixed in some fashion to the transport incubator to prevent disconnection from the patient.

The development of portable, low-energy transcutaneous PO_2 ($TcPO_2$) monitors provides the capability of continuously monitoring arterial PO_2 during transport.[16,38] Pulse oximetry and

$TcPO_2/CO_2$ monitors are also available and, though not extensively evaluated during transport, may be useful adjuncts for monitoring intra-transport ventilatory support.

No matter what type of equipment is purchased, maintenance and servicing are important

---

TABLE 1-4

Volume and Flow Duration of Oxygen in Two Sizes of Cylinders

	FULL		¾ FULL		½ FULL		¼ FULL	
Reading on cylinder pressure gauge								
Pressure (lb/in²)	244		183		122		61	
Cylinder type	E	H	E	H	E	H	E	H
Contents (ft³)	22	244	16.5	183	11	122	5.5	61
(liters)	622	6900	466	5175	311	3450	155	1725
Approximate number of hours of flow								
Cylinder type	E	H	E	H	E	H	E	H
Flow rate (liters/min)								
2	5.1	56	3.8	42	2.5	28	1.3	14
4	2.5	28	1.8	21	1.2	14	0.6	7
6	1.7	18.5	1.3	13.7	0.9	9.2	0.4	4.5
8	1.2	14	0.9	10.5	0.6	7	0.3	3.5
10	1.0	11	0.7	8.2	0.5	5.5	0.2	2.7
12	0.8	9.2	0.6	6.7	0.4	4.5	0.2	2.2
15	0.6	7.2	0.4	5.5	0.3	3.5	0.1	1.7

From Segal S: Transport of high risk newborn infants, Canadian Pediatric Society, 1972.

TABLE 1-5

Effective FIo_2 Delivery from Various Combinations of Air and Oxygen Flow*

		$\dot{V}Io_2$ V (OXYGEN FLOW IN LITERS/MIN)								
		1	2	3	4	5	6	7	8	9
$\dot{V}_{air}$ (air flow in liters/min)	10	0.93	0.87	0.82	0.77	0.74	0.70	0.67	0.65	0.63
	9	0.92	0.86	0.80	0.76	0.72	0.68	0.65	0.63	0.61
	8	0.91	0.84	0.76	0.74	0.70	0.66	0.63	0.61	0.58
	7	0.90	0.82	0.76	0.71	0.67	0.64	0.61	0.58	0.56
	6	0.89	0.80	0.74	0.68	0.64	0.61	0.57	0.55	0.53
	5	0.87	0.77	0.70	0.65	0.61	0.57	0.54	0.51	0.49
	4	0.84	0.74	0.66	0.61	0.56	0.53	0.50	0.47	0.45
	3	0.80	0.68	0.61	0.55	0.51	0.47	0.45	0.43	0.41
	2	0.74	0.61	0.53	0.47	0.44	0.41	0.39	0.37	0.35
	1	0.61	0.47	0.41	0.37	0.34	0.32	0.30	0.30	0.29

From Ferrara A and Harin A: Emergency transfer of the high-risk neonate, St Louis, 1980, The CV Mosby Co.

$$*FIo_2 = \frac{0.21\ \dot{V}Io_2 + \dot{V}_{air}}{\dot{V}_{air} + \dot{V}Io_2}$$

considerations. A few key principles to remember are:

1. Replacement parts should be readily available.
2. Local equipment representatives should be available to service the equipment and provide technical updates to the transport team.
3. Warranty and maintenance contracts should be easily obtained.
4. Loan equipment should be available when major equipment is being repaired.
5. Hospital biomedical engineers should be familiar with the equipment and provide routine preventive and reparative maintenance.

A list of commonly used equipment and supplies for neonatal transport is provided below:

I. Equipment
   A. Battery operated
      1. Transport incubator
      2. Cardiorespiratory monitor
      3. Blood pressure monitor
      4. Suction apparatus
      5. Thermometer with skin probe
      6. Oxygen analyzer
      7. IV infusion pump
      8. Laryngoscope with blades (various sizes)
      9. Transcutaneous oxygen monitor
      10. Pulse oximeter
   B. Suction catheters (no. 6, no. 8, and no. 10 Fr)
   C. Bulb/ear syringe
   D. Feeding tubes (no. 5 and no. 8 Fr)
   E. Umbilical arterial catheters (no. 3.5, no. 5, and no. 8 Fr)
   F. Thoracostomy tubes (Red Robinson catheters)
   G. DeLee suction catheters
   H. Three-way stopcocks
   I. Needle (blunt) catheter adapters (18- to 20-gauge)
   J. Scalp vein needles (21-, 23-, and 25-gauge)
   K. Intracaths (22- to 24-gauge)
   L. IV pump tubing
   M. Alcohol swabs
   N. Skin prep swabs (benzoin)
   O. Povidone-iodine (Betadine) swabs
   P. Umbilical ligature
   Q. 4-0 silk suture with cutting needle
   R. Tape (½ inch and 1 inch)
   S. Povidone-iodine (Betadine) solution
   T. Dextrostix (Ames Laboratories)
   U. Lancets
   V. Capillary tubes
   W. Culture bottles (aerobic, anaerobic)
   X. Syringes (various sizes)
   Y. Needles (various sizes)
   Z. Gauze pads (2 by 2 inch, 4 by 4 inch)
   AA. Monitor (ECG) leads
   BB. IV filters
   CC. Blood pressure transducers with domes
   DD. Sterile water vials
   EE. Bacteriostatic saline bottles (30 ml)
   FF. Endotracheal tubes (2.5, 3, 3.5, and 4 mm)
   GG. Stylets for endotracheal tubes
   HH. Heimlich valves
   II. Flashlight batteries (extras)
   JJ. Laryngoscope bulbs
   KK. Y-connectors
   LL. Oxygen tubing
   MM. Diapers
   NN. Blanket
   OO. Umbilical catheter tray
   PP. Plastic bag
   QQ. Oxygen face masks (sizes 0, 1, and 2)
   RR. Self-inflating resuscitation bag
   SS. Oxygen hood
   TT. Nebulizer
   UU. Flashlight or outdoor light source
   VV. Oxygen and air cylinders
   WW. Stethoscope

II. Drugs
   A. 25% albumin
   B. 5% albumin
   C. Atropine multidose vial
   D. Calcium gluconate, 10% solution
   E. 10% dextrose in water ($D_{10}W$), 250 ml
   F. D_5W, 250 ml

G. Digoxin, 0.5 mg ampule

H. Heparin, 1000 units/ml

I. Isoproterenol (Isuprel), 0.5 mg ampule

J. Tolazoline (Priscoline), 25 mg/ml

K. Furosemide (Lasix), 20 mg ampule

L. Lidocaine multidose vial

M. Naloxone (Narcan), 0.2 mg ampule

N. Sodium bicarbonate, 0.5 mEq/ml

O. Diazepam (Valium), 10 mg vial

P. Phenobarbital, 120 mg vial

Q. Ampicillin

R. Gentamicin

S. Phytonadione (Aquamephyton), 10 mg ampule

T. Dopamine vial

U. Pancuronium (Pavulon)

V. Epinephrine, 1:10,000

W. Ringer's lactate, 250 ml

X. Heparinized flush solution (5% dextrose, 0.16 M 20% sodium lactate, heparin sodium, 2 units/ml)

Y. Prostaglandin (pediatric), 500 μg/ml

IV solutions should be carried in plastic IV bags rather than glass containers. It is useful to have a single case in which to carry the consumable and smaller supplies. At the completion of each transport, the equipment should be checked, batteries charged, and supplies restocked. A checklist of these functions kept with the transport equipment can help ensure timely completion and preparation for the next call.

Mode of transport

Maternal and neonatal transports are most commonly accomplished by either ground ambulance or aircraft. Selection of the mode is based on careful consideration of a number of variables.

DISTANCE

Within a 100-mile radius, the use of surface vehicles seems most appropriate. Very little time is gained by the use of aircraft in this range. Transferring the team and equipment from aircraft to ambulance to hospital at both ends of the transport consumes any time saved in travel. Between 100 and 250 miles, the helicopter is most expedient. Allowing for certain technical difficulties in transport, the helicopter's ability to land near the hospital can still save considerable ground time. Beyond a 250-mile radius, fixed-wing aircraft are probably the vehicles of choice.[42]

LOCAL FACILITIES

The location of landing sites with reference to the referring hospital is an important consideration in air transports. Newer hospitals or recently constructed additions frequently have helicopter landing sites near or on the buildings. If no close landing site is available, the 100-mile-radius guideline for ground transport may have to be disregarded. Fixed-wing aircraft will require some sort of general aviation facility for landing. The landing's proximity to the hospital must be determined, not because it affects the mode of transport, but because of the need for a timely and coordinated ground transfer from plane to hospital.

CREW AVAILABILITY

The availability of ambulance drivers, pilots, and air crews will depend on the relationship between the perinatal center and the ambulance service. Without previous arrangements, ambulances or aircraft may not always be available. If transport volume is large enough, service contracts with carriers may be one solution. Major metropolitan hospitals may even own some of their own ambulance services. For the smaller or less frequent user, availability can be a problem. Alternative plans must frequently be developed for each transport. In this latter system it may not always be possible to immediately respond to or accept a request for referral until a carrier has been identified.

WEATHER

Weather is a factor of primary concern to air transport, although in certain climates extremes of weather may interfere with any form of transport. Weather conditions at the point of origin and destination must be assessed. In case of rapidly changing weather fronts, the projected duration of the trip should be known. For air transports, the decision to fly in difficult weather conditions should be left to the pilot. Regardless of the patient's condition, he or she and the team are safer in the local hospital than on an uncertain flight.

TERRAIN

Local geography is generally a problem in selecting the mode of transport only for the shorter (ambulance or helicopter) trips. The use of aircraft, especially a helicopter, may be advantageous on very short trips when the terrain would not allow a reasonably expedient ground trip. Obstacles such as large bodies of water, mountains, or traffic jams in urban areas are commonly encountered problems.

PATIENT'S CONDITION

Regardless of the mode of transport selected, there must be ample room to care for the patient. Smaller aircraft and low-topped ambulances frequently do not afford this capability. Helicopters have a major disadvantage in this area. Once aboard a helicopter, the team and patient are exposed to an unusual amount of noise, vibration, and rotational forces. Evaluation and monitoring of a patient may be almost impossible. On flights after dusk, lighting in the patient area may interfere with the pilot's night vision. If the mother and/or infant are not adequately stabilized before lift-off, they will not likely become so in flight. For patients whose condition is tenuous or who require constant attention, another mode of transport may be advisable.

Finally, there are a few miscellaneous cautions about selecting the transport vehicle. Never initiate a transfer with a crew that is unfamiliar with the craft. The FAA and many state or county health agencies have certifying procedures for ambulance or aircraft personnel. The regional center should always be sure that the patient and transport team are in the best possible hands for travel.

For each transport, alternative referral sites or temporary stops should be identified. Regardless of the amount of preparation, the possibility of vehicle malfunction or patient deterioration always exists. It may be necessary to stop temporarily for equipment or vehicle repair or for stabilization of the patient.

By whatever means the team is traveling, they should always have access to communication with the center. The center should be kept informed of their progress, the estimated time of arrival, any changes in the patient's condition, and the patient's anticipated needs on arrival. The center should set up a communication relay with the referring hospital to transmit similar information. Should the team be delayed, management advice can be given continually.

Cost, although not necessarily one of the last considerations, is not a prime consideration; however, when all other variables are considered, cost should be kept to a minimum. Generally this is well addressed by tailoring the transport service to the needs of each patient. A properly planned transport should be able to fairly accurately predict its needs.

Stabilization of the infant

The transition from the uterine to extrauterine environment requires a series of complex physiologic changes affecting virtually every organ of the infant's system. How well the infant tolerates the pregnancy, labor, and delivery can have a direct bearing on how smoothly this transition goes. Stabilization involves monitoring the infant throughout the transitional period and treating any abnormalities that, if left unattended, can result in deterioration of the infant's condition. The process can begin during the antepartum period with careful monitoring of the fetus and continue through the early neonatal period. In the infant stabilization focuses attention on six basic physiologic areas:

1. Thermal support (see Chapter 5)
2. Oxygenation and ventilation (see Chapter 17)

3. Acid-base balance (see Chapter 8)
4. Vascular volume and fluid therapy (see Chapters 3 and 10)
5. Metabolic (glucose) support (see Chapter 11)
6. Vital signs (see Chapter 6)

Care of the parents

The advent of regionalization and perinatal transport has brought many new problems. One of the most frequent is the alteration in family ties. The emotional impact resulting from the birth of an ill infant interrupts the normal bonding or attachment of the mother, family, and infant. Transferring the infant to a distant hospital adds an element of physical separation that may greatly aggravate the problem. Parents often feel as though they have lost control of the situation; they may have difficulty understanding all that is happening. They continually fear the worst—their infant has died or will die. Parental attachment becomes difficult. The hospital staff must realize this potential problem and not conclude that the parents are completely indifferent. It is important for nurses and physicians to understand the processes of attachment and grieving, since these processes often intermingle. There are a number of things that hospital staff can do to help parents cope with their relationship with the infant, with each other, and with the staff.

As soon as conditions permit, the parents need to be informed in an honest and forthright manner of their infant's health status. A verbal description of the infant and of the equipment being used is often helpful. As soon as possible, the parents should be allowed to visit their child. Physical contact between parents and infant should be encouraged. Seeing, touching, and talking to their baby can add a measure of reality to allay their fears or fantasies. If the parents cannot visit, self-developing snapshots of the baby can provide alternative contact for the parents.

When both mother and infant have been transported, the normal family support mechanisms for dealing with crisis are disrupted. It is the cen-

ter's responsibility to at least provide alternate mechanisms, such as clergy, social workers, and special parent support groups.

Depending on the distance from the parent's home to the center, lodging and financial assistance may be required. The referral hospital should maintain a listing and provide information about community groups that could be helpful. Every attempt should be made to keep the parents informed, available, and involved in their child's care.

SUMMARY

Perinatology has been one of the most rapidly growing areas of clinical medicine. It now involves a degree of technical and physical sophistication not previously experienced in pediatrics or obstetrics. As a result the limited financial and human resources must be used in an efficient and effective manner. This requires cooperation and coordination between health providers not only locally, but also regionally. This chapter has attempted to provide some basis for the scope of activities encompassed in transport for perinatal care. The elements touched on here represent key features to the success of a very expensive and constantly changing area of care for the mother and her infant.

REFERENCES

1. American Medical Association: Centralized community or regionalized perinatal intensive care (Report J). Adopted by the AMA House of Delegates, June 1971.
2. American Medical Association: Availability of health services in rural areas. Adopted by the AMA House of Delegates, Dec 1975.
3. American Medical Association Committee on Maternal and Child Care: Action guide for maternal and child care committees, Chicago, 1974, American Medical Association.
4. Amil-Tison C: Neurologic evaluation of the maturity of newborn infants, Arch Dis Child 43:89, 1969.
5. Avery GB: Neonatology, ed 2, Philadelphia, 1981, JB Lippincott Co.
6. Ballard JL: A simplified assessment of gestational age, Pediatr Res 11:374, 1977.
7. Barth J: Staff preparation and training for high-risk neo-

natal transport. In Graven S, editor: Newborn air transport, Evansville, Ind, 1978, Mead Johnson.

8. Battaglia FC and Lubchenco LO: A practical classification of newborn infants by birth weight and gestational age, J Pediatr 71:159, 1967.

9. Bellig LL: The expanded nursing role in the neonatal intensive care unit, Clin Perinatol 7:59, 1980.

10. Bowes WA and Merenstein GB: Recommendations and guidelines for the transport of high risk obstetrical patients, Colorado Perinatal Care Council Transport Committee, March 1978.

11. Brann AW: Perinatal health care in Mississippi 1973. In Sunshine P, editor: Regionalization of perinatal care: report of the Sixty-sixth Ross Conference on Pediatric Research, Columbus, Ohio, 1974, Ross Laboratories.

12. Brown FB: The management of high-risk obstetric transfer patients, Obstet Gynecol 51:674, 1978.

13. Butterfield LJ: Newborn Country U.S.A., Clin Perinatol 3:281, 1976.

14. Butterfield LJ: Organization of regional perinatal programs, Semin Perinatol 1:217, 1977.

15. Chance GW, O'Brien MJ, and Swyer PR: Transport of risk infants 1972: unsatisfactory aspect of medical care, Can Med Assoc J 109:847, 1973.

16. Clarke TA et al: Transcutaneous oxygen monitoring during neonatal transport, Pediatrics 65:884, 1980.

17. Day RL: What evidence exists that intensive care has changed survival? In Lucey JF, editor: Problems of neonatal intensive care units: report of the Fifty-ninth Ross Conference on Pediatric Research, Columbus, Ohio, 1969, Ross Laboratories.

18. Dubowitz LMS, Dubowitz V, and Goldberg C: Clinical assessment of gestational age in the newborn infant, J Pediatr 77:1, 1970.

19. Ferrara A and Harin A: Emergency transfer of the high-risk neonate, St Louis, 1980, The CV Mosby Co.

20. Goodwin JW, Dunne JT, and Thomas BW: Antepartum identification of the fetus at risk, Can Med Assoc J 101:458, 1969.

21. Greene WT: Organization of neonatal transport services in support of a regional referral center, Clin Perinatol 7:187, 1980.

22. Hackel A: An organization system for critical care transport, Int Anesthesiol Clin 25:1, 1987.

23. Harris HB et al: Reorganization of regional newborn transport to allow reallocation of medical personnel time, Pediatr Res 11:383, 1977.

24. Harris TR, Isaman J, and Giles HR: Improved survival in very low birth weight premature and postmature neonates through maternal transport, Clin Perinatol 26:180, 1976.

25. Hobel CJ: Perinatal health care in Mississippi 1973. In Sunshine P, editor: Regionalization of perinatal care: report of Sixty-sixth Ross Conference on Pediatric Research, Columbus, Ohio, 1974, Ross Laboratories.

26. Hobel CJ et al: Perinatal and intrapartum high risk screening: prediction of the high risk neonate, Am J Obstet Gynecol 117:1, 1973.

27. Infant death: an analysis by maternal risk and health care, Washington, DC, 1973, Institute of Medicine, National Academy of Sciences.

28. Klaus MH and Kennel JH: Parent-infant bonding, St Louis, 1982, The CV Mosby Co.

29. Ledger WJ: Identification of the high risk mother and fetus: does it work? Clin Perinatol 7:125, 1980.

30. Lubchenco LO: The high risk infant, Philadelphia, 1976, WB Saunders Co.

31. Lubchenco LO, Hansman C, and Boyd E: Intrauterine growth in length and head circumference as estimated from live births from 26-42 weeks, Pediatrics 47:831, 1971.

32. Lubchenco LO, Searls DT, and Brazie JV: Neonatal mortality rate: relationship to birth weight and gestational age, J Pediatr 81:814, 1972.

33. McCarthy JT et al: Who pays the bill for neonatal intensive care? J Pediatr 95:755, 1979.

34. Merenstein GB et al: An analysis of air transport results in the sick newborn. II. Antenatal and neonatal referrals, Am J Obstet Gynecol 128:520, 1977.

35. Merkatz IR and Johnson KG: Regionalization of perinatal care for the United States, Clin Perinatol 3:271, 1976.

36. Meyer HBP: Transportation of high risk infants in Arizona. In Regionalization of perinatal care: report of the Sixty-sixth Ross Conference on Pediatric Research, Columbus, Ohio, 1974, Ross Laboratories.

37. Meyer HBP: Regional care for mothers and their infants, Clin Perinatol 7:205, 1980.

38. Miller C et al: Control of oxygenation during the transport of sick neonates, Pediatrics 66:117, 1980.

39. Mitchell RG and Farr V: The meaning of maturity and the assessment of maturity at birth. In Dawkins M and MacGregor WG, editors: Gestational age, size and maturity, London, 1965, William Heinemann, Ltd.

40. Modenlow HD: Antenatal versus neonatal transport to a regional perinatal center: a comparison between matched pairs, Obstet Gynecol 53:725, 1979.

41. Pettett G: Outcome of maternal air transport. In Graven S, editor: Maternal air transport, Evansville, Ind, 1979, Mead Johnson.

42. Pettett G et al: An analysis of air transport results in the sick newborn infant. I. The transport team, Pediatrics 55:774, 1975.

43. Reynolds EOR and Taghizadeh A: Improved prognoses of infants mechanically ventilated for hyaline membrane disease, Arch Dis Child 49:505, 1974.

44. Ross Planning Associates: Referral centers providing perinatal and neonatal care, Columbus, Ohio, 1979, Ross Laboratories.

45. Ryan GM Jr: Toward improving the outcome of pregnancy, Am J Obstet Gynecol 46:375, 1975.

46. Ryan GM Jr: Regional planning for maternal and perinatal health services, Semin Perinatol 1:255, 1977.

47. Schneider JM: Developmental and educational aspects of a regionalized program. In Sunshine P, editor: Regionalization of perinatal care: report of the Sixty-sixth Ross Conference on Pediatric Research, Columbus, Ohio, 1974, Ross Laboratories.

48. Segal S: Transport of high risk newborn infants, 1972, Canadian Pediatric Society.

49. Sobol RJ et al: Clinical application of high risk scoring on an obstetric service, Am J Obstet Gynecol 134:904, 1979.

50. Stahlman MT: What evidence exists that intensive care has changed the incidence of intact survival. In Lucey JF, editor: Problems of neonatal intensive care units: report of the Fifty-ninth Ross Conference on Pediatric Research, Columbus, Ohio, 1969, Ross Laboratories.

51. Stahlman MT et al: A six year followup of clinical hyaline membrane disease, Pediatr Clin North Am 20:433, 1973.

52. Stewart AL and Reynolds EOR: Improved prognosis for infants of very low birth weight, Pediatrics 54:724, 1974.

53. Swyer P: The regional organization of special care for the neonate, Pediatr Clin North Am 17:761, 1970.

54. Usher RH: Changing mortality rates with perinatal intensive care and regionalization, Semin Perinatol 1:309, 1977.

CHAPTER 2

Prenatal environment: impact on neonatal outcome

JOANNE BARTRAM · WILLIAM H. CLEWELL

The human fetus develops within a complex setting. Structurally defined by the intrauterine/intraamniotic compartment, the character of the prenatal environment is largely determined by maternal variables. The fetus is absolutely dependent on the maternal host for respiratory and nutritive support and is significantly influenced by maternal metabolic, cardiovascular, and environmental factors. In addition, the fetus is limited in its ability to adapt to stress or modify its surroundings. This creates a situation in which the prenatal environment exerts a tremendous influence on fetal development and well-being. This influence lasts well beyond the period of gestation, often affecting the newborn in ways that have profound significance for both immediate and long-term outcome. There is great utility in the identification of maternal factors that adversely impact on the condition of the fetus. Providers of obstetric care have long used this information to identify the "at-risk" population and design interventions that prevent or reduce the occurrence of fetal and neonatal complications. It is equally important that neonatal care providers obtain a clear picture of the prenatal environment and use this information prior to delivery to anticipate the newborn's immediate needs and make appropriate preparations for resuscitation and initial nursery care. Following delivery, an awareness of the likely sequelae of environmental compromise helps to focus ongoing assessment and aids in clinical problem solving.

The purpose of this chapter is to help the neonatal care provider to evaluate maternal influences on the prenatal environment, identify significant environmental compromise, and anticipate the associated neonatal problems. Information on the assessment and treatment of specific neonatal problems is provided throughout this text and is not repeated here. For a more extensive discussion of perinatal physiology and the complicated pregnancy, refer to the references cited within this chapter.

PHYSIOLOGY

Two variables have a critical influence on fetal well-being throughout gestation: placental function and the inherent maternal resources. The interplay of these factors is the major determinant of fetal oxygenation, metabolism, and growth.

The placenta has a dual role in providing nutrients and metabolic "fuels" to the fetus. First, placental secretion of endocrine hormones, chiefly human chorionic somatomammotropin (HCS), increases throughout pregnancy, causing progressive changes in maternal metabolism. The net effect of these changes is an increase in maternal glucose and amino acids available to the fetus, especially in the second half of pregnancy. Second, the placenta is instrumental in the transfer of these (and other) essential nutrients from the maternal to the fetal circulation and, conversely, of metabolic wastes from the fetal to the maternal system.

Fetal "respiration" is also dependent on adequate placental function. Respiratory gases (oxygen and carbon dioxide) readily cross the placental membrane by simple diffusion, with the rate of diffusion determined by the PO_2 (or PCO_2) differential between maternal and fetal blood.

Although the placenta mediates the transport of respiratory gases, carbohydrates, lipids, vitamins, minerals, and amino acids, it is the maternal "reservoir" that is their source. Maternal-fetal transfer depends on the characteristics and absolute content of substances within the maternal circulation, the relative efficiency of the maternal cardiovascular system in perfusing the placenta, and the function of the placenta itself.[108] The fetal environment can be disrupted by inappropriate types or amounts of substances in the maternal circulation, decreases or interruptions in placental blood flow, or abnormalities in placental function.

THE COMPROMISED FETAL ENVIRONMENT
Compromise due to preexisting maternal disease
DIABETES

Despite major reductions in mortality over the past several decades, the infant of a diabetic mother (IDM) continues to have a considerable perinatal disadvantage. The physiologic changes in maternal glucose utilization that accompany pregnancy, coupled with either a preexisting hyperglycemia (as found in type I and II diabetes) or an inability to mount an appropriate insulin response (as seen in the gestational diabetic), results in a fetal environment that is markedly abnormal as a result of the increased level of maternal glucose available to the fetus. Early in pregnancy this environment may actually have a teratogenic effect on the embryo, accounting for the dramatic

increase in congenital malformations in the offspring of diabetic women.[28] During the second and third trimesters the mechanics of placental transport dictate that fetal glucose levels are dependent on, but slightly less than, maternal levels.[87] Assuming adequate placental function and perfusion, elevations in maternal glucose lead to fetal hyperglycemia and increased fetal insulin production. Repeated or continued elevations in blood glucose result in fetal hyperinsulinism, alterations in the utilization of glucose and other nutrients, and altered growth patterns.[41,87]

In addition to the basic metabolic disturbances, diabetes predisposes the woman to a number of other complications, including hypertension, renal disease, and vascular compromise (these additional complications are often described by the use of White's classification system for diabetes in pregnancy). **The various complications of diabetes are also associated with fetal and neonatal problems, including prematurity, growth retardation, chronic hypoxia, and intrauterine demise.[21,85,87] In terms of predicting perinatal morbidity and mortality, the "Prognostically Bad Signs of Pregnancy," first identified by Pedersen in the 1960s, are especially significant. The occurrence of any of these signs, which include diabetic ketoacidosis, pregnancy-induced hypertension, pyelonephritis, and maternal noncompliance, continue to be useful predictors of increased fetal and neonatal risk.[21]**

In preparing for the delivery of an infant of a diabetic mother, the neonatal team should consider the classification of maternal diabetes (type I, II, or gestational diabetes mellitus [GDM]), the quality of glucose control throughout the pregnancy, maternal complications, and the duration of the pregnancy, along with indicators of fetal growth and well-being. Table 2-1 summarizes key maternal factors, their environmental implications, and the fetal and neonatal outcomes associated with diabetes in pregnancy.

TABLE 2-1

Maternal Diabetes, the Prenatal Environment, and Perinatal Outcome

MATERNAL FACTORS	ENVIRONMENTAL IMPLICATIONS	FETAL AND NEONATAL CONSEQUENCES
Hyperglycemia		
Early	Exposure to elevated glucose levels during organogenesis	Increased incidence of congenital anomalies
Late	Availability of excess glucose leads to fetal hyperinsulinism, abnormal growth, and delayed surfactant production	Macrosomia, organomegaly, trauma during delivery, neonatal hypoglycemia, increased incidence of respiratory distress syndrome (RDS), polycythemia secondary to hypoxemia
Ketoacidosis	Fetal exposure to excess glucose and ketones can result in fetal diabetic ketoacidosis[41]	Fetal hypoxemia, intrauterine fetal demise
Hypertension, cardiovascular, and renal disease	Placental insufficiency secondary to vascular compromise results in diminished fetal oxygenation and nutrition	Growth retardation, fetal asphyxia, intrauterine fetal demise, prematurity
	Increased incidence of maternal urinary tract infections	Prematurity, RDS, sepsis

THYROID DISEASE

The thyroid hormones triiodothyronine (T_3), thyroxine (T_4), and thyroid-stimulating hormone (TSH) generally do not cross the placental barrier. The fetal thyroid concentrates iodine and synthesizes its own hormones as early as 10 weeks gestation; this is totally independent of maternal thyroid function.[25] As a result, maternal hypothyroidism does not inhibit fetal thyroid function and generally poses little threat to the fetus. For the same reason, treatment with replacement hormone is also well tolerated.[70,76,88]

Maternal hyperthyroidism presents a totally different situation. Thyroid-stimulating antibodies, commonly found in patients with Grave's disease, as well as many of the drugs used to treat hyperthyroidism, do cross the placenta and can have a significant effect on the fetus. Antibodies, including long-acting thyroid stimulant (LATS) and thyroid-stimulating immunoglobulin (TSI), can cause an increase in fetal thyroid hormone

production. High levels are associated with fetal and neonatal hyperthyroidism.[70,115] Untreated maternal thyrotoxicosis may be associated with an increased incidence of nonspecific congenital defects; the mechanism for this is unclear, and the effect is sporadic.[75] In rare cases the offspring of women with Grave's disease may themselves be afflicted with this condition. In the fetus and newborn, this is evidenced by elevations in heart rate, growth retardation, goiter, and congestive heart failure. Perinatal mortality is high.[42,88] Administration of antithyroid medication to the mother can decrease thyroid hormone production in both the mother and the fetus but may result in fetal hypothyroidism and goiter.

Another maternal antibody, TSH-binding inhibitor immunoglobulin, also crosses the placenta and can prevent the expected fetal thyroid response to TSH. The result is a transient fetal and neonatal hypothyroidism.[70,66,115] Iodine deficiency in the mother is another cause of fetal/

neonatal hypothyroidism and, in its severe form, cretinism because of the fetus's dependence on maternal iodine reserves.[39]

PHENYLKETONURIA

Phenylketonuria (PKU) is a genetic disorder in which an enzymatic defect precludes the conversion of the essential amino acid phenylalanine to tyrosine. This metabolic derangement is evidenced by the accumulation of excessive amounts of phenylalanine in the blood and its subsequent excretion in the urine of affected persons. Historically, PKU resulted in virtually certain mental retardation; affected individuals were often institutionalized and rarely reproduced. With the advent of widespread neonatal screening and effective dietary treatment to prevent hyperphenylalaninemia during infancy and early childhood, genetically affected persons may now avoid the devastating effects of this disease, develop normally, and become pregnant. However, even in women who were treated in childhood and are developmentally normal, maternal PKU poses a significant environmental risk for the fetus. The care of these women and their infants presents a unique perinatal challenge.

The offspring of women with PKU are frequently microcephalic and retarded. They also have an increased incidence of growth retardation and congenital cardiac defects regardless of whether they are themselves affected with PKU.[54,55] The problem arises because most phenylketonurics remain on a low-phenylalanine diet only through early childhood. After that time they can tolerate high levels of phenylalanine without significant mental deterioration. However, during pregnancy elevated levels of phenylalanine in the mother are associated with fetal hyperphenylalaninemia. This prenatal exposure to excessive phenylalanine appears to be the primary mechanism of fetal injury. Maternal diet therapy offers the best hope for an unimpaired infant. **Phenylalanine levels drop quickly once dietary restrictions are instituted, and there is a strong correlation between maternal blood levels and** neonatal outcome.[58,98] **As with diabetes, control is ideally achieved before conception. Several studies have identified improved long-term outcomes when desirable phenylalanine levels (less than 2 to 8 mg/dl) are achieved prior to or early in pregnancy and maintained throughout.**[19,55,98]

RENAL DISEASE

Maternal adaptation to pregnancy involves significant changes in renal function and structure. Plasma volume increases, as does renal blood flow and the glomerular filtration rate (GFR). There is increased retention of sodium and water. These changes place unique demands on the urinary tract; women with preexisting renal disease are often unable to tolerate this stress and may experience a deterioration in function. Furthermore, renal dysfunction complicates pregnancy and increases fetal risk.

Renal disease in pregnancy may occur as a result of urinary tract infections, glomerular disease, or as a complication of systemic diseases including diabetes and systemic lupus erythematosus (SLE). **Regardless of the underlying etiology, pregnancy outcome relates most closely to two factors: the presence of hypertension and the degree of renal insufficiency that existed before the pregnancy.**[3,48,105] Many women with renal disorders are hypertensive prior to pregnancy, and they often develop a superimposed pregnancy-induced hypertension (preeclampsia). Even those with previously normal blood pressures run an increased risk of developing hypertension during pregnancy.[3,37,43] The presence of hypertension in these pregnancies represents a significant risk to the fetus and is strongly associated with intrauterine growth retardation, preterm delivery, and perinatal loss.[6,29,48,105] Drug therapy to control chronic hypertension has been shown to have a beneficial effect on fetal outcome and is generally continued throughout pregnancy. Renal insufficiency, as measured by creatinine clearance or serum creatinine level, also has implications for fetal outcome. Mild to moderate renal insufficiency (serum creatinine <1.5 mg/dl) is associated with a generally favorable outcome, whereas severe insufficiency (serum creatinine >1.6 mg/dl) often carries an increased risk for perinatal death.[3,43,48,63] As a rule, the number of preterm deliveries and growth-retarded infants increases with increasing blood pressure and decreasing renal function.[20]

Two special circumstances that merit brief mention are dialysis during pregnancy and pregnancy following renal transplantation. Women undergoing dialysis rarely become pregnant. When pregnancy does occur, it is associated with significant perinatal morbidity and mortality. Uteroplacental insufficiency may result from maternal hypotension during treatment; growth retardation and prematurity are common.[29,37,63] Pregnancy following transplantation is more common but also carries significant fetal risk. Penn et al.[89] report an extremely high rate of preterm delivery and an overall 30% rate of neonatal complications. These complications include RDS, congenital anomalies, adrenocortical insufficiency, hyperviscosity, seizures, and overwhelming septicemia. The criteria used to predict fetal outcome with other renal patients (i.e., hypertension and renal insufficiency) also have predictive value in posttransplantation pregnancies.

NEUROLOGIC DISORDERS

Neurologic disorders such as epilepsy, multiple sclerosis (MS), and myasthenia gravis generally have little effect on fertility; pregnancy can, and does, occur. The risks that accompany such pregnancies vary according to the individual disease entity and pertain to both the course of the mother's disease and the pregnancy outcome.

Maternal seizure disorders have been associated with increased fetal and neonatal risks, including prematurity, congenital defects, intrauterine demise, neonatal depression and drug withdrawal, and neonatal hemorrhage.* These risks are in part attributable to the alterations in

*References 4, 5, 52, 77, 80, 84.

the fetal environment that occur as a result of either the seizure disorder itself or the administration of anticonvulsant drugs to the mother. An epilepsy-related genetic predisposition to certain major congenital defects may also be a factor.[46,84] A significant number of women experience an increase in seizure activity during pregnancy. This is most likely due to decreased compliance with medication regimens, physiologic changes associated with pregnancy, and gestational changes in plasma levels of anticonvulsant drugs.[52,84,100,103] There is evidence that maternal seizures compromise fetal oxygenation, possibly because of diminished placental blood flow or maternal hypoxemia secondary to postseizure apnea.[107] There are also data linking seizure activity during pregnancy to an increased incidence of poor pregnancy outcome.[77,80] For these reasons, control of maternal seizure activity is one of the primary goals of prenatal care. This is accomplished through the use of a variety of anticonvulsant medications. Unfortunately, anticonvulsant therapy is not without its own risk to the fetus.

Placental transport of anticonvulsants does occur, resulting in fetal levels that approximate or in some cases exceed maternal levels.[78,103] Several studies have demonstrated an increased incidence of congenital defects in the offspring of epileptic women treated with anticonvulsants.[46,80,84,103] These anomalies are most likely attributable in part to drug teratogenicity, but the influence of the seizure disorder itself, as well as genetic makeup, may also be a factor. The specific teratogenic potential of several drugs has been identified. Two, trimethadione and valproic acid, are associated with major defects. Trimethadione is considered to be a potent teratogen, and its use is contraindicated in pregnancy. It is associated with craniofacial anomalies, intrauterine growth retardation, hypoplasia of the fingers and nails, congenital heart defects, and mental retardation.[17,77,103,114] Valproic acid is associated with neural tube defects, craniofacial abnormalities, and several minor malformations.[17,78,106] Other anticonvulsants, including hydantoins, primidone, and barbiturates, have been implicated in minor birth defects but appear to be far less powerful teratogens than trimethadione or valproic acid.

Infants born to mothers treated with anticonvulsants, especially barbiturates, may exhibit signs of generalized depression, including decreased respiratory effort, poor muscle tone, and feeding difficulties.[84] They may also have symptoms indicative of drug withdrawal. These symptoms usually present in the first week of life and include tremors, restlessness, hypertonia, and hyperventilation.[5] In addition, there have been reports of abnormal clotting and hemorrhage in the offspring of women treated with phenytoin, phenobarbital, and primidone.[4,103] This appears to be due to a decrease in vitamin K–dependent clotting factors. Hemorrhage usually starts within the first 24 hours, is often severe, and may result in death. Infants born to these mothers should have cord blood clotting studies done, vitamin K prophylaxis on admission to the nursery, and close observation.

MS frequently strikes women during their reproductive years. The onset of MS is usually insidious; the course is marked by a seemingly capricious cycle of exacerbations and remission. A wide range of sensory, motor, and functional changes are associated with this disease; the type and severity of symptoms vary dramatically from one individual to another and in any one patient over time. The etiology of the disease is not well understood. Genetic, environmental, and immunologic mechanisms have been implicated; viral factors have also been suggested.[68] Pregnancy is usually well tolerated; however a higher than expected number of relapses has been identified in the first 6 months after delivery.[93]

In women with MS, the disease process itself is generally not considered a threat to fetal or neonatal well-being. No increases in perinatal morbidity, mortality, or in the incidence of congenital defects have been demonstrated.[68,93,94] **The priority for neonatal care providers is to determine the extent of the mother's disability, in-cluding her level of fatigue, and her ability to care for her infant. The availability of appropriate support systems, both personal and professional, should be assessed, and needed follow-up and referrals made.**

Even though the prognosis for these infants is excellent, there are some factors associated with MS that are potentially problematic. Bladder dysfunction, common in women with MS, often results in urinary tract infections during pregnancy. Associated fetal/neonatal problems include preterm delivery and sepsis. Early identification and prompt treatment with appropriate antibiotics should minimize these risks. An additional area of concern is the variety of drugs administered to MS patients. Immunosuppressants are frequently used during severe exacerbations. The placental transport, and fetal risk, varies with the individual agent used. Prednisone is generally considered safe for use in pregnancy; the safety of azathioprine is still in question.[8,53,68] Although there have been reports of healthy infants born following maternal azathioprine therapy, there have also been reports of fetal complications, including hypoplasia of the thymus, immunoglobulin deficiency, decreases in cortisol levels, and transient chromosomal abnormalities.[53] Cyclophosphamide has been associated with skeletal defects.[8,68] Both azathioprine and cyclophosphamide are best avoided during pregnancy. Several drugs are used to ameliorate the bladder dysfunction of MS patients, including baclofen, dantrolene, propantheline, ditropan, and diazepam. Baclofen and dantrolene are a teratogen and a carcinogen, respectively, in animal studies. Little is known about the effects of propantheline and ditropan; diazepam has been associated with congenital anomalies.[68] A final consideration is a long-term one: the incidence of MS in the offspring of a parent with the disease is higher than the incidence in the general population.[64,68]

Myasthenia gravis is an autoimmune disorder in which a dearth of acetylcholine receptor (AChR) results in neuromuscular dysfunction.[97] Antibodies to AChRs have been found in most affected persons.[59] Distinguishing features include generalized weakness and muscle fatigue with activity. Persons with myasthenia gravis may also experience respiratory compromise and difficulty swallowing. In some cases pregnancy leads to deterioration; maternal deaths related to post-delivery myasthenic crisis have occurred.[92] **Infants born to myasthenic mothers are also at risk. They may be affected by maternal drug therapy; an increased rate of preterm delivery has also been reported.[92] An additional risk stems from transplacentally acquired anti-acetylcholine receptor antibodies, which cause approximately 12% of these newborns to experience a transient, self-limited course of myasthenia gravis.[22,97] It is difficult to predict which pregnancies will result in an affected infant, although infants born to women with very high AChR antibody titers may be at highest risk. Affected infants usually present at birth, or within the first 24 hours of life, with generalized weakness, diminished suck and swallow, and a decreased respiratory effort that may require mechanical support.**

HEART DISEASE

Marked changes in cardiovascular function accompany normal pregnancy. Plasma and red blood cell volumes rise, heart rate and cardiac output increase, and peripheral vascular resistance falls. These changes facilitate increased uterine blood flow, placental perfusion, and fetal oxygenation and growth; they also increase maternal oxygen consumption and cardiovascular work load and can further compromise the cardiovascular status of women with preexisting serious heart disease.[71] Pregnancy also creates a risk for maternal cardiovascular complications, including an increased incidence of thromboembolism and sudden death.[67] In some cases, such as Eisenmenger's syndrome, pulmonary hypertension, and Marfan's syndrome, the risk to maternal survival is so great that pregnancy is contraindicated.[113] In general, how well the woman with heart disease tolerates pregnancy depends on the specific dis-

ease process and the degree to which her cardiac status is compromised.[49,71,111]

Maternal heart disease also impacts the fetus. Fetal risks stem from three main sources: genetic factors, alterations in placental perfusion and exchange, and the impact of maternally administered drugs. The genetic risk is demonstrated by the increased incidence of congenital heart defects that occurs in the offspring of parents who have such a defect. The exact risk depends on the specific parental lesion, mode of inheritance, and exposure to environmental triggers.[11,83]

Alterations in placental perfusion and gas exchange occur when the mother's condition involves chronic hypoxemia or a significant decrease in cardiac output. These factors increase the threat to the fetus, with fetal risk increasing as maternal cardiac status declines.[71] Chronic maternal hypoxemia results in a decrease in oxygen available to the fetus and is associated with fetal loss, prematurity, and intrauterine growth retardation.[111] Significant reductions in maternal cardiac output create decreased uterine blood flow and diminished placental perfusion with a resulting impairment in the exchange of nutrients, oxygen, and metabolic wastes.[2,71,113] Possible fetal and neonatal consequences include spontaneous abortion, intrauterine growth retardation, neonatal asphyxia, central nervous system (CNS) damage, and intrauterine demise.[32,113]

A wide variety of drugs are used in the management of maternal cardiovascular disease. Although it is sometimes difficult to differentiate drug effects from the effects of the underlying disease, some associations between drug administration and fetal outcomes can be made. Anticoagulants are used to decrease the risk of thromboembolism, especially in women with artificial valves, a history of thrombophlebitis, or rheumatic heart disease.[36,112] Oral anticoagulants, specifically warfarin (coumarin) have been associated with fetal malformations, including nasal hypoplasia and epiphyseal stippling, when administered during the first trimester. They have also been associated with eye and CNS abnormalities when administered later in pregnancy.[36] The incidence of warfarin embryopathy is estimated at 15% to 25%; an additional 5% to 10% of these pregnancies are complicated by perinatal hemorrhage with an associated risk of fetal death, prematurity, and neonatal hemorrhage.[104] Heparin has been used in place of warfarin for anticoagulation during pregnancy and is generally considered the preferable agent. Heparin does not cross the placenta and so does not result in fetal anticoagulation or neonatal hemorrhage (although maternal hemorrhage may still occur), nor has it been associated with congenital defects.[109]

Antiarrhythmic medications and cardiac glycosides used during pregnancy cross the placenta to varying degrees. They have not been implicated in fetal malformations and, although several have been associated with other complications, are generally considered safe for use in pregnancy.[99,109] Reported complications include uterine contractions (quinidine, disopyramide), decreased birth weights (digoxin, disopyramide), and maternal hypotension with a sudden decrease in placental perfusion (verapamil).

Antihypertensives and diuretics have also been used in the treatment of cardiovascular disease during pregnancy. Propranolol, a beta-blocker commonly used to treat both hypertension and dysrhythmias, acts as a uterine stimulant and is a possible cause of preterm labor.[71] It is also associated with neonatal depression, including decreased respiratory effort and bradycardia at the time of delivery, as well as with hypoglycemia, polycythemia, and hyperbilirubinemia in the newborn period.[71,99,112] Atenolol and metoprolol, selective beta-blockers that can also be used to treat chronic hypertension, appear to have fewer adverse consequences for the neonate and are preferable agents.[99,109] Diuretic use in pregnancy remains an area of some controversy.[109] Fetal and neonatal compromise can result from diuretic-induced electrolyte and glucose imbalance and decreased placental perfusion secondary to maternal hypovolemia. The use of thiazide diuretics has been linked to neonatal liver damage and

thrombocytopenia. In general, diuretic use is restricted to women with pulmonary edema or acute cardiac or renal failure.[71,109] Although a great number of possible complications have been listed here, it is important to remember that with few exceptions most of the drugs used in the treatment of maternal heart disease can be used in pregnancy if the maternal condition warrants it.

Compromise due to maternal behavior
SMOKING

The link between maternal smoking and diminished fetal growth has been well established. Smoking is associated with dose-related reductions in both birth weight and length, as well as with an increase in the incidence of birth weights below 2500 g.[73] The exact mechanism by which fetal growth is retarded is not entirely clear, but reductions in placental blood flow secondary to vasoconstriction, elevated carbon monoxide levels, and chronic fetal hypoxia may all play a role.[10,40,74] Maternal smoking is also associated with placental dysfunction, an increased incidence of placental abruptions and previas, premature and prolonged rupture of the membranes, and intrauterine fetal demise.[73] Fetal risk seems to increase with increasing maternal age and parity, maternal anemia, previous poor perinatal outcome, and low socioeconomic status.[72] **There is evidence that eliminating or reducing smoking can improve fetal growth; women should be counseled to do so even relatively late in pregnancy.**[101]

SUBSTANCE ABUSE

Maternal drug and alcohol abuse places the fetus and newborn at risk for a plethora of structural, functional, and developmental problems. Perinatal morbidity is related to the direct effects of the abused substance on the developing fetus, its sudden "withdrawal," the interactions of multiple abused substances, the nutritional effects of addiction on the mother, and/or the social and health care implications of substance abuse.

Alcohol is one of the most commonly abused

substances during pregnancy. Alcohol in the maternal circulation crosses the placenta, resulting in direct fetal exposure to alcohol and its metabolites.[1] The exposed fetus may suffer a wide range of effects, including craniofacial malformations, growth retardation, CNS dysfunction, and organ or joint abnormalities.[1,44] The mechanism of fetal injury is not entirely clear but is likely related to three main factors: a teratogenic effect, hypoxia as a result of increased oxygen consumption, and a diminished ability to use amino acids in protein synthesis.[1] The expression of fetal alcohol effects ranges from subtle to extreme and depends on the timing of exposure, the dose, and the genetic response of the mother and fetus to the effects of alcohol. Secondary factors, such as maternal age, nutritional status, general health, and the interactive effects of other abused substances may also influence the outcome.[1] When the more severe effects are exhibited, the condition is known as fetal alcohol syndrome (FAS). FAS occurs only in the offspring of chronic alcoholics and is defined by a triad of defects consisting of intrauterine growth retardation with microcephaly, characteristic facial anomalies (small palpebral fissures, low nasal bridge, indistinct philtrum, thin upper lip, shortened lower jaw), and CNS dysfunction, including mental retardation.[44] These infants may also exhibit tremors, irritability, and hypertonus related to alcohol withdrawal.[91] The effects of prenatal alcohol exposure may be seen in postnatal life as continued abnormalities in motor, behavioral, and intellectual development.

Drug use and addiction in pregnancy is a complex problem. Maternal reporting of drug use is often unreliable; frequently more than one substance is involved; and there may be a cycle of drug use and periodic abstinence during pregnancy.[116] In addition, a host of medical and social problems are associated with maternal drug abuse. These women have generally poor health; infectious diseases, including pneumonia, sexually transmitted disease, urinary tract infections, and hepatitis, are common; anemia is frequently seen; and nutrition is often inadequate.[24,116] The exact

TABLE 2-2

The Addicted Newborn: Withdrawal Symptoms

Changes in tone	Tremors
	Marked flexor rigidity; resistance to extension
	Exaggerated reflexes (Moro)
Changes in state	Irritable
	Shortened sleep periods
	Frequent crying; cry may be high pitched
	Frantic movement, rooting, or fist sucking
	Seizures
Changes in feeding behavior and gastro-intestinal function	Poor feeding
	Vomiting
	Diarrhea
Miscellaneous changes	Tachypnea
	Temperature instability
	Yawning, sneezing
	Sweating, mottling
	Fever

fetal and neonatal effects vary with the specific drug(s) used; however, several generalizations can be made. The majority of drugs used by the mother, including narcotics, stimulants, and depressants, cross the placenta and have an effect on the fetus; fetal risks include intrauterine growth retardation, malformations, intrauterine demise, prematurity, asphyxia, and CNS dysfunction; fetal addiction does occur and is associated with neonatal abstinence (withdrawal) syndrome[24,44,69,116] (Table 2-2).

Maternal cocaine use merits special mention. Cocaine is a CNS stimulant that produces vasoconstriction, tachycardia, and hypertension in both the mother and fetus, often with devastating consequences. Its use during pregnancy has been linked to placental abruption and fetal cerebral infarcts, as well as to impaired performance on the Brazelton Neonatal Behavioral Assessment tool.[13]

NUTRITION

Fetal nutrition is linked to maternal intake during pregnancy and to the existent maternal stores of various nutrients, as well as to placental function. In general, poorly nourished mothers have more perinatal losses and give birth to smaller babies; this is especially true of the markedly underweight woman who fails to gain adequate weight during the course of pregnancy.[18,32,56,110] However, it is difficult to draw direct correlations between poor maternal diet and fetal growth unless the nutritional disturbances are severe. Many fetuses grow well despite suboptimal maternal nutrition, in part because of the complexities of placental transport and the ability of the fetus to be preferentially supplied with some nutrients.[18]

While reduced birth weight is associated with inadequate carbohydrate, protein, and total caloric intake, inappropriate amounts of other nutrients may also affect the fetus. Vitamin and mineral deficiencies have been linked to spontaneous abortion (vitamin C), congestive heart failure (thiamine), megaloblastic anemia (folic acid, B_{12}), congenital anomalies (folic acid, zinc, copper), and skeletal abnormalities (vitamin D, calcium).[110] Vitamin overdosage, especially of the fat-soluble vitamins, has also been implicated in fetal abnormalities; vitamin A overdose has been associated with kidney malformations, neural tube defects, and hydrocephalus, and vitamin D overdose with cardiac, neurologic, and renal defects.[62,110]

Nutritional deficiencies (or excesses) should be identified prior to or early in pregnancy, and both weight gain and fetal growth should be monitored throughout gestation. When problems are identified, individualized intervention strategies should be implemented in an attempt to increase birth weights and improve perinatal outcome.

Compromise due to obstetric complications
ANTEPARTUM BLEEDING

Maternal cardiovascular support is crucial to fetal well-being. Chronic blood loss can lead to maternal anemia and a related decrease in oxygen-carrying capacity. Uncompensated acute bleeding results in diminished blood volume, decreased systolic pressure, decreased cardiac output, and ultimately to decreased placental perfusion.[9] The net effect on the fetus is decreased oxygenation and impaired nutrient delivery.

The most common causes of hemorrhage late in pregnancy include placental abruption and placenta previa. In an abruption, a normally implanted placenta separates from the uterine wall before the time of delivery, resulting in maternal bleeding and a functional decrease in uteroplacental size.[95] The separation may be partial or complete, involving peripheral and/or central portions of the placenta. Fetal compromise relates to the extent of the separation and to the frequent need for preterm delivery. When the abruption is small and bleeding minimal, the pregnancy may continue without marked fetal compromise; however, it is important to remember that the decrease in uteroplacental surface area is irreversible and reduces the absolute placental capability. As the fetus grows or experiences additional stressors, its ability to tolerate the abruption may change. Extensive abruptions are poorly tolerated by both fetus and mother; the resulting maternal hemorrhage and decreased placental function lead to fetal asphyxia and, without immediate intervention, to intrauterine demise.

A placenta previa exists when the placenta lies abnormally low in the uterus and to some extent covers or encroaches on the internal cervical os. In the latter part of pregnancy, the normal elongation of the lower uterine segment and changes in the cervix disrupt the attachment of the overlying placenta. This generally presents as episodic painless maternal bleeding, often accompanied by preterm labor.[95] Fetal compromise relates to the extent of the previa, severity of maternal hemorrhage, degree of the resulting fetal hypoxia, and gestational age at delivery.

PREGNANCY-INDUCED HYPERTENSION

Pregnancy-induced hypertension (PIH) is a condition in which hypertension, accompanied by proteinuria and edema, develops during the second half of pregnancy in women without preexisting hypertensive disease. It is most common in primigravidas, in women younger than 16 or older than 35, in multiple gestations and molar pregnancies, and in women with a family history of PIH.[14] As a perinatal complication, PIH is significant because of its high toll in terms of both maternal and fetal well-being.

Pregnancy is normally associated with vasodilation and decreased peripheral vascular resistance. The net effect is that even though there is a significant increase in blood volume, maternal blood pressure does not increase during pregnancy.[30] In contrast, pregnancy-induced hypertension is associated with vasoconstriction and an increase in vascular resistance and arterial pressure. The result is a reduction in blood flow to the vital organs, including the kidney, liver, brain, and uterus; reduced maternal blood volume; and a host of maternal hepatic, CNS, and coagulation abnormalities.[23,30,32] The major impact on the intrauterine environment is placental insufficiency due to significant reductions in uteroplacental blood flow and the development of placental vascular abnormalities.[30] Associated fetal and neonatal risks include intrauterine growth retardation, perinatal asphyxia, and polycythemia.[6,23,102] Prematurity, with all of its attendant risks, is common; the risk of placental abruption is also increased.[30] The risk to the infant increases with earlier onset and increasingly severe maternal disease. Maternal seizures (eclampsia) further compromise the fetus by promoting hypoxemia and acidosis, often resulting in intrauterine demise.[23,30]

Drugs commonly used to treat pregnancy-induced hypertension include magnesium sulfate and hydralazine (Apresoline). Magnesium sulfate is used to prevent maternal seizures; reported neonatal side effects include hypotonia and CNS depression; however, it is not clear if these effects are due to maternal magnesium administration or to other complications such as prematurity and asphyxia.[35] Hydralazine is used in the treatment of severe maternal hypertension; its actions include relaxation of the arterial bed, decreased vascular resistance, and decreased blood pressure. Maternal response to hydralazine administration must be carefully monitored, since precipitous decreases in blood pressure reduce placental perfusion and further compromise the fetus.

PRETERM LABOR

Preterm birth, defined as any birth before 37 weeks gestation, poses an unparalleled threat to neonatal survival and well-being. Its cost, both human and economic, is staggering, and its prevention is a primary focus of modern obstetric care. Prevention is best accomplished through an aggressive effort to identify women at risk and close follow-up to achieve early recognition and appropriate intervention should preterm labor occur.[61] Unfortunately, many women continue to receive inadequate prenatal care, or no care at all. Even women who obtain early and ongoing care often fail to recognize the signs of preterm labor, and delay reporting symptoms until intervention is difficult if not impossible.

Although in many specific instances a definitive cause cannot be identified, it is possible to identify several factors that are generally associated with preterm labor and delivery.[32,34,47] These factors are summarized in Table 2-3. When preterm labor cannot be halted, it culminates in the delivery of a physiologically immature infant. The result is a host of neonatal problems that relate largely to the degree of immaturity, but also to compounding problems such as infant anomalies or maternal disease, as well as to the events that led to the preterm delivery (e.g., asphyxia secondary to placenta previa). Problems commonly encountered in preterm infants include respiratory distress, asphyxia, hyperbilirubinemia, metabolic disturbances, fluid and electrolyte imbalance, neurologic and behavioral problems, infection, nutritional deficits and feeding problems, ineffective thermoregulation, cardiovascular disturbances, chronic respiratory disease, and hematologic disturbances.[32,51]

Beta-sympathomimetic agents, such as ritodrine hydrochloride and terbutaline sulfate, are commonly used as a means of interrupting pre-

TABLE 2-3

Factors Associated with Preterm Labor and Delivery

Maternal history	Chronic disease
	Diabetes
	Renal disease
	Cardiovascular disease
	Respiratory disease
	In utero exposure to diethylstil-bestrol (DES)
	Reproductive tract anomalies
	Underweight (prior to pregnancy)
	Smoking
	Age extremes (below 18, above 40)
	Previous preterm labor
This pregnancy	Inadequate weight gain
	Acute maternal illness
	Pregnancy-induced hyper-tension
	Urinary tract infection
	Chorioamnionitis, vaginal infection
	Antepartum hemorrhage
	Isoimmunization
	Premature rupture of membranes (PROM)
	Multiple gestation
	Polyhydramnios
	Retained IUD
Fetal factors	Fetal anomalies
	Intrauterine fetal demise
	Infection

term labor. They achieve their tocolytic action by stimulating $beta_2$-receptors in the uterus with a resulting decrease in uterine smooth muscle contractility.[61] While these drugs are effective in prolonging gestation, they are also associated with maternal, fetal, and neonatal complications.[7,12,60,61,96] Mothers may experience tachycardia and arrhythmias, hyperglycemia, hypokalemia, anxiety, nausea, and vomiting. The fetus may also develop tachycardia and hyperglycemia. **Neonates born after beta-sympathomimetic therapy may develop a rebound hypoglycemia in response to in utero hyperglycemia and overproduction of insulin. No long-term problems have been identified.**

Magnesium sulfate has also been employed as a tocolytic. Magnesium sulfate decreases muscle contractility, thereby inhibiting uterine activity and effectively interrupting preterm labor.[90] **Neonatal consequences of maternal magnesium administration include decreased muscle tone and drowsiness, as well as decreases in serum calcium levels.[35,90]**

Prostaglandins play an important role in the onset of labor. Prostaglandin synthetase inhibitors, such as indomethacin, are a class of pharmacologic agents that interfere with the body's synthesis of prostaglandin, thereby inhibiting prostaglandin-mediated uterine contractions. These drugs have been used as an experimental means of interrupting preterm labor. Animal studies suggest the potential for in utero constriction, or closure, of the ductus arteriosus with resulting development of fetal pulmonary hypertension and congestive heart failure.[57,80,81] This problem has not been clearly demonstrated in humans. Other neonatal risks include decreased platelet activity and gastrointestinal irritation.[81]

Calcium antagonists, such as nifedipine, also have a demonstrated ability to interfere with the labor process. Uterine contractility is directly related to the presence of free calcium; increased calcium concentration enhances muscle contractility, whereas decreased calcium levels inhibit contractility.[26] Calcium antagonists block the entry of calcium into cells and inhibit uterine muscle contraction. No serious fetal or neonatal side effects have been linked to the maternal administration of calcium antagonists; continued clinical investigation is warranted.[26]

ENVIRONMENTAL EFFECTS OF LABOR ON THE FETUS
Effects of contractions

During labor the dynamics of uterine contractions alter the intrauterine environment and influence the fetus. The "healthy" fetus is equipped to withstand the challenge of labor; but when the fetus is compromised or the labor dysfunctional, the fetus can be taxed beyond its capacity, placing it at risk for further compromise, asphyxia, and/or intra-uterine death.

Strong uterine contractions are characterized by decreased blood flow through the intervillous spaces in the placenta.[15,95] As blood flow decreases, there is a corresponding decline in placental gas exchange, and the fetus must depend on its existing reserves to maintain oxygenation until placental blood flow is reestablished. The net effect is that fetal PaO_2 decreases as the consequence of uterine contraction. In the fetus with adequate reserves, the fall in PaO_2 is not drastic; the fetus remains adequately oxygenated and so is able to tolerate the stress of labor.

Fetal reserve

The factors that influence fetal reserve fall into two general categories: those that diminish reserves and those that exhaust reserves. When fetal oxygen reserves are diminished, the fetus has less than optimal oxygenation at the onset of a contraction. This may occur as a consequence of any condition that decreases placental exchange, including reduced placental surface area due to abruption, previa, or an abnormally small placenta[15]; decreased placental perfusion due to maternal hypotension or hypertension; or maternal hypoxemia. Oxygen reserves can also be diminished as a result of a reduction in fetal oxygen-carrying capacity, as in severe anemia or acute fetal hemorrhage.

A fetal reserve that is adequate at the onset of labor can be exhausted by factors that place unusual demands on the fetus. Exhaustion of reserves occurs with contractions that last for a prolonged period of time, that are of extremely high intensity, or that occur with increased frequency and without an adequate recovery period between individual contractions.[15] This is often a consequence of the use of oxytocics to induce or augment labor.

Fetal response to contraction-induced hypoxia

When the fetal oxygen reserve is diminished or exhausted, uterine contractions can precipitate a marked fall in PaO_2. The fetus is quite limited in its ability to compensate for this hypoxemia. The adult mechanism, which involves increasing total cardiac output by increasing heart rate, does not play a major role in the fetal response.[33] Instead, the fetus responds with a redistribution of cardiac output as a means of maintaining critical function; blood flow to the brain and heart increases while perfusion of less critical organs is reduced.[2,33] This mechanism enables the fetus to survive brief episodes of hypoxia, but severe and prolonged hypoxic episodes are poorly tolerated.

Acute hypoxemia leads to the development of acidosis and also produces a reflex bradycardia secondary to vagal stimulation, both of which further compromise fetal oxygenation. In addition, myocardial hypoxia has a direct bradycardic effect.[2] These mechanisms give rise to one of the classic signs of fetal distress, the late deceleration, in which the peak of uterine pressure, which also represents the nadir of intervillous blood flow and the onset of fetal hypoxia, is followed by a decline in fetal heart rate.[15,33,95] Late decelerations are significant in that they help to identify the fetus unable to tolerate labor because of inadequate oxygen reserves, and they allow for the implementation of measures to enhance fetal reserve, improve placental perfusion, or interrupt labor. It must be remembered, however, that gestational age may also influence how the fetus responds to hypoxemia and how well the fetus tolerates this condition. The preterm infant who develops late decelerations with hypoxemia seems to tolerate longer periods of distress than does the term infant, whereas the postterm infant is uniquely fragile and may be in significant distress without displaying this characteristic fetal heart rate pattern.[15]

Other factors that evoke a fetal response during labor
HEAD COMPRESSION

Pressure on the fetal head during labor, especially with pushing efforts in the second stage, also produces a vagal response and a reflex slowing of the fetal heart rate.[15,32] In general, this does not indi-

TABLE 2-4

Fetal and Neonatal Effects of Maternal Analgesia and Anesthesia during Labor

DRUG	*POSSIBLE FETAL AND NEONATAL SIDE EFFECTS*
Barbiturates	CNS depression
	Respiratory depression
	Slowed metabolism
	Lethargy, decreased tone, and feeding difficulties
Narcotics	Fetal and neonatal effects are related to the dose, route, and timing of maternal administration and may be reversed by the administration of a narcotic antagonist (naloxone); they include:
	CNS depression
	Fetal bradycardia
	Depressed respiratory effort
	Decreased muscle tone and reflexes
	Decreased responsiveness
Tranquilizers	Fetal tachycardia and decreased beat to beat variability
	Depressed respiratory effort; apnea
	Decreased muscle tone and reflexes
	Impaired thermoregulation
	Feeding difficulties
Paracervical block	Fetal bradycardia and asphyxia related to decreased uterine blood flow and direct fetal myocardial depression
Epidural and spinal block	Fetal bradycardia and asphyxia related to maternal hypotension
	Fetal neonatal toxicity
General (inhalation) anesthesia	Fetal and newborn effects relate to the duration and depth of maternal anesthesia and include:
	CNS depression
	Respiratory depression
	Decreased responsiveness

cate hypoxia or fetal compromise and is often seen in the healthy fetus. The deceleration that accompanies head compression, also referred to as an early deceleration, is differentiated from the late deceleration of fetal asphyxia by its timing in relation to a contraction. In early deceleration the heart rate begins to fall as a contraction builds, reaching its lowest point as the contraction peaks. As the contraction subsides, the heart rate returns to baseline. The result is a uniformly shaped dip that mirrors the shape of the contraction. In comparison, a late deceleration also has a uniform shape but lags behind the contraction, with the fall in heart rate beginning at or slightly after the contraction peak and continuing to fall as the contraction subsides. With a late deceleration the heart rate does not return to baseline until well after the contraction has ended.

CORD COMPRESSION

Compression of the umbilical cord can occur when the cord is looped around fetal body parts or is knotted, as a result of cord prolapse, or when there is scant amniotic fluid. During labor, cord compression may be exacerbated by contractions and by descent of the fetus, resulting in varying degrees of occlusion of the umbilical vessels and diminutions of blood flow. Partial venous occlusion may be manifested by fetal tachycardia, whereas significant occlusion precipitates a rapid fall in heart rate, caused at least in part by vagal reflex.[15,45] The deceleration pattern associated with cord compression varies in terms of its onset in relation to contractions and the overall shape of the dip; hence the term *variable* deceleration. Variable decelerations are identified by a decline in heart rate that generally begins before the contraction peaks but, unlike early decelerations, falls rapidly and does not mirror the shape of the contraction. Typically, recovery of the heart rate is also rapid. However, when the occlusion is severe or of long duration, or the fetus has diminished oxygen reserves, recovery may be slow, indicating fetal hypoxia and in essence incorporating a component of late deceleration within the variable deceleration.[15]

MATERNAL PAIN MEDICATION

Many drugs have been used to provide pain relief to laboring women or anesthesia for operative deliveries. Most of those have the potential to affect the infant, either during labor and delivery or in the newborn period. The risk is increased if the fetus is preterm or otherwise compromised. This is not to say that there is no place for these drugs in obstetric care, only that they must be used judiciously, and with a clear understanding of the risks and benefits involved. Table 2-4 summarizes the effects of commonly used analgesic and anesthetic agents on the fetus and the newborn.[31,50,79]

ASSESSMENT OF FETAL WELL-BEING

Over the past 20 years the ability to assess fetal well-being has advanced from simple auscultation of the fetal heart to direct physiologic and biochemical measurement of fetal status. With these advances an appreciation of the similarities between the fetus and the newborn, as well as a more complete understanding of the unique features of fetal life, have become evident. This knowledge reinforces the importance of viewing fetal physiology as a precursor of neonatal function, and especially as a significant influence on the success with which the fetus will complete the adaptations required by the birth process.

The clinical problem posed by an adverse prenatal environment involves determining when the environment is so adverse that delivery of the fetus is indicated. This problem is relatively simple when the fetus is close to term, at which time any evidence of a hostile environment is justification for delivery. The further one is from term, the more difficult decision making becomes. As is evident from the earlier discussion, many maternal conditions can adversely affect the fetus very early in gestation. When compromise is suspected in the immature fetus, the clinician must weigh the relative risks and advantages of preterm delivery versus continued intrauterine development. A variety of tests of fetal well-being have been developed in an attempt to aid in such decision making. No one test has been shown to be clearly superior to the others in any single circumstance. The tests in use today share one characteristic limitation: while they are very good at detecting fetal well-being, they are relatively poor at predicting fetal compromise. In other words, a "reassuring" test result is quite reliable for almost all of the tests, but a "nonreassuring" result does not reliably identify fetal compromise. The clinician faced with a "nonreassuring" antepartum test usually must perform additional tests to confirm that the fetus is indeed in jeopardy before proceeding to delivery.

The first test that was widely used in clinical practice was the contraction stress test (CST), which grew out of the use of fetal heart rate monitoring during labor. The principle behind the CST is that uterine contractions cause a transient interruption in uteroplacental perfusion.[27] With normal placental reserve, this intermittent interruption is well tolerated. With inadequate or exhausted reserve, late fetal heart rate decelerations appear. Since late decelerations during labor had been associated with fetal hypoxia and acidosis, it was reasoned that similar interpretations could be applied to contractions induced in the antepartum patient. Thus the CST is considered a test of uteroplacental reserve.

As initially carried out, the CST entailed an intravenous (IV) infusion of oxytocin to induce uterine contractions (hence the term *ocytocin challenge test* or OCT). The rate of infusion of oxytocin was increased until three contractions occurred within a 10-minute period. The fetal heart rate pattern was then analyzed. Variable or early heart rate decelerations during a CST were interpreted as equivocal signs of fetal compromise. If late decelerations were observed, the test was considered positive and fetal compromise assumed to be present. However, follow-up studies showed that one half of the fetuses with positive CST results could be delivered in good condition, without further evidence of fetal hypoxia, following induction of labor. This calculates to a 50% false-positive rate for the test. On the other hand, most studies showed that negative ("reassuring") test results were associated with less than a 1% incidence of intrauterine fetal death within 1 week of the test, a very low rate of false-negative test results.

The requirement of an IV infusion of oxytocin makes this test both expensive and time consuming. The fact that nipple stimulation triggers the release of endogenous oxytocin from the posterior pituitary has been used to advantage in the development of the nipple stimulation CST. In this procedure the patient massages first one and then both breasts to induce uterine contractions. The fetal heart rate is recorded and interpreted exactly as if the test were performed with an IV infusion of oxytocin. The CST performed in this manner is simpler and less expensive than the OCT and seems to be as safe and reliable.

After the introduction of the CST into clinical practice, it became apparent that the normal fetus exhibited fetal heart rate variations, or "reactivity," in response to movement. That is, when fetal movement was perceived, there was an acceleration in the fetal heart rate.[86] This reactivity is a characteristic of the mature fetus and may be absent in the relatively immature fetus (>32 weeks). This test, since it does not require stressing the fetus by inducing contractions, has been designated the *nonstress test* (NST). The test was formalized by requiring two episodes of fetal heart rate accelerations of at least 15 beats/min within a 20-minute period. Such a test result is considered "reactive" and a sign of fetal well-being. Fetuses not demonstrating heart rate accelerations with movement are considered "nonreactive" and suspect for fetal jeopardy.

There has been some debate as to which is more sensitive to fetal hypoxia, the CST or the NST. In fact, these two tests evaluate slightly different aspects of fetal well-being. The CST evaluates uteroplacental reserve, whereas the NST seems to reflect the state of fetal CNS oxygenation at the time of the test. The NST has certain specific advantages over the CST. Since it does not entail the production of uterine contractions, there are fewer potential problems or contraindications to the NST. It is also usually quicker and easier to conduct. For these reasons, it is often the first-line screening test of fetal well-being. Its disadvantages are that it does not evaluate uteroplacental reserve and that it has a higher false "abnormal" rate than the CST.

With the ready availability of real-time ultrasound equipment, the ability to observe fetal behavior in more detail has been used to assess fetal well-being. The biophysical profile (Table 2-5) was introduced to take advantage of this capability and hopefully to refine fetal assessment. The biophysical profile is in reality a fetal behavioral assessment tool, evaluating parameters such as fetal breathing movements, gross body movement, and fetal muscle tone, in conjunction with amniotic fluid volume and neurologic integrity (via the NST).[65] Its principal value is in the further (and more comprehensive) evaluation of the fetus with a nonreactive NST result, but with contraindications to a CST (e.g., premature rupture of membranes, preterm labor, or multiple gestation). In these circumstances the clinician can use the biophysical profile to confirm or rule out fetal compromise and to make a decision to either continue the pregnancy or deliver the fetus.

The biophysical profile is only one way in which the use of ultrasound has changed fetal evaluation. A long and growing list of fetal conditions

TABLE 2-5

Biophysical Profile Scoring

BIOPHYSICAL VARIABLE	NORMAL (2)	ABNORMAL (0)
1. Fetal breathing—At least one episode of at least 30 seconds during 30-minute observation	Present	Absent
2. Gross body movement—At least three body/limb movements during 30-minute observation	>3	2 or less
3. Fetal tone—One episode of extension/flexion of limbs or trunk during 30-minute observation	Present	Absent or sluggish movements
4. Reactive NST—At least two episodes of 15 beats/min fetal heart rate accelerations during 30-minute observation	Yes	No
5. Amniotic fluid volume—At least one pocket of at least 1 by 1 cm in two directions	Present	Absent

NORMAL SCORE: 8-10

can be detected by real-time ultrasound. Most of these conditions involve anatomic abnormalities, but functional abnormalities are being recognized with increasing frequency. When real-time ultrasound is combined with Doppler assessment of fetal blood flow velocity, one begins to look at fetal physiology in real-time. At this time fetal Doppler blood flow velocimetry is largely an experimental tool; however, it seems likely that it soon will find a place in the clinical evaluation of the fetus.

The dramatic improvement in ultrasound image quality over the past 10 years has also made it possible to directly sample fetal blood and tissue. The technique of percutaneous umbilical blood sampling (PUBS) has given the obstetrician access to the fetal circulation with relative safety for both the fetus and the mother.[16] In this procedure real-time ultrasound is used to guide the insertion of a needle into the umbilical vein or artery. Samples of fetal blood can be obtained or, as in the case of red cell isoimmunization, transfusions carried out. Thousands of such procedures have been done in many centers. The fetal risk appears to be in the neighborhood of 1% to 2% per procedure. Normal values for many substances in fetal blood at various gestational ages are now know. Among these are the respiratory gases. It seems likely that soon these may be used in selected cases to assess fetal well-being.

SUMMARY

In summary, a host of maternal conditions and behaviors have the potential to create a less than optimal environment for fetal development and thereby adversely impact fetal well-being. The degree of fetal compromise varies with the specific maternal condition, but devastating fetal injury and lifelong disability, as well as fetal or neonatal demise, can result from maternal disease or behavior. The role of perinatal care providers involves the early detection and appropriate management of the complicated pregnancy, skillful assessment of fetal well-being, timely delivery, comprehensive assessment of the newborn and appropriate intervention, follow-up of both the infant and the mother's conditions, as well as family support and counseling. In addition, the role of the clinician as an educator is instrumental in preventing avoidable complications and achieving the optimal outcome.

REFERENCES

1. Abel EL: Consumption of alcohol during pregnancy: a review of effects on growth and development of offspring, Hum Biol 54:421, 1982.
2. Battaglia FC and Meschia G: An introduction to fetal physiology, Orlando, Fla, 1986, Academic Press, Inc.
3. Benedetti RG and Berl T: Renal disease. In Abrams RS and Wexler P, editors: Medical care of the pregnant patient, Boston, 1983, Little, Brown & Co, Inc.

4. Bleyer WA and Skinner AL: Fatal neonatal hemorrhage after maternal anticonvulsant therapy, JAMA 235:626, 1976.

5. Bossi L et al: Plasma levels and clinical effects of anti-epileptic drugs in pregnant epileptic patients and their newborns. In Johannessen SI et al, editors: Antiepileptic therapy: advances in drug monitoring, New York, 1980, Raven Press.

6. Brazy JE, Grimm JK, and Little VA: Neonatal manifestations of severe maternal hypertension occurring before the thirty-sixth week of pregnancy, J Pediatr 100:256, 1982.

7. Brazy JE, Little VA, and Grimm JK: Isoxsuprine in the perinatal period. II. Relationships between neonatal symptoms, drug exposure, and drug concentration at the time of birth, J Pediatr 98:146, 1981.

8. Briggs G: Drugs in pregnancy and lactation: a reference guide to fetal and neonatal risk, Baltimore, 1983, Williams & Wilkins.

9. Bucheit K and Price J: Obstetrical hemorrhage emergency care. In Perez RH, editor: Protocols for perinatal nursing practice, St Louis, 1981, The CV Mosby Co.

10. Bureau MA et al: Maternal cigarette smoking and fetal oxygen transport: a study of P50,2,3-diphosphoglycerate, total hemoglobin, hematocrit, and type F hemoglobin in fetal blood, Pediatrics 72:22, 1983.

11. Burns J: Congenital heart disease: risk to offspring, Arch Dis Child 58:947, 1983.

12. Caritis SN et al: Pharmacodynamics of ritodrine in pregnant women during preterm labor, Am J Obstet Gynecol 147:752, 1983.

13. Chasnoff IJ et al: Perinatal cerebral infarct and maternal cocaine use, J Pediatr 108:456, 1986.

14. Chesley LC: Hypertensive disorders in pregnancy, J Nurse Midwifery 30:99, 1985.

15. Cibils LA: Electronic fetal-maternal monitoring, Littleton, Mass, 1981, PSG Publishing Co, Inc.

16. Daffos F, Capella-Pavlovsky M, and Forestier F: Fetal blood sampling during pregnancy with use of a needle guided by ultrasound: a study of 606 consecutive cases, Am J Obstet Gynecol 153:655, 1985.

17. Dalessio DJ: Seizure disorders and pregnancy, N Engl J Med 312:559, 1985.

18. Dancis J: Fetomaternal interaction. In Avery GB, editor: Neonatology: pathophysiology and management of the newborn, ed 3, Philadelphia, 1987, JB Lippincott Co.

19. Davidson DC et al: Outcome of pregnancy in a phenylketonuric mother after low phenylalanine diet introduced from the ninth week of pregnancy, Eur J Pediatr 137:45, 1982.

20. Davison JM, Katz AL, and Lindheimer MD: Kidney disease and pregnancy: Obstetric outcome and long-term renal prognosis, Clin Perinatol 12:497, 1985.

21. Diamond MP et al: Reassessment of White's classification and Pedersen's prognostically bad signs of diabetic pregnancies in insulin-dependent diabetic pregnancies, Am J Obstet Gynecol 156:599, 1987.

22. Donaldson JO et al: Antiacetylcholine receptor antibody in neonatal myasthenia gravis, Am J Dis Child 135:222, 1981.

23. Feinberg LE: Hypertension and preeclampsia. In Abrams RS and Exler P, editors: Medical care of the pregnant patient, Boston, 1983, Little, Brown & Co, Inc.

24. Finnegan LP: Drugs and other substance abuse in pregnancy. In Stern L, editor: Drug use in pregnancy, Balgowlah, NSW, Australia, 1984, ADIS Health Science Press.

25. Fisher DA and Klein AH: Thyroid development and disorders of thyroid function in the newborn, N Engl J Med 302:702, 1981.

26. Forman A, Anderson KE, and Ulmsten U: Inhibition of myometrical activity by calcium antagonists, Semin Perinatol 5:288, 1981.

27. Freeman R: Contraction stress testing for primary fetal surveillance in patients at high risk for uteroplacental insufficiency, Clin Perinatol 9:265, 1982.

28. Fuhrmann K et al: Prevention of congenital malformations in infants of insulin-dependent diabetic mothers, Diabetes Care 6:219, 1983.

29. Gabert HA and Miller JM: Renal disease in pregnancy, Obstet Gynecol Sur 40:449, 1985.

30. Gant NF and Worley RJ: Hypertension in pregnancy: concepts and management, New York, 1980, Appleton-Century-Crofts.

31. Gibbs CP: Anesthetic management of the high-risk patient. In Warshaw JB and Hobbins JC, editors: Principles and practice of perinatal medicine, maternal-fetal and newborn care, Menlo Park, Calif, 1983, Addison-Wesley Publishing Co, Inc.

32. Gilbert ES and Harmon JS: High-risk pregnancy and delivery: nursing perspectives, St Louis, 1986, The CV Mosby Co.

33. Gimovsky ML and Caritis SN: Diagnosis and management of hypoxic fetal heart rate patterns, Clin Perinatol 9:313, 1982.

34. Gravett MG: Causes of preterm delivery, Semin Perinatol 8:246, 1984.

35. Green KW et al: The effects of maternally administered magnesium sulfate in the neonate, Am J Obstet Gynecol 142:29, 1983.

36. Hall JG, Pauli RM, and Wilson KM: Maternal and fetal sequelae of anticoagulation during pregnancy, Am J Med 68:122, 1980.

37. Hayslett JP: Interaction of renal disease and pregnancy, Kidney Int 25:579, 1984.

38. Reference deleted in galleys.

39. Hetzel BS: Iodine deficiency disorders (IDD) and their eradication, Lancet 2:1126, 1983.

40. Hoff C et al: Trend associations of smoking with maternal, fetal, and neonatal morbidity, Obstet Gynecol 68:317, 1986.

41. Hollingsworth DR: Pregnancy, diabetes and birth: a management guide, Baltimore, 1984, Williams & Wilkins.

42. Hollingsworth DR and Mabry C: Congenital Graves disease, Am J Dis Child 130:148, 1976.

43. Hou SH, Grosman SD, and Madias NE: Pregnancy in women with renal disease and moderate renal insufficiency, Am J Med 78:185, 1985.

44. Hutchings DE: Drug abuse during pregnancy: embryopathic and neurobehavioral effects. In Braude MC and Zimmerman AM: Genetic and perinatal effects of abused substances, Orlando, Fla, 1987, Academic Press, Inc.

45. James LS, Yeh MN, and Morishima HO: Umbilical vein occlusion and transient acceleration of the fetal heart rate, Am J Obstet Gynecol 126:276, 1976.

46. Janz D: Antiepileptic drugs and pregnancy: altered utilization patterns and teratogenesis, Epilepsia 23 (suppl):S53, 1982.

47. Kaltreider DF and Kohl S: Epidemiology of preterm delivery, Clin Obstet Gynecol 23:17, 1980.

48. Katz AI et al: Pregnancy in women with kidney disease, Kidney Int 18:192, 1980.

49. Katz M et al: Outcome of pregnancy in 110 patients with organic heart disease, J Reprod Med 31:343, 1986.

50. Keller B: Control of pain in labor. In Perez RH, editor: Protocols for perinatal nursing practice, St Louis, 1981, The CV Mosby Co.

51. Korones SB: High risk newborn infants. The basis for intensive nursing care, ed 4, St Louis, 1986, The CV Mosby Co.

52. Krumholz A: Epilepsy and pregnancy. In Goldstein PJ: Neurological disorders of pregnancy, Mt Kisco, NY, 1986, Futura Publishing Co, Inc.

53. Lavin JP Jr: Pharmacologic therapy for chronic medical disorders during pregnancy. In Rayburn WF and Zuspan FP, editors: Drug therapy in obstetrics and gynecology, ed 2, Norwalk, Conn, 1986, Appleton-Century-Crofts.

54. Lenke RR and Levy HL: Maternal phenylketonuria and hyperphenylalaninemia: an international survey of the outcome of untreated and treated pregnancies, N Engl J Med 303:1202, 1980.

55. Lenke RR and Levy HL: Maternal phenylketonuria—results of dietary therapy, Am J Obstet Gynecol 142:548, 1982.

56. Leonard LG: Pregnancy and the underweight woman, MCN 9:331, 1984.

57. Levin DL: Effects of inhibition of prostaglandin synthesis in fetal development, oxygenation and the fetal circulation, Semin Perinatol 4:35, 1980.

58. Levy HL and Waisbren SE: Effects of untreated maternal phenylketonuria and hyperphenylalaninemia on the fetus, N Engl J Med 309:1269, 1983.

59. Lindstrom JM et al: Antibody to acetylcholine receptor in myesthenia gravis, Neurology 26:1054, 1976.

60. Lipshitz J: Beta-adrenergic agonists, Semin Perinatol 5:252, 1981.

61. Lirette M, Holbrook RH, and Creasy RK: Management of the woman in preterm labor, Perinatol Neonatol 10:30, 1986.

62. Luke B: Megavitamins and pregnancy: a dangerous combination, MCN 10:18, 1985.

63. MacCarthy EP and Pollack VE: Maternal renal disease; effect on the fetus, Clin Perinatol 8:307, 1981.

64. MacKay RP and Myrianthopoulos N: Multiple sclerosis in twins and their relatives, Arch Neurol 15:449, 1966.

65. Manning FA et al: Fetal assessment based on fetal biophysical profile scoring: experience in 12,620 referred high risk pregnancies. I. Perinatal mortality by frequency and etiology, Am J Obstet Gynecol 151:343, 1985.

66. Matsuura N et al: Familial neonatal transient hypothyroidism due to maternal TSH-binding inhibitor immunoglobulins, N Engl J Med 303:738, 1980.

67. McAnulty JH, Metcalfe J, and Ueland K: General guidelines in the management of cardiac disease, Clin Obstet Gynecol 24:773, 1981.

68. McArthur JC and Young F: Multiple sclerosis and pregnancy. In Goldstein PJ: Neurological disorders of pregnancy, Mt Kisco, NY, 1986, Futura Publishing Co.

69. Merker L, Higgins P, and Kinnard E: Assessing narcotic addiction in neonates, Pediatr Nurs 11:177, 1985.

70. Mestman JH: Thyroid disease in pregnancy, Clin Perinatol 12:651, 1985.

71. Metcalfe J, McAnulty JH, and Ueland K: Heart disease and pregnancy: physiology and management, ed 2, Boston, 1986, Little, Brown & Co, Inc.

72. Meyer MB, Jonas BS, and Tonascia JA: Perinatal events associated with maternal smoking during pregnancy, Am J Epidemiol 103:464, 1976.

73. Meyer MB and Tonascia JA: Maternal smoking, pregnancy complications, and perinatal mortality, Am J Obstet Gynecol 128:494, 1977.

74. Mochizuki M et al: Effects of smoking on fetoplacental-maternal system during pregnancy, Am J Obstet Gynecol 149:413, 1984.

75. Momotani N et al: Maternal hyperthyroidism and congenital malformation in the offspring, Clin Endocrinol 20:695, 1984.

76. Montoro M et al: Successful outcome of pregnancy in women with hypothyroidism, Ann Intern Med 94:31, 1981.

77. Nakane Y et al: Multi-institutional study in the teratogenicity and fetal toxicity of antiepileptic drugs: a report of a collaborative study group in Japan, Epilepsia 21:663, 1980.

78. Nau H et al: Valproic acid and its metabolites: placental transfer, neonatal pharmacokinetics, transfer via mother's milk and clinical status in neonates of epileptic mothers, J Pharmacol Exp Ther 219:768, 1981.

79. Naulty JS: Obstetric anesthesia. In Avery GB, editor: Neonatology: pathophysiology and management of the newborn, ed 3, Philadelphia, 1987, JB Lippincott Co.

80. Nelson KB and Ellenberg JH: Maternal seizure disorder, outcome of pregnancy and neurologic abnormalities in the children, Neurology 32:1247, 1982.

81. Niebyl JR: Prostaglandin synthetase inhibitors, Semin Perinatol 5:274, 1981.

82. Niebyl JR and Johnson JWC: Inhibition of preterm labor, Clin Obstet Gynecol 23:115, 1980.

83. Nora JJ, Nora AH, and Wexler P: Hereditary and environmental aspects as they affect the fetus and newborn, Clin Obstet Gynecol 24:851, 1981.

84. Noronha A: Neurological disorders during pregnancy and the puerperium, Clin Perinatol 12:695, 1985.

85. Ogata ES: Diabetes-related problems of the newborn, Perinatol Neonatol 8:48, 1984.

86. Paul RH: Evaluation of antepartum fetal well-being using the non-stress test, Clin Perinatol 9:253, 1982.

87. Pedersen J: The pregnant diabetic and her newborn, ed 2, Baltimore, 1977, Williams & Wilkins.

88. Pekonen F et al: Women on thyroid hormone therapy: pregnancy course, fetal outcome, and amniotic fluid thyroid hormone level, Obstet Gynecol 63:635, 1984.

89. Penn I, Makowski EL, and Harris P: Parenthood following renal transplantation, Kidney Int 18:221, 1980.

90. Petrie RH: Tocolysis using magnesium sulfate, Semin Perinatol 5:266, 1981.

91. Pierog S, Chandarasu O, and Wexler I: Withdrawal symptoms in infants with the fetal alcohol syndrome, J Pediatr 90:630, 1977.

92. Plauche WC: Myasthenia gravis, Clin Obstet Gynecol 26:592, 1983.

93. Poser S and Poser W: Multiple sclerosis and gestation, Neurology 33:1422, 1983.

94. Poser S et al: Pregnancy, oral contraceptives and multiple sclerosis, Acta Neurol Scand 59:108, 1979.

95. Pritchard JA, MacDonald PC, and Gant NF: Williams' obstetrics, ed 17, East Norwalk, Conn, 1985, Appleton-Century-Crofts.

96. Procianoy RS and Pinheiro CEA: Neonatal hyperinsulinism after short term maternal beta sympathomimetic therapy, J Pediatr 101:612, 1982.

97. Repke JT and Klein VR: Myasthenia gravis in pregnancy. In Goldstein PJ: Neurological disorders of pregnancy, Mt Kisco, NY, 1986, Futura Publishing Co.

98. Rohr FJ et al: New England maternal PKU project: prospective study of untreated and treated pregnancies and their outcomes, J Pediatr 110:391, 1987.

99. Rotmensch HH, Elkayam U, and Frishman W: Anti-arrhythmic drug therapy during pregnancy, Ann Intern Med 98:487, 1983.

100. Schmidt D et al: Change in seizure frequency in pregnant epileptic women, J Neurol Neurosurg Psychiatry 46:751, 1983.

101. Sexton M and Hebel JR: Clinical trial of change in maternal smoking and its effect on birth weight, JAMA 251:911, 1984.

102. Sibai BM et al: Maternal-fetal correlations in patients with severe preeclampsia/eclampsia, Obstet Gynecol 62:745, 1983.

103. Stempel LE and Rayburn WF: Anticonvulsant therapy during pregnancy. In Rayburn WF and Zuspan FP, editors: Drug therapy in obstetrics and gynecology, ed 2, Norwalk, Conn, 1986, Appleton-Century-Crofts.

104. Stevenson RE et al: Hazards of oral anticoagulants during pregnancy, JAMA 243:1549, 1980.

105. Surian M et al: Glomerular disease and pregnancy, Nephron 36:101, 1984.

106. Tein I and MacGregory DL: Possible valproate teratogenicity, Arch Neurol 42:291, 1985.

107. Teramo K et al: Fetal heart rate during a maternal grand mal epileptic seizure, J Perinat Med 7:3, 1979.

108. Tropper PJ and Petrie RH: Placental exchange. In Lavery JP, editor: The human placenta, clinical perspectives, Rockville, Md, 1987, Aspen Publishers, Inc.

109. Ueland K et al: Special considerations in the use of cardiovascular drugs, Clin Obstet Gynecol 24:809, 1981.

110. Wall RE: Nutritional problems during pregnancy. In Abrams RS and Wexler P, editors: Medical care of the pregnant patient, Boston, 1983, Little, Brown & Co, Inc.

111. Whittemore R: Congenital heart disease: its impact on pregnancy, Hosp Pract 18:65, 1983.

112. Witter FR, King TM, and Blake DA: Adverse effects of cardiovascular drug therapy on the fetus and neonate, Obstet Gynecol 58 (suppl):100S, 1981.

113. Wolf PS: Cardiovascular disorders. In Abrams RS and Wexler P: Medical care of the pregnant patient, Boston, 1983, Little, Brown & Co, Inc.

114. Zackai EJ et al: The fetal trimethadione syndrome, J Pediatr 87:280, 1975.

115. Zakarija M and McKenzie M: Pregnancy-associated changes in the thyroid-stimulating antibody of Graves' disease and the relationship to neonatal hyperthyroidism, J Clin Endocrinol Metab 57:1036, 1983.

116. Zuspan FP and Rayburn WF: Drug abuse during pregnancy. In Rayburn WF and Zuspan FP, editors: Drug therapy in obstetrics and gynecology, East Norwalk, Conn, 1986, Appleton-Century-Crofts.

CHAPTER 3

Delivery room care

STEPHEN M. GOLDEN · DOLORES Y. PETERS

The primary goal of immediate delivery room care is to support the newborn's respiratory and circulatory functions during the transition from fetal to neonatal life. Normal physiologic changes at birth include lung expansion with initiation of air exchange and closure of circulatory shunts that were necessary during intrauterine life. These processes may be profoundly affected by intrapartum complications, such as asphyxia and shock, causing the distressed newborn's survival and well-being to depend on steps taken to support bodily functions in the first few minutes after birth. Neonatal resuscitative techniques include stimulation, assisted ventilation, cardiac massage, and the use of volume expansion and medications. Information in this chapter will provide the reader with a clearer understanding of the physiologic and pathophysiologic events that take place in the distressed neonate and the techniques and equipment used in delivery room resuscitation.

PHYSIOLOGY

Physiologic transition from an intrauterine to an extrauterine existence must be made by the neonate at birth. Effective rhythmic respirations should be initiated within 30 to 45 seconds after birth. Environmental factors such as a relatively cool ambient temperature and tactile stimulation assist in initiating respiration. In addition, clamping of the umbilical cord with immediate changes in PaO_2 and $PaCO_2$ affects chemoreceptors and aids in the reflexive initiation of respiration. The initial breath may generate from 20 to 70 cm H_2O of negative intrathoracic pressure to expand the collapsed alveoli. A rapid decrease in pulmonary vascular resistance and increase in pulmonary circulation occur following lung expansion, allowing the pulmonary perfusion required for extrauterine life. Removal and absorption of intrauterine lung fluid is also necessary, and this is affected by two factors: (1) in a vaginal delivery pressures applied to the infant's chest may "squeeze" fluid from the respiratory tract, and (2) after delivery, colloid osmotic pressure and hydrostatic pressure of blood within the pulmonary circuit assist in absorbing alveolar fluid. After this fluid is absorbed, closure of fetal right-to-left shunts is necessary (Figure 3-1 and Table 3-1).

ASPHYXIA AND APNEA

Neonatal asphyxia and intrauterine asphyxia occur when there is inadequate cellular perfusion and oxygenation. Hypoxic tissues begin anaerobic metabolism, producing metabolic acids that are initially buffered by bicarbonate. When the bicarbonate supply fails, acidosis ($\downarrow$ pH) occurs. Initially, acidosis and hypoxia result in reflexive, compensatory changes. After an initial tachycardia, cardiac output decreases and a generalized peripheral vasoconstriction occurs to maintain a blood pressure adequate for perfusion of vital organs. Conversion from aerobic to anaerobic glycolysis takes place with the accumulation of lactate and the development of metabolic acidosis.

Intrauterine asphyxia may result in fetal respiratory movements, alterations in fetal heart rate patterns, and the passage of meconium. In animal experiments the temporary cessation of respirations following an acute asphyxic episode is called

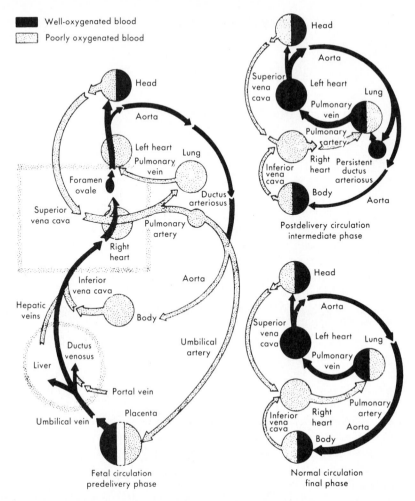

Well-oxygenated blood

Poorly oxygenated blood

Figure 3-1. Blood circulation before and after birth. (From Babson SG, Pernoll ML, and Benda GI: Diagnosis and management of the fetus and neonate at risk: a guide for team care, ed 4, St Louis, 1980, The CV Mosby Co.)

primary apnea (Figure 3-2). If the asphyxic insult progresses 1 to 2 minutes further in utero, the heart rate falls and a series of spontaneous deep gasps occurs. Gasping will continue but become weaker and finally cease (secondary apnea).

The longer artificial ventilation is delayed after an infant's last gasp, the longer the time required for the infant's first spontaneous gasp after resuscitation. For every 1-minute delay, the time to the first gasp is increased by about 2

minutes, and the time to the onset of spontaneous breathing is delayed by more than 4 minutes.

Clinically, in utero asphyxia causes the fetus to have tachycardia, loss of baseline variability, late decelerations, or prolonged bradycardia. Infants born with primary apnea may have cyanosis and bradycardia but can have good capillary filling and some muscle tone. Spontaneous respirations may be induced by sensory

TABLE 3-1

Comparison of Vascular and Pulmonary Functions before and after Birth

FETAL FUNCTION	BODY STRUCTURE	EXTRAUTERINE FUNCTION
Shunts most of the oxygenated blood from placenta to inferior vena cava	Ductus venosus	Disappears within 2 weeks after birth; becomes ligamentum venosum
Connects right and left atria; permits oxygenated blood from right atrium to bypass right ventricle and pulmonary circuit and go directly into left atrium	Foramen ovale	Functionally closes soon after birth; anatomically seals during childhood
Shunts blood from pulmonary artery directly into aorta	Ductus arteriosus	Functionally closes soon after birth; eventually becomes ligamentum arteriosum
Carries blood to and from placenta, the organ of respiration before birth	Umbilical arteries and veins	Clamped at birth, obliterating placenta connections; become ligaments
Carries oxygenated and deoxygenated blood from left ventricle and pulmonary arteries	Aorta	Carries oxygenated blood from left ventricle into systemic circulation
Collapsed; minimal pulmonary circulation; fetal respiratory movements	Lungs	Expanded and aerated; pulmonary circulation allows CO_2 and O_2 exchange; organ of respiration

stimuli (e.g., vigorous drying or positive-pressure ventilation).

Infants born with secondary apnea appear bradycardic (heart rate <60 beats/min), pale, and flaccid. Spontaneous respirations can no longer be induced by sensory stimuli because of the profound circulatory, biochemical, and neurologic changes that have occurred. If secondary apnea is not treated by immediate resuscitation, brain damage or death can result. Profound fetal and neonatal asphyxia adversely affect physiologic transitions to extrauterine life. As previously indicated, onset of rhythmic breathing is delayed by neurologic depression, resulting from intrauterine hypoxia and acidosis. After delivery, the baby's ineffective respiratory efforts and decreased cardiac output will result in progressive biochemical deterioration:

- A plasma PO_2 of 0 in less than 5 minutes
- An increase in PCO_2 of 8 mm Hg/min
- A decrease in pH of 0.04 units/min
- A decrease in bicarbonate of 2 mEq/min

The normally high fetal pulmonary vascular re-

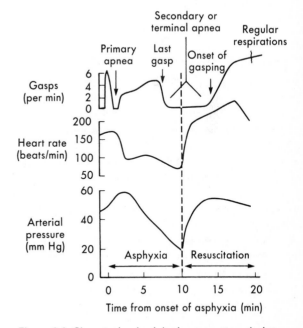

Figure 3-2. Changes in physiologic parameters during asphyxiation and resuscitation of Rhesus monkey fetus at birth. (From Klaus MH and Fanaroff AA: Care of the high-risk neonate, ed 2, Philadelphia, 1979, WB Saunders Co.)

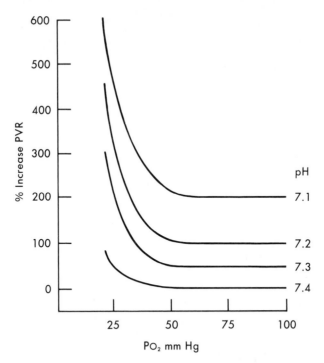

Figure 3-3. Pulmonary vascular resistance in calf. *PVR,* Pulmonary vascular resistance. (From Rudolph AM and Yuan S. Reproduced from The Journal of Clinical Investigation, 1966, 45:399, by copyright permission of the American Society for Clinical Investigation.)

sistance may not decrease in the presence of persistent acidosis and hypoxia, and consequently the pulmonary circuit continues to carry low volumes of blood and remains hypoperfused (Figure 3-3). Lung fluid clearance may also be delayed because of pulmonary hypoperfusion. Additionally, intraalveolar fluid may accumulate as a result of leakage from damaged pulmonary capillaries. Normal closure of fetal shunts is delayed by pulmonary hypoperfusion, hypoexpansion, and hypoxia, thus resulting in persisting right-to-left shunting.

Prevention, treatment, and intervention

Birth asphyxia is a medical emergency, requiring immediate and proper intervention to prevent infant mortality or morbidity.

High-risk factors during the mother's pregnancy and problems or abnormalities during labor may be used to identify the infant prone to neonatal asphyxia (see pp. 11-12). Any "normal" pregnancy, however, may become "high risk" with the onset of previously unexpected or undetected complications during the intrapartum phase (e.g., maternal hemorrhage, prolapsed cord, and meconium staining).

Prevention, detection, and treatment of fetal asphyxia is the responsibility of the obstetric team. Once diagnosed, therapeutic intervention should be coordinated between the obstetric and neonatal services to allow for a timely delivery and effective, coordinated resuscitation.

The basic goals of resuscitation are:
1. **To expand the lungs and maintain adequate ventilation and oxygenation**

2. To maintain adequate cardiac output and tissue perfusion
3. To maintain normal core temperature and avoid hypoglycemia while stabilizing the infant for transport to the nursery

To achieve these goals, resuscitation procedures should be *simple*, with established procedures and protocols; *organized*, with a minimum of two people (with clearly understood and preassigned functions); and *effective*, with continuous observation and assessment to individualize treatment for each neonate's particular needs.

Anticipation and preparation are the key concepts inherent in delivery room resuscitation techniques (Table 3-2). Physicians and nursing personnel skilled in neonatal resuscitation, functional equipment (Table 3-3), and emergency medications should be immediately available (Table 3-4).

The pediatric staff should be familiar with the prenatal and intrapartum history of the

---

TABLE 3-2

Conditions that May Require Availability of Skilled Resuscitation at Delivery

1. Fetal distress
    a. Persistent late decelerations
    b. Severe variable decelerations without baseline variability
    c. Scalp pH <7.25
    d. Meconium-stained amniotic fluid
    e. Cord prolapse
2. Operative delivery
3. Third-trimester bleeding
4. Multiple births
5. Low birth weight infant
6. Prematurity
7. Breech presentation
8. Prolonged, unusual, or difficult labor
9. Insulin-dependent diabetes
10. Severe isoimmunization
11. Suspected maternal infection

Modified from American Academy of Pediatrics and American College of Obstetricians and Gynecologists: Guidelines for perinatal care, ed 2, Evanston, Ill, 1988, American Academy of Pediatrics and American College of Obstetricians and Gynecologists.

TABLE 3-3

Equipment Used during Neonatal Resuscitation

Required materials
Stethoscope
Laryngoscope (with extra batteries)
No. 0 and no. 1 blades (with extra bulbs)
Ventilator bag (100% oxygen capability; in-line manometer preferable)
Suction apparatus (bulb, DeLee or wall vacuum, sterile catheters)
Neonatal face masks
Endotracheal tubes (2.5, 3, 3.5, and 4 mm)
Oxygen source (tank or wall outlet; regulator, blender, heated nebulizer)
Radiant heat source (servocontrol, flat bed)

Additional materials
Catheterization tray
IV solutions (i.e., $D_{10}W$)
Resuscitative drugs (see Table 3-5)
Blood administration set

Miscellaneous equipment
Warm blankets and towels
Cord clamps
Sterile gloves
Procedure lights
Tape, gauze, alcohol swabs, skin prep (e.g., benzoin)
Antiseptic spray, syringes
Needles, IV catheter and tubing

Optional equipment
Oxygen analyzer
Neonatal oropharyngeal airway
Cardiorespiratory monitor
Wall clock or stopwatch

TABLE 3-4

Emergency Neonatal Resuscitation Drugs and Dosages*

DRUG OR THERAPEUTIC INTERVENTION	HOW TO PREPARE			CLINICAL INDICATIONS	PRECAUTIONS
	SHELF CONCENTRATION	DOSE			
Volume expanders				Shock, hypotension, blood loss, volume depletion	Monitor blood pressure.
Whole blood	Hct 35-45	10 ml/kg increments			
Packed RBCs	Hct 70-80	10 ml/kg increments			
0.9% NaCl	0.9% NaCl	10-20 ml/kg increments			
5% salt-poor albumin	5% in 0.9% NaCl	10-20 ml/kg increments			
Plasmanate	5% in 0.9% NaCl	10-20 ml/kg increments			
Epinephrine 1:10,000	1:1000 1:10,000	10 μg (0.1 ml)/kg IV, ET tube		Bradycardia, asystole	Never give into artery. Administer rapidly; do not mix with $NaHCO_3$ (inactivation).
Atropine	0.1 mg/ml (prefilled syringe)	0.01 mg (0.1 ml)/kg IV, ET tube		Bradycardia (vagal nerve blocker)	Administer rapidly. Neonatal vagolytic dose unknown; hyperthermia.
Neonatal naloxone (Narcan)	0.02 mg/ml	0.005-0.01 mg/kg (0.25-0.5 ml)/kg IV IV, ET tube		Respiratory depression as a result of maternal narcotics	Give only in presence of narcotic depression. Do not give to infants of drug-dependent mothers. Repeat 2-3 doses every 30-90 min, if necessary.
Dextrose	10% (100 mg/ml)	2 ml/kg (200 mg/kg)		Hypoglycemia	Administer alone or as diluent. Monitor for glucosuria. Follow Dextrostix.
Sodium bicarbonate ($NaHCO_3$)	44 mEq/50 ml 50 mEq/50 ml 0.5 mEq/1 ml	1-2 mEq/kg IV (½ mEq/ml)		Metabolic acidosis (persistent pH <7.25)	Administer only with adequate ventilation. Administer slowly (2 ml/min). Diluted forms remain hypertonic.

*Although intrauterine asphyxia can cause cardiogenic shock, the most common causes of cardiovascular insufficiency are hypoxia and acidosis. Drugs should be administered only if the infant fails to respond to endotracheal intubation and ventilation using 100% oxygen, cardiac massage, and volume expansion. Drugs are the last treatment of choice and are only administered if the infant's heart rate remains less than 100 beats/min despite all previous interventions. Intracardiac epinephrine should be avoided and used only in extremis.

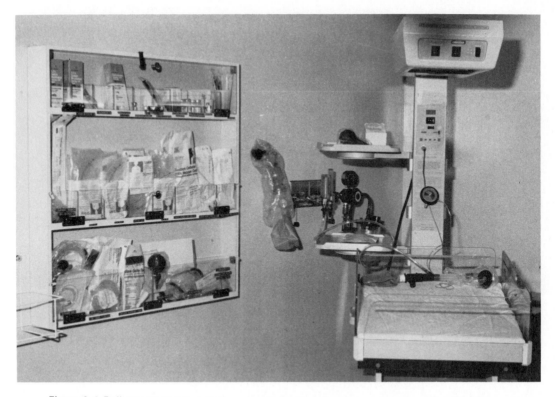

Figure 3-4. Delivery room resuscitation area consisting of radiant warmer, anesthesia-style ventilator bag with manometer, wall oxygen and suction outlets, backup self-inflating hand ventilator, and easily accessible resuscitation drugs and equipment located in wall unit. Umbilical catheterization tray and additional supplies are kept in storage area of radiant warmer.

mother and fetus, since these data will affect the initial level of resuscitation preparation.

Resuscitation equipment and drugs should always be readily available, portable, functional, and assembled for immediate use in a specific location, ideally in a specific area of the delivery room. Consumable supplies and small equipment can be stored on specially constructed wall shelves or on a radiant warmer intensive-care bed equipped with easily accessible shelves (Figures 3-4 and 3-5).

Prepare for resuscitation by performing the following:

- Preheat the transport incubator; assure that the battery pack is fully charged.
- Be certain that the portable oxygen tanks are filled.
- Preheat the radiant warmer.
- Turn on the oxygen flow to the ventilation bag and check all connections, pop-off control valves, manometer function, and face masks.
- Check suction equipment for function, and set the wall vacuum regulator control at less than or equal to 60 mm H_2O.
- Check the laryngoscope for a bright light

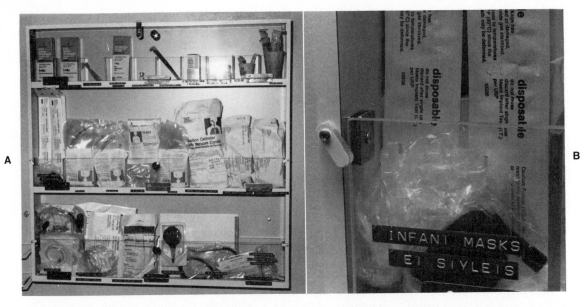

Figure 3-5. **A,** Wall-mounted storage bin. Unit consists of three Plexiglas shelves; each shelf is divided by Plexiglas into smaller compartments. Each compartment is labeled. Shelves can be opened for cleaning. Each shelf is held in place by hinge and magnet. **B,** Hinge and magnet device used to ensure closure of Plexiglas shelves.

source and appropriate blades (size no. 0 for premature infants and size no. 1 for term infants); tighten the bulb.

- **Check for availability of endotracheal tubes.**
- **Check for ancillary equipment (i.e., sterile trays, intravenous [IV] solutions, drugs).**
- **If the clinical situation warrants it, draw up emergency medications for ready administration and obtain O negative packed red blood cells for emergency transfusion.**
- **Check availability and cleanliness of stethoscopes.**

Apgar score

The Apgar scoring system, developed by Dr. Virginia Apgar in 1952, provides an objective, quantitative measure of the infant's condition shortly after birth (Figure 3-6). Although used as an indicator of the need and extent for resuscitation, intervention should not be stopped or delayed to determine the Apgar score. The Apgar score also may be used to objectively assess an infant's response to resuscitative measures. Although degrees of asphyxia may be qualitatively associated with Apgar scores as indicated below, it is possible for an infant to have a low Apgar score without having asphyxia. For example, an infant born to a mother who received general anesthesia may be flaccid, have depressed reflexes, and poor respiratory efforts. The heart rate of such an infant should be greater than 100 beats/min, and the Apgar score should be between 2 and 3. These infants usually respond rapidly to bag and mask ventilation, and no further intervention is necessary. Conversely, an infant may have an Apgar score of 2 as a result of intrauterine asphyxia and require prolonged resuscitative efforts. Likewise, an infant with a midrange Apgar score between 6 and 7 may be using all of his or her homeostatic

SIGN		SCORE		
		0	1	2
A	Appearance (color)	Blue, pale	Body pink Extremities blue	Completely pink
P	Pulse (heart rate)	Absent	Below 100	Above 100
G	Grimace (reflex, irritability to suctioning)	No response	Grimace	Cough or sneeze
A	Activity (muscle tone)	Limp	Some flexion	Well flexed
R	Respiration (breathing efforts)	Absent	Weak, irregular	Strong cry

Figure 3-6. Practical epigram of Apgar score. (From Butterfield J and Covey M: JAMA 181:353, 1962. Copyright 1962, American Medical Association.)

mechanisms to maintain an adequate central blood pressure and cardiac output.

Physicians and nursing personnel must recognize that the Apgar score does not reflect the eventual state of an infant's well-being. A low score, however, requires that life support be initiated.

NO ASPHYXIA (APGAR SCORE BETWEEN 8 AND 10)

If a neonate has an Apgar score between 8 and 10, perform the following steps:

- Place the neonate in a radiant warmer in a Trendelenburg position to drain mucus, and rapidly dry the infant with warm towels to prevent heat loss.
- Suction the nose and oropharynx with a bulb syringe.
- If the heart rate is greater than 120 beats/min, the oropharynx and stomach may be suctioned with a catheter.
- Monitor the heart rate and discontinue suctioning if a vagal bradycardia is elicited.
- Minimize needless body exposure.
- Clamp the umbilical cord.
- After the infant is stabilized and vigorous, perform elective procedures, such as applying ophthalmic prophylaxis or weighing.

- Wrap the infant in a blanket or place next to the mother's skin. (A vigorous, crying, well-oxygenated infant may be safely held and/or nursed by the parents after delivery.)
- Prepare the infant for transport to the nursery in a warmed transport incubator.

MILD ASPHYXIA (APGAR SCORE BETWEEN 5 AND 7)

If the neonate has an Apgar score between 5 and 7, perform the following steps:

- Place the neonate in a radiant warmer in a Trendelenburg position.
- Suction the nose and oropharynx with a bulb syringe to clear secretions.
- Provide quick, gentle stimulation while drying the infant with warmed towels.
- Monitor the heart rate, respiratory rate, and general appearance.
- Provide warmed, humidified oxygen by face mask.
- If spontaneous respirations are delayed, administer intermittent positive-pressure breathing with a bag and mask using 20 to 25 cm H_2O pressure at 30 to 40 breaths/min. (Deliver constant positive airway pressure with 8 to 10 cm H_2O if available.)

Adequate ventilation and pink central color should be established with these interventions.

- Clamp the umbilical cord.
- After the infant is stabilized and vigorous, elective procedures may be performed.

MODERATE ASPHYXIA (APGAR SCORE BETWEEN 3 AND 4)

If the neonate's Apgar score is between 3 and 4, perform the following steps:

- Place the neonate in a radiant warmer in a Trendelenburg position.
- Suction the nose and oropharynx with a bulb syringe.
- Dry the newborn off quickly with warmed towels.
- Monitor the heart rate, respiratory rate, and general appearance.
- Begin bag and mask ventilation with 100% oxygen at pressures of 20 to 25 cm H_2O and a rate of 30 to 40 breaths/min initially. (NOTE: Higher pressures of 30 to 40 cm H_2O may be required to open collapsed alveoli. Proceed cautiously to avoid pneumothorax.)
- Observe chest wall movement, quality of breath sounds, skin color, and muscle tone.

Once the neonate begins spontaneous respirations, continue oxygen administration until acyanotic. If the heart rate is less than 60 beats/min, begin cardiac resuscitation measures. Three attendants are required for optimal resuscitation to (1) manage the airway and ventilation, (2) monitor the heart rate and peripheral pulses, and (3) prepare and administer emergency drug therapy and record the time and dose given.

Although a stethoscope is adequate for monitoring the heart rate, electronic cardiorespiratory monitoring is useful for the patient requiring prolonged, continuous, assessment. Heart rate monitoring, however, should not be delayed to set up equipment and attach leads, especially since self-adhesive leads often fall off a newborn's moist, vernix-covered skin, unless time is taken to properly cleanse and dry contact surfaces. The heart rate may also be obtained by palpating the umbilical cord pulse. The individual assessing the heart rate should indicate each pulse by tapping the thumb and index finger together. If the heart rate continues to be less than 100 beats/min and there is poor peripheral perfusion, begin circulatory support measures. (Refer to the section on circulatory support and Table 3-4.)

Although these infants are usually acidotic at birth, they will usually correct their acidotic state spontaneously once ventilation is well established. Metabolic correction of the pH balance is a slow process, taking several hours, and treatment with $NaHCO_3$ is not mandated without prior blood gas analysis.

Monitor blood pressure, hematocrit (Hct), and blood gases. If necessary, provide volume expansion with fluids or blood by an umbilical venous catheter or IV (see Table 3-4). If the infant has a persistent requirement for oxygen, insert an umbilical artery catheter for periodic arterial blood gas assessments. Transfer the neonate to the nursery in a warmed transport incubator with required support measures. Delay elective procedures until the infant is physiologically stable.

SEVERE ASPHYXIA (APGAR SCORE BETWEEN 0 AND 2)

If the neonate's Apgar score is less than 3, perform the following steps;

- Start immediate, vigorous resuscitation using at least three trained people working together as a swift, efficient team. (Responsibilities should be assigned and understood before the infant is received to ensure efficient clinical intervention.)
- Place the baby in a radiant warmer in a Trendelenburg position.
- Quickly suction the airway with a bulb syringe.
- Dry off the trunk quickly with warmed towels and keep warm.

- Monitor the heart rate and other vital signs.
- Immediately begin bag and mask ventilation or promptly intubate and ventilate with 100% oxygen at 25 to 35 cm H_2O at 30 to 40 breaths/min. (The infant initially may require higher pressures.)
- Immediately begin coordinated external cardiac massage at a rate of 100 to 120 compressions/min.
- Perform endotracheal intubation and continue artificial ventilation.
- Place an umbilical venous catheter for required administration of volume expansion fluids and drugs. (Refer to Table 3-4.)
- Monitor the time of the baby's first respiratory effort and response to resuscitative efforts, adjusting therapeutic interventions as needed.
- When stabilized, transport the infant to the nursery as soon as possible for follow-up treatment and observation.
- Defer all elective procedures until the infant is stable.
- If the infant has no vital signs after 20 minutes of vigorous, appropriate resuscitative interventions and drug therapy, consider discontinuing life support measures.

Figure 3-7 shows a logical progression of resuscitative procedures.

Transport from delivery room to nursery

1. Transport should not interfere with ongoing care and monitoring.
2. A warmed transport incubator should be used.
3. The heart rate should be monitored with a stethoscope or electronic monitor.
4. The infant should not be moved until adequate spontaneous or controlled ventilation is established, the heart rate is at least 80 beats/min, and the infant is dried and protected from excessive heat loss.

BAG AND MASK VENTILATION

Effective ventilation can be maintained using a bag and face mask. Ventilation should be initiated with inspiratory pressures of 20 to 30 cm H_2O and a rate of 30 to 40 breaths/min. Infants with collapsed or fluid-filled alveoli may occasionally require inspiratory pressures of 40 to 60 cm H_2O. The adequacy of ventilation must be continuously assessed by auscultating and visualizing chest wall movement, monitoring heart rate, and observing skin color. Peak inspiratory pressure should be limited to that which is necessary to visualize chest wall movement and auscultate breath sounds. Inspiratory pressures cannot be judged clinically, and all bags should be fitted with an in-line pressure manometer. Use 100% oxygen for all resuscitations requiring mechanical ventilation. Oral airways are usually not needed for bag and mask ventilation.

RESUSCITATION BAGS

Anesthesia bags. Anesthesia bags contain an inflatable gas reservoir that is refilled between breaths.

Advantages. Advantages include:
1. The ability to deliver 100% oxygen and any desired inspiratory pressure
2. The ability to maintain a positive end expiratory pressure
3. Can easily be fitted with an in-line manometer

Disadvantages. Disadvantages include:
1. Dependence on an external oxygen supply
2. Requires practice and experience for efficient and safe use
3. Can deliver very high inspiratory pressures with risk of pneumothorax

Self-inflating bags. Self-inflating bags fill with ambient air and are independent of an external oxygen or a compressed air source.

Advantages. Advantages include:
1. Simplicity of use
2. Self-inflation (useful backup system in case compressed oxygen source fails)

Disadvantages. Disadvantages include:
1. The maximum pressure–limiting pop-off value, usually set by the manufacturer at 30 to 35 cm H_2O, will preclude adequate ventilation in a noncompliant lung. (Some models have a manual override device

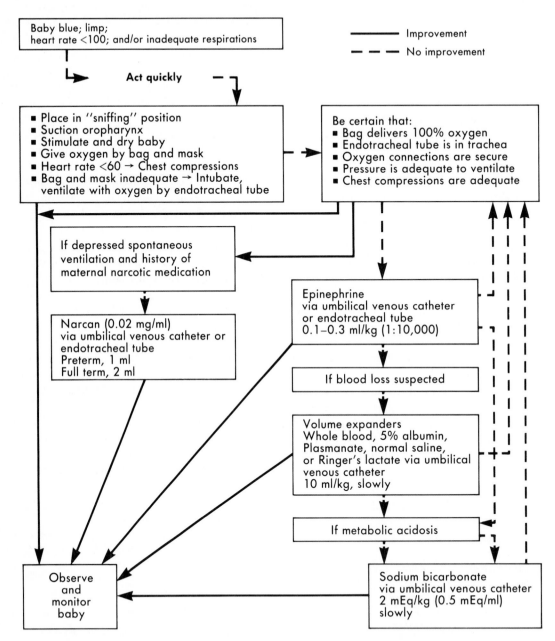

Figure 3-7. Neonatal resuscitation flow chart. (Redrawn from Unit 6, Neonatal Resuscitation, Perinatal Continuing Education Program, 1989 edition, University of Virginia, Charlottesville.)

that will allow increased inspiratory pressures.)

2. A reservoir must be attached to deliver 100% oxygen.

3. The bags cannot deliver end expiratory pressure, and it is difficult to retrofit them with an in-line manometer.

Pressure face masks. Pressure face masks consist of a face mask and a gas-releasing trigger; they are supplied with many infant warming units marketed for delivery room use. Pressure face masks should not be used in lieu of a resuscitation bag, because peak inspiratory pressures are difficult to control, excessive pressures are easily delivered, tidal volume and inspiratory times are difficult to maintain, and changes in the lung and airway compliance cannot be judged.

BAG AND MASK TECHNIQUE

- Rapidly clear the mouth and pharynx of debris and fluid.
- Slightly extend the head into a neutral "sniffing" position. (Avoid hyperextension.)
- Place a proper-size face mask over the infant's nose and mouth (size 0 for infants <2000 g and size 1 for infants >2000 g).
- Maintain a tight seal between the face and mask using the thumb, index finger, and fleshy portion of the palm between the thumb and index finger.
- Place remaining fingers at the angle of the mandible and along the length of the mandible, and exert an upward and outward pressure to counteract the downward pressure on the face mask and maintain the head in a slightly extended position (Figure 3-8).
- Ventilate with 100% oxygen.

ENDOTRACHEAL INTUBATION

A noncuffed, uniform-diameter endotracheal (ET) tube should be used for intubation. A variety of ET tube sizes should always be available, since the initial estimate of the tracheal diame-

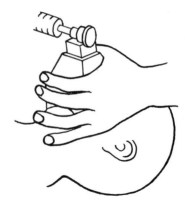

Figure 3-8. Position for bag and mask ventilation.

ter may be incorrect. Orotracheal intubation is recommended over nasotracheal intubation during acute resuscitation because it can be performed rapidly without stylets and forceps. A stylet can facilitate intubation by providing extra rigidity and a fixed curvature, but the stylet tip should end no less than 1 cm from the end of the ET tube to prevent trauma to the pharyngeal and tracheal structures. A suction apparatus should be readily available.

INTUBATION TECHNIQUE

- Lay the infant on a flat, unobstructed and slightly extended "sniffing" position.
- Hold the laryngoscope handle in the left hand.
- Using a no. 0 or no. 1 straight blade, insert the laryngoscope blade into the right corner of the infant's mouth.
- With a smooth, sweeping motion, push the tongue to the left, using the vertical side of the laryngoscope blade. This should allow visualization of the midline glottic opening (Figure 3-9).
- If the epiglottis is not seen, slowly withdraw the laryngoscope blade until the epiglottis is seen.
- Position the tip of the blade into the vallecula or under the end of the epiglottis. (The laryngoscope blade is usually in one of

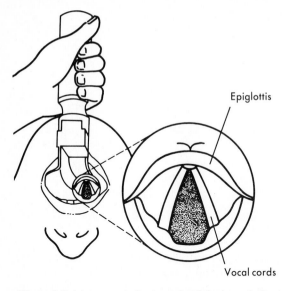

Figure 3-9. Laryngoscopic view of epiglottis and glottis.

these two positions when the epiglottis is visualized.) (Figure 3-10)

- Using the junction of the laryngoscope blade and handle as a fixed fulcrum point, gently tip the laryngoscope back until the glottic opening is clearly seen.
- Avoid applying pressure on the upper gingiva.
- Applying a gentle, downward external pressure on the trachea may help visualize the glottis. (This can be performed by the intubator or by an assistant.) (Figure 3-10)
- Insert the ET tube from the right corner of the mouth.
- Constantly observe the ET tube during its approach to and entry into the trachea.
- The ET tube should lay above the carina. Evaluate the tube position by auscultation for bilaterally equal breath sounds and symmetric chest wall movement.

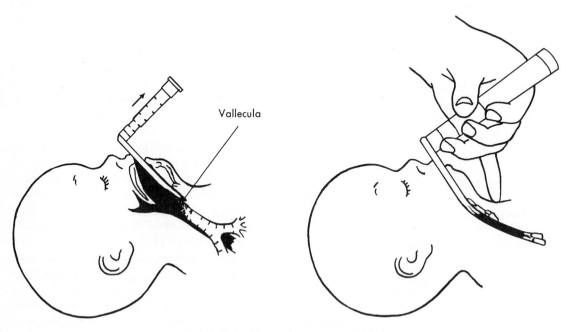

Figure 3-10. Positions of laryngoscope blade.

- **Dry and prep the infant's face with benzoin. Tape the ET tube into position and confirm the location by chest x-ray film.**
- **Avoid excessive motion of the infant's head after intubation because flexion tends to push the ET tube farther into the trachea, and extension may dislodge the tube from the trachea.**
- **Monitor the infant's heart rate during intubation efforts. Severe bradycardia may be a reason to cease intubation and resume bag and mask ventilation with 100% oxygen until the heart rate returns to baseline values.**

CIRCULATORY SUPPORT OF THE INFANT IN SHOCK

Resuscitation of an asphyxiated or depressed infant must be performed rapidly to prevent or limit tissue injury because of hypoxia, acidosis, and hypoglycemia. Delay in appropriate therapy may exacerbate cellular injury in all organ systems and result in long-term morbidity or mortality. The immediate physiologic goal of resuscitation is to remove cellular waste products and restore oxygen and glucose delivery to all tissues. After establishing an airway and pulmonary ventilation, cardiac output and blood pressure must be maintained to perfuse tissues. Lack of response to proper ventilation, such as persistent bradycardia or evidence of poor peripheral perfusion, should be considered a harbinger of shock, and the infant must be treated in a rapid, systematic manner (see Figure 3-7).

Persistent peripheral vasoconstriction temporarily maintains systemic blood pressure but results in inadequate tissue perfusion with progressive cellular hypoxia and acidosis. Circulating volume and cardiac output are gradually reduced by third-space leakage from damaged capillaries. Persistent hypoxia and acidosis will eventually result in irreversible cellular damage refractory to all therapy.

The overlapping symptomatology of the multiple causes of low Apgar scores in the delivery room makes the precise diagnosis of shock difficult (see outlines on pp. 66-68). Common symptoms of shock seen in older infants and children, such as oliguria, tachycardia, cyanosis, and hypothermia, are unreliable indicators of shock in infants.

Common clinical symptoms of shock in the delivery room include (1) poor peripheral perfusion, pallor, and decreased capillary filling; (2) hypotension; and (3) bradycardia. Although metabolic acidosis is always present in shock, none of the previously mentioned symptoms alone or in combination is an absolute indicator of shock in the delivery room. The diagnosis is often retrospective and determined by the infant's response to resuscitative measures, the eventual clinical course, and perinatal history. Management and prevention of shock require maintaining cardiac output, blood pressure, and adequate circulating volume.

External cardiac compression

External cardiac compression is indicated when the heart rate is equal to or less than 60 beats/min or less than 80 beats/min with effective ventilation being given. To perform the technique of external cardiac compression:

1. **Draw an imaginary line between the baby's nipples, and place your index and middle fingers on the midsternum, which should be about one finger's width below the imaginary line. To effectively use this technique, the infant must be lying on a firm surface, and you must be cautious of the amount of force applied (Figure 3-11).**
2. **Using your fingertips, compress the midsternum vertically ½ to 1 inch, but not more than two thirds of the baby's anteroposterior diameter, at a rate of 100 compressions/min (five in 3 seconds or less).**
3. **The infant should be ventilated between every fifth compression, although absolute coordination between ventilation and compression is not mandatory. A small di-**

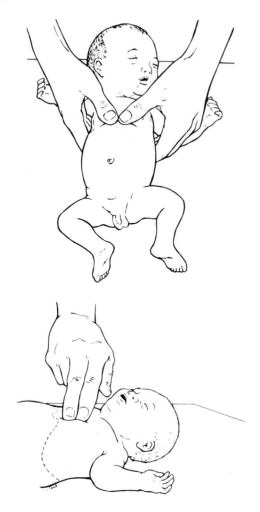

Figure 3-11. Position for cardiac massage. (From Whaley LF and Wong DL: Nursing care of infants and children, St Louis, 1979, The CV Mosby Co.)

aper roll or towel may be placed beneath the baby's neck to help maintain airway patency for ventilation during cardiac compressions.

Complications

Excessively vigorous compressions or compressions over the xyphoid process can result in a fractured xyphoid process, liver or spleen lac-

eration, or cardiac rupture. Evaluation of the therapy should include a determination of the adequacy of external cardiac compression by palpating the femoral, brachial, or carotid pulses and by observing capillary filling. A member of the resuscitation team should check for all common causes of failure to respond to ventilation and external cardiac compression:

1. Is the ET tube in proper position or obstructed, causing inadequate ventilation?
2. Is the oxygen supply functioning and are all the lines connected?
3. Are other therapeutic modalities indicated, such as drugs and volume expansion? (See Figure 3-7 and Tables 3-3 to 3-6.)

Common causes of intrauterine shock

I. Hypovolemia
   A. Abruptio placentae
   B. Acute fetal-maternal bleeding
   C. Umbilical cord tear
   D. Twin-to-twin transfusion
II. Asphyxia neonatorum
III. Hypoxic-induced myocardial dysfunction
IV. Sepsis
V. Hydrops fetalis
VI. Intrauterine paroxysmal supraventricular tachycardia
VII. Intrauterine closure of patent ductus arteriosus
VIII. Intrauterine adrenal insufficiency

Extrauterine causes of neonatal shock

I. Delayed institution of resuscitation
   A. Improper technique
   B. Equipment malfunction
II. Inadequate pulmonary ventilation
   A. Intrinsic lung disease
      1. Respiratory distress syndrome
      2. Hypoplastic lungs
      3. Pneumonia
   B. Extrinsic airway obstruction
      1. Meconium aspiration
      2. Tension pneumothorax
      3. Diaphragmatic hernia
      4. Choanal atresia
      5. Laryngeal web
      6. Tumor

TABLE 3-5

Complications during and after Resuscitation

PROBLEM	CAUSE	DIAGNOSIS	REMEDIES
Persistent cyanosis	Inadequate FIo_2		Always administer 100% O_2
	Disconnected O_2 line	Check all connections and flow meters	Reconnect line
	Empty O_2 cylinder	Check O_2 source	Start new O_2 cylinder
	Inadequate ventilation		
	Malpositioned ET tube	Check tube position with laryngoscope	Reinsert ET tube into trachea
		Check breath sounds	Adjust tube so that breath sounds are bilaterally equal
			Tape ET tube in place
	Pneumothorax	Check breath sounds	Decompress tension pneumothorax
		Check for asymmetry of chest	
		Transillumination	
		Chest x-ray examination	
	Improper bag and mask ventilation		
	Insufficient insufflation pressure	Diminished breath sounds; little chest wall movement	Increase insufflation pressure until breath sounds are audible and chest movement seen
	Compression of airway	Diminished breath sounds; little chest wall movement	Apply upward force to mandible to counteract downward force holding face mask in place; tilt head backward
	Inadequate face mask seal	Diminished breath sounds; little chest wall movement; air leak around face mask	Readjust face mask; seal tightly against skin
Bradycardia	Same as cyanosis	Auscultation; electronic monitor or palpation	See above for cyanosis
			External cardiac compression if heart rate <80 beats/min with effective ventilation followed by drugs (see Table 3-4)
	Perinatal myocardial ischemia	Diagnosis is often retrospective and based on lack of response to oxygenation and ventilation	Same as above
Hypothermia	Evaporative heat loss; conductive heat loss	Specific symptoms overlap those of asphyxia and shock	Dry off infant
		Low core temperature	Keep under radiant warmer
Hypoglycemia	Using glucose stores before birth or during resuscitation	Specific symptoms overlap those of asphyxia and shock	Infusion of $D_{10}W$ at 100 ml/kg/24 hr
		Dextrostix	
Disconnected venous line or arterial line	Inadequately secured IV/IA line	Hemorrhage	Keep all IV connection sites in plain view
			During transport, tape IV/IA connections to tongue blade
			Tape UAC/UVC in place in addition to suturing lines

*TABLE 3-6*_____

Solutions Suitable for Volume Expansion

SOLUTION	ADVANTAGES	DISADVANTAGES
Whole blood or packed red blood cells	Isotonic Oncotic properties of plasma	Expensive Time delay inherent in obtaining blood from blood bank NOTE: "On call" O negative washed cells reconstituted with plasma from AB donor will eliminate time delay in typing and cross-matching blood against mother Risk of hepatitis, CMV, HIV
Heparinized cord blood (2.5 U heparin/ml)	Same as above Immediately available in delivery room	Sample not always sterile Danger of heparinization of infant
Isotonic, isooncotic solutions, such as Plasmanate, fresh frozen plasma, and balanced electrolyte solution with 5% albumin	Immediately available in delivery room Oncotic properties	Lack of O_2 transport and buffering capacity
Crystalloid and glucose solutions, such as lactated Ringer's, NaCl, D_5W, and $D_{10}W$	Immediately available in delivery room Can be rapidly formulated with $NaHCO_3$ for buffering capacity	Will rapidly dissipate out of intravascular space unless albumin is added to solution Lack of O_2 transport capacity Most solutions will become hypertonic with addition of $NaHCO_3$

III. Blood loss
    A. Cord tear
    B. Fetal-maternal transfusion
    C. Twin-to-twin transfusion
    D. Abruptio placentae
    E. Neonatal hemorrhage
IV. Intraventricular hemorrhage
V. Hypothermia
VI. Hypoglycemia
VII. Subdural hematoma

Volume expansion

Expansion of the plasma and blood volumes may be required to maintain the cardiac output, blood pressure, and peripheral perfusion of infants who require resuscitation. Volume expansion should be considered when there is (1) acute blood loss with shock or pallor (e.g., abruptio placentae, umbilical cord tear or rupture, acute fetal-to-maternal bleeding, and acute neonatal hemorrhage); (2)

hypotension and poor capillary filling unresponsive to oxygen and assisted ventilation; (3) bradycardia unresponsive to oxygen, ventilation, maintenance of neutral thermal environment, glucose, and resuscitative drugs; and (4) cardiac arrest.

PROPERTIES OF VOLUME-EXPANDING FLUIDS

COLLOID OSMOTIC PRESSURE (ONCOTIC PRESSURE). IV fluids rapidly dissipate out of the vascular space and equilibrate among the extravascular space, thereby limiting the effective time of volume expansion and potentially contributing to peripheral and pulmonary edema. This diffusion can be limited by the fluid-retaining force of large macromolecules, such as albumin and globulin. Each gram of albumin retains approximately 14 ml of fluid, and each gram of dextran retains 20 ml of fluid. Albumin

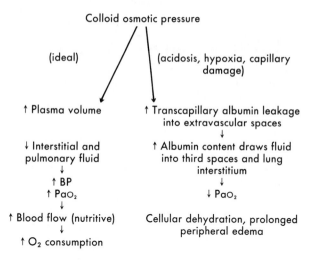

Colloid osmotic pressure

(ideal)   (acidosis, hypoxia, capillary
                                        damage)

↑ Plasma volume   ↑ Transcapillary albumin leakage
                              into extravascular spaces
                                          ↓
↓ Interstitial and   ↑ Albumin content draws fluid
pulmonary fluid   into third spaces and lung
        ↓   interstitium
      ↑ BP   ↓
      ↑ PaO₂   ↓ PaO₂
        ↓
↑ Blood flow (nutritive)   Cellular dehydration, prolonged
        ↓   peripheral edema
   ↑ O₂ consumption

Figure 3-12. Benefits and side effects of colloid infusions.

exerts the major portion of the colloid osmotic pressure (COP) in plasma. A 5% albumin solution has the same COP as serum in the full term infant. The fluid-retaining force of large macromolecules is the COP or "oncotic" pressure and is described by Starling's hypothesis:

$$F = k_f [(P_c - P_{isf}) - (\pi pl - \pi isf)]$$

Where

F = Net capillary filtration
k_f = Capillary filtration or membrane permeability coefficient
P = Hydrostatic pressure
π = Colloid osmotic pressure
c = Capillary
pl = Plasma
isf = Interstitial fluid

The actual flux of fluids across a capillary bed is also affected by other factors not described in Starling's hypothesis, such as blood flow, arteriolar dilator and constrictor phases, local tissue Po_2 and Pco_2, lymph flow, tissue distensibility, elastic recoil, and endothelial cellular integrity.

Albumin infusion in high-risk newborns has been shown to increase the serum COP, cir-

culating blood volume, and glomerular filtration rate but has not improved the long-term outcome.

Proteins normally "leak" from vascular to extravascular spaces. Healthy, full-term infants have a transcapillary escape rate (TCER) of 18%/hr, whereas preterm infants of 28 to 36 weeks gestation have had TCERs measured up to 29.6%. These high TCERs may be partly responsible for adverse effects of albumin infusion. For example, oxygen toxicity causes ultrastructural abnormalities in the alveolar pulmonary capillary membrane and resultant pulmonary edema. Albumin leakage into the pulmonary interstitial spaces may be responsible for worsening arterial/alveolar Po_2 ratios reported in some infants after albumin infusion (Figure 3-12). Albumin infusion may have no effect in restoring blood pressure in infants whose hypotension is not a result of hypovolemia.

OSMOLALITY AND OSMOLAL TOXICITY

Normal full-term serum osmolality ranges from 275 to 295 mOsm/kg. A gradient of 5 to 6 mOsm between plasma water and extracellular fluid will cause water movement out of cells to eliminate the gradient. The osmolality of 10% dextrose in water ($D_{10}W$) is twice that of normal serum, and molar sodium bicarbonate (8%) has an osmolality of nearly 2000 mOsm/kg. Infusion of 3 to 5 mEq/kg of sodium bicarbonate for a 5-minute period has been shown to raise serum osmolality up to 64 mOsm/kg over the initial preinfusion values. The hyperosmolar state caused by $NaHCO_3$ infusion is transient

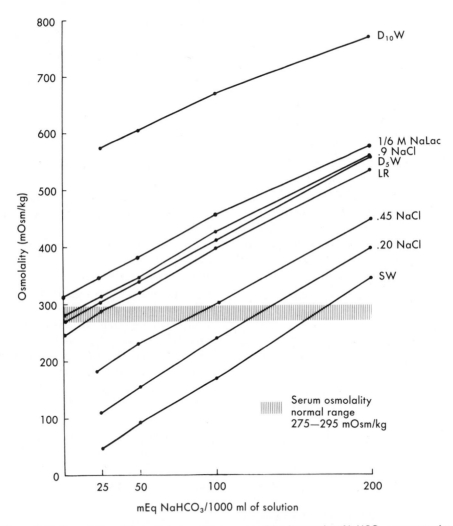

Figure 3-13. Osmolality of formulated solutions caused by increasing $NaHCO_3$ concentrations. Isotonic solutions can be rapidly formulated in delivery room. Using 10 ml volumes, each $NaHCO_3$ concentration is 0.25, 0.5, 1, and 2 mEq $NaHCO_3$/10 ml. *$D_{10}W$*, 10% dextrose in water; *D_5W*, 5% dextrose in water; *⅙ M NaLac*, ⅙ molar sodium lactate; *NaCl*, sodium chloride; *LR*, lactated Ringer's; *SW*, sterile water. (From Golden S, Monaghan WP, and Steenbarger J: Crit Care Med 12:86, 1982.)

and usually lasts less than 3 minutes, although the effect on plasma volume and hematocrit lasts more than 30 minutes. These acute iatrogenic osmotic gradients between plasma and cells may cause the immediate adverse effects of therapeutically induced hyperosmolar states such as pulmonary and intraventricular hemorrhage.

Consequently, if volume-expanding fluids are administered, isotonic solutions should be infused to diminish the changes of iatrogenic tissue damage. Figure 3-13 shows the resultant osmolality of a variety of common crystalloid and glucose solutions containing $NaHCO_3$ concentrations ranging from 25 to 200 mEq/L. Adding albumin to a solution to formulate a 5% albumin mixture will ot significantly alter the initial solution's osmolality.

VOLUME EXPANSION AND INTRAVENTRICULAR HEMORRHAGE

Rapid volume expansion with an acute elevation of the systolic blood pressure has been implicated as an etiologic factor in neonatal intraventricular hemorrhage. Distressed newborns have impaired autoregulation of cerebral blood flow, with the blood flow directly related to the systolic blood pressure. Increased cerebral blood flow and elevated systolic pressures may be responsible for intraventricular hemorrhage in the presence of a capillary bed insulted by acidosis and hypoxia. Autopsy studies also suggest that increased cerebral venous capillary pressure can initiate intraventricular hemorrhage (Figure 3-14). Because of the potential hazard of intraventricular hemorrhage associated with acute increases in systolic blood pressure, volume expansion should be performed cautiously in asphyxiated infants, infusing 10 ml/kg aliquots of fluid over a 5- to 10-minute period and evaluating the patient's response before administering repeated aliquots of fluid. The exception to this rule is the infant who has experienced acute perinatal hemorrhage and who should have the circulation fluid volume restored as rapidly as possible.

Normal neonatal blood pressures are shown in Figures 3-15 and 3-16. The lower portion of the 95% confidence limits should be used as a guide when attempting to elevate systolic blood pressure during resuscitative efforts to decrease the risk of intraventricular hemorrhage. Table 3-6 lists the advantages and disadvantages of various solutions used for volume expansion. The clinical response to volume expansion should be evaluated by assessing blood pressure, peripheral pulses and circulation, heart rate, respiratory status, and central venous pressure. If there is no clinical response after volume expansion and drug administration, the efficacy of the ventilation and oxygen delivery must be quickly evaluated.

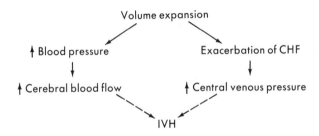

Figure 3-14. Potential adverse effects of rapid volume expansion.

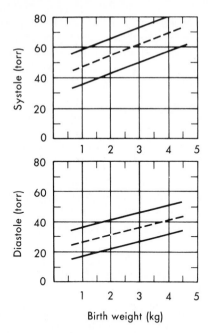

Figure 3-15. Mean aortic and pulse pressures during first 12 hours after birth. Linear regressions (*broken lines*) and 95% confidence limits (*solid lines*) on birth weight in healthy newborn infants. (From Versmold H et al: Pediatrics 67(5):607, 1981. Reproduced by permission of Pediatrics.)

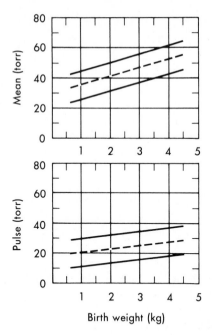

Figure 3-16. Aortic blood pressure during first 12 hours after birth. Linear regressions (*broken lines*) and 95% confidence limits (*solid lines*) of systolic and diastolic blood pressures on birth weight in healthy newborn infants. (From Versmold H et al: Pediatrics 67(5):607, 1981. Reproduced by permission of Pediatrics.)

COMMON DELIVERY ROOM COMPLICATIONS REQUIRING SPECIALIZED RESUSCITATION TECHNIQUES
Meconium-stained amniotic fluid

Meconium-stained amniotic fluid most often occurs in infants older than 34 weeks gestational age, particularly in postterm neonates (>42 weeks gestational age) and is associated with asphyxia. Meconium aspiration can sometimes be avoided if the obstetrician vigorously suctions the mouth and pharynx of an infant on delivery of the head, before respiration begins. It is important to distinguish between discolored amniotic fluid (with meconium finely dispersed throughout) and fluid containing particulate meconium that could block airways if aspirated. Infants born with meconium-stained amniotic fluid who cry immediately after birth, are acyanotic, and not in respiratory distress with clear lungs may require no special care. The trachea may be visualized on an elective basis to confirm the absence of meconium.

Infants born through thick, particulate meconium must have the oropharynx and mouth suctioned immediately after delivery. Thick, viscous meconium in the trachea must be removed by intubating the trachea and applying suction direction to the ET tube with appropriate barrier precautions for the health care provider. If the infant is apneic, bradycardic, or has poor respiratory efforts, assisted ventilation with 100% oxygen should be instituted as soon as possible after suctioning by either a face mask or an orotracheal tube. Although it is important to remove particulate meconium before ventilation, care must be taken to avoid worsening the asphyxiated state or even losing the heart rate during prolonged suctioning. If the infant is severely asphyxiated, early institution of ventilation may have to take precedence over thorough oral and tracheal suctioning.

Diaphragmatic hernia

A diaphragmatic hernia should be suspected when there is a scaphoid abdomen and respiratory distress.

- Intubate immediately and ventilate by an ET tube only. (Bag and mask positive-pressure ventilation will distend the gastrointestinal tract and further tamponade the lungs.)
- Insert an orogastric tube to decompress the gastrointestinal tract.
- Prepare for surgical intervention.

Bilateral choanal atresia

Bilateral choanal atresia should be suspected with dyspnea and cyanosis, which increases when the mouth is closed.

- Insert an oropharyngeal airway or intubate.
- Keep the airway clear of mucus and prepare for surgical intervention.

Tension pneumothorax

Tension pneumothorax may be characterized by sudden cyanosis, a shift of the cardiac point of maximal intensity, and muted heart and/or breath sounds. There may be unilaterally diminished breath sounds, hypotension, and bradycardia.

- Check the ET tube placement and equipment function.
- Confirm the diagnosis of pneumothorax by auscultation or transillumination.
- Perform emergency decompression using a 21-gauge needle in the lateral third intercostal space and aspirate air with a stopcock and syringe.
- Connect to underwater seal drainage.
- Insert a chest tube if the air leak persists or if the infant remains symptomatic.

PARENT TEACHING

Encouraging the presence of the father or of a mature support person in the delivery room is becoming common obstetric practice. The Lamaze method of delivery even encourages the presence of a labor coach in the delivery room. Although the decision to allow these individuals in the delivery room lies with the obstetrician, their presence should not pose any problems to the pediatric staff. Ideally, the pediatrician or pediatric nurse should introduce himself or herself to the parents before the delivery. Parents have a great deal of anxiety concerning the procedures performed on their newborn, and a few moments spent describing these procedures will help allay their fears and avoid their misinterpretation of routine procedures, such as suctioning, as indicative of a medical problem. If no problems are expected, it is usually sufficient to describe the routine procedures followed after a birth. When an infant is "at risk," a more detailed explanation of neonatal assessment and life support measures is necessary. While this explanation may increase parental anxiety, the knowledge that the medical staff has expected and is prepared to care for possible problems can help relieve their concerns. Care must be taken, however, to avoid instilling undue alarm. Nonverbal cues such as tone of voice, body language, and comments to other staff members often give the parents a different message from the spoken word. One should be able to explain emergency medical procedures in a calm, professional, and reassuring manner.

If an infant requires resuscitation or prolonged physiologic assessment, the attending staffs' primary obligation is to immediately administer this care. The presence of the father or a support team must not be allowed to interfere with or delay the delivery of care; however, the pediatric staff should tell the parents what is happening at the earliest possible opportunity. The lack of communication while the medical staff hovers over the infant causes moments of prolonged agony for the parents. A few brief statements to explain the procedure can relieve the anguish of silence.

•   •   •

Prevention and immediate treatment of neonatal hypoxia and asphyxia at birth can significantly reduce infant morbidity and mortality. Resuscitation techniques are designed to facilitate adaptation to extrauterine life and help establish effective ventilation, increase pulmonary blood flow, eliminate and clear lung fluid, and close fetal circulatory shunts for all infants, whether or not they are compromised by asphyxia. Professionals responsible for resuscitation of neonates should be thoroughly trained in theoretical knowledge and clinical skills related to life support techniques to perform in an effective and efficient manner.

SELECTED READINGS

Adamsons K et al: Resuscitation by positive ventilation and tris-hydroxy-methyl-aminomethane of rhesus monkeys asphyxiated at birth, J Pediatr 65:807, 1964.

Avery GB: Delivery room management of the newborn. In Phibbs RH: Neonatology: pathophysiology and management of the newborn, ed 3, Philadelphia, 1986, JB Lippincott Co.

Babson SG et al: Resuscitation and stabilization of the depressed infant. In Babson SG et al, editors: Diagnosis and management of the fetus and neonate at risk: a guide for team care, ed 4, St Louis, 1980, The CV Mosby Co.

Carson BS et al: Combined obstetric and pediatric approach to prevent meconium aspiration syndrome, Am J Obstet Gynecol 126(6):712, 1976.

Clotherty JP and Stark AR: Resuscitation in the delivery room. In Clotherty JP and Stark AR: Manual of newborn care, Boston, 1980, Little, Brown & Co.

Dawes GS, Hibbard E, and Windle WF: The effect of alkali and glucose infusion on permanent brain damage in rhesus monkeys asphyxiated at birth, J Pediatr 65(6):801, 1964.

Finberg I: The relationship of intravenous infusions and intracranial hemorrhage: a commentary, J Pediatr 91:777, 1977.

Fox W, Gutsche B, and Devore J: Delivery room approach to meconium aspiration syndrome, Clin Pediatr 16(4):325, 1977.

Goldberg RN et al: The association of rapid volume expansion and intraventricular hemorrhage in the preterm infant, J Pediatr 96:1060, 1980.

Gruber UF and Messmer K: Colloids for blood volume support, Prog Surg 15:49, 1977.

Harper RG and Yoon JJ: Delivery room resuscitation procedures. In Harper RG and Yoon JJ: Handbook of neonatology, Chicago, 1974, Year Book Medical Publishers, Inc.

James LS: Emergencies in the delivery room. In Fanaroff AA and Martin RJ: Neonatal-perinatal medicine, St Louis, 1987, The CV Mosby Co.

Kattwinkel J et al: Resuscitating the newborn infant. In Kattwinkel J et al: Perinatal continuing education program, Book 1, Fetal education, Charlottesville, Va, 1979, University of Virginia Medical Center.

Kehrberg DD: Immediate care. In Streeter NS, editor: Neonatal care, Aspen, Colo, Aspen Publications, 1986.

Klaus MH and Fanaroff AA: Resuscitation of the newborn infant. In Klaus MH and Fanaroff AA: Care of the high-risk neonate, ed 3, Philadelphia, 1986, WB Saunders Co.

Korones SB: Evaluation and management of the infant immediately after birth. In Korones SB: High-risk newborn infants: the basis for intensive nursing care, ed 4, St Louis, 1986, The CV Mosby Co.

Loe HC, Lassen NA, and Friis-Hansen B: Impaired autoregulation of cerebral blood flow in the distressed newborn infant, J Pediatr 94:118, 1979.

Miller FC et al: Significance of meconium during labor, Am J Obstet Gynecol 122:573, 1975.

Patel HB and Tsu FY: Resuscitation. In Tsu FY, editor: Drug therapy in the neonate and small infant, Chicago, 1985, Year Book Medical Publishers, Inc.

Philip AGS: The delivery room. In Philip AGS: Neonatology: a practical guide, New York, 1980, Medical Examination Publishing Co, Inc.

Raju TNK and Vidyasagar D: Neonatal resuscitation. In Aladjem S, Brown AK, and Sureau C, editors: Clinical perinatology, ed 2, St Louis, 1980, The CV Mosby Co.

Rave MI and Arango A: Colloid versus crystalloid resuscitation in experimental bowel obstruction, J Pediatr Surg 11:635, 1976.

Sheldon RE: Management of perinatal asphyxia and shock, Pediatr Ann 6:227, 1977.

Shussman LC: Pathophysiology and prevention of meconium aspiration syndrome, J Fam Pract 10:987, 1980.

Skillman JJ: The role of albumin and oncotically active fluids in shock, Crit Care Med 4:55, 1976.

Standards and Guidelines for Cardiopulmonary Resuscitation (CPR) and Emergency Cardiac Care (ECC). National Convention on Cardiopulmonary Resuscitation (CPR) and

Emergency Cardiac Care (ECC) 1985, Part VI. Neonatal advanced life support, JAMA 255:2905, 1986.

Textbook of advanced cardiac life support, Dallas, American Heart Association, 1981.

Ting P and Brady J: Tracheal suctioning in meconium aspiration, Am J Obstet Gynecol 122:767, 1975.

Weisberg HF: Osmotic pressures of the serum proteins, Ann Clin Lab Sci 8:155, 1978.

Wigglesworth JS et al: Hyaline membrane disease, alkali, and intraventricular hemorrhage, Arch Dis Child 51:755, 1976.

CHAPTER 4

Initial nursery care

CYNDI J. LEPLEY · SANDRA L. GARDNER · LULA O. LUBCHENCO

This chapter teaches the basis of newborn care in the first hours of life. The neonate must demonstrate a condition of well-being before being considered a normal low-risk infant. It is essential for health professionals involved in neonatal intensive care to understand the normal neonate to care for the sick neonate. This chapter provides an understanding of the initial assessment, transitional period, gestational age, and how these apply to initial nursery care.

Physical changes occur so rapidly after birth that the newborn examination can be divided into four time periods. Apgar defined the first evaluation in terms of seconds "exactly 60 *seconds* after birth" and the next evaluation in minutes. The transition period is considered in hours, and the hospital stay in days. If one continues this logarithmic time span for newborns, one uses weeks for the first few follow-up visits, then months, and eventually one speaks of the child's age in years.

Each of these four newborn examinations has a specific purpose. One should consider these examinations in relation to the *age* of the infant rather than to the *location* of the mother and infant in the hospital—or to arbitrary nursery routines (delivery room versus birthing room, transition nursery versus mother's recovery room, rooming-in versus low-risk nursery, etc.). The examination at delivery is aimed at detecting life-threatening emergencies. The examination during the next few hours (transition period) is used to evaluate the infant's adjustment to extrauterine life and to estimate and anticipate likely morbidities. The complete newborn examination, at about 24 hours, is an important examination, since

many findings can be treated or complications avoided. It should be as thorough as possible. The discharge examination is geared toward helping the parents establish a lasting relationship with their baby and in understanding the child's individual nature. This is done by demonstrating the baby's unique abilities and answering questions raised during the examination, which need not be as detailed as the 24-hour examination. At this time it is advisable to ask a series of simple questions aimed at detecting problems in the parent-infant relationship.

EXAMINATION AT DELIVERY

Before the delivery occurs, one should obtain pertinent facts regarding the pregnancy, such as parity, gravidity, fetal losses, estimated birth weight and gestational age of the fetus, and, of course, any problems present in the current pregnancy.

During labor one can observe the frequency and duration of contractions and the mother's reaction to contractions. Passage of meconium, rupture of membranes, fetal distress, etc., will alert the attendants to impending problems. At birth the amount and distribution of vernix should be noted, since it is quickly wiped off. The initial cry and tone, part of the Apgar evaluation, are noted even before 60 seconds, since one does not wait for the 1-minute Apgar to begin resuscitative procedures if the infant is limp and not breathing. If the baby is vigorous, the obstetrician may elect to place the baby on the mother's abdomen or in her arms—the Apgar score can just as well be done there as in a bassinet or warmer.

The score is repeated at 5 minutes. Under

some conditions, such as prolonged asphyxia and resuscitation, it is helpful to have a score at 10 or 15 minutes. Between the 1- and 5-minute Apgar, one systematically evaluates the baby for potential or apparent medical emergencies. Cardiac and respiratory problems were identified before the 60-second Apgar. One has noted size and approximate gestational age from the physical appearance. A further glance after turning the infant to a prone position will reveal congenital abnormalities such as spina bifida, imperforate anus, skeletal abnormalities, and/or genital defects. Even internal abnormalities may be suspected if there is an "empty" or scaphoid abdomen (diaphragmatic hernia) or profuse oral or nasopharyngeal mucus (TE fistula). Choanal atresia may present as apnea after respirations have been established. One may test for choanal atresia by closing the infant's mouth, since newborns are obligate nasal breathers. Examination of the umbilical cord and vessels may give a clue to other abnormalities. The size and amount of Wharton's jelly, especially if the cord is thin, suggests problems in intrauterine nutrition. Persistent pulsation of the umbilical cord, best felt in the skin-covered stump, suggests inadequate ventilation (fetal circulation). A single umbilical artery may be a clue to other anomalies.

PHYSIOLOGY
Transitional phases and significance

With the first breath of life and the cutting of the umbilical cord, all neonates begin the transition from intrauterine to extrauterine life. The neonate is to be considered a recovering patient, similar to a patient recovering from anesthesia. The transitional phase of the neonate is closely monitored to recognize any abnormalities, initiate appropriate measures for referral, and screen the neonate for common problems in early neonatal life.

In 1966 Desmond et al.[6] described temporal changes occurring in the behavior and physiology of the infant during the first few hours after birth. Figure 4-1 gives a summary of the physical findings noted during the first 10 hours of extrauterine life in a representative high-Apgar-score infant delivered with the mother under spinal anesthesia without prior medication. Vital signs, including the heart rate, temperature, and blood pressure, are so closely related to age after birth that the examiner can almost estimate the age of the infant from them when there are no problems in the transition to extrauterine life. Vital signs thus alert one to problems if the heart rate, respirations, temperature, and blood pressure do not follow the usual time course.

A heart rate of 160 beats/min at any time other than the first hour after birth would alarm the observer. And, of course, if this rate persisted, it would indicate some serious problem. In the healthy infant shown on this graph, the rate falls to a more usual rate seen in newborns. Equally disturbing is the respiratory rate after birth. When one considers the pulmonary adjustments the infant must make immediately after birth, it is not surprising to see tachypnea, but it is disturbing to see barreling of the chest, which is usually indicative of extraalveolar air. The improvement, spontaneously, is just as surprising and gives us even greater respect for the ability of the newborn organism.

The temperature fall shown in Figure 4-1 (which was made many years ago) may well be iatrogenic. It adds a stress to the infant already stressed by birth and all the adjustments he or she must make. Cold stress requires the infant to use sources of energy that are easily depleted, and if feeding is delayed, hypoglycemia may occur. Hypoglycemia is especially critical in the small-for-gestational-age infant, whose stores of glycogen and fat are limited.

Behavior in terms of awake-sleep states are equally significant. The infant is usually awake and alert for the first hour after birth and often indicates hunger by mouthing movements or hand-to-mouth contact. If fed at this time, the infant nurses well; then sleep ensues. The infant can be aroused from sleep and will come to an alert state if no problems exist. If there are medical problems, the infant will fluctuate between

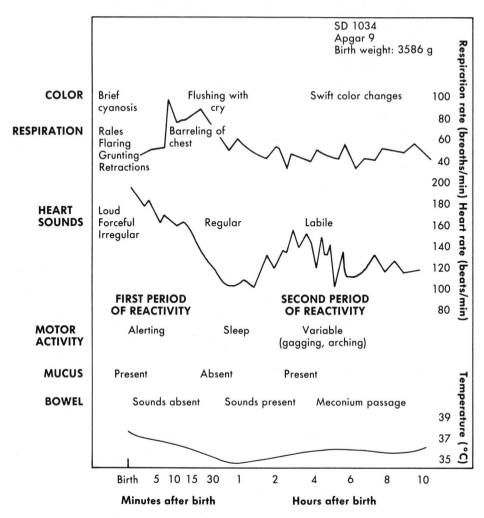

Figure 4-1. Neonatal transitional period. (From Desmond M et al: Pediatr Clin North Am 13:656, 1966.)

sleep and crying without an alert period in between. Feeding during a drowsy or fussing state will therefore be unsatisfactory and gives us one of the earliest signs of illness—"poor feeding." More subtle signs of distress in the infant are also being recognized (e.g., closed eyes with hands tightly fisted and arms extended rather than kept toward the midline, peripheral or circumoral cyanosis, and regurgitation). Attempts by the infant to alleviate distress and quiet himself or her-

self can be observed when the infant brings the hands to the face or mouth.

During these first hours one can begin to assess the risk of the infant for various morbidities. Again, this exercise is aimed at anticipating or preventing problems that interfere with the infant's adjustment to extrauterine life. Warmth and comfort measures are, of course, indicated throughout this transition period.

Because the newborn infant tends to respond

to illness or stress by "turning off" his reactions, recognition of illness is made even more difficult. Furthermore, when one suspects illness, there are very few clues as to the specific problem. For instance, illness is suspected when the infant is hypotonic, does not feed well, or is difficult to arouse or bring to an alert state. These signs are the same whether the infant has hypoglycemia, polycythemia, or sepsis. Illness may be suspected, but it requires laboratory documentation to determine the cause. Hence, many nurseries have adopted routines that include blood glucose determinations, hematocrit counts, x-ray films, etc., for the most common problems (blood pressure, heart rate, and respiratory rate are already routine). Blood and other cultures, blood typing, screening for congenital infections, and other tests may be indicated depending on the pregnancy history.

BOWEL ACTIVITY

Bowel sounds are absent until about 1 hour of age. In some babies bowel sounds will occur earlier, especially if they were stressed during labor or delivery and passage of meconium occurred at this time. Auscultate the abdomen for the presence or absence of bowel sounds.

TEMPERATURE

The infant's temperature drops rapidly after delivery and may not begin to stabilize for several hours unless appropriate intervention is made. A newborn needs to be dried off immediately after delivery to prevent heat loss caused by evaporation. Until the temperature has stabilized, a radiant heater, incubator, or maternal skin contact should be used to maintain thermoneutrality (see Chapter 5). Obviously, bathing should be deferred until a normal transition has been achieved.

PULSE AND RESPIRATIONS

As the cardiopulmonary system changes from fetal to neonatal circulation, the transition from intrauterine to extrauterine life begins (see Chapter 3). Initially the neonate may exhibit grunting, flaring, retracting, and cyanosis that resolves in the first hour of life (see Figure 4-1). Also, rales may be heard in the normal newborn's chest. As lung fluid is absorbed, the chest sounds clear. Observe, evaluate, and record the infant's respiratory rate and effort. A normal respiratory rate is 30 to 60 beats/min without grunting, flaring, or retracting. Auscultate and record the apical pulse. A normal pulse rate is 120 to 160 beats/min.

MOTOR ACTIVITY

A full-term infant who has not been subjected to medications or stress during labor and delivery will be awake and alert immediately after delivery. Observe, evaluate, and record the baby's state and activity.

FIRST PERIOD OF REACTIVITY. The first period of reactivity occurs during the first 1 to 2 hours after birth. This is an excellent time for parents to be with their baby and begin the bonding process. Although the neonate may be physiologically unstable, it is safe to allow the mother and baby to be together under the close observation of the professional staff.

SLEEP PERIOD. The baby becomes hungry, will nurse, and then fall asleep after an initial awake period and will sleep for several hours. Care providers should avoid disturbing the baby at this time with laboratory work, physical examinations, or feedings so that the infant can recover from the stress of labor and birth. Bathing should be postponed until the baby is awake and the temperature has stabilized.

SECOND PERIOD OF REACTIVITY. A second period of reactivity occurs between 4 to 6 hours of age. The infant frequently has significant mucoid secretions. The baby will awaken, begin to cry, and demand feeding. Suction secretions as needed.

AWAKE AND SLEEP STATES. Awake and sleep states affect the neonate's behavior and ability to respond to the environment. The newborn may go from one state to another quite frequently in the nursery and at home. Listed below are six states of consciousness of the newborn°:

Sleep states
1. Deep sleep—Hard to awaken the baby, eyes closed, some jerky movements
2. Light sleep—Eyes closed, moves from deep to light sleep, light sleep to drowsy state; there may be sucking present

Awake states
3. Drowsy or semidozing—Eyes open or closed, reacts to sensory stimuli (occasionally with a delayed response), some fussing
4. Quiet alert—Focuses on stimuli source, minimal motor activity, eyes with a bright look
5. Active alert—Much motor activity, increased startles or activity in relation to stimuli, may or may not be fussing
6. Crying—Difficult to get a response to stimuli; will need to bring infant down to state 5 to elicit response to stimuli or to feed baby

ETIOLOGY

Failure to make a normal transition to extrauterine life may be the result of obstetric anesthesia or analgesia, neonatal illness, or stress such as perinatal asphyxia and its sequelae. If the infant's pulse, respirations, color, and activity have not stabilized within the normal ranges after 1 hour of life, a problem should be suspected and investigated.

PREVENTION

Knowledge of the normal vital processes of an infant's first 24 hours of life assists the care provider in early recognition of deviations from normal extrauterine life and in early initiation of corrective interventions.[8,14] Delay in recognizing and initiating therapy increases morbidity and mortality.[21]

°Adapted from Brazelton TB: Neonatal behavioral assessment scale, Philadelphia, 1973, JB Lippincott Co/Spastics International Medical Publishers.

DATA COLLECTION
History

Good perinatal care requires the identification of social, demographic, and medical-obstetric risk factors that correlate with fetal outcome. This must be an ongoing process, since high-risk patients may be identified on the first prenatal visit, during follow-up prenatal visits, or not until the intrapartum and postpartum periods. Review of the perinatal history is important in determining significant factors for neonatal health management. Identification of an at-risk maternal situation is essential in order to plan and organize care for the at-risk neonate. Review of the perinatal history includes antepartum and intrapartum events (see section on maternal referrals in Chapter 1) and events of the neonatal course such as normal or abnormal transition, timing and onset of symptoms, and the ability to feed.

Signs and symptoms

Unlike the verbalizing adult patient, the nonverbal neonate communicates needs primarily by behavior. Through objective observations and evaluations the neonatal care provider interprets this behavior into information about the individual infant's condition. Assessment of the neonate includes:
1. Estimation of gestational age
2. Physical examination
3. Neurologic examination
4. Brazelton's examination

All care providers must not only be familiar with these tools, but also be proficient in performing and interpreting them.

Assessment of gestational age

An assessment of gestational age should be done on all newborns to assign a newborn classification, to determine their neonatal mortality risk, to generate a problem list of potential morbidities, and to quickly initiate appropriate screening procedures and/or interventions for recognized morbidities.[17,20] Gestational age can be assessed by obstetric methods and by pediatric methods.

The obstetric methods for determining maturity will have already been performed by the time the newborn reaches the nursery. However, the newborn's care providers should be familiar with dating a pregnancy. Dating the last menstrual period (LMP) could be the most accurate method, if the mother is sure of the dates of her last menstrual period. Some women will have spotting or even a light period after becoming pregnant, making them unsure of the time of conception. The use of birth control pills may also make the time of ovulation and conception unknown; therefore pregnancy tests are useful in confirming the pregnancy and the time of conception. Although amniotic fluid analysis is used for gestational assessment, ultrasound examination is preferred because it confirms conception, assesses gestation, and evaluates fetal growth. Office ultrasound examination has improved the obstetrician's ability to assess the duration of gestation. The pregnancy can also be dated by examining for the presence of fetal heart tones, measuring fundal height, and by quickening.

Pediatric methods of gestational age are based on physical characteristics and neurologic examination. On admission to the nursery, every newborn should have an assessment of gestational age by physical characteristics. Numerous tables, charts, and graphs are available for determining gestation. Some tables are more subjective than others, but at least one form should be used by all nurseries caring for babies.

Three of the available charts for determining gestational age by physical characteristics are shown in Figures 4-2, 4-3, and 4-4. Figure 4-2 does not place much emphasis on the neurologic assessment, which may not be valid in the first 24 hours because of birth recovery.[3] To use this chart, an X or " " is placed in each appropriate slot. Then an age is assigned according to a line drawn through the point where most of the marks have been placed. The disadvantage of this system is the subjectivity of the chart; the advantage is that items relate to gestational age, not a score. Therefore the examiner must be experienced to offset the possibility for error in the chart.

Figure 4-4 incorporates physical maturity and neuromuscular maturity on an equal basis. An X is placed in the appropriate box for each category. The score for the neuromuscular and physical maturity is added and noted under the maturity rating column. Weeks of gestation are assigned according to the maturity rating score.

To accurately use these charts, the following physical characteristics must be assessed.[17,20]

VERNIX

At 20 to 24 weeks vernix is produced by sebaceous glands. Note the amount and distribution of vernix on the baby's skin (best done in the delivery room). It is high in fat content and protects the skin from the aqueous amniotic fluid and bacteria. At 36 weeks the white, cheeselike material begins to decrease and disappears by 41 weeks.

SKIN

In early gestation the skin of the fetus is very transparent, and veins are easily seen. As gestation progresses, the skin becomes tougher, thicker, and less transparent. By 37 weeks very few vessels are visible. From 36 weeks to delivery, fat deposits begin to form and grow. In the postterm infant, desquamation will be prominent at the ankles, wrists, and possibly palms and soles. As gestation progresses, the loss of vernix and subcutaneous tissue causes wrinkling. Note skin turgor, color, texture, and the prominence of vessels, especially on the abdomen.

LANUGO

At 20 weeks fine downy hair, lanugo, appears over the entire body of the fetus. At 28 weeks it begins to disappear around the face and ante-

CLINICAL ESTIMATION OF GESTATIONAL AGE
An Approximation Based on Published Data

⌂ Examination First Hours

PHYSICAL FINDINGS	WEEKS GESTATION																												
	20	21	22	23	24	25	26	27	28	29	30	31	32	33	34	35	36	37	38	39	40	41	42	43	44	45	46	47	48
VERNIX		APPEARS					COVERS BODY, THICK LAYER												ON BACK, SCALP, IN CREASES		SCANT, IN CREASES			NO VERNIX				
BREAST TISSUE AND AREOLA			AREOLA & NIPPLE BARELY VISIBLE NO PALPABLE BREAST TISSUE												AREOLA RAISED			1-2 MM NODULE	3-5 MM	5-6 MM		7-10 MM					?12 MM		
EAR — FORM					FLAT, SHAPELESS											BEGINNING INCURVING SUPERIOR		INCURVING UPPER 2/3 PINNAE					WELL-DEFINED INCURVING TO LOBE						
EAR — CARTILAGE							PINNA SOFT, STAYS FOLDED								CARTILAGE RETURNS SLOWLY FROM FOLDING		THIN CARTILAGE SPRINGS BACK FROM FOLDING					PINNA FIRM, REMAINS ERECT FROM HEAD							
SOLE CREASES							SMOOTH SOLES ? CREASES						1-2 ANTERIOR CREASES		2-3 AN-TER-IOR CREASES		CREASES ANTERIOR 2/3 SOLE			CREASES INVOLVING HEEL			DEEPER CREASES OVER ENTIRE SOLE					
SKIN — THICKNESS & APPEARANCE			THIN, TRANSLUCENT SKIN, PLETHORIC, VENULES OVER ABDOMEN EDEMA													SMOOTH THICKER NO EDEMA		PINK			FEW VESSELS	SOME DES-QUAMATION PALE PINK	THICK, PALE, DESQUAMATION OVER ENTIRE BODY						
NAIL PLATE	AP-PEAR												NAILS TO FINGER TIPS									NAILS EXTEND WILL BEYOND FINGER TIPS						
HAIR		APPEARS ON HEAD				EYE BROWS & LASHES				FINE, WOOLLY, BUNCHES OUT FROM HEAD						SILKY, SINGLE STRANDS LAYS FLAT							RECEDING HAIRLINE OR LOSS OF BABY HAIR SHORT, FINE UNDERNEATH						
LANUGO	AP-PEARS					COVERS ENTIRE BODY									VANISHES FROM FACE			PRESENT ON SHOULDERS					NO LANUGO					
GENITALIA — TESTES									TESTES PALPABLE IN INGUINAL CANAL								IN UPPER SCROTUM				IN LOWER SCROTUM							
GENITALIA — SCROTUM														FEW RUGAE				RUGAE, ANTERIOR PORTION			RUGAE COVER				PENDULOUS			
GENITALIA — LABIA & CLITORIS												PROMINENT CLITORIS LABIA MAJORA SMALL WIDELY SEPARATED					LABIA MAJORA LARGER NEARLY COVERED CLITORIS					LABIA MINORA & CLITORIS COVERED						
SKULL FIRMNESS					BONES ARE SOFT						SOFT TO 1" FROM ANTERIOR FONTANELLE					SPONGY AT EDGES OF FON-TANELLE CENTER FIRM			BONES HARD SUTURES EASILY DISPLACED					BONES HARD, CANNOT BE DISPLACED					
POSTURE — RESTING		HYPOTONIC LATERAL DECUBITUS				HYPOTONIC					BEGINNING FLEXION THIGH		STRONGER HIP FLEXION		FROG-LIKE		FLEXION ALL LIMBS				HYPERTONIC				VERY HYPERTONIC			
RECOIL - LEG					NO RECOIL											BEGIN FLEXION NO RE-COIL		PROMPT RECOIL MAY BE INHIBITED					PROMPT RECOIL					
ARM						NO RECOIL														PROMPT RECOIL					PROMPT RECOIL AFTER 30" INHIBITION				
	20	21	22	23	24	25	26	27	28	29	30	31	32	33	34	35	36	37	38	39	40	41	42	43	44	45	46	47	48

Figure 4-2. Clinical estimation of gestational age: examination in first hour. (Reproduced, with permission, from Kempe CH, Silver HK, and O'Brien D: Current pediatric diagnosis and treatment, 3rd edition, copyright Lange Medical Publications, 1974.)

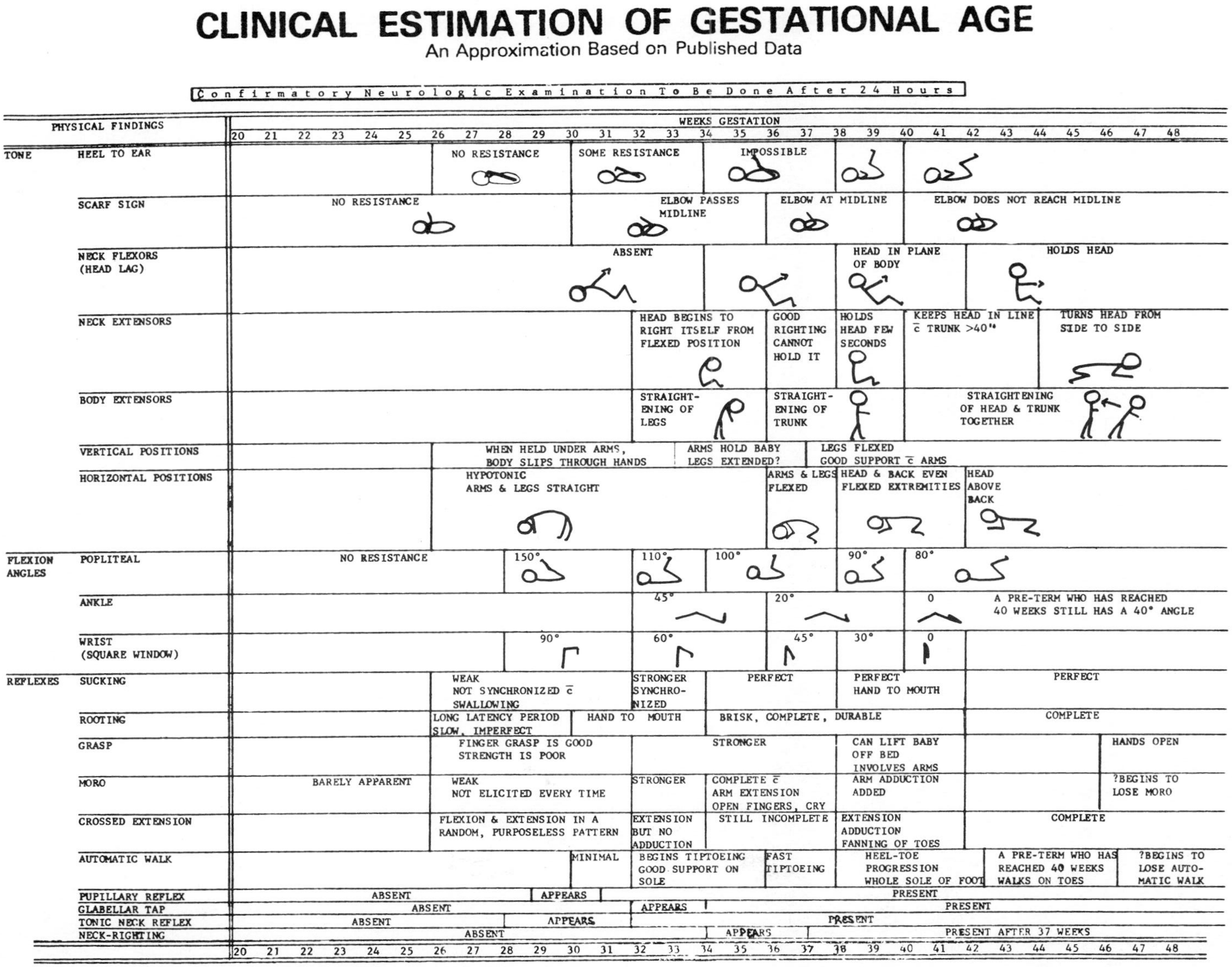

CLINICAL ESTIMATION OF GESTATIONAL AGE

An Approximation Based on Published Data

Figure 4-3. Clinical estimation of gestational age: examination after first 24 hours. (Reproduced, with permission, from Kempe CH, Silver HK, and O'Brien D: Current pediatric diagnosis and treatment, 3rd edition, copyright Lange Medical Publications, 1974.)

NEWBORN MATURITY RATING
and
CLASSIFICATION

ESTIMATION OF GESTATIONAL AGE BY MATURITY RATING
Symbols: X - 1st Exam   O - 2nd Exam

NEUROMUSCULAR MATURITY

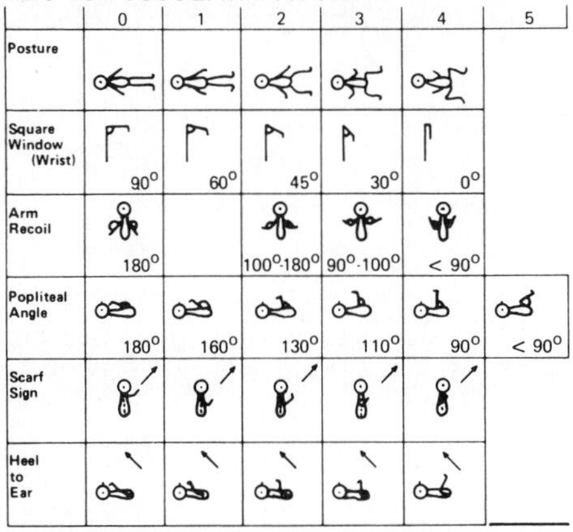

	0	1	2	3	4	5
Posture						
Square Window (Wrist)	90°	60°	45°	30°	0°	
Arm Recoil	180°	100°-180°	90°-100°	< 90°		
Popliteal Angle	180°	160°	130°	110°	90°	< 90°
Scarf Sign						
Heel to Ear						

PHYSICAL MATURITY

	0	1	2	3	4	5
SKIN	gelatinous red, transparent	smooth pink, visible veins	superficial peeling &/or rash, few veins	cracking pale area, rare veins	parchment, deep cracking, no vessels	leathery, cracked, wrinkled
LANUGO	none	abundant	thinning	bald areas	mostly bald	
PLANTAR CREASES	no crease	faint red marks	anterior transverse crease only	creases ant. 2/3	creases cover entire sole	
BREAST	barely percept.	flat areola, no bud	stippled areola, 1–2 mm bud	raised areola, 3–4 mm bud	full areola, 5–10 mm bud	
EAR	pinna flat, stays folded	sl. curved pinna, soft with slow recoil	well-curv. pinna, soft but ready recoil	formed & firm with instant recoil	thick cartilage, ear stiff	
GENITALS Male	scrotum empty, no rugae		testes descending, few rugae	testes down, good rugae	testes pendulous, deep rugae	
GENITALS Female	prominent clitoris & labia minora		majora & minora equally prominent	majora large, minora small	clitoris & minora completely covered	

Gestation by Dates _____ wks

Birth Date _____ Hour _____ am / pm

APGAR _____ 1 min _____ 5 min

MATURITY RATING

Score	Wks
5	26
10	28
15	30
20	32
25	34
30	36
35	38
40	40
45	42
50	44

SCORING SECTION

	1st Exam=X	2nd Exam=O
Estimating Gest Age by Maturity Rating	_____ Weeks	_____ Weeks
Time of Exam	Date _____ am / pm Hour _____	Date _____ am / pm Hour _____
Age at Exam	_____ Hours	_____ Hours
Signature of Examiner	_____ M.D.	_____ M.D.

Scoring system: Ballard JL, *et al*: A Simplified Assessment of Gestational Age. Pediatr Res 11:374, 1977. Figures adapted from "Classification of the Low-Birth-Weight Infant" by AY Sweet in Care of the High-Risk Infant by MH Klaus and AA Fanaroff, WB Saunders Co, Philadelphia, 1977, p. 47.

Figure 4-4. Clinical estimation of gestational age according to newborn maturity rating and classification. (Courtesy Mead Johnson & Co., Evansville, Ind. Scoring section adapted from Ballard JL et al: Pediatr Res 11:374, 1977. Figures adapted from Sweet AY: Classification of the low-birth-weight infant. In Klaus MH and Fanaroff AA: Care of the high-risk infant, Philadelphia, 1977, WB Saunders Co.)

rior trunk. At term a few patches of lanugo may still be present over the shoulders. Note the distribution of lanugo, first on the face and anterior trunk, then on the rest of the body.

SOLE CREASES

Sole creases develop from toe to heel, progressing with gestational age. An infant with intra- uterine growth retardation and early loss of vernix may have more sole creases than expected. By 12 hours after birth, the skin has dried to a point that sole creases are no longer a valid indicator of gestational age. Note the development of sole creases as they progress from the superior to inferior aspect of the foot (Figure 4-5).

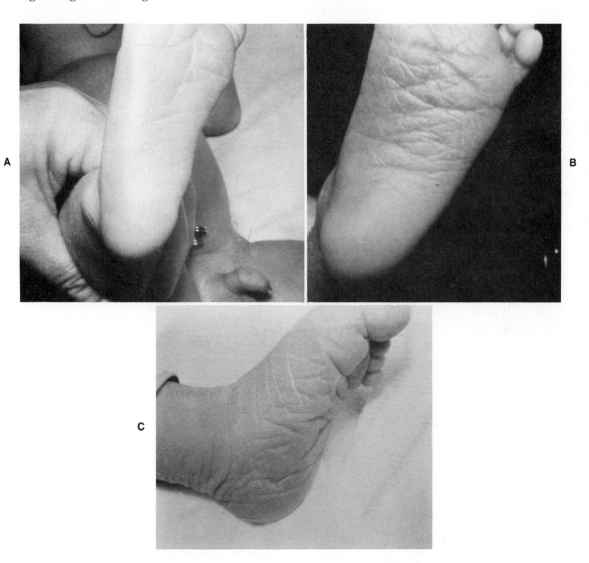

Figure 4-5. Sole creases at different gestational ages. **A,** Age 31 to 33 weeks. **B,** Age 34 to 38 weeks. **C,** Term.

HAIR ON THE HEAD

Hair appears on the head at 20 weeks. At 20 to 23 weeks the eyelashes and eyebrows develop. From 28 to 34 or 36 weeks the hair is fine and woolly and sticks together. It appears disheveled and sticks out in bunches from the head. At term the hair lies flat on the head, it feels silky, and single strands are identifiable. Note the quality and distribution of the hair and feel its texture.

EYES

In the third month of fetal life the eyelids fuse. At 26 to 30 weeks they reopen.

From 27 to 34 weeks of gestation, examination of the anterior vascular capsule of the lens

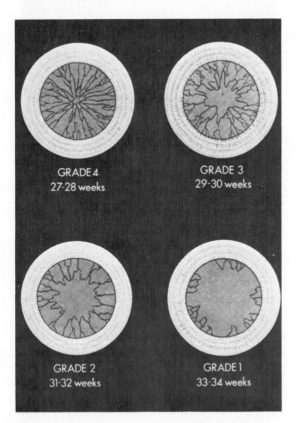

Figure 4-6. Anterior vascular capsule and gestational age. (From Hittner H et al: J Pediatr 91:455, 1977.)

is useful in assessing gestational age. Gestational age is determined by assessing the level of remaining embryonic vessels on the lens (Figure 4-6). Before 27 weeks the hazy cornea prevents visualization of the vascular system. After 34 weeks only remnants of the vascular system are visible. Since rapid atrophy occurs in the vascular system, an ophthalmoscopic examination should be performed during the first physical examination or within 24 to 48 hours after birth.

EARS

Before 34 weeks the pinna of the ear is a slightly formed, cartilage-free double thickness of skin. When it is folded, it remains folded. As gestation progresses, the pinnas develop more cartilage, resulting in better form so that they recoil when folded (Figure 4-7). Check ear recoil by folding the ear in half or into a three-corner-hat shape. Consistently folding it the same way helps the care provider develop a baseline for judging maturity. Note the form and cartilage development of the ear. Examine both ears to be sure they are the same and without defects.

BREAST DEVELOPMENT

Breast development is the result of the growth of glandular tissue related to high maternal estrogen levels and fat deposition. The areola is raised at 34 weeks. Note the size, shape, and placement of both breasts. Palpate the breast nodule and determine its size. If the infant is growth retarded, breast size may be less than expected at term.

GENITALIA

MALE GENITALIA. At 28 weeks the testes begin to descend from the abdomen. By 37 weeks they are high in the scrotum. By 40 weeks the testes are completely descended, and the scrotum is covered with rugae. As gestation progresses, the scrotum becomes more pendulous (Figure 4-8). Note the presence of rugae on the

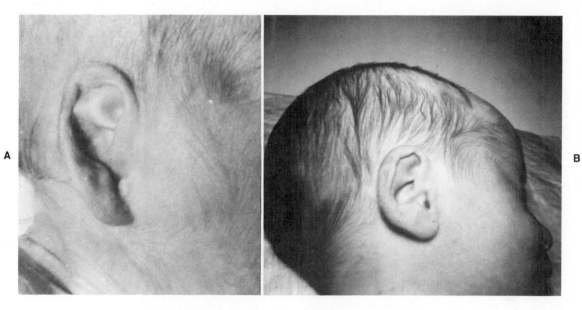

Figure 4-7. Ear form and gestational age. **A,** Age 34 to 38 weeks. **B,** Term.

scrotum and its size in relation to the position of the testes. When examining the baby for descended testes, put the fingers of one hand over the inguinal canal to prevent the testes from ascending into the abdominal cavity and palpate the scrotal sac with the other hand.

FEMALE GENITALIA. Early in the female's gestation the clitoris is prominent with small and widely separated labia. By 40 weeks the fat deposits have increased in size so that the labia majora completely cover the labia minora (Figure 4-9). Note the labial development in relation to the prominence of the clitoris.

NEWBORN CLASSIFICATIONS

The clinical estimate of gestation is defined by weeks of gestation into the following categories (Figures 4-10 and 4-11):

Preterm (PR)	Through 37 completed weeks
(Full) term (F)	38 through 41 completed weeks
Postterm (PO)	42 weeks or more

Intrauterine growth curves for the 10th and 90th percentiles are represented in Figures 4-10 and 4-11. Small-for-gestational-age (SGA) infants are those below the 10th percentile. Appropriate-for-gestational-age (AGA) infants are those between the 10th and 90th percentiles. Large-for-gestational-age (LGA) infants are above the 90th percentile. Based on birth weight the infant's intrauterine growth will be either SGA, AGA, or LGA.

Using the clinical estimate of gestational age (in weeks) and the birth weight (in grams), the newborn's classification is determined. Combining gestational age and weight criteria in Figure 4-11 forms nine possible newborn classifications: preterm, full-term, and postterm, large-for-gestational-age (PRLGA, FLGA, and POLGA); preterm, full-term, and postterm, appropriate-for-gestational-age (PRAGA, FAGA, and POAGA); and preterm, full-term, and postterm, small-for-gestational-age (PRSGA, FSGA, and POSGA).

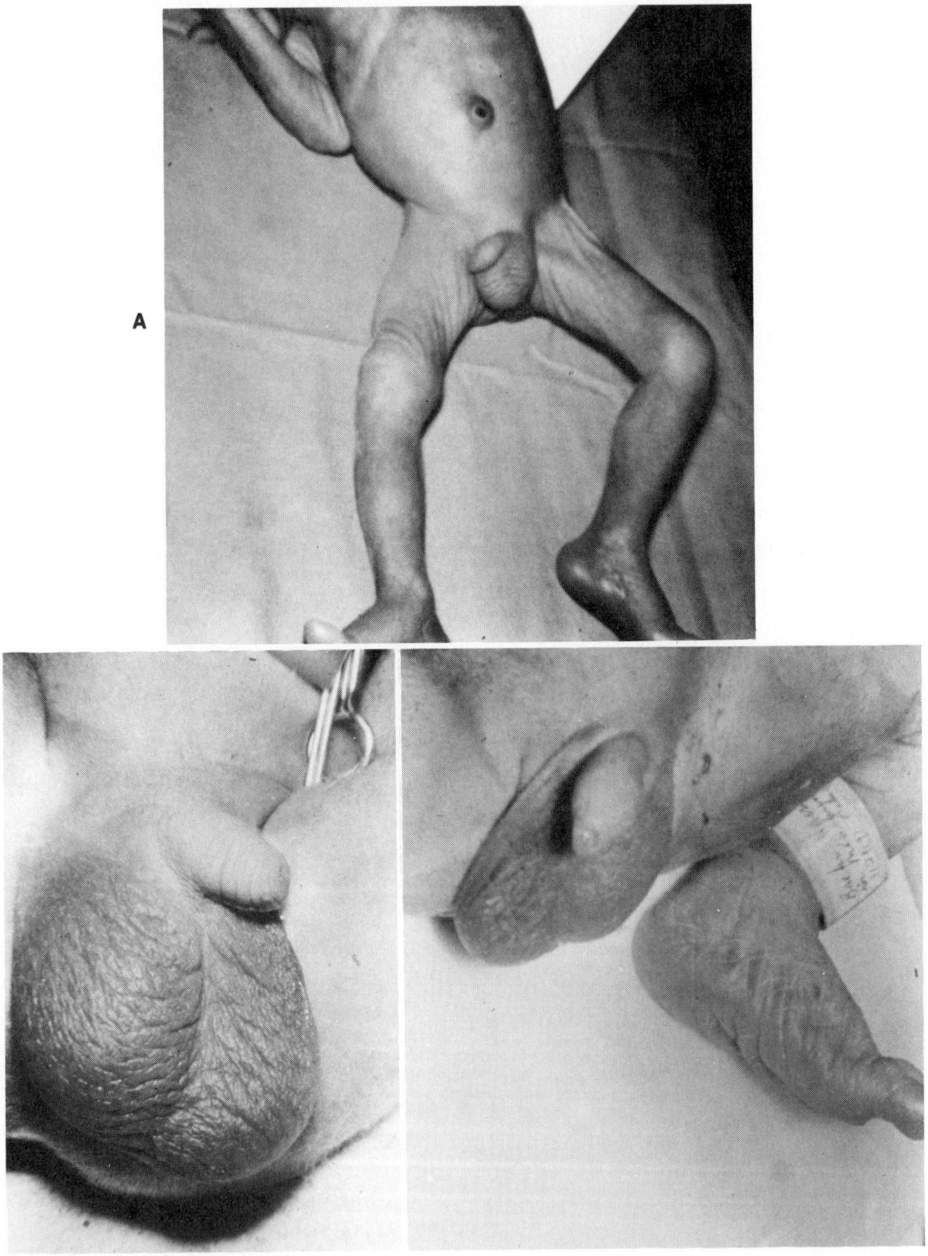

Figure 4-8. Male genitalia and gestational age. **A**, Age 28 to 35 weeks. **B**, Term. **C**, Age 42 or more weeks.

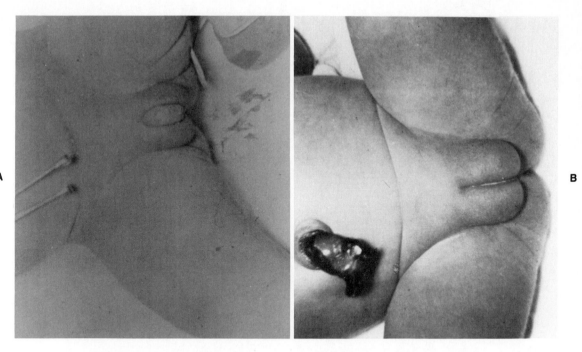

Figure 4-9. Female genitalia and gestational age. **A,** Age 30 to 36 weeks. **B,** Term.

Using Figure 4-11, plot the newborn weight in grams against the clinical gestational age and mark an X on the chart. Determine to which of the nine categories the baby belongs. Then classify and note the newborn's classification on the record.

NEONATAL MORTALITY RISK. Neonatal mortality risk (NMR), the chance of dying in the neonatal period, can be determined from graphs such as those shown in Figures 4-10 and 4-11 and is based on birth weight and gestational age. On both charts the area of least risk is the FAGA infant. Deviations from this area of least risk in relation to either weight or gestational age increase the newborn's mortality risk.

Both charts are included here to illustrate the change in mortality over time because of an increasingly physiologic basis of care (Figure 4-11) coupled with sophisticated professional care, technology, transport systems, and aggressive management to handle increasingly at-risk populations (Figure 4-10). NMR graphs are useful in making decisions about potential viability and the appropriate level of care.[13] Babies with greater than 10% risk will usually require level II or III care. Note the infant's NMR on the chart (Figure 4-11) and record in the newborn record. NOTE: To determine the appropriate NMR, read to the right of the vertical lines and above the horizontal line.

Examination of NMR on Figure 4-10 also reveals that two infants with the same birth weight but with different gestational ages may have very different risks of death. For example, *infant A* may have a birth weight of 3000 g and a gestational age of 33 weeks. Plotting these values on Figure 4-10, the NMR for this infant is

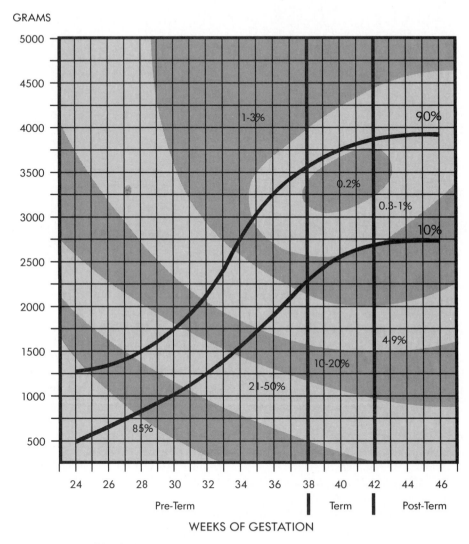

Neonatal Mortality Risk
by Birthweight and Gestational Age

GRAMS

Figure 4-10. Neonatal mortality risk by birth weight and gestational age. (From Lubchenco LO et al: J Pediatr 81:814, 1972. © 1982 Mead Johnson & Co.)

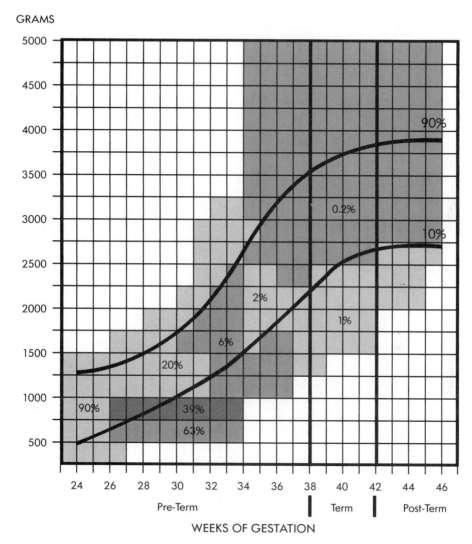

Neonatal Mortality Risk
by Birthweight and Gestational Age

1974-1980 BASED ON 14,413 LIVEBIRTHS AT UNIVERSITY OF COLORADO
HEALTH SCIENCES CENTER

Figure 4-11. Neonatal mortality risk by birth weight and gestational age. (From Koops BL et al: J Pediatr 101:969, 1982. © 1982 Mead Johnson & Co.)

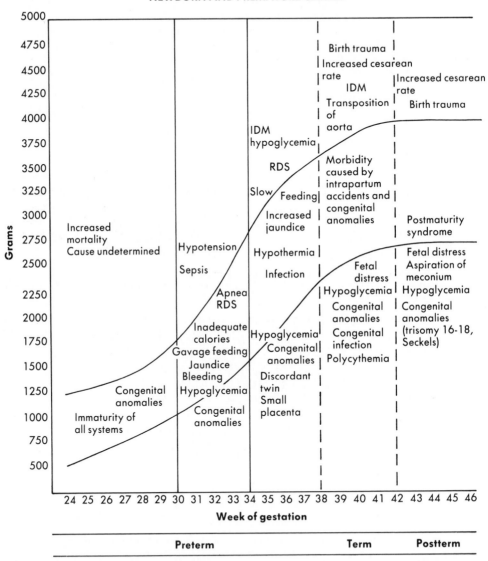

Figure 4-12. Specific neonatal morbidity by birth weight and gestational age. (From Lubchenco LO: The high risk infant, Philadelphia, 1976, WB Saunders Co.)

2%. *Infant B*, on the other hand, may also weigh 3000 g but have a gestational age of 40 weeks. The infant's risk is only 0.2%. *Infant A* thus has a mortality risk 10 times greater than *infant B*, even though they have the same birth weight.

NEONATAL MORBIDITY RISK. Neonatal morbidity risk (Figure 4-12) is determined by deviations of intrauterine growth and newborn classification. Classification of the newborn assists in identification, observation, screening, and treatment of the most commonly occurring problems. For every newborn, formulate a problem list based on the morbidities common to the newborn classification. Observe, screen, intervene, and refer as necessary to prevent complication.

The order of the first, thorough examination is done using the least stressful items first to obtain optimal information on organ systems. However, the examination is usually recorded in an orderly manner from head to toe.

When one appreciates how stressful it is to the newborn to be undressed, it becomes obvious that as much as possible should be done without exposing the infant. Warm hands and instruments are essential, and a warm environment helps. Before touching the infant or removing any covers, observe the face, head, and hands as they appear.

Physical examination

The purpose of the physical examination is (1) to discover common variations of normal and/or obvious defects, (2) to quickly initiate intervention or referral for deviations from normal, and (3) to establish a data base for serial observations and comparisons. The best data are obtained from the neonate when the physical examination is organized to limit stress, maximize interaction with the examiner, and not overwhelm the newborn. To maximize data and minimize stress, the physical examination should entail observation, quiet examination, and head-to-toe examination.

OBSERVATION

Observation of the neonate provides pertinent data without touching the newborn. General condition, anomalies, resting posture, and respirations of the infant should be observed.

GENERAL CONDITION. The general condition of the infant should be assessed by noting the color, activity and neonatal state, and crying of the child.

Color. The color of the newborn is normally pink. Acrocyanosis, peripheral cyanosis of the hands and feet, is commonly present in the first 24 hours of life and may be due to immature circulation or cold stress. Ecchymotic areas, especially on the presenting part, are common; however, they may be confused with cyanosis. To differentiate the two, apply pressure to the area. An ecchymotic area remains blue with pressure, whereas a cyanotic area will blanch.

General cyanosis and central cyanosis of the lips, mouth, and mucous membranes may indicate central nervous system (CNS), heart, or lung disease. Jaundice appearing at birth or within the first 12 hours of life is abnormal. Physiologic jaundice appears after 24 hours, but jaundice may indicate other abnormalities. Pallor at or directly after birth is a sign of circulatory failure, anoxia, edema, or shock. Pallor of anoxia is associated with bradycardia, and the pallor of anemia with tachycardia. Plethora, a beef-red color, may indicate polycythemia. It is confirmed by hemoglobin and hematocrit determinations. However, lack of plethora does not rule out polycythemia or hyperviscosity.

Activity and neonatal state. Activity and the neonatal state at the beginning of the examination and appropriate changes throughout the examination should be observed. If the infant is asleep, is it quiet or rapid-eye-movement (REM) sleep? Spontaneous, symmetric movements are normal. Tremors and twitching movements of short duration are normal in relation to states of coldness or startling. Good muscle tone is established with adequate oxygenation soon after birth.

Flaccidity, floppiness, or poor muscle tone should be noted. Spasticity, hyperactivity, opisthotonos, twitching, hypertonicity, tremors, or convulsions may be indicative of CNS damage. Asymmetry may result from intrauterine pressure or birth trauma. No crying or lack of evasive behaviors in response to the manipulations of a physical examination are not normal.

Crying. The infant's cry should be lusty at birth. Note the character of the cry. Attempts to calm and console the crying infant during this part of the examination assist in better data collection during the quiet examination. It has been suggested in recent research that crying may "compromise psychosocial development through contributing to poor eye contact and unsuccessful breastfeeding." It may also delay the successful transition from the fetal to the adult circulatory pattern. Observe the infant's ability to quiet himself or herself when crying.

A high-pitched cry suggests increased intracranial pressure. Weak crying, no crying, or constant, irritable crying may indicate brain injury. Hoarse cries or crowing inspirations result from laryngeal inflammation or anomalies. A weak, groaning cry or expiratory grunt is indicative of respiratory disease.

ANOMALIES. Obvious bodily malformations such as omphalocele, cleft lip and palate, imperforate anus, syndactyly, polydactyly, spina bifida, or myelomeningocele should be observed and recorded as anomalies. Odd facies or body appearances that are often associated with specific syndromes should also be noted.

RESTING POSTURE. Resting posture should be observed while the infant is quiet and not disturbed. The infant may take a position of comfort assumed in utero. The infant's posture systematically develops according to gestational age. It develops first from extension to flexion of the lower extremities, and then to flexion of the upper extremities. Asymmetry may result from intrauterine pressure or birth trauma.

RESPIRATIONS. Respirations should be evaluated while the infant is at rest and before any manipulation. The normal rate is 30 to 60 breaths/min. Count the respiratory rate and rhythm, noticing the infant's use of accessory muscles. Respiration is normally abdominal or diaphragmatic.

After the first hour of life a respiration rate of more than 60 breaths/min indicates tachypnea. It is the earliest sign of many neonatal respiratory, cardiac, metabolic, and infectious illnesses. Tachypnea, apnea, dyspnea, or cyanosis may indicate cardiorespiratory distress. Labored respirations include retractions, flaring nares, and expiratory grunt.

If the infant is swaddled, the observation examination will not be as extensive as is possible when the infant is unclothed in an incubator or under a radiant warmer. If the infant is swaddled, unwrap gently so that observations of the thorax, abdomen, genitalia, and extremities may also be done during this phase of the examination.

Without touching the baby, one can rule out a multitude of conditions. In fact, over 80% of the newborn examination is made through observation and palpation.

QUIET EXAMINATION

Quiet examination is defined as any part of the examination in which data are best collected from the quiet, cooperative newborn. The heart, lungs, head and neck, scalp and skull, abdomen, eyes, and blood pressure are areas that should be checked during the quiet examination. Using pacifiers, warming hands and stethoscopes, and holding and gently manipulating the infant are ways to avoid overwhelming the baby and prevent crying.

AUSCULTATION

Heart. Auscultation of the heart, lungs, and abdomen is most effective when the infant is quiet. When the infant is quiet and at rest, auscultate the heart rate, rhythm, and regularity at the apex. The normal rate is 120 to 160 beats/min at a regular rhythm. Sinus arrhythmia is normal and may be heard. The point of maximal intensity (PMI) of the neonatal heart is lateral to the midclavicular line at the third to fourth interspace. Note the PMI.

A rate of less than 120 beats/min is bradycardia that may be associated with anoxia, cerebral defects, or increased intracranial pressure. A rate greater than 160 beats/min is tachycardia that may be associated with respiratory problems, anemia, or congestive heart failure when accompanied by cardiomegaly, hepatomegaly, and generalized edema.

Murmurs are noted for loudness, quality, location, and timing. They are best auscultated at the base of the third or fourth interspace. Note dextrocardia—heart sounds audible on the right side of the chest. Pneumothorax, pneumomediastinum, dextrocardia, or diaphragmatic hernia result in muffled heart sounds or a shift in PMI.

Lungs. Normally the lungs and chest are resonant after birth, and fine rales may be present for the first few hours. Auscultation reveals bronchial breath sounds bilaterally. Air entry should be good, particularly in the midaxilla. A normal respiratory rate is 30 to 60 breaths/min.

Hyperresonance suggests pneumomediastinum, pneumothorax, or diaphragmatic hernia. Decreased resonance is a result of decreased aeration—atelectasis, pneumonia, or respiratory distress syndrome. Expiratory grunt suggests difficulty in aeration and oxygenation. Peristaltic sounds heard in the chest may be caused by a diaphragmatic hernia.

Abdomen. Also, peristalsis is normally heard shortly after birth.

PALPATION. Palpation of the fontanels and abdomen is best accomplished before the infant begins crying, since guarded muscles and the normally tense fontanels of the crying baby give little useful data.

Head and neck. The head and neck of the newborn make up 25% of the total body surface. The head is usually 2 cm larger than the newborn's chest. Normal head circumference

ranges between 32 and 38 cm for an FAGA infant. Note the size, shape, symmetry, and general appearance.

Microcephaly is characterized by a small head size in proportion to body size. Craniosynostosis is a small head size caused by early closure of suture(s). Hydrocephalus is a condition in which an increase in cerebrospinal fluid creates an abnormally large and growing head.

Scalp and skull. Temporary deformation of the head is caused by pressures during labor and delivery. The head circumference measurements may be altered so that the occipitofrontal circumference (OFC) on the first day of life may be smaller than on the second or third. Caput succedaneum is an edematous area over the presenting part of the scalp that extends across suture lines and resolves in 24 to 48 hours. Cephalhematoma is a soft mass of blood in the subperiosteal space on the surface of the skull bone. The blood mass does not extend across suture lines and resolves in 6 to 8 weeks.

Deviating from the normal, skull fractures may be linear or depressed, palpable or nonpalpable.

The anterior fontanel, a diamond-shaped space normally measuring from 1 to 4 cm, may be gently palpated at the junction of the sagittal suture and coronal suture and between the two parietal bones. Normally the anterior fontanel softly pulsates with the infant's pulse, becomes slightly depressed when the infant sits upright and is quiet, and may bulge when the infant cries. Within 24 to 48 hours after birth, the initial molding of the head and overlap of the suture resolve, resulting in a larger fontanel and in suture lines that should be palpated as depressions.

The posterior fontanel, formed at the juncture of the sagittal suture and the lambdoidal suture, is palpated between the occipital and parietal bones. Normally it is triangular shaped and barely admits a fingertip.

A bulging, tense, or full fontanel may be associated with increased intracranial pressure caused by birth injury, bleeding, infection, or hydrocephalus. A depressed fontanel, a very late sign in the newborn, may indicate dehydration. A third fontanel, located along the sagittal suture between the anterior and posterior fontanels, may be a sign of an at-risk infant, of Down's syndrome, or of a normal variant.

Sutures are palpable ridges between skull bones. The coronal suture is located between the frontal and two parietal bones. The sagittal suture intersects the two parietal bones, and the lambdoidal suture lies between the occipital and the two parietal bones. With increasing gestational age, the suture edges become firmer. Evaluate with gentle palpation. Sutures may be open to a varying degree or may be overlapped because of molding. Lack of normal expansion may indicate microcephaly or craniosynostosis. Abnormally rapid expansion indicates hydrocephalus or increased intracranial pressure. They are palpable as hard ridges.

Abdomen. The abdomen will appear slightly scaphoid at birth but will become distended as the bowel fills with air. Gentle palpation of the abdomen for organs or masses reveals that the spleen tip can be felt from the infant's left side and is sometimes 2 to 3 cm below the left costal margin. The liver is palpable 1 to 2 cm below the right costal margin. Superficial veins over the abdominal wall may be prominent.

A markedly scaphoid abdomen coupled with respiratory difficulty may indicate a diaphragmatic hernia. Abdominal distention and lack of bowel sounds may occur because of intestinal obstruction, paralytic ileus, ascites, imperforate anus, meconium plug, peritonitis, omphalocele, Hirschsprung's disease, or necrotizing enterocolitis. The infant should be observed for abdominal wall defects such as umbilical hernia; omphalocele, a herniation into the base of the umbilical cord; and gastroschisis, a defect of the abdominal wall.

The umbilical cord may also be observed and inspected while the abdomen is being palpated. The diameter of the cord varies depending on the amount of Wharton's jelly present. Two arteries and one vein are normally present in the umbilical cord. The umbilical cord begins to dry soon after birth, becomes loose from the skin by 4 to 5 days, and falls off by 7 to 10 days.

A single umbilical artery, rather than the common two arteries, is a congenital vascular malformation that may be associated with congenital anomalies of the cardiovascular, gastrointestinal, and urinary systems. Redness, foul odor, or wetness of the cord may indicate omphalitis.

INSPECTION

Eyes. Inspection of the infant's eyes is best accomplished when the infant is found in the quiet alert state or when the infant has been aroused to wakefulness during the examination. The eyes cannot be observed while the baby is crying. Tipping the baby backward and raising him or her slowly or shading the infant's eyes from bright light often causes the eyes to open.

The newborn's eyes open spontaneously, look toward a light source, fix, focus, and follow. Uncoordinated eye movements are common. Subconjunctival or scleral hemorrhages are a common result of the pressures of labor and birth. The size, shape, and structure of the eye should be noted.

The pupils of the normal newborn respond to light by constricting. Red reflex is normally present and indicates an intact lens. Tears are not normally produced until 2 months of age. The iris is usually dark blue until 3 to 6 months of age. Doll's eye maneuvers are normally associated with eyes that follow movement of the head, often with a lag and/or nystagmus.

Discharge from the eyes may represent irritation or infection. A lateral upward slope of the eyes with an epicanthal fold may indicate syndromes of mental, physical, or chromosomal aberrations. The absence of red reflex may indicate tumors or congenital cataracts accompanying rubella, galactosemia, or disorders of calcium metabolism. Chorioretinitis is often found in congenital viral diseases such as cyto-megalovirus and toxoplasmosis. White speckles on the iris known as Brushfield's spots are associated with Down's syndrome and mental retardation or are a normal variant. Scleral blueness is associated with osteogenesis imperfecta and scleral yellowness with jaundice. Brain injury may be indicated by a constricted pupil, unilaterally dilated fixed pupil, nystagmus, or strabismus.

BLOOD PRESSURE. Blood pressure with non-invasive Doppler devices are best accomplished before the infant is upset. The blood pressure should be checked in all four extremities of the infant's body to screen for coarctation of the aorta. Since the blood pressure proximal to the area of obstruction is higher than the blood pressure distal to the area of obstruction, blood pressure in the upper extremities is higher (>15 mm Hg) than in the lower extremities (see Figures 3-14 and 3-15).

HEAD-TO-TOE EXAMINATION

The infant's crying will not affect the data to be gathered in the head-to-toe examination.

SKIN. As each body part is examined, the skin is also inspected. Vernix, a white, cheeselike material, normally covers the body of the fetus and decreases with increased gestational age. Discoloration of the vernix occurs with intrauterine distress, postmaturity, hemolytic disease, and breech presentations.

The color of the skin is normally pink. Mongolian spots caused by the presence of pigmented cells may cover the sacral-gluteal areas of black infants or Asian infants. The degree of generalized pigmentation varies and is less intense in the newborn period than later in life. Nevi may be present at the nape of the neck or on the eyelids.

Note the size, shape, color, and degree of ecchymosis, erythema, petechiae, or hemangiomas. Meconium staining suggests prior fetal distress and anoxia. Erythema toxicum appears as a generalized red rash in the first 3 days of life. Milia caused by retained sebum are pinpoint white spots on the cheeks, chin, and bridge of the nose.

The normal texture of the neonate's skin is soft. A preterm infant's skin is more translucent than a term infant's skin. Slight desquamation may occur as skin becomes dry. Moderate to severe desquamation occurs in postterm infants with intrauterine growth retardation. Puffy, shiny skin is symptomatic of edema. Localized edema of a presenting part is caused by trauma and is only temporary. Edema should be distinguished from increased subcutaneous fat. Lanugo coverage decreases with increasing gestational age.

Tissue turgor is the sensation of fullness derived from the presence of hydrated subcutaneous tissue and intrauterine nutrition. Test the elasticity of the skin by grasping a fold of skin between the thumb and forefinger. When released, the skin should promptly spring back to the surface of the body. A loss of normal skin turgor resulting in peaking of the skin is a late sign of dehydration. A generalized hardness of the skin is a sign of sclerema that occurs in debilitated, stressed infants.

EARS. Cartilage development and ear form progress according to gestational age. Observe the external ears for size, shape, and position. The angle of placement of the ears is almost vertical. If the angle of placement is greater than 10 degrees from vertical, it is abnormal. The level of placement is determined by drawing an imaginary line from the outer canthus of the eye to the occiput. If the ear intersects the line, it is placed normally. Slapping hands or other sharp noises will normally elicit a twitching in the eyelid or a complete Moro reflex.

Malformed or malpositioned (lowset or rotated) ears are often associated with renal and chromosomal abnormalities and other congenital anomalies. Abnormalities such as skin tags or sinuses may be associated with renal problems or hearing loss. Forceps or difficult deliveries may injure the outer ear. Congenital deafness is suspected if the infant does not respond to noise. It is confirmed by standardized hearing screening tests and follow-up.

NOSE. Note the shape and size of the nose. Deformities caused by intrauterine pressure may be temporary. Neonates are obligatory nasal breathers and must have patent nasal passages. Check the patency of the alae nasi by (1) obstructing one nostril, closing the mouth, and observing breathing from the open nostril; (2) placing a stethoscope under the nostrils that will "fog" the diaphragm and auscultate breathing; or (3) passing a soft catheter if necessary.

Abnormal configuration may be associated with congenital syndromes. Obstructions can be caused by drugs, infections, tumors, nasal discharge, and mucus. Choanal atresia, a membranous or bony obstruction in the nasal passage, may be unilateral or bilateral. Choanal atresia is characterized by the noisy breathing, cyanosis, and apnea of the quiet infant (mouth closed), as opposed to the pink color of the same crying infant (mouth open).

MOUTH. Examination of the mouth may be done here or at the end of the examination when the infant is crying loudly with a wide, open mouth. At birth the normal infant is able to suck and swallow (develops at 32 to 34 weeks gestation) and root and gag (develops at 36 weeks gestation). Elicit each.

Lips and mucous membranes are normally pink. Observe the lips and mucous membranes for pallor and cyanosis. If the infant is well hydrated, the membranes should be moist. Open the mouth to look for anomalies. Palpate the hard and soft palate for a membranous cleft or submucous cleft. Epithelial pearls are common along the gum margins and the palate.

Natal teeth may be present and require removal to prevent aspiration. A large tongue (macroglossia), cleft lip or palate (including submucous cleft), or high-arched palate may be associated with abnormal facies or be an isolated finding. Esophageal atresia and tracheo-

esophageal fistula are often present with drooling or distress in feeding.

THORAX. Conformation of the newborn chest is cylindric with an anteroposterior ratio of 1:1. Note the shape, symmetry, position, and development of the thorax. Asymmetry of the chest may be caused by diaphragmatic hernia, paralysis of the diaphragm, pneumothorax, emphysema, pulmonary agenesis, or pneumonia. Fullness of the thorax caused by increased anteroposterior diameter occurs with an overexpansion of the lung. Retractions, inward pulls of the soft parts of the chest while inhaling, indicate air-entry interference or pulmonary disease.

BREASTS. Breast tissue systematically develops according to gestational age. Enlargement of breasts because of maternal hormones occurs in either sex on the second or third day. Milky secretions may be present. Unilateral redness or firmness indicates infection.

CLAVICLES. Observe and palpate the area above each clavicle. A fracture of the clavicle is evidenced by a palpable mass, crepitation, tenderness at the fracture site, and limited arm movements on the affected side.

GENITALIA. Male and female genitalia systematically develop according to gestational age.

Male. Inspect the genitalia for the presence and position of the urethral opening. Palpate the testes either in the inguinal canal or scrotum. The scrotum appears large and pendulous with the presence of descended testes. A tight prepuce may be found. In dark-skinned races darker pigmentation of the genitalia is normal. Hypospadias exists if the urethral opening is on the ventral surface of the penis. Epispadias exists if the opening is on the dorsal surface.

Female. Inspect the genitalia for the presence and position of the urethral opening. The introitus is posterior to the clitoris. A vaginal skin tag is a visible hymenal ring.

Edema of the genitalia in both sexes is common in breech deliveries. Note the presence of a hydrocele or hernia. Fecal urethral discharge may indicate rectourethral fistulas. Note femoral pulses.

Rectum. Visualize and check the patency of the anal opening by gently inserting a soft rubber catheter (do not use rigid objects such as glass rectal thermometers). Observe the anatomy and feel the muscle tone. Meconium is normally present during the first days of life.

Imperforate anus, irritation, or fissures may be present. Meconium passage before birth suggests fetal intrauterine distress. Failure to pass meconium within 48 hours suggests obstruction. Meconium ileus is associated with cystic fibrosis.

Back. Place the infant in a prone position and observe for a flat and straight vertebral column. Separate the buttocks to observe the coccygeal area. To check incurving reflex, stroke one side of the vertebral column. The baby will turn the buttocks toward the side stroked. Deviations from normal include curvature of the vertebral column, pilonidal dimple, pilonidal sinus, spina bifida, or myelomeningocele.

EXTREMITIES

Upper extremities. Note the size, shape, and symmetry of the arms and hands. Observe and feel for fractures, paralysis, and dislocations. Count and inspect the fingers. The hands are normally clenched into fists. The infant is capable of adduction, flexion, internal rotation, extension, and symmetry of movement. Note the tone of the muscles. Flexion develops with increasing gestational age.

Simian creases may indicate chromosomal abnormalities that are frequent causes of deformity. Polydactyly and syndactyly of the fingers may be found. Osteogenesis imperfecta is characterized by multiple fractures and deformities. Palsies caused by fractures, dislocations, or injury to the brachial plexus are recognized by limited movement of the extremity. Fractures may also be present with edema and palpable crepitus.

Lower extremities. Note the size, shape, and symmetry of the feet and legs. Note the normal position of flexion (develops according to gestational age) and abduction. Note symmetry of movement, thigh folds, and gluteal folds. A full range of motion is possible, including the "frog position," a rotation of the thighs with the knees flexed. Observe and feel for fractures, paralysis, and dislocations. Palpate femoral pulses.

Polydactyly and syndactyly of the toes may exist. Osteogenesis imperfecta results in multiple fractures and deformities. Paralysis of both legs is caused by severe trauma or congenital anomaly of the spinal cord. A unilaterally or bilaterally dislocated hip (more common in females) causes a hip click when the baby's legs are abducted into the "frog" position. Although soft clicks are common, a sharp click indicates dislocation. Fractures may be present and are characterized by limited movement and edematous, crepitant areas. Chromosomal abnormalities are frequent causes of deformity.

Recoil is a test of flexion development and muscle tone. It systematically develops as flexion develops in the lower extremities first and then in the upper extremities. Extend the legs and then release. Both legs should return promptly to the flexed position in accordance with the gestational age of the infant. Extend the arms alongside the body. On release, prompt flexion should occur at the elbows.

Hypotonia causes the infant to become limp and "floppy" with little control. The extremities fall without resistance when the infant is raised off the bed. Recoil may be partial or absent. Hypertonia causes the infant to tremble and startle easily. The fists are tightly clenched, arms flexed, and legs stiffly extended.

Neurologic examination

Clinical, electric, and anatomic studies of the nervous systems of premature and full-term neonates have confirmed the belief that the CNS of the human fetus matures at a fairly constant rate. Neurologic findings, clinical signs, and electroencephalogram (EEG) findings specifically correlating to gestational age have been established.[7,12] However, there are recognized limitations in clinical applications of the neurologic evaluation. The evaluation is of little value in the first 24 hours of life unless there is an obvious palsy or seizure. Since the newborn is recovering from the stress of birth, the neurologic examination is not valid until after the infant has successfully completed the transition to extrauterine life. Therefore the neurologic examination should be performed after the first 24 hours of life (see Figure 4-3). If the infant is ill or has obstetric anesthesia or analgesia, the neurologic examination may not be valid even after 24 hours.

Brazelton examination

The Neonatal Behavioral Assessment Scale[3] assesses the interactive behavior of the newborn. This psychologic scale for the neonate enables assessment of the infant's individual capabilities for social relationships. Clinical application of the Brazelton scale includes neonatal research and evaluation of infant capabilities after illness, prematurity, or maternal medications. A modified version of the Brazelton examination is useful in teaching parents about their individual infant's patterns of behavior, temperament, and states.[4,9,18]

By understanding the uniqueness of their infant, parents may more intelligently assess and interpret their baby's cues for interaction and distance. If the parents know their infant's individual strengths and weaknesses, they will be more capable of realistically reacting to their infant. It is important for the care provider to elicit the parents' assessment of their infant's behavior and responsiveness. Unrealistic expectations or incorrect parental perceptions may exist. The care provider therefore uses this opportunity for parent teaching, counseling, and possibly referral.[5]

The Brazelton examination is usually performed at 2 to 3 days of life, at discharge, or on the first follow-up visit at 1 to 2 weeks. This examination assesses the infant's best performance in response to stimulation and handling by the examiner. For research purposes, the scoring technique by a certified examiner is required. For clinical use, knowledge of the specific techniques and interpretation of results is all that is required.[5] Since the state of consciousness influences the newborn's reactions, the most important variable in the examiner's observation is knowledge of the infant's state (see section on awake and sleep states in this chapter). Performing the examination with the parents present provides the opportunity for parental participation and observation of their infant's response. Selected maneuvers and ratings of good and poor performances are outlined in Table 4-1. Average performance falls along the continuum between these two points.

Laboratory data

See screening tests for hypoglycemia, polycythemia, and hyperviscosity under the interventions section.

INTERVENTIONS

After the newborn has been examined and assessed, certain admission procedures should be performed. Vital signs should include pulse, respirations, skin or axillary temperature (never rectal), and blood pressure. During the transitional period, vital signs should be recorded frequently enough to monitor the infant's condition and provide appropriate care:

1. If the infant is distressed (elevated heart rate or respiratory rate, retracting and/or nasal flaring), vital signs may be required every ½ to 1 hour.

2. If the baby's vital signs are normal on admission (120 to 160 heart rate, 30 to 60 respiratory rate, 36° to 36.5° C [97.8° to 98.6° F] temperature, and blood pressure 50), they may be recorded once or twice during the transition.

TABLE 4-1

Brazelton's Neonatal Behavioral Assessment: Clinical Clusters and Performance Descriptions

Interactive ability
Alertness
Length of time neonate able to maintain alert state without becoming tired or overstimulated (good—30 minutes; poor—only brief intervals)

Orientation
Good—able to elicit; poor—unable to elicit
1. Visual animate: alert, focuses and follows face
2. Visual inanimate: alert, focuses and follows object (ball, rattle)
3. Auditory animate: alert, searches and turns toward voice
4. Auditory inanimate: alert, searches and turns toward objects (bell, rattle, music box)
5. Visual and auditory animate: alert, focuses, and follows human voice and face

Consolability
Good—may quiet self with hand-to-mouth behavior; responds to adult attempts to console (talking, touching, rocking bed)
Poor—may not be consoled until held and rocked

Motor ability
Tone
Good—normal reflexes, moderate activity level, good tone with handling; relaxed when handling ceases
Poor—hypotonia or hypertonia

Activity
Good—spontaneous and elicited movements are smooth and coordinated; controls head; moderate startles, hand-to-mouth behaviors
Poor—uncoordinated movements, hypotonic or hypertonic reflexes; little activity or constant, unconsolable activity

Organization—state control
Habituation
Good—alerts to stimuli and gradually decreases bodily response to repeated stimuli
Poor—inability to decrease response to intrusive stimuli

State lability
Good—few state swings and easy transition from state to state
Poor—frequent state swings; depressed, unarousable baby

Irritability
Good—able to quiet self and lower irritability
Poor—unable to quiet self; early, prolonged irritability; unable to arouse to irritable state with intrusive stimuli

Organization—physiologic response
Skin color
Degree of color change and frequency during examination
Good—some flushing or mottling, but normal color quickly returns
Poor—profound mottling, central or peripheral cyanosis with slower recovery of normal color

Startles and tremors
Good—more startles or tremors at beginning of examination
Poor—frequent startles and tremulous responses with little decrement

Modified from Als H et al: Specific neonatal measures: the Brazelton neonatal behavioral assessment scale. In Osofsky JD, editor: Handbook of infant development, New York, 1979, John Wiley & Sons, Inc.

3. Vital signs should be recorded at least once every 8 hours.

4. Blood pressure in the arm and leg should be taken on admission and at discharge to rule out possible coarctation of the aorta.

5. Rectal temperatures are contraindicated in the newborn infant because of the risk of rectal perforation (see Chapter 5).

Weight, length, and head circumference should be graphed on the appropriate intra-

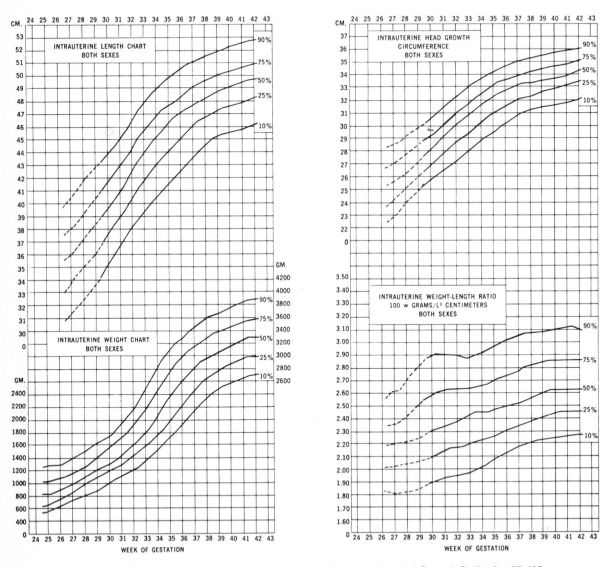

Figure 4-13. Colorado intrauterine growth charts. (From Lubchenco LO et al: Pediatrics 37:403, 1966. Original art published by Ross Laboratories, Columbus, Ohio. Reproduced by permission of Pediatrics.)

uterine growth chart to show in which percentile the baby falls. The parameters should be set at less than 10%, between 10% and 90%, and greater than 90%. Determine the weight/length ratio (Figure 4-13). The weight/length ratio normally increases with fetal age. The baby becomes heavier for length as term approaches. In intrauterine growth retardation the weight/length ratio decreases as the rate of growth in weight is affected more than length. Severe and prolonged intrauterine malnutrition may affect head, weight, and length ratios.

Blood sugar levels

At birth the blood glucose of the normal, healthy neonate is approximately 60% to 70% of the simultaneous maternal value. Over the next several hours, glucose normally falls to a level of 35 to 40 mg/dl and by 6 hours of age rises to 45 to 60 mg/dl (Figure 4-14).

A blood-glucose test (Dextrostix) should be done on admission, at 4 hours of age, and more often if the infant is in an at-risk group (LGA [insulin-dependent mother], SGA, or PRAGA). Hypoglycemia in SGA infants calls for prompt

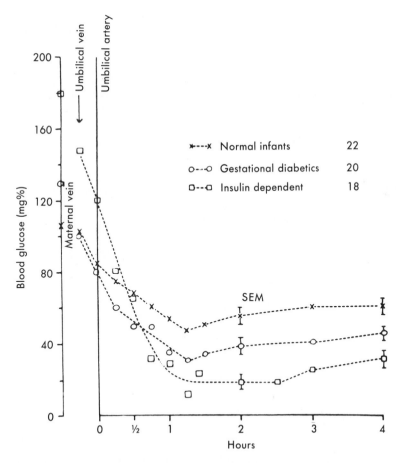

Figure 4-14. Blood glucose changes after birth in normal infant and infants of gestational and insulin-dependent diabetic mothers. (From Cornblath M and Schwartz R: Disorders of carbohydrate metabolism, Philadelphia, 1976, WB Saunders Co.)

action, since these infants lack stores of fat or glycogen to mobilize glucose. Stressed infants are also at risk for the development of hypoglycemia. Stress may include perinatal asphyxia, cold stress, maternal disease such as maternal diabetes, or any acute illness in the infant (see Chapter 11).

Hematocrit

A hematocrit determination is performed to rule out the possibility of blood loss or polycythemia. A peripheral or central hematocrit should be done during the newborn's transitional period. If the peripheral hematocrit is greater than 65 or less than 45, a central hematocrit is drawn (see Chapter 14).

COMPLICATIONS

Complications of common morbidities (Figure 4-12) are prevented by classification, assessment, and screening of all newborns at birth. Complications of the morbidities in Figure 4-12 are thoroughly discussed in the appropriate chapters.

PARENT TEACHING

Transitional care, neonatal assessment, and initial care need not take place in a nursery where the newborn and family are isolated from each other. Alternative settings for initial care include birthing rooms, recovery rooms where family and baby are kept together, or in the mother's postpartum room. In fact, keeping the family together not only facilitates bonding, but also provides unique opportunities for teaching parents about the uniqueness and individuality of their newborn. At this time, parents are most receptive to information about the baby, who is the center of attention.

The initial assessment of gestational age and physical condition is best performed with the mother and father in attendance so that deviations from normal such as caput, cleft lip, cleft palate, or clubfoot can be explained. Performing screening procedures such as Dextrostix

and hematocrit with the parents present provides an opportunity to explain the procedure and why it is necessary for their baby. Eliciting parental cooperation is important. For example, when the major concern is whether or not the procedure "will hurt," a response such as, "it is routine," will not comfort and reassure well-informed, noninterventionist consumers. Rather, a more physiologically oriented explanation about the condition being screened, why their particular infant is at increased risk, and what interventions are available encourages parental cooperation.

Professional care providers are only temporary caretakers. It is the care providers' responsibility to help parents become confident, primary caretakers of their own infants. Actively involving parents in the treatment of their newborn further solidifies their position as primary caretakers. Encouraging active parental involvement enhances the parents' self-esteem and confidence in their abilities[8]; thus the care providers' actions must tell the parents, "You are able to care for this baby."

At discharge, performing the physical examination in the room with the parents offers a final opportunity to teach, counsel, and advise them before they take their new baby home. Information about feeding, cord care, bathing, elimination patterns, safety, signs of illness, medications, and the importance of follow-up care is essential for parents of a full-term, healthy newborn and for parents taking home an infant after prolonged hospitalization. In addition, a modified version of Brazelton's examination on all neonates enables parents to become familiar with a newborn's competencies for reacting to and shaping his or her environment and with strategies for parental intervention. Developing written materials for parents about normal newborn care and documenting teaching sessions and return demonstrations ensure that no important information is forgotten.[5,19] Figures 4-15 and 4-16 illustrate teaching guides for basic neonatal care.

University of Colorado Health Sciences Center
University Hospital
Department of Nursing Service

Standards of Care

Basic Neonatal Care

S.O. = Significant other   Date initiated _____

| | Date and initial | | |
	Instructed in newborn class	Instructed individually	Understands S.O.
Patient outcome criteria			
I. Has knowledge of breast-feeding technique and formula preparation			
A. Frequency and length of breast-feeding A			
B. Type of formula to be used and resource for purchase B			
C. How to dilute chosen formula and how long it may be refrigerated C			
D. How often to feed baby D			
E. How much to feed baby			
1. Per feeding 1			
2. Per day 2			
II. Have knowledge of the physical care needed by the infant			
A. Frequency that cord care is needed A			
B. Care of the circumcised penis B			
C. Care of diaper rash			
1. Expose buttocks to air 1			
D. Cause and care of cradle cap			
1. Wash hair with bath 1			
III. Have knowledge of home safety and car safety			
A. Prevention of falls A			
B. Prevention of choking B			
C. Knowledge of recommended car seats C			
IV. Has knowledge of signs of illness			
A. Has instruction on taking axillary temperature and what is an elevated temperature A			
B. Has instruction about normal patterns in sleep, feeding, urine and stool, and fussiness B			
C. Awareness that changes in above may indicate signs of illness C			

Continued.

Figure 4-15. Standards of care: basic neonatal care, Denver, 1982, University of Colorado Health Sciences Center.

	Date and initial		
	Instructed in newborn class	Instructed individually	Understands S.O.
V. Parents have knowledge of what sibling rivalry is and how to deal with it			
A. Expected behavior in a sibling who is jealous of newborn — A			
B. Ways to help sibling who is jealous of newborn — B			
VI. Have knowledge of normal awake/ sleep patterns for age of their newborn and the need for stimulation when awake			
A. Normal number of hours the newborn sleeps per day — A			
B. Whether baby can and/or should sleep through the night — B			
C. Ways to stimulate baby's senses (sight, hearing, touch, taste) — C			
D. Behavior modifications program, if applicable — D			
VII. Have knowledge of importance of follow-up care			
A. Can identify a clinic or physician to do follow-up care — A			
B. Verbalizes that an appointment has been made for 1 to 2 weeks after discharge with appropriate clinic — B			
C. Verbalizes that a public health nurse will make a home visit — C			
VIII. Administers medications safely			
A. Demonstrates safe administration of medication — A			
B. Can identify purpose and side effects of medication — B			
C. Verbalizes understanding of or can read instructions of discharge medications (name, route, dose, length of course of medication) Name of medication			
1. _____ — 1			
2. _____ — 2			
3. _____ — 3			
4. _____ — 4			

The above information was discussed with

_____   _____
(Name)   (Relationship)

_____ Nurse's signature and initials

Figure 4-15, cont'd. For legend see p. 105.

ST. FRANCIS REGIONAL MEDICAL CENTER, DIVISION OF NURSING
Nursing Standards

DIAGNOSIS: Neonate
DRG: 391

NURSING DIAGNOSIS	TIME LINE	NURSING INTERVENTIONS	DESIRED OUTCOMES
Health maintenance, potential alteration in	0-2 hours 0-2 hours 0-6 hours 1-3 hours 2-4 hours 1-2 days	1. Perform initial assessment and estimate gestational age per routine nursing procedure. 2. Provide warmth until temperature is stable. 3. Hourly vital signs for first 6 hours or as ordered by physician. 4. Initiate feedings within 3 hours after delivery. 5. Perform initial bath. 6. Perform routine genetic screening after 48 hours of age or before dismissal.	1. Mother and/or significant other will verbalize understanding of continuing care needs and available resources.
Sensory/perceptual alterations ☐ Visual	1-2 days	1. Establish eye-to-eye contact. 2. Place black and white patterns in crib at eye level. 3. Dim lights at night.	1. Neonate demonstrates en face position with health professionals and/or parents. 2. Neonate maintains fixation for at least 3 seconds. 3. Neonate establishes day and night.
☐ Auditory	1-2 days	1. Encourage mother and father to talk to neonate. 2. Play music at night (lullaby, Bach, Brahms, or Beethoven). 3. Encourage calling neonate by name. 4. Encourage use of adult speech.	1. Neonate's head turns to locate sound. 2. Neonate demonstrates quiescent behavior (snuggles or nests). 3. Neonate orients to sound and name by turning head, brightening face, and dilating pupils. 4. Neonate vocalizes and initiates rhythmic movements to voices.
☐ Olfactory	1-2 days	1. Provide mother's milk if breast-feeding. 2. Provide article of mother's clothing of her preference if not nursing.	1. Neonate demonstrates response to specific olfactory stimulation.
☐ Gustatory	1-2 days	1. Encourage neonate's hand in mouth or pacifier in mouth.	1. Neonate demonstrates increased self-regulated sucking and saliva production.

Continued.

Figure 4-16. Standards of care. (Courtesy St. Francis Regional Medical Center.)

Nursing Standards

DIAGNOSIS: Neonate
DRG: 391

NURSING DIAGNOSIS	TIME LINE	NURSING INTERVENTIONS	DESIRED OUTCOMES
☐ Vestibular	1-2 days	1. Encourage use of rocking chair when holding neonate. 2. Encourage lifting and lateral positioning for up-and-down and side-to-side sensations for neonate. 3. Encourage passive flexion and extension exercises of the upper and lower extremities of neonate. 4. Encourage placing small objects in hand of neonate (ball, toy, pacifier).	1. Neonate demonstrates flexion, quiescence, visual attentiveness, improved muscle tone, and grasp reflex.
Nutrition, potential alteration in ☐ Breast ☐ Formula	1-2 days	1. Provide neonate with feedings every 3-4 hours or on demand during day and evening. 2. Provide feeding at least one time during night or on demand. 3. Provide supplemental feedings as indicated. 4. Burp during and after feeding.	1. Neonate is provided with optimal nutrition and fluid intake.
Elimination, potential alteration in ☐ Bowel	1-2 days	1. Record eliminations and note variations. 2. Note stool color.	1. Neonate demonstrates normal bowel functions.
☐ Urine	1-2 days	1. Record eliminations and note variations. 2. Note urine color.	1. Neonate demonstrates normal urinary output.
Skin integrity, impairment of: potential ☐ Circumcision care ☐ Umbilical cord care	1-2 days	1. Provide routine circumcision care when applicable. 2. Provide routine umbilical cord care.	1. Minimal irritation and/or bleeding. 2. Absence of infection observed. 3. Observation of initial healing process.
Home maintenance management	1-2 days	1. Provide mother and/or significant other with educational materials concerning neonate. 2. Provide mother and/or significant other with available referral services. 3. Encourage mother and/or significant other to continue with follow-up care.	1. Mother and/or significant other will verbalize understanding or continuing care needs and resources.

Figure 4-16, cont'd. For legend see p. 107.

Equipping parents for the discharge of a baby with special care needs is discussed in the parent teaching section of several chapters, such as Chapter 15.

Understanding the transition of the neonate from intrauterine to extrauterine life is essential.

Since the implementation of diagnostic related groups (DRGs) and capitation for hospital stays, the length of hospital stay for a normal mother and baby continues to decrease. The national average length of stay for normal deliveries has fallen since 1982 from 3 days to 2 days, with a trend toward discharge at 1 day postpartum. It is anticipated that in the near future most obstetric care will take place on an outpatient basis (less than 24 hours total in-hospital time), with accompanying excellent home care services and support for the family.

A recent study conducted in a semirural county in upstate New York shows that a model program of prenatal and postnatal home visits can be instrumental in preventing health and developmental problems in both mother and baby. Hospital nurses need to be astutely aware that a new mother cannot learn until she is ready and is motivated by need. Early discharge may preclude the mother or father's being able to learn newborn care. Providing for home health care, having parents return to the hospital for classes, and use of a telephone advice service are measures that may promote education and learning as readiness occurs.

REFERENCES

1. Als H et al: Specific neonatal measures, the Brazelton neonatal behavioral assessment scale. In Osofsky JD, editor: Handbook of infant development, New York, 1979, John Wiley & Sons, Inc.
2. Barness LA: Manual of pediatric physical diagnosis, ed 5, Chicago, 1981, Year Book Medical Publishers, Inc.
3. Brazelton TB: Neonatal behavioral assessment scale, Philadelphia, 1973, JB Lippincott Co/Spastics International Medical Publishers.
4. Buckner EB: Use of Brazelton neonatal behavioral assessment in planning care for parents and newborns, JOGN Nurs 12:26, 1983.
5. Cagan J and Meier P: A discharge planning tool for use with families of high risk infants, JOGN Nurs 8:146, 1979.
6. Desmond M et al: The transitional care nursery, Pediatr Clin North Am 13:656, 1966.
7. Dubowitz LMS, Dubowitz V, and Goldberg C: Clinical assessment of gestational age in the newborn infant, J Pediatr 77:1, 1970.
8. Galloway K: Early detection of congenital anomalies, JOGN Nurs 2:37, 1973.
9. Gardner SL: Mothering, the unconscious conflict between nurses and new mothers, Keep Abreast J 3:192, 1978.
10. Gibes RM: Clinical uses of the Brazelton neonatal behavioral assessment scale in nursing practice, Pediatr Nurs 7:23, 1981.
11. Gill NE et al: Transitional newborn infants in a hospital nursery: from first oral cue to first sustained cry, Nurs Management 33(4):213, 1984.
12. Koeningsberger R: Judgment of fetal age. I. Neurologic evaluation, Pediatr Clin North Am 13:823, 1966.
13. Koops BL et al: Neonatal mortality risk in relation to birthweight and gestational age; update, J Pediatr 101:969, 1982.
14. Lubchenco LO: Watching the newborn for disease, Pediatr Clin North Am 8:471, 1961.
15. Lubchenco LO: The high risk infant, Philadelphia, 1976, WB Saunders Co.
16. Lubchenco LO et al: Intrauterine growth in length and head circumference as estimated from live births at gestational ages from 26-42 weeks, Pediatrics 37:403, 1966.
17. Lubchenco LO et al: Neonatal mortality risk: relationship to birthweight and gestational age, J Pediatr 81:84, 1972.
18. Nugent JK: The Brazelton neonatal behavioral assessment scale: implications for interventions, Pediatr Nurs 7:18, 1981.
19. Schmidt J: Using a teaching guide for better postpartum and infant care, JOGN Nurs 7:23, 1978.
20. Usher R et al: Judgement of fetal age. II. Clinical significance of gestational age and an objective method for its assessment, Pediatr Clin North Am 13:835, 1966.
21. Van Leewan G: The nurse in prevention and intervention in the neonatal period, Nurs Clin North Am 8:509, 1973.
22. Wald MK: Problems in metabolic adaptation: glucose, calcium and magnesium. In Klaus MH and Fanaroff AA, editors: Care of the high risk neonate, ed 2, Philadelphia, 1979, WB Saunders Co.

SELECTED READINGS

Adreoli KG et al: Major trends shaping the future of neonatal nursing, J Neonatal Nurs 6(4):325, 1986.
American Academy of Pediatrics, Committee on Drugs and Committee on Fetus and Newborn: Prophylaxis and treatment of neonatal gonococcal infections, Pediatrics 65:1047, 1980.

American Academy of Pediatrics and American College of Obstetricians and Gynecologists: Guidelines for perinatal care, ed 2, Evanston, Ill, 1988, American Academy of Pediatrics and American College of Obstetricians and Gynecologists.

Ballard JL et al: A simplified assessment of gestational age, Pediatr Res 11:374, 1977.

Battaglia F and Lubchenco L: Practical classification of newborn infants by weight, J Pediatr 71:159, 1967.

Butterfield P and Emde R: Effects of silver nitrate on initial visual behavior, Am J Dis Child 132:426, 1978.

Chinn P and Leitch C: Child health maintenance: a guide to clinical assessment, ed 2, St Louis, 1979, The CV Mosby Co.

Emde R et al: Human wakefulness and biologic rhythms after birth, Arch Gen Psychiatry 32:780, 1975.

Hittner H et al: Assessment of gestational age by examination of the anterior vascular capsule of the lens, J Pediatr 91:455, 1977.

Klaus MH and Fanaroff AA editors: Care of the high-risk neonate, ed 2, Philadelphia, 1986, WB Saunders Co.

Koops BL and Battaglia FC: The newborn infant. In Kempe CH, editor: Current pediatric diagnosis and treatment, ed 9, Altos, Calif, 1986, Lange Medical Books.

Lipsitt L and Field TM: Perinatal influences on the behavior of full-term newborns. In Lipsitt L and Field TM, editors: Infant behavior and development: perinatal risk and newborn behavior, Norwood, NJ, 1982, Ablex Publishing Corp.

Ludington SM: Infant stimulation, 1987, A comprehensive course of study in infant growth, development and enhancement, Symposia Medicus, Walnut Creek, Calif.

March of Dimes Birth Defects Foundation: Nursing staff modules. Module 4: Assessment of risk in the newborn. Part A: Evaluation during the transitional period, Part B: Birth injuries, Part C: Congenital anomalies, Part D: Neonatal growth and maturity, 1982, March of Dimes Birth Defects Foundation.

Merenstein GB: Rectal perforation by thermometer, Lancet 1:1007, 1970.

Olds DL et al: Improving the delivery of prenatal care and outcomes of pregnancy: a randomized trial of nurse home visitation, Pediatrics 77:16, Jan 1986.

The perinatal assessment of maturation: pediatric, newborn series, S-2819, Washington DC, 1979, The National Audiovisual Center.

CHAPTER 5

Heat balance

GERALD B. MERENSTEIN · SANDRA L. GARDNER · W. WOODS BLAKE

When it was noted by Villermi and Milne-Edwards in the early nineteenth century that infant mortality in France was higher during the colder months, interest in proper warming of neonates first appeared in the medical literature. Attempts to maintain warmth in premature infants demonstrated the first widespread efforts to salvage babies who had seldom survived before. During the last half of the nineteenth century, several devices were constructed for the sole purpose of warming small neonates and improving their survival. Since these first incubators were developed, a great deal of information about the physiology of heat balance has been learned, and technical advancements in equipment have been made. Research continues today to further determine the best methods for maintaining the optimal temperature of the tiniest newborn infants.

The purpose of this chapter is to present the reader with current knowledge of the physiology and pathophysiology of neonatal thermoregulation and its application in neonatal care.

PHYSIOLOGY

Excessive cooling or heating is detrimental to neonates, and extreme environmental temperature could have serious consequences and even lead to death. The neutral thermal environment is one in which an infant's body temperature remains normal with minimal metabolic effort and therefore minimal oxygen consumption. Factors such as ambient air temperature, humidity, air velocity, and the temperature of objects in direct contact with the infant or surfaces involved with radiant heat exchange should be considered as part of the environment. Likewise, the *neutral thermal skin temperature* is the skin temperature (usually measured over the abdomen) at which oxygen consumption is minimal. The range of thermal neutrality is narrow for the naked infant, and there is a critical temperature below this range where oxygen consumption increases in an attempt to maintain a normal body temperature. Overheating also causes an increase in oxygen consumption. An abnormal body temperature may mean that the thermal stress from an inappropriate environmental temperature has overwhelmed the infant's thermoregulatory mechanisms.

CAUTION: **All studies used to develop Figures 5-1 and 5-2 have been done under specific, controlled environments that may not exist in the clinical setting. The ideal temperature varies with the particular baby and environmental variables, such as relative humidity, type of incubator used, and use of clothing.**

Heat balance is a function of heat production (metabolic activity of the baby), heat loss, and heat supplied from external sources. Although shivering is a major means of heat production in adults, neonates do not shiver but depend mainly on the metabolism of *brown fat* located around the great vessels, kidneys, scapulas, axilla, and nape of the neck. This nonshivering thermogenesis is initiated by stimulation of thermal receptors in skin, primarily in the face. It is controlled by the sympathetic nervous system through the release of norepinephrine, which stimulates the hydrolysis of brown fat triglycerides into nonesterified free fatty acids and glycerol. Further

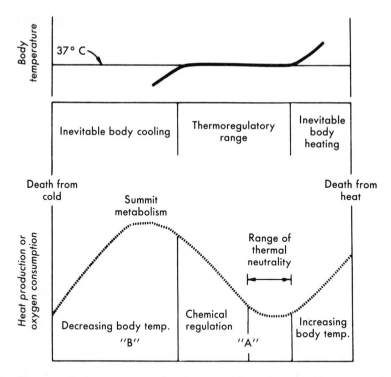

Figure 5-1. Temperature versus oxygen consumption. Effect of environmental temperature on oxygen consumption and body temperature. (From Klaus M and Fanaroff A: Care of the high-risk neonate, ed 2, Philadelphia, 1979, WB Saunders Co.)

metabolism of the fatty acids produces heat, but the entire thermogenic process also requires oxygen and glucose. The increased oxygen demand in a baby with accompanying respiratory compromise leads to increased anaerobic metabolism, producing metabolic acidosis, pulmonary acidosis, and ultimately death. Hypoglycemia is frequently seen with hypothermia and may be the result of rapid use of carbohydrate stores for the metabolism of brown fat by lipolysis or by the inhibition of glycolysis. Furthermore, the increased circulating nonesterified free fatty acids compete with bilirubin for albumin-binding sites, thus possibly increasing the risk for kernicterus, especially in the presence of acidosis.

Heat loss by the infant must first reach the body surface and then dissipate to the environment.

Heat generated from the metabolic process reaches the body surface by direct conduction through the body tissues or the bloodstream to the skin. The infant's vasomotor responses to either heat or cold stress play an important role in thermoregulation. The expiration of warm, moist air is also a source of heat loss for the infant.

The cold that stresses a newborn may increase the axillary temperature because of its close proximity to brown fat stores, even though the abdominal skin temperature is decreased. Vasodilation in response to overheating causes an increase in skin temperature. Therefore if servocontrol is used, the heat output will decrease, causing a reduction in the incubator temperature. Vasoconstriction in response to cold stress causes a decrease in skin

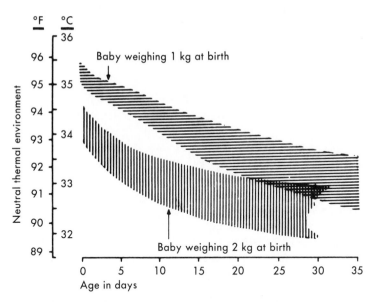

Figure 5-2. Thermal neutral environments. Range of temperature to provide neutral environmental conditions for baby lying naked on warm mattress in draft-free surroundings of moderate humidity (50% sat.) when mean radiant temperature is same as air temperature. Hatched area shows average neutral temperature range for healthy baby weighing 1 kg (≡) or 2 kg (▥) at birth. Optimal temperature probably approximates to lower limit of neutral range as defined here. Approximately 1° C (34° F) should be added to these operative temperatures to derive appropriate neutral air temperature for single-walled incubator when room temperature is less than 27° C (80° F), and more if room temperature is much less. (From Katz G and Hey EN: Arch Dis Child 45:328, 1970.)

temperature; therefore an increased heat output through the incubator's servocontrol mechanism subsequently increases the incubator temperature.

Heat exchange from warmer to cooler objects takes place between the infant's body surface and the environment as a function of the physical principles of radiation, evaporation, conduction, and convection. *Radiation* is the transfer of heat from the baby's skin to cooler surrounding surfaces not in contact with the infant. The increased relative surface area of the neonate, especially a low birth weight infant, makes this the major source of heat loss in the newborn. *Evaporation* causes heat loss from the mucosa of the respiratory tract and from skin and is most pronounced in the delivery room. Adequate environmental humidity minimizes evaporative losses from the lungs and skin surfaces. *Conduction* is the transfer of heat between two surfaces in direct contact with each other. *Convection* involves heat loss from the moving air at the skin surface. The actual amount of heat loss depends primarily on the velocity of airflow and the air temperature. The neonate's surface area exposed to the airflow and cold air blown in the neonate's face also cause convective heat loss and are stimuli for increased oxygen consumption. Swaddling prevents contact of the neonate's skin with the cooler room air.

The neonate radiates heat to the cooler walls of the incubator, which are affected by the room temperature. Therefore incubators should be moved from cold sources, such as windows, drafts, and air conditioning outlets. A heat shield or the inner wall of a double-walled incubator, which is the same temperature as the ambient air inside the incubator, decreases radiant heat loss, since the temperature gradient between the infant and the shield or inner wall is small.

To decrease evaporative heat loss, dry the infant immediately on delivery and wrap in a warm blanket as soon as it is feasible. Because the head makes up one fourth of the neonate's body surface, covering the head may decrease heat loss. Keep the skin dry. An environmental relative humidity of at least 50% decreases evaporative losses. Drying and placing the healthy neonate in direct skin contact with the mother and wrapping both in a warm blanket causes the mother's body warmth to be conducted to the skin of her infant and helps keep the baby warm, although swaddling decreases direct observation. NOTE: Before wrapping the infant in insulating material such as a bubble wrap or foil, the infant must be warm since wrapping the infant in these devices retains body warmth and does not generate heat.

Normally a mattress or piece of clothing has low conductivity and poses an insignificant source of heat loss. A cool, solid, and more conductive surface, such as a scale or a cold hand, however, may cause cold stress, and contact of these surfaces with the newborn should be avoided.

Drafts and cool air temperatures should be avoided to minimize convective heat loss. The convective currents in an incubator increase heat loss only to a small degree because the velocity is low and the air temperature is relatively high.

Oxygen delivered to the neonate by either an ET tube or blown into a head box should be warmed to between 31° and 34° C (88° and 93° F). Hyperthermia or hypothermia could be induced if the supplied gas were too warm (>34° C or >93° F) or too cool (<31° C or <88° F).

Body temperature has long been recognized as an indicator of health and should routinely be monitored in neonates. The deep body ("core") temperature may be measured by determining the esophageal or tympanic membrane temperature using flexible, specialized probes or measuring the rectal temperature using thermometers or thermistors that must be inserted at least 5 cm to obtain a stable core temperature. This insertion depth, however, risks perforating the rectum in the neonate. The mortality from rectal perforation in the neonate is approximately 70% in reported cases.

A safer and more practical way to measure temperature is by firmly holding a thermometer in the axilla for 3 minutes, providing an accurate equivalent of deep body temperature in the neonate.

The skin temperature is routinely measured over the abdomen for consistency. Vasoconstriction may cause skin temperature to fall and therefore is an early indication of cold stress. The deep body temperature may not fall unless heat-producing mechanisms can no longer compensate for heat loss and oxygen consumption has already markedly increased.

Measuring the esophageal and tympanic membrane temperatures on a routine basis is impractical. Measuring rectal temperature is unsafe, since the sigmoid colon makes a right angle to itself at a depth of 3 cm; insertion less than 3 cm will not perforate the rectum but will not accurately reflect the core temperature. Since the risks outweigh the benefits, measuring rectal temperatures (with either a glass rectal thermometer or an electronic probe) is contraindicated on a routine basis in the neonate.

Often when initial temperatures are taken rectally, the rationale is to diagnose an imperforate anus. An alternative and less dangerous mode of establishing rectal patency is inserting a lubricated, soft, red rubber catheter than can maneuver around the angulation of the colon and avoid perforation.

Measuring the axillary temperature is the

safest and most practical means of monitoring deep body temperature in the neonate, but in the cold-stressed infant, the metabolism of axillary brown fat may make this temperature measurement misleadingly high (Figure 5-3).

In a cold-stressed infant the skin temperature usually decreases first because of peripheral vasoconstriction. If the cold stress progresses, the infant will no longer be able to compensate, and the core temperature as mea-

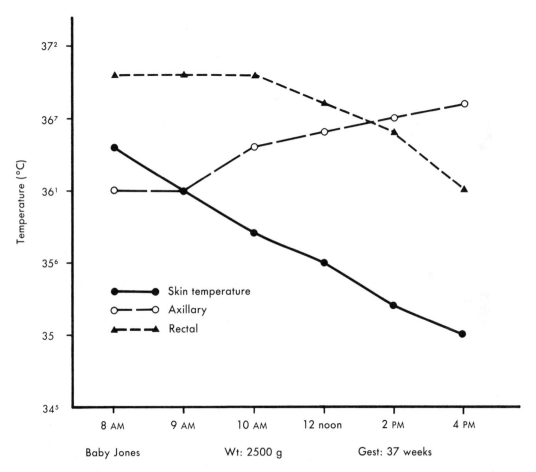

Baby Jones   Wt: 2500 g   Gest: 37 weeks

Figure 5-3. Temperature measurement at various sites during cold stress. In environment that is less than thermal neutral, cold stress begins as skin temperature decreases (*9 AM*) because of vasoconstriction of skin. *10 AM*, Axillary temperature increases as infant burns brown fat to keep warm; rectal temperature is unchanged, since core temperature is maintained. *Noon*, Infant is still cold stressed (skin temperature is down); axillary temperature is up as infant continues to compensate (burns brown fat); rectal temperature is still in normal range. *2 to 4 PM*, Skin temperature reflects severe cold stress; axilla is warm but baby is cold; rectal (core temperature) falls as body decompensates—severe cold stress.

sured in the rectum or esophagus will fall. The axillary temperature, however, may still be normal because of the close proximity to axillary brown fat that is being metabolized (Figure 5-3).

Early detection and appropriate response to cold stress prevent the neonate from facing the additional stress of decompensation in an attempt to maintain heat balance.

ETIOLOGY

Recognizing the risk factors is essential in planning the prevention of thermal stress to neonates. Hypothermia in the preterm, low birth weight infant is the result of several factors:

1. Preterm infants have a high surface area–to–body mass ratio when compared with older children and adults, and therefore have a relatively high surface area from which to lose heat.
2. They have thin skin, decreased amounts of subcutaneous tissue, brown fat, and glycogen stores.
3. They have an immature central nervous system (CNS).
4. They require frequent manipulation and intervention by health care providers.

Older children decrease the surface area exposed to a cool environment by flexing their extremities to their trunk. Preterm infants lack good flexion development and therefore lie primarily in extension, thus exposing a greater surface area to the environment. Less time in utero means less time for the accumulation of subcutaneous tissue, which acts as an insulation between the body core and the surface, and for the accumulation of substantia available for thermogenesis from the metabolism of brown fat. The preterm infant's response to cold stress is muted and immature, which is related to a diminished norepinephrine response to cold stress. The procedures necessary for the care of sick preterm infants increase their general stress and increase the possibility of exposure

to a cold delivery room or nursery environment.

Hypothermia in the term but small-for-gestational-age (SGA) infant also is related to several factors that contribute to hypothermia in premature infants:

1. SGA infants have a higher surface area–to–body mass ratio and a relatively high surface area in which to lose heat.
2. Decreased subcutaneous tissue, brown fat, and glycogen stores may all pose problems for the SGA infant.
3. Decreased placental flow, frequently present in SGA infants, may cause chronic hypoxia and is detrimental to fetal brain development.
4. SGA infants often require frequent manipulation and intervention because they are often ill.

Although small, the SGA infant is mature and has good flexion development that decreases the exposed surface area from which heat can be lost. The loss of subcutaneous tissue, brown fat, and glycogen used in utero for survival leaves little insulation or fuel for metabolic thermogenesis after birth. Depressed CNS function further impairs the response to cold stress. Manipulation and intervention increase the risks of cold stress for the same reasons as in preterm infants.

Birth asphyxia or drug narcosis may interfere with the infant's ability to respond to cold stress. Sepsis and intracranial hemorrhage affect the infant's response to temperature stress.

Hyperthermia in neonates may be iatrogenic or an indication of a disease process. The most common cause of hyperthermia in the neonate is use of extra heat sources, but sepsis may also cause hyperthermia in the neonate. Since adequate fluid volume is necessary to regulate body temperature, dehydration can contribute to hyperthermia.

Drugs received either transplacentally or after delivery may have a sedative effect that depresses the infant's response to cold stress. The ability of the CNS to adequately respond to cold stress is impaired with asphyxia at birth, and therefore the effects of cold stress are more detrimental in the infant with intracranial pathologic conditions, such as asphyxia, hemorrhage, meningitis, or developmental anomalies. Either congenital or acquired sepsis may be first evidenced by a decrease in body temperature. When an infant is in a servocontrolled environment with normal skin temperature, fever may be noted by a drop in incubator temperature. Excessive clothing and blankets in a warm room and temperature settings on incubators or radiant warmers that are inappropriate for the infant's needs frequently cause overheating. Placing an incubator in sunshine may create a "greenhouse effect" within the incubator, causing the infant to become too warm. Increased fluids are required in the following situations where dehydration may occur:

1. In low birth weight infants who have an increased skin permeability and therefore an increased insensible water loss
2. When using phototherapy or radiant warmers, which also increase insensible water loss
3. When there is abnormal fluid loss such as nasogastric suction, ostomy drainage, vomiting, or diarrhea.

PREVENTION

The goals of preventing heat imbalance and its sequelae are to maintain a neutral thermal environment and to block the avenues of heat loss from the infant. The neutral thermal environment minimizes the oxygen consumption for heat production, while the deep body temperature stays within the normal range ($36.5°$ to $37.5°$ C) ($97.7°$ to $99.5°$ F). The neutral thermal environment for newborns is $32.5° \pm 1.4°$ C ($90.5° \pm 2.6°$ F) for larger babies and $35.4° \pm 0.5°$ C ($95.7° \pm 0.9°$ F) for smaller babies (Table 5-1). Newborns in the 500 to 800 g range are not adequately addressed in currently available tables but should have a starting environmental temperature setting of $36.5°$ C ($97.7°$ F).

A neutral thermal environment may be maintained with either servocontrolled or manually adjustable heating equipment. Servocontrolled heating units are frequently used to automatically adjust heat output so that the infant's skin temperature is maintained at a preset level. If the thermistor attached to the skin indicates a temperature below the "set point," heat production will increase until the skin temperature reaches the set point. If the skin temperature rises above that point, heat output decreases until the skin temperature falls to the "set point."

When using servocontrolled heating units, attach the skin probe with tape to the upper right quadrant of the abdomen. If a radiant heater is used, a deflecting metal or foam pad should cover the probe. Set the servomechanism to the desired skin temperature between $36°$ and $36.5°$ C ($96.8°$ to $97.7°$ F). Newer incubators also offer the capability of air temperature servocontrol, so that heat output fluctuates to maintain a set air temperature within the incubator. Observe and chart temperatures from the skin probe (the neonate's skin temperature), the ambient air in the incubator, and the axillary temperature (the neonate's deep body temperature). Problems associated with equipment malfunction should be avoided by checking that the alarms are set in the "on" position for high and low temperature limits.

Without servocontrol, the heating device must be regulated manually to maintain a neutral thermal environment. The warming device should be set at the neutral thermal environmental temperature desired (see Table 5-1).

EXAMPLE: An infant weighing 1 kg who is 2 days old should be placed in an incubator whose temperature is $34°$ C ($93.2°$ F). Approximately $1°$ C ($1.8°$ F) should be added to this operative temperature when the

TABLE 5-1

Neutral Thermal Environmental Temperatures

AGE AND WEIGHT	STARTING TEMPERATURE (°C)	RANGE OF TEMPERATURE (°C)
0-6 hours		
Under 1200 g	35.0	34.0-35.4
1200-1500 g	34.1	33.9-34.4
1501-2500 g	33.4	32.8-33.8
Over 2500 g (and >36 weeks)	33.9	32.0-33.8
6-12 hours		
Under 1200 g	35.0	34.0-35.4
1200-1500 g	34.0	33.5-34.4
1501-2500 g	33.1	32.2-33.8
Over 2500 g (and >36 weeks)	32.8	31.4-33.8
12-24 hours		
Under 1200 g	34.0	34.0-35.4
1200-1500 g	33.8	33.3-34.3
1501-2500 g	32.8	31.8-33.8
Over 2500 g (and >36 weeks)	32.4	31.0-33.7
24-36 hours		
Under 1200 g	34.0	34.0-35.0
1200-1500 g	33.6	33.1-34.2
1501-2500 g	32.6	31.6-33.6
Over 2500 g (and >36 weeks)	32.1	30.7-33.5
36-48 hours		
Under 1200 g	34.0	34.0-35.0
1200-1500 g	33.5	33.0-34.1
1501-2500 g	32.5	31.4-33.5
Over 2500 g (and >36 weeks)	31.9	30.5-33.3
48-72 hours		
Under 1200 g	34.0	34.0-35.0
1200-1500 g	33.5	33.0-34.0
1501-2500 g	32.3	31.2-33.4
Over 2500 g (and >36 weeks)	31.7	30.1-33.2
72-96 hours		
Under 1200 g	34.0	34.0-35.0
1200-1500 g	33.5	33.0-34.0
1501-2500 g	32.2	31.1-33.2
Over 2500 g (and >36 weeks)	31.3	29.8-32.8

From American Academy of Pediatrics and American College of Obstetricians and Gynecologists: Guidelines for perinatal care, ed 2, Evanston, Ill, 1988, American Academy of Pediatrics and American College of Obstetricians and Gynecologists. Data from Scopes JW and Ahmed I: Minimal rates of oxygen consumption in sick and premature infants, Arch Dis Child 41:407, 1966; Scopes JW and Ahmed I: Range of critical temperatures in sick and premature newborn babies, Arch Dis Child:417, 1966. For their table, Scopes and Ahmed had the walls of the incubator 1° to 2° warmer than the ambient air temperatures. Generally speaking, the smaller infants in each weight group require a temperature in the higher portion of the temperature range. Within each time range, the younger the infant, the higher the temperature required.

TABLE 5-1—cont'd

Neutral Thermal Environmental Temperatures

AGE AND WEIGHT	STARTING TEMPERATURE (°C)	RANGE OF TEMPERATURE (°C)
4-12 days		
Under 1500 g	33.5	33.0-34.0
1501-2500 g	32.1	31.0-33.2
Over 2500 g (and >36 weeks)		
4-5 days	31.0	39.5-32.6
5-6 days	30.9	29.4-32.3
6-8 days	30.6	29.0-32.2
8-10 days	30.3	29.0-31.8
10-12 days	30.1	29.0-31.4
12-14 days		
Under 1500 g	33.5	32.6-34.0
1501-2500 g	32.1	31.0-33.2
2-3 weeks		
Under 1500 g	33.1	32.2-34.0
1501-2500 g	31.7	30.5-33.0
3-4 weeks		
Under 1500 g	32.6	31.6-33.6
1501-2500 g	31.4	30.0-32.7
4-5 weeks		
Under 1500 g	32.0	31.2-33.0
1501-2500 g	30.9	29.5-32.2
5-6 weeks		
Under 1500 g	31.4	30.6-32.3
1501-2500 g	30.4	29.0-31.8

room temperature is less than 27° C (80.6° F) and a single-walled incubator is being used.

Monitor temperature and maintain the tele-thermometer with the skin probe between 36° and 36.5° C (96.8° to 97.7° F) and axillary temperature between 36.5° and 37.5° C (97.7° to 99.5° F).

When cared for by experienced nurses, infants can be appropriately managed in incubators using skin temperature servocontrol, air temperature servocontrol, or manual adjustments.

By blocking avenues of heat loss through radiation, evaporation, convection, and conduction, the risks of cold stress can be minimized. Radiant heat loss represents the greatest loss of heat from the neonate. Heat radiates from the neonate to the incubator walls, which radiate heat to surrounding cooler objects, such as windows and walls in the room. Evaporative heat loss occurs from the skin and respiratory mucosa. Its greatest effect is in the delivery room before the infant's skin is dried. Wet linens and wet skin increase evaporative heat loss. Evaporative loss from the respiratory mucosa is dependent on the rate of ventilation and the humidity of the environment. Adequate humidity decreases evaporative losses. Conductive heat loss is generally minimal, since objects that usually touch the infant (clothing and bed linens) have poor conductance. Convective heat loss is caused by air currents. Air that is delivered to the infant can cause cold stress if it is too cool or

hyperthermia if it is too warm. Swaddling decreases heat losses from radiation, evaporation, and convection.

Controversy continues regarding the optimal method of maintaining appropriate heat balance in newborn infants. The use of radiant heaters, convectively heated incubators, conductive heat sources, and combinations of these have been studied. As with many treatment modalities in neonates, the benefits of one modality often require compromise of the benefit of another modality. The effects of changing many thermal variables have been discovered, but the best combinations for specific neonates is still not known. The primary advantage of radiant warmers is the easy access they give to neonates needing procedures, especially in the delivery room, and for initial admission to the nursery. Since warmth is maintained by pumping a large amount of infrared light energy into the infant's skin, wide swings in heat balance will occur when the operator's hands, head, or drapes block the heat source from the infant. A major disadvantage with radiant warmers is the increased insensible water loss necessitating meticulous monitoring of water balance and a 40% to 100% increase in the volume required. The oxygen consumption and cardiac output of infants nursed under radiant heaters are greater than those of infants nursed in incubators, but the clinical significance of this is unknown. Plastic blankets or shields can be used to effectively decrease evaporative and convective heat loss but must be moved to allow procedures, causing wide swings in environmental conditions. Radiant warmers must be servocontrolled to a set skin temperature, although the optimal skin temperature for control remains unknown. Incubators can be servocontrolled to skin or air temperature or may be manually set to a particular temperature.

Humidity can be supplemented to the environment within the incubator, thus reducing evaporative heat loss and insensible water loss. If, however, the skin is used for servocontrol, the metabolic rate is increased at both low and high humidity because of changes in the partition of heat loss. When neutral air temperature is maintained, relative humidity has little or no effect on the metabolic rate or total heat balance. Infants benefit from high humidity in subthermoneutral conditions because of the reduced net heat loss. Heat shields in incubators tend to decrease evaporative and radiant heat loss, but with skin servocontrol this is offset by an increased nonevaporative heat loss as the incubator cools in response to warmer skin. Likewise, when double-walled incubators are used with skin servocontrol, there is a decreased radiant heat loss but the air temperature requirement is also decreased, so that the net thermal balance is unchanged.

When the air temperature is servocontrolled and not disturbed, a double-walled incubator offers no advantage over a single-walled incubator, since the air temperature in the latter would increase to compensate for increased radiant heat loss. Double-walled incubators maintain a more steady temperature when exposed to a colder environment such as transport, or when the doors are opened for procedures.

In summary, much investigation remains to be done regarding the optimal methods of temperature control to minimize metabolic requirements for thermoregulation. Both incubators and radiant heaters are widely used, and both have a role in the care of the newborn. The skill and experience of nurses with each method will to some extent also influence which is better for a specific neonate. Other factors such as clothing and head covering, nursery temperature, and lighting also affect heat balance in particular instances and must also be considered. There may also be a role for conductive heat sources such as heating pads in both incubators and radiantly heated beds, although care must be taken to avoid thermal burns.

Radiant heat loss can be diminished primarily in two ways: (1) a heat shield or the inner wall of a double-walled incubator is warmed by the heated ambient air in the incubator; and (2) because the temperature gradient between the infant and this interposed surface is much less than the difference between the infant and the

cooler, outer incubator wall, the radiant heat lost by the infant is less.

The incubator should be kept away from cool influences such as air-conditioning ducts or cool windows, and the ambient nursery room temperature should be kept between at least 22.2° and 24.4° C (72° to 76° F). To decrease evaporative heat loss, every effort should be made to dry the infant's skin quickly after delivery and to keep it dry. Bed linens should be checked frequently and kept dry, and air and oxygen administered to the infant should be humidified (50%).

Cold examiner hands, scales, treatment tables, x-ray plates, and stethoscopes are good conductors and pose a risk of significant cold stress if allowed to contact the infant's skin. Drafts over an infant's body surface may be avoided by decreasing unnecessary opening of portholes, organizing care, placing open warmers away from drafts, and not blowing oxygen or air directly into the infant's face.

Oxygen and air administered to the neonate should be 32° to 36° C (90° to 97° F) at delivery, and not as it leaves the nebulizer, since cooling occurs in the tubes. Gases delivered directly by an ET tube should be warmed to 35° to 36° C (95° to 97° F). A thermometer in the Oxyhood measures the air temperature as it is delivered to the infant.

Swaddling materials include various types of infant wrappings from a warm blanket to clothing, and from foil to plastic, but using swaddling materials makes observing the infant more difficult and may block heat from the overhead radiant warmers. Check that infants are warmed before applying a foil wrap, because they cannot be readily warmed with radiant heat or warmed ambient air in an incubator, and the low temperature of the infant will be maintained in the foil.

DATA COLLECTION
History

The prenatal history and early neonatal evaluation are essential for the anticipation and prevention of problems, and clinical signs and symptoms can give early clues to thermal instability.

Review the prenatal history for the expected date of confinement (EDC), agents such as drugs, the possibility of congenital infection, and CNS depressants, such as analgesics or tranquilizers, that may blunt the infant's thermoregulatory response.

Evidence of perinatal asphyxia, such as the resuscitation required or the need for invasive procedures, indicates the stress endured and the baby's ability to respond. Ischemic injury to the CNS may cause a muted response to temperature stress. Preterm infants and term or postterm SGA infants are at the greatest risk for developing hypothermia. Exposure to infections in the perinatal period may include vaginal or cervical colonization, prolonged rupture of membranes, invasive resuscitative procedures, use of ventilator equipment, inadequate hand washing by nursery staff, or infectious nursery outbreaks such as necrotizing enterocolitis.

The temperature recorded must document not only the infant's axillary and skin temperature, but also environmental temperatures such as the ambient air temperature in an incubator or heat output from a radiant warmer. Temperature determinations should be made on a schedule, such as every 1 to 2 hours in low birth weight and sick neonates, every 2 to 3 hours during the neonatal transition period, and every 3 to 4 hours in healthy, term neonates.

Signs and symptoms

Hypothermic infants frequently feel cold to the touch. This may be a result of a decrease in "core" temperature or an early vasoconstrictive response to cold stress. Immediately check the temperature if the neonate's hands, feet, or trunk feel cold.

"Poor feeding" is common in infants with thermal instability and may manifest itself as poor sucking, decreased volume of food intake, increased gastric residuals, apathy toward feedings, abdominal distention, or vomiting.

An astute observer watches for the following minor behavioral changes:

- Poor feeding
- Increased or decreased spontaneous activity
- Weak cry
- Decreased muscle tone
- Difficult arousal with pleasant or unpleasant stimulus
- Irritability
- Lethargy

Since color change may be a clue to thermal instability, observe for the following symptoms:

- A bright red color present after the failure of oxyhemoglobin dissociation at low temperatures or overheating
- Cyanosis of the lips, extremities, mucous membranes, or central cyanosis
- Pallor

Thermal instability may cause apnea, bradycardia, or respiratory distress. Hyperthermic infants usually feel hot because of vasodilatory efforts to dissipate heat. Any neonate who feels hot to the touch should have his or her temperature checked immediately. Be alert for the following subtle behavioral changes:

- Poor feeding
- Increased or decreased activity
- Irritability
- Lethargy
- Hypotonia
- Weak or absent crying

Watch for (1) a bright red skin color after peripheral vasodilation and (2) sweating, which is limited in the newborn and absent before 32 weeks gestation.

Laboratory data

Laboratory data should evaluate metabolic derangements that are frequently associated with thermal instability. Suspect and test for the following disorders:

1. Metabolic acidosis (serum pH)
2. Hypoglycemia (blood glucose or Dextrostix)
3. Hyperkalemia (electrolytes)
4. Elevated blood urea nitrogen (BUN)

TREATMENT AND INTERVENTION
Hypothermia

Initiate corrective measures by supplying extra heat to the neonate. Rewarming too quickly, however, may be hazardous to the already compromised cold-stressed infant, and cause apnea. Oxygen consumption is minimal when the difference between the skin and the ambient air temperature is less than 1.5° C (35° F). Block avenues of heat loss, monitor temperatures, and search for and treat any underlying pathologic or iatrogenic causes of hypothermia.

If hypothermia is mild, slow rewarming is preferred. External heat sources should be set slightly warmer than the skin temperature and increased every 2 to 3 hours until the infant's temperature is within the neutral thermal range. Efforts to block radiant, convective, conductive, and evaporative heat loss should be made as described earlier. Skin, axillary, and incubator environmental temperatures should be measured and recorded every 30 minutes during the rewarming period.

Hyperthermia

The usual approach to treating the hyperthermic infant is to cool by removing external heat sources and by removing anything blocking heat loss while monitoring skin, deep body, and environmental temperatures.

A practical approach to cooling the hyperthermic infant includes (1) checking that the environmental temperature is appropriately set and functioning; (2) removing the crib or incubator from extra heat sources, such as sunlight, bilirubin lights, or heaters; and (3) removing blankets, swaddling, and swaddling materials. During stabilization, monitor and record axillary, skin, and environmental temperatures every 30 minutes. Nonenvironmental causes of hyperthermia, such as infection, dehydration, or disorders of the CNS should be considered.

CONSEQUENCES
Hypothermia

Hypoglycemia may result from an increased use of carbohydrate stores in an effort to maintain the "core" temperature. Vasoconstriction in an attempt to conserve heat may further necessitate anaerobic metabolism, which is already present because of increased oxygen demands to generate heat and decreased oxygen presented in the tissues. The resultant metabolic acidosis causes pulmonary vasoconstriction that further perpetuates the hypoxia-acidosis cycle, inhibits lecithin formation, and increases the severity of respiratory distress syndrome.

There may be an increased risk of kernicterus at lower bilirubin levels, since fatty acids from brown fat metabolism compete with bilirubin for binding sites on albumin. Albumin has a decreased affinity for bilirubin in the presence of acidosis, and brain mitochondrion has an increased attraction for bilirubin in the presence of acidosis.

The blood-brain barrier is also altered in the face of acidosis, increasing the risk for passage of bilirubin to brain tissue.

During the rewarming process in the treatment of hypothermia, several complications can arise, including hypotension from peripheral vasodilation associated with rewarming too rapidly. Seizures with rewarming may be the result of ischemic brain insult from low blood flow following peripheral vasodilation, although this consequence is not well understood.

Apnea may be caused by hypoxia or another unknown central mechanism. Dehydration can become a significant problem, since insensible water loss may increase by three to four times the hypothermic level when the baby is rewarmed.

Hyperthermia

Hypotension because of peripheral vasodilation may be seen in a heat-stressed infant. Seizure activity may be caused by "overheating" effects on the CNS, much like febrile convulsions. Apnea may be a complication of hyperthermia, and dehydration may develop as a result of the threefold to fourfold increase in insensible water loss with hyperthermia.

Hypothermia

During the rewarming process, complications should be observed by frequently checking vital signs and urine output and continuous cardiorespiratory monitoring. Volume expanders may be needed to maintain an adequate blood pressure.

Determination of the blood glucose level should be made every hour until the infant is stable. Dextrose in the form of intravenous 10% dextrose in water (IV $D_{10}W$) should be supplied if the serum glucose is less than 45 mg/dl. Observe for the following clinical signs and symptoms of hypoglycemia:

- Tremors or jitteriness
- Respiratory difficulty or apnea
- Lethargy
- Seizures
- Irritability

Arterial blood gases should be monitored closely, and every effort should be made to prevent hypoxia and acidosis. Serum bilirubin becomes a greater concern at lower levels, and phototherapy should be used more readily.

Hyperthermia

Evaluating skin turgor, mucous membrane moisture, urine output, arterial blood pressure, activity level, and body weight are satisfactory ways in which to clinically assess the degree of hydration. This should be suspected in hyperthermic infants, and blood pressure, urine output, and capillary filling should be monitored frequently. Volume expanders may be required to maintain an adequate blood pressure. Infants should be maintained with continuous cardiorespiratory monitoring, and resuscitative equipment should be kept at the baby's bedside. Seizure activity may be quite subtle in the neonate and may manifest itself as tremors, jitteriness, opisthotonus, hypotonia, chewing motions, "boxing" motions, apnea, or staring facial expressions. Seizure-control medication should be readily available for all hyperthermic infants, and the physician should be notified of any behavioral changes.

PARENT TEACHING

Stimulate parent-infant interaction by encouraging the parents to touch or hold their infant, but preserve the infant's thermal stability. Instruct the parents in the proper technique for taking the infant's temperature at home and for maintaining a comfortable environmental temperature for the infant.

Check the incubator and infant temperatures carefully when parents have the portholes open to touch the infant.

When the parents hold the infant outside the incubator, check the infant's temperature before removal from the incubator and monitor the temperature continuously with a telethermometer while the infant is outside the incubator. Keep the infant wrapped in warm blankets and provide extra heat with a portable radiant warmer if necessary. Demonstrate the proper temperature-taking technique and explain why only the axillary temperature is to be taken at home. A written instruction sheet should also be given to the parents.

Request that the parents demonstrate the proper technique for taking the neonate's temperature. Stress the "range of normal temperatures" concept. During the first 2 months a physician should be notified if the temperature is below 36° C (96.8° F) or above 37.8° C (100° F).

Generally a room temperature that is comfortable for the parents is desirable for the infant. The infant should be dressed in clothing suitable for the room temperature. Usually parents overheat the room or overdress the infant and cause heat stress. The parents should receive written instructions regarding a comfortable environment for infants.

CONCLUSION

The neonate's thermal balance is frequently precarious because of the tremendous flux of heat to and from the newborn. Meticulous attention to detail is most important in managing all the variables of neonatal thermoregulation, and care must be taken in extrapolating even satisfactory laboratory studies to the clinical setting. No one should attempt to care for neonates without a thorough understanding of heat balance and the functions of the equipment used to maintain that balance.

SELECTED READINGS

Agate FJ and Silverman WA: The control of body temperature in the small newborn infant by low energy infrared radiation, Pediatrics 31:725, 1963.

American Academy of Pediatrics and American College of Obstetricians and Gynecologists: Guidelines for perinatal care, ed 2, Evanston, Ill, 1988, American Academy of Pediatrics and American College of Obstetricians and Gynecologists.

At what temperature should you keep a baby? (editorial). Lancet 2:556, 1970.

Baumgart S: Reduction of oxygen consumption, insensible water loss, and radiant heat demand with use of a plastic blanket for low birth weight infants under radiant warmers, Pediatrics 74:1022, 1984.

Bell EF: Infant incubators and radiant warmers, Early Hum Dev 8:351, 1983.

Bell EF: Incubators v. radiant warmers: clinical perspective, AAMI Technology Assessment Report TAR No 9, 1984.

Bell EF and Rios G: Air versus skin temperature servocontrol of infant incubators, J Pediatr 103:954, 1983.

Bell EF and Rios G: A double-walled incubator alters the partition of body heat loss of premature infants, Pediatr Res 17:135, 1983.

Bell EF, Weinstein MR, and Oh W: Heat balance in premature infants: comparative effects of convectively heated incubator and radiant warmer, with and without plastic heat shield, J Pediatr 94:460, 1980.

Cone TE: History of the care and feeding of the premature infant, Boston, 1985, Little, Brown & Co.

Committee on Environment Hazards: Infant radiant warmers, Pediatrics 61:113, 1978.

Committee on Fetus and Newborn: Standards and recommendations for hospital care of newborn infants, ed 6, Evanston, Ill, 1977, American Academy of Pediatrics.

Day RL: Maintenance of body temperature of premature infants, Pediatrics 31:717, 1963.

Du JNH and Oliver TK: The baby in the delivery room, JAMA 207:1502, 1969.

Fanaroff AA and Martin RN: Neonatal-perinatal medicine, ed 4, St Louis, 1987, The CV Mosby Co.

Gandy GM et al: Thermal environment and acid-base homeostasis in human infants during the first few hours of life, J Clin Invest 43:751, 1964.

Hey EN: The relationship between environmental temperature and oxygen consumption in the newborn baby, J Physiol 200:589, 1969.

Hey EN and Katz G: The optimal thermal environment for naked babies, Arch Dis Child 45:328, 1970.

Hey EN and Mount LE: Heat losses from babies in incubators, Arch Dis Child 42:75, 1967.

Hey EN and O'Connell B: Oxygen consumption and heat balance in the cotnursed baby, Arch Dis Child 45:335, 1970.

Kanto WP and Calvert LJ: Thermoregulation of the newborn, Am Fam Physician 16:157, 1977.

Karlberg P: The significance of depth of insertion of the thermometer for recording rectal temperatures, Acta Paediatr 38:359, 1949.

Klaus MH and Fanaroff AA: Care of the high-risk neonate, ed 3, Philadelphia, 1986, WB Saunders Co.

LeBlanc MH: Relative efficacy of an incubator and an open warmer in producing thermoneutrality for the small premature infant, Pediatrics 69:439, 1982.

Marks KH, Nardis EE, and Momin M: Energy metabolism and substrate utilization in low birth weight neonates under radiant warmers, Pediatrics 78:456, 1986.

Marks KH et al: Thermal head wrap for infants, J Pediatr 107:956, 1985.

Mayfield SR et al: Temperature measurement in term and preterm neonates, J Pediatr 104:271, 1984.

Mayfield SR et al: Tympanic membrane temperature of term and preterm neonates, Early Hum Dev 9:241, 1984.

Merenstein GB: Rectal perforation by thermometer, Lancet 1:1007, 1970.

Pearlsten PH: Games with children, Pediatrics 61:666, 1978.

Rogers MC, Greenberg M, and Albert JJ: Cold injury of the newborn, N Engl J Med 285:332, 1971.

Scopes JW and Ahmed I: Range of critical temperature in sick and premature newborn babies, Arch Dis Child 41:417, 1966.

Silverman WA, Agate FJ, and Fertig JW: A sequential trial of the nonthermal effects of atmospheric humidity on survival of newborn infants of low birth weight, Pediatrics 31:719, 1963.

Silverman WA, Fertig JW, and Berger A: Influences of the thermal environment upon survival of newly born premature infants, Pediatrics 22:876, 1958.

Silverman WA and Sinclair JC: Temperature regulation in the newborn infant, N Engl J Med 274:92, 1966.

Sinclair JC: Thermal control in premature infants, Ann Rev Med 23:129, 1972.

Stephenson JM et al: The effect of cooling on blood gas tensions in newborn infants, J Pediatr 76:848, 1970.

Topper WH and Stewart TP: Thermal support for the very-low-birth-weight infant: role of supplemental conductive heat, J Pediatr 105:810, 1984.

Torrance JT: Temperature readings of premature infants, Nurs Res 17:312, 1978.

Walther FJ et al: Cardiovascular changes in preterm infants nursed under radiant warmers, Pediatrics 80:235, 1987.

Williams PR and Oh W: Effects of radiant warmers on insensible water loss in newborn infants, Am J Dis Child 128:511, 1974.

CHAPTER 6

Physiologic monitoring

JOHN R. PIERCE · BARBARA S. TURNER

Since the clinical usefulness of the umbilical vessels was first demonstrated by Diamond in 1947 when exchange transfusions were being performed to prevent kernicterus, many advances have taken place. In most nurseries it is a matter of routine to use the umbilical artery for monitoring blood gas status and arterial blood pressure. Because of the frequency and clinical significance of complications, alternatives to indwelling artery catheters have been sought vigorously. The development of transcutaneous oxygen monitoring has been a major step toward this goal.

The purpose of this chapter is to review the procedures for using indwelling umbilical catheters and to look at technical advances in physiologic monitoring.

PHYSIOLOGY
Pulmonary

Gas exchange takes place in the alveolus of the lung. Ventilation is the movement of air in and out of these air spaces. Diffusion is the movement of oxygen from the alveolar space into the pulmonary capillary and the movement of carbon dioxide from the pulmonary capillary into the alveolar space for eventual exhalation. Pulmonary perfusion is the flow of blood through the pulmonary capillaries that surround the alveolar spaces. Once oxygen diffuses through the alveolar lining cells and into the capillaries, it is bound to hemoglobin within the red blood cell.

□ The opinions and assertions in this chapter are those of the authors and do not necessarily represent those of the Department of the Army or the Department of Defense.

Oxygen content in the arterial blood is the sum of the amount of oxygen dissolved in the plasma and the amount bound to hemoglobin. Approximately 3% of the oxygen content is dissolved in the plasma, with the remaining 97% bound to hemoglobin. PaO_2 is the partial pressure of the oxygen dissolved in the plasma. Fetal hemoglobin has a higher affinity for oxygen than does adult hemoglobin; therefore at any given PaO_2 more oxygen is bound to fetal hemoglobin than is bound to adult hemoglobin (Figure 6-1). Oxygen saturation (SaO_2) is the percentage of oxygen bound to hemoglobin.

Transcutaneous blood gas monitoring

Oxygen normally diffuses from the skin capillaries through the dermis to the surface of the skin. To measure this amount of oxygen, it is necessary to heat the skin. Heating the skin has three effects:

1. Heating changes the lipid structure of the stratum corneum, allowing oxygen to diffuse through the skin faster.
2. Tissue and blood beneath the electrode are heated slightly, decreasing oxygen solubility and shifting the oxygen-hemoglobin dissociation curve to the right.
3. Heat dilates the local capillaries and arterializes the capillary blood.

Carbon dioxide diffuses through the skin in a manner similar to that of oxygen. Although carbon dioxide can be measured transcutaneously without heating the skin, the reading is more accurate if the skin is heated.

Noninvasive oxygen saturation monitoring relies on a pulsating arteriolar vascular bed between

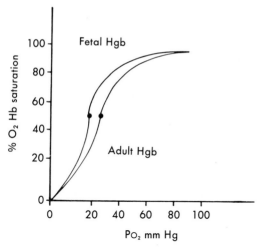

Figure 6-1. Oxygen dissociation curve for fetal hemoglobin (Hgb) (*left*) and adult hemoglobin (*right*).

a dual light source and a photoreceptor. As blood passes between the light source and the photoreceptor, different amounts of red and infrared light are absorbed, depending on the percentage of oxygen saturation. This difference in light absorption is electronically processed and displayed by the monitor as arterial hemoglobin oxygen saturation.

Cardiorespiratory monitoring

The electrical activity of the infant's heart is picked up by chest leads (usually three) placed on the infant and is recorded by the cardiorespiratory monitor. The recording is displayed on a visual screen as the infant's electrocardiographic pattern. The infant's respiratory pattern is also recorded, because the chest leads electronically detect movement of the infant's chest with each respiration.

Blood pressure monitoring

Systolic blood pressure (measured in millimeters of mercury) is the pressure at the height of the arterial pulse and coincides with left ventricular systole. Diastolic blood pressure (measured in millimeters of mercury) is the lowest point of the

arterial pulse and coincides with left ventricular diastole. Mean arterial pressure is the diastolic pressure plus one third the pulse pressure. Central venous pressure is the blood pressure in the right atrium and may be approximated by the blood pressure in any of the large central veins.

DATA COLLECTION

The indications for using the various techniques for physiologic data collection depend on the infant's clinical situation.

Umbilical artery catheters

An umbilical artery catheter is placed in those infants requiring frequent blood gas determinations. Infants who are candidates for indwelling catheters are those suffering from congenital heart disease or disorders that cause respiratory insufficiency, such as surfactant deficiency, meconium aspiration syndrome, persistent pulmonary hypertension, and diaphragmatic hernia. Although use of an indwelling umbilical artery catheter allows arterial pressure monitoring and accessibility for parenteral infusions, it is not acceptable to place an umbilical artery catheter for these indications alone.

Umbilical vein catheters

Umbilical vein catheters are used to deliver emergency fluids or chemicals in delivery room resuscitation. Exchange transfusions remove sensitized red blood cells and decrease serum bilirubin. Partial exchange transfusions are used in cases of polycythemia and hyperviscosity. Central venous pressure may also be monitored.

Noninvasive oxygen monitoring

Oxygen monitoring is indicated in the infant receiving oxygen for any reason. Acute monitoring is used in management of acute respiratory disorders. Chronic monitoring is used to wean infants with chronic lung disease from oxygen. During transportation of infants, noninvasive oxygen monitoring is useful. Carbon dioxide monitoring is useful in the infant with a respiratory disease in

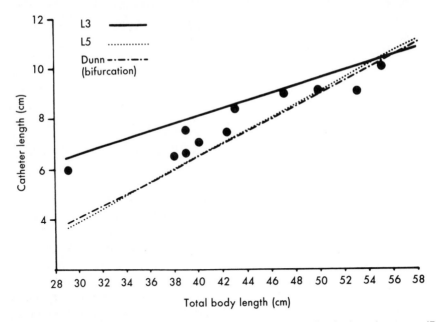

Figure 6-2. Graph for distance of catheter insertion from umbilical ring for low placement. (From Rosenfeld W et al: J Pediatr 96:735, 1980.)

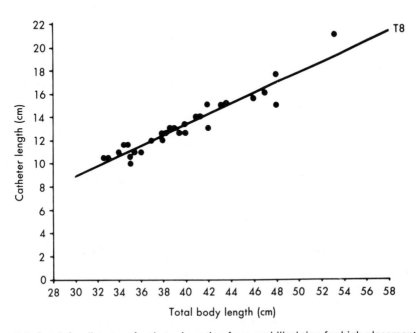

Figure 6-3. Graph for distance of catheter insertion from umbilical ring for high placement (T8). (From Rosenfeld W et al: J Pediatr 98:627, 1981.)

which retention of carbon dioxide may become clinically significant.

Cardiorespiratory monitoring

Cardiorespiratory monitoring should be used in any infant who requires intensive or intermediate care and in any infant at risk for apnea.

Blood pressure monitoring

Blood pressure monitoring should be used in the infant requiring surgery and in the infant acutely ill with cardiorespiratory distress or with any other illness in which hypotension may be a significant contributor to the pathologic state. Central venous pressure should be monitored in infants who potentially may experience an excess or loss of blood volume.

INTERVENTIONS
Umbilical artery catheters

Determine the size and length of the catheter to be inserted. For infants weighing more than 1250 g use a no. 5 Fr catheter, and for infants weighing less than 1250 g use a no. 3.5 Fr catheter. (Refer to Figures 6-2 and 6-3, which correlate total body length to the length of the catheter to be inserted.) Place the infant in a supine position on a radiant heater or in an incubator. Skin temperature should remain between 36° to 37° C (96.8° to 98.6° F). Provide appropriate oxygenation and ventilation. Restrain the infant's hands and feet. This prevents the infant from contaminating the sterile field and interfering with the placement procedure. Wash hands before and after the procedure. Put on a gown and globes. Open the catheterization tray. Catheterization tray contents are shown in Figures 6-4 and 6-5. Supplementary needs that are not shown are a tape measure, twelve 4- by 4-inch gauze pads, and two towel drapes. Prepare the catheter by flushing it with a flush solution. Prepare the cord and base of the umbilicus with povidone-iodine (Betadine) and then alcohol. Infants weighing less than 1000 g may experience iodophor skin burns; therefore an excess of povidone-iodine should be avoided

so that the infant is not lying in the solution during the procedure. Any residual iodophor should be carefully washed off the infant after the procedure is completed. Drape the infant by placing an eye sheet over the umbilicus. Use additional sterile drapes as necessary. Ensure that the infant's head and feet remain visible during the procedure to assess the infant's color. A small eye drape with adhesive backing (Steri-Drape) has the advantage of being transparent so that the infant's color can be seen and temperature maintained. Towel drapes may interfere with a radiant heat source used for temperature regulation.

Since the tie will be left in place, umbilical tape should be tied around the base of the cord to ensure that the tape is not around skin. The tape is used to control bleeding. A single overhand knot that allows tightening as needed is preferred. Using tissue forceps, pick up the cord and cut it with a scalpel about 1 to 1.5 cm above the base. Arterial spasm allows only minimal bleeding. Identify the vessels. There are usually two arteries and one vein. The arteries are small, thick-walled, and constricted. The vein is larger, thin-walled, and usually gaping open. If the vein is at the 12 o'clock position, the arteries are usually at the 4 and 8 o'clock positions (Figure 6-6). Stabilize the umbilical stump by grasping the cord between the thumb and index finger or grasping the edge of the stump with a mosquito hemostat. Ensure that the hemostat does not crush the umbilical vessels. With iris forceps dilate one of the arteries by placing the tips of the forceps in the artery and gently allowing them to spring open. This procedure may need to be repeated several times. While grasping one side of the wall of the dilated artery, gently insert the catheter or insert the catheter between the open prongs of the forceps, dilating the artery. Instructional aids such as Baby Umbi° and the Umbilical Ar-

°Medical Plastics Laboratory, Inc., P.O. Box 38, Gatesville, Tex. 76528.

tery Catheterization Slide-Tape Neonatal Educational Program° are helpful. As the catheter passes into the artery, resistance may be met at several different points:

1. At the umbilical tape—The tape may be tied too tightly. Loosen slightly.

°Charles R. Drew Postgraduate Medical School, 1621 E. 120th Street, Los Angeles, Calif. 90059.

2. At the point where the umbilical artery turns downward (caudal) into the abdomen—Steady gentle pressure is important, since forceful pressure may cause the catheter to perforate the artery wall and create a false channel.

3. At the point where the umbilical artery joins the external iliac artery—Once again, steady gentle pressure is important.

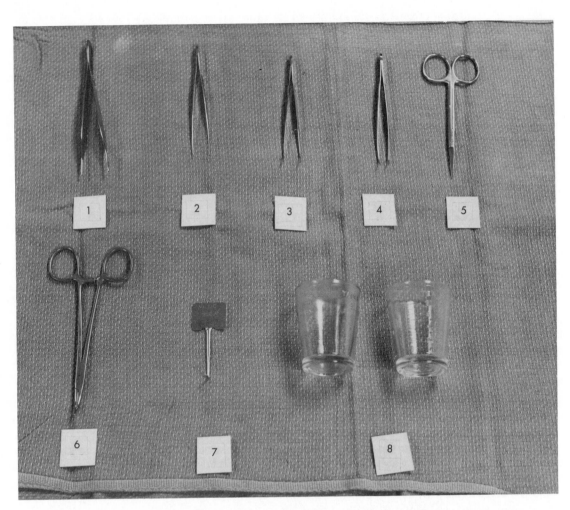

Figure 6-4. Mini umbilical vessel catheterization tray. *1,* Adson's tissue forceps; *2,* straight iris forceps without teeth; *3,* half-curved forceps with teeth; *4,* full-curved forceps without teeth; *5,* iris scissors; *6,* curved mosquito clamp; *7,* vein flag; *8,* two containers for antiseptic.

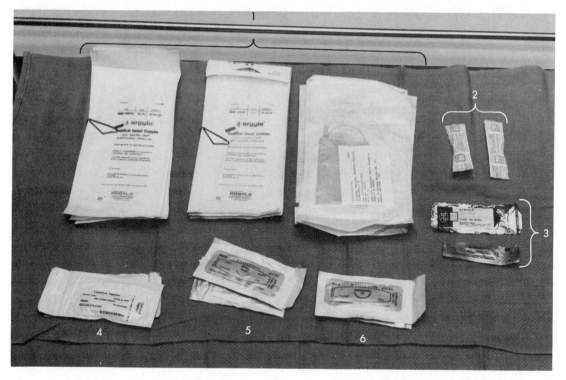

Figure 6-5. Supplemental sterile equipment for umbilical vessel catheterization. *1,* Umbilical vessel catheters, sizes 3.5, 5, and 8 Fr; *2,* Luer stub adapters, 18- and 20-gauge; *3,* knife blades, sizes 15 and 20; *4,* umbilical ligature; *5,* silk suture on curved needle; *6,* chromic suture on curved needle.

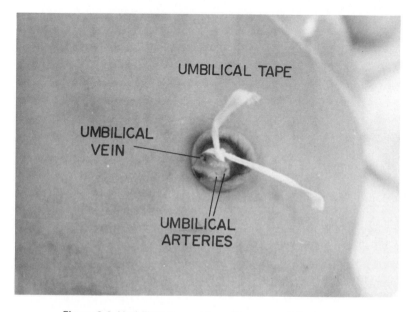

Figure 6-6. Umbilical tape and position on umbilical vessels.

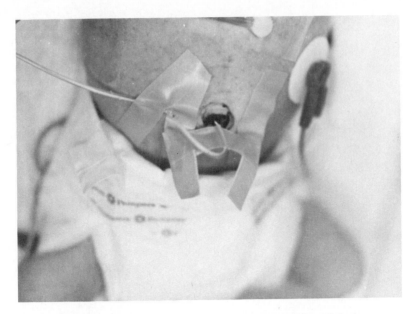

Figure 6-7. Umbilical artery catheter secured in "goalpost" design.

Insert the catheter to the predetermined length. Aspiration on the syringe should provide immediate blood return. Lack of blood return may indicate that:

1. The catheter is not inserted far enough. Insert farther.
2. The vessel wall has been perforated, or a false channel has been created. If the catheter has pierced through the vessel wall, repeat the procedure using the other artery.
3. The catheter is kinked. Pull back slightly and then advance.
4. The stopcock is turned off. Correct the stopcock position. Return aspirated blood to the infant and flush until the catheter clears.

Observe the feet, legs, and buttocks of the infant for signs of vascular compromise. If any blanching or blueness occurs, follow the steps outlined under complications. Secure the catheter by making a "goalpost," using benzoin on the skin (Figure 6-7). Properly secured by the "goalpost" taping method, the catheter is secure, and foreign bodies such as sutures are avoided. (Many centers, however, use sutures to secure the catheter.) Connect the stopcock to the intravenous (IV) solution and set an appropriate infusion rate. Ensure that no air is in the tubing, stopcock, or catheter. All connections must be secure. A tongue blade may be used to stabilize and secure this connection. Automatic infusion pumps must be used for umbilical artery catheters. Determine catheter placement by an abdominal x-ray examination. Figure 6-8 shows how the umbilical artery catheter will appear on lateral x-ray film. Note that the catheter enters the umbilicus and travels inferiorly before turning superiorly. This "leg loop" is characteristic of an arterial catheter. Optimal placement is L3-4 for a low catheter and T8 for a high catheter. Figure 6-9 shows high catheter placement, and Figure 6-10 shows low catheter placement. If the catheter is

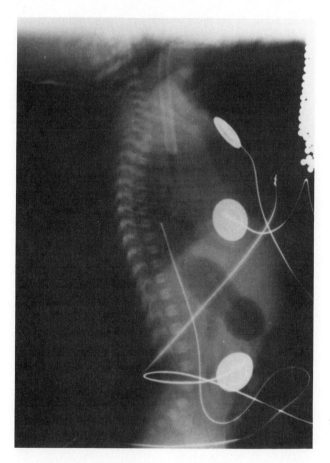

Figure 6-8. High catheter demonstrating "leg loop."

too high, measure on the x-ray film the distance from the tip of the catheter to the desired level and pull the catheter back the appropriate distance. Some clinicians multiply this length times 0.8 to account for radiographic magnification. If the catheter is placed too low, the catheter cannot be advanced but must be removed because the external portion of the catheter is no longer sterile.

TEACHING MODEL

The umbilical cord can be used for teaching the procedure of both arterial and venous catheter-

ization. Many of the steps can be effectively carried out using a fresh placenta.

Special umbilical artery catheters and monitors are available for continuous Po_2 and/or oxygen saturation monitoring.

NURSING CARE AND USE OF UMBILICAL ARTERY CATHETERS

Infants can be positioned on their sides or their backs. The abdominal position is avoided, since accidental slipping, kinking, and removal of the catheter may occur without being immediately apparent. Care needs to be taken that the in-

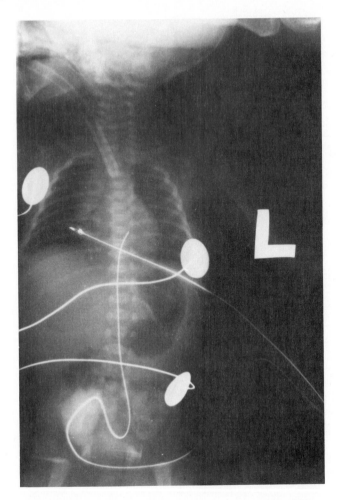

Figure 6-9. Umbilical artery catheter in high position (T8).

fant is adequately restrained so that the catheter cannot be accidentally removed. Soft wrist restraints that restrict the range of movement will prevent the infant's fingers from grasping the catheter or connections. Diapers are an effective mechanism for preventing the feet and toes from becoming entangled in the catheter. The diaper is folded below the umbilicus. If the infant is receiving phototherapy and thus not diapered, leg restraints may be indicated. A dressing over the umbilicus is unnecessary.

Dressings inhibit inspection of the umbilicus and evaluation of the catheter. The IV tubing, connecting tubing, and stopcock should be changed daily. Clots form in the stopcock, so changing it daily prevents the likelihood of emboli forming. Blood backing into the catheter can be caused by:

1. Increased intraabdominal pressure commonly caused by the infant crying vigorously
2. Disconnection of tubing

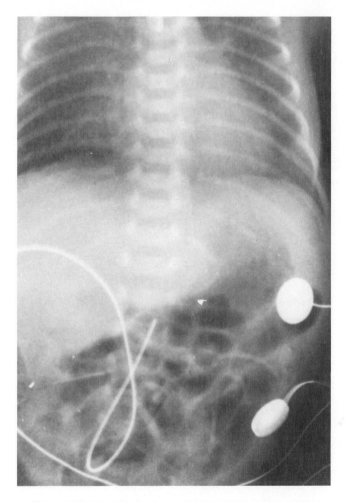

Figure 6-10. Umbilical artery catheter in low position (L3).

3. Stopcock turned in wrong direction
4. Infusion pump malfunction
5. Leak in filter or tubing

The procedure for drawing blood gases from an umbilical catheter must be kept sterile. It requires one person and three syringes: one dry, one with heparin, and one filled with flush solution. Syringes are used for aspirating fluid and blood from the line, collecting blood gas samples, and flushing the line.

PROCEDURE FOR DRAWING BLOOD GAS

Turn the stopcock so that the IV solution stops flowing. Aspirate 1 to 2 ml from the catheter into the dry syringe (Figure 6-11). The IV fluid is prevented from infusing, and aspiration clears the catheter of its IV fluid. Turn the stopcock to the neutral position (Figure 6-12), remove the syringe, and replace it with the heparinized syringe. The neutral position of the stopcock prevents contaminating the sam-

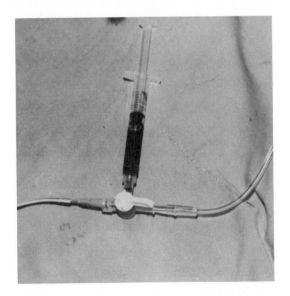

Figure 6-11. Stopcock off to IV solution; 1 to 2 ml aspirated into syringe.

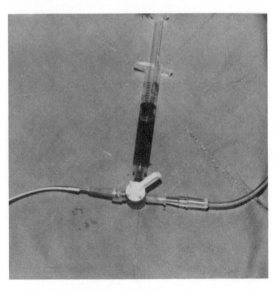

Figure 6-12. Stopcock in neutral position.

ple with IV fluid and prevents blood loss from the infant. CAUTION: Never allow blood to drip from an open stopcock. Using steady, even pressure, aspirate blood into the heparinized syringe. Turn the stopcock to the neutral position and remove the syringe (Figure 6-13). Remove the air from the syringe, cap the end, and chill it to preserve values. Usually 0.2 to 1 ml of blood is needed, depending on the laboratory requirements. Replace the syringe that has the aspirated blood in it with the syringe filled with flush solution. Turn off the stopcock to the IV. Slightly aspirate to remove any air in the stopcock and slowly insert it. After infusing the flush solution, return the stopcock to the neutral position. Record the amount of blood removed from the infant. Replace the syringe filled with flush solution with a clean, dry syringe. Turn the stopcock so that the IV can be infused.

To ensure the integrity of all connections, the stopcock and other connections must be visible at all times. Do not place the stopcock and other connections under linen, because this would hamper the immediate detection of an accidental disconnection that would cause severe blood loss in the infant. Immediately remove any air in the tubing or catheter, because air is a potential embolus. It is best removed through the stopcock. If the air has passed the stopcock, it can be easily aspirated back into a syringe.

Umbilical vein catheter placement procedure

A no. 5 Fr catheter is normally used in the umbilical vein catheter placement procedure. To determine the length of the catheter to be inserted, the distance from the umbilicus to the sternal notch should be measured and multiplied by 0.6. Complete steps for the placement procedure are found in this chapter's section on umbilical artery catheters. The only difference is that the vein is used instead of the artery up to the point of stabilizing the cord. The vein is usually gaping open and does not require dila-

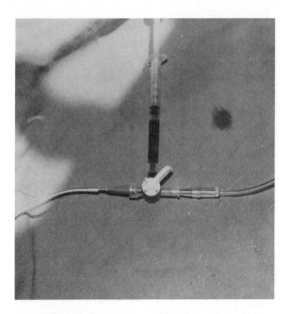

Figure 6-13. After blood is aspirated into heparinized 1 ml syringe, stopcock is placed in neutral position before syringe is removed.

tion. The catheter can be easily advanced to the desired position. The catheter should lie in the inferior vena cava that is above the diaphragm but below the heart on x-ray film. Umbilical vein catheters do not have the "leg loop" found on the lateral x-ray film of the umbilical artery catheters. The catheter should be taped in the same manner as an umbilical artery catheter.

Transcutaneous oxygen/carbon dioxide monitoring

Skin oxygen tension ($TcPO_2$) and carbon dioxide tension ($TcPCO_2$) are measured by using one or two electrodes, depending on the model and brand of the monitor. The electrode(s), once positioned on the skin, heat the area under the probe and cause certain physiologic changes as previously discussed. Oxygen and carbon dioxide that diffuse through the heated skin are measured by the electrode, and the value is

digitally displayed on the monitor. Many models have strip chart recorders that allow continuous tracings of the infant's values. If intervals between calibration are longer than 4 hours, the readings are subject to drift. $TcPO_2$ monitors are calibrated to barometric pressure. $TcPCO_2$ monitors require calibration to high and low carbon dioxide gas concentrations. The calibration procedures vary with the instruments used. Inherent in the calibration process is the necessity to change the position of the skin electrode on the infant. At the time of each calibration the membrane should be checked for wrinkles, air bubbles under the membrane, and the presence of foreign bodies, all of which can be a source of error in the transcutaneous readings. In the clinical setting the correlation of the $TcPO_2$ and PaO_2 has been reported to vary from $r = .84$ to as low as $r = .16$. Better correlations are found when the instrument is calibrated every 4 hours and the temperature is set correctly. If the temperature of the probe cannot be maintained at 43° to 44° C, a lower temperature should be selected to avoid possible burns. At a lower temperature the $TcPO_2$ monitor can be used to monitor trends but should not be interpreted as actual arterial PaO_2 values. The transcutaneous monitors may underestimate the PaO_2 when the infant is hypoxemic, when the infant is poorly perfused or in shock, and when the patient is beyond the neonatal period.

Clinical use of transcutaneous blood gas monitors includes rapid and continuous determination of the best oxygen concentration and/or ventilator settings for a critically ill newborn, clinical management of infants with chronic lung disease, and determination of right-to-left shunting through a patent ductus arteriosus. In an infant with suspected significant right-to-left shunting through a patent ductus arteriosus such as persistent pulmonary hypertension, two transcutaneous electrodes can be placed on the infant: one preductally (right shoulder) and the other postductally (lower abdomen or legs).

Significant right-to-left shunting through the patent ductus arteriosus is present when the preductal oxygen tension is significantly higher than the postductal oxygen tension.

When comparing the arterial PO_2 readings with $TcPO_2$ readings, both values must be obtained from either above or below the ductus arteriosus for valid comparisons. If a goal of therapy is to prevent hyperoxia to the eyes, then the $TcPO_2$ monitor should be routinely placed above the ductus until it is proved that the ductus has closed.

The disadvantages to the use of transcutaneous monitoring are that the instrument requires frequent calibration, requires the use of a heated electrode, requires a 15-minute period after calibration to heat the skin to the correct temperature, and has a 15- to 20-second delay in the readings as compared with the patient's real time values. The advantages are that it is not invasive, does not require the removal of blood for analysis, and displays a continuous readout of skin oxygen/carbon dioxide tensions.

NURSING CARE OF INFANTS WITH TRANSCUTANEOUS MONITORS

The electrode can be placed on any portion of the infant's body as long as good contact between the electrode and the skin is maintained. Uneven areas of skin such as skin over bones should be avoided because of poor contact between the membrane and the skin surface. The infant should not lie on the electrode. Placing the infant on top of the electrode increases the pressure on the underlying capillaries, thus affecting the flow of blood under the probe and resulting in a drop in $TcPO_2$ values. Because of the heat generated by the electrode (43° to 44° C), small red areas are produced on the infant's skin. To minimize trauma to the infant's skin, the electrode should be repositioned every 2 to 4 hours depending on the infant's skin sensitivity. Activities that produce a rise or fall in the transcutaneous oxygen should be noted and incorporated into the nursing plan for the infant. Such procedures as positioning (right versus left), suctioning, postural draining, handling, blood sampling, and nonnutritive sucking may have an effect on the readings. Grouping of nursing interventions has resulted in minimizing the time that the infant receives less than optimal oxygenation.

Oxygen saturation monitoring

Oxygen saturation is monitored by placing a small sensor on the infant in such a manner that the infant's finger, toe, foot, or wrist comes between the light source and the photoreceptor. The light source and receptor must be directly opposite each other to have a pulse detected.

The monitor does not require any heat source or warm-up period; nor does it require calibration or changing of the probe position. Oxygen saturation monitoring provides the care provider with continuous and instantaneous readout of the oxygen saturation of the infant. In comparison with a blood gas analyzer, which calculates the relative oxygen saturation based on established nomograms, the oxygen saturation monitor measures the actual saturation of the hemoglobin. Calculated values using standard nomograms do not reflect shifts in the affinity of oxygen for hemoglobin based on changes in the patient's temperature, pH, PCO_2, or 2,3-DPG.

The oxygen saturation monitor relies on adequate perfusion to the site and the ability to detect arterial pulsations; thus if it is placed distal to a blood pressure cuff, there will be an inaccurate reading while the cuff is inflated. There may be incorrect readings when the probe is placed under or near infrared heat lamps and under phototherapy lamps. The light from these external sources interferes with the light receptor on the infant's extremity. Newer neonatal probes have built-in external light source protectors that are not found on adult probes.

Oxygen saturation is more indicative of the total oxygen content of the blood than is PaO_2 and is the most sensitive to hypoxemia when it is on the steep part of the oxygen dissociation curve (see Figure 6-1). Keeping the SaO$_2$ at 90% to 92% will keep the infant in a normoxemic state under most conditions.

There are no complications associated with the use of oxygen saturation monitoring other than the potential for skin trauma due to the adhesive on the probe. Newer probes, held in position by gentle elastic pressure, have no adhesive touching the infant's skin.

Cardiorespiratory monitoring

The chest leads are applied in a triangular pattern on the infant's chest. Integrity of the leads must be ensured. Allowing the contact gel to dry or inadvertently dislodging the lead during procedures such as x-ray examination, echocardiography, and lumbar puncture may account for inaccurate tracings. Various components of the electrocardiogram (ECG) pattern may be diagnostically helpful. The QRS complex should be monitored for baseline height. A sudden decrease in QRS complex height that is not caused by artifact may be an indication of pneumothorax. The QT interval is helpful in diagnosing hypocalcemia in some infants. Other portions of the strip may be evaluated for electrolyte imbalance and possible cardiac ischemia. Changes registered on the visual display or strip recorder should be verified by a 12-lead ECG.

Blood pressure monitoring

Arterial pressure monitoring may be accomplished via the umbilical artery catheter attached to a transducer and monitor. Newer transducers require calibration only once daily. Central venous pressure monitoring may be carried out in the same manner. The same transducers may be used for either arterial or venous pressure recording.

COMPLICATIONS

Umbilical artery catheters act as foreign bodies, causing fibrin deposition and thrombus formation around the catheter. Although most catheters are associated with thrombus formation, it is of clinical significance in less than 10% of patients. The most common problem associated with major complications of umbilical artery catheters is ischemic disease resulting from emboli or spasms. In such cases the catheter should be removed immediately and heparin therapy considered. Although vasospasm is quite common, usually it does not require immediate removal of the catheter. Blue discoloration is seen rather than blanching. Obviously a hemorrhage may occur when the catheter slips out or when any of the various connections loosen. For reasons such as these, umbilical artery catheters require constant attention.

Umbilical vein catheters may cause thrombi. Clots may form in the portal vessels, resulting in portal hypertension. Hepatic necrosis, gut ischemia, and hemorrhage have been associated with umbilical vein catheters.

Transcutaneous blood gas monitoring may cause burns to the skin.

If the extremities or buttocks blanch, the catheter should be removed immediately and heparin therapy considered. To prevent bleeding once the catheter is removed, pressure should be applied immediately below the umbilicus. When the color has returned to the affected area and the infant is stable, replacement of the catheter can be considered. If vasospasm occurs in one leg or foot, apply warm wraps (diapers wet with warm water) to the opposite leg or apply wraps to the upper extremities, thereby producing a reflex vasodilation to the legs. Inherent in this action, though, is the hazard of obscuring recognition of compromise in that extremity. The wraps need to be reheated every 10 to 15 minutes until the spasm has resolved. The skin temperature of the infant must be greater than 36° C for wraps to be effective. Infants with umbilical artery catheters need blood available for immediate transfusion.

CONTROVERSIES

Complications involving high catheter placement (T8) are fewer but more severe than the complications involving low catheter placement

(L3-4). Prophylactic antibiotic agents are not indicated. Use of the umbilical artery catheter for infusion of antibiotic agents, calcium, hyperalimentation solutions, or blood varies, and no definite studies are available. Blood cultures drawn from the umbilical artery catheter are accurate for 6 hours after insertion. The use of heparin in the infusate is controversial. Practices vary widely, and definite studies are lacking; however, it appears safe to feed infants enterally with an umbilical artery catheter in place. Routine monitoring on all infants is the standard of care. Indwelling catheters for blood pressure monitoring have the advantage of continuous readout, but external cuffs are less invasive.

PARENT AND FAMILY TEACHING

As for the many other invasive procedures in neonatology, permission is obtained from the parents for umbilical vessel catheterization. This may be the clinician's first contact with the family and thus sets the atmosphere for future contacts. Although parents are initially hesitant about umbilical catheter placement, they are generally comforted to learn that it will result in a painless way of drawing blood. Before visiting the infant, parents need to be told what the umbilical catheter, transcutaneous monitors, cardiorespiratory monitors, and blood pressure monitors look like in place and what they are registering. Often parents are confused as to where the catheter goes once it enters the umbilicus and what the purpose of other monitoring devices is. Some parents are uncomfortable with the arm and leg restraints on their infant. It may be unwise for parents to hold their infant while an umbilical catheter is in place because manipulating the infant may accidentally dislodge the catheter, and subsequently the infant may lose blood. Also, when the infant is being held out of the incubator and is wrapped in blankets, the integrity of the catheter and connections cannot be evaluated.

SUMMARY

Physiologic monitors and their applications to neonatal intensive care have been an unchallenged success in the management of the sick neonate. Despite all the benefits, there remain risks that have implications for the infant, the family, and all health care providers.

SELECTED READINGS

Boyle R and Oh W: Erythema following transcutaneous pO_2 monitoring, Pediatrics 65:333, 1980.

Henrickson P, Wesstrom G, and Hedner U: Umbilical artery catheterization in newborns, Acta Paediatr Scand 68:719, 1979.

Jennis MS and Peabody JL: Pulse oximetry: an alternative for the assessment of oxygenation in newborn infants, Pediatrics 79:524, 1987.

Kitterman JA, Phibbs RH, and Tooley WH: Catheterization of umbilical vessels in newborn infants, Pediatr Clin North Am 17:895, 1970.

Long JG, Philip AGS, and Lucey JF: Excessive handling as a cause of hypoxemia, Pediatrics 65:203, 1980.

Morohisky ST et al: Low positioning of umbilical artery catheters increases associated complications in newborn infants, N Engl J Med 299:561, 1978.

Rome ES et al: Limitations of transcutaneous Po_2 and Pco_2 monitoring in infants with bronchopulmonary dysplasia, Pediatrics 74:217, 1984.

Rooth G, Hych A, and Huch R: Transcutaneous oxygen monitors are reliable indicators of arterial oxygen tension (if used correctly), Pediatrics 79:283, 1987.

Rosenfeld W et al: A new graph for insertion of umbilical artery catheters, J Pediatr 96:735, 1980.

Rosenfeld W et al: Evaluation of graphs for insertion of umbilical artery catheters below the diaphragm, J Pediatr 98:627, 1981.

Speidel BD: Adverse effects of routine procedures on preterm infants, Lancet 1:864, 1978.

Stairs RL and Krauss AN: Complications of neonatal intensive care, Clin Perinatol 7:107, 1980.

Symansky MR and Fox HA: Umbilical vessel catheterization: indications, management and evaluation of technique, J Pediatr 80:820, 1972.

Wesstrom G and Finnstrom O: Umbilical artery catheterization in newborns: infections in relation to catheterization, Acta Paediatr Scand 68:713, 1979.

Wesstrom G, Finnstrom O, and Stenport G: Umbilical artery catheterization in newborns: thrombosis in relation to catheter type and position, Acta Paediatr Scand 68:575, 1979.

CHAPTER 7

Pharmacology in neonatal care

M. GAIL MURPHY · BARBARA S. TURNER

Individual infants given an identical dosage regimen of a drug exhibit a variety of clinical responses. There are many factors that influence either the intensity or the duration of a drug's effect. In some cases measurable characteristics that relate to the aging process (i.e., changes in maturation of the liver and kidney or changes in body weight and composition) result in predictable changes in drug disposition. Since much drug variability remains unexplained, it is increasingly important to monitor adequately for both desirable and toxic effects.

PHYSIOLOGY

Neonates show dramatic differences in the way they respond to drugs as compared with older children and adults. Variability in the dose-response relationship is attributed to differences in "what the body does to the drug" (*pharmacokinetics*) or "what the drug does to the body" (*pharmacodynamics*) (Figure 7-1). Pharmacokinetics is the study of drug disposition (i.e., an overview of a drug's concentration in the body over time). *Disposition* can be classified into four processes: *drug entry* (absorption), *distribution, biotransformation,* and *elimination*. Pharmacodynamics refers to the study of the relationship between drug concentration and drug effect. Recognition of the essential role of drug concentration in linking

---

☐ The opinions and assertions in this chapter are those of the authors and do not necessarily represent those of the Department of the Army or the Department of Defense.

dose to response enables an understanding of potential causes of variability in the dose-response relationship. The apparent increase in response, reflected in the statement, "Infants are more sensitive to the effects of drugs," might be attributed to differences in pharmacokinetics or pharmacodynamics.

The drug-receptor theory is the unifying principle of drug therapy. At the site of action of a drug, the time course of drug concentration at the receptor strongly influences the time course of drug effect. Unfortunately, most drug receptors are in tissues that are clinically inaccessible for routine monitoring. For many commonly used drugs, after an initial short distribution phase, the rate of change of the plasma drug concentrations will parallel the rate of change of the drug concentration at the receptor (Figure 7-2). This is the least complex model of drug movement in the body. Dose design and modification with drugs that follow this model are expressed mathematically in a straightforward fashion with disposition parameters, such as clearance, volume of distribution, and half-life, and can be solved with a four-function calculator.

Initially the clinician's choice of a dose regimen is based on data relating the dose with the incidence of therapeutic response and toxic effect in the average patient. When therapeutic drug monitoring is appropriate, a similar choice is made for the target plasma concentration at steady state (Css). During maintenance therapy, steady state occurs when the input of a

ABBREVIATIONS

C	Drug concentration (plasma or serum)	mg/L
Css	Steady state concentration (average)	mg/L
MEC	Minimum effective concentration	mg/L
MSC	Maximum safe concentration	mg/L
F	Extent of drug availability (0 to 1); how much active drug gets to the systemic circulation	unitless
V	Volume of distribution; relates to loading dose	L/kg
Cl	Clearance; relates to maintenance dose	L/kg/hr
$t_{1/2}$	Drug elimination half-life; relates to the time course of changes in drug concentration	hours

NOTE: L = liter = 1000 milliliters
      mg = milligram = 1000 micrograms

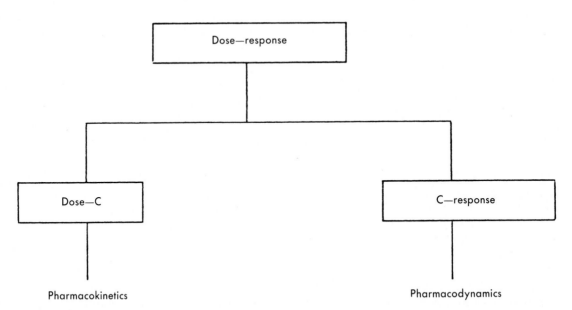

Figure 7-1. Variability in dose-response relationship can be due to differences in pharmacokinetics or pharmacodynamics. *C,* Drug concentration (plasma or serum).

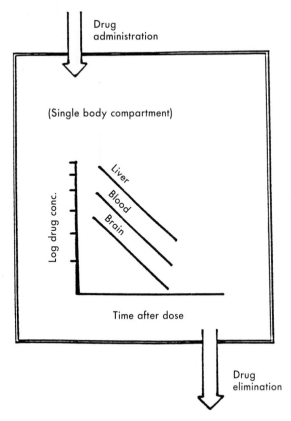

Drug
administration

(Single body compartment)

Log drug conc.

Liver

Blood

Brain

Time after dose

Drug
elimination

Figure 7-2. Representation of single-compartment drug disappearance curves. (From Roberts RJ: Principles of neonatal pharmacology. In Avery ME and Taeusch HW Jr, editors: Schaffer's diseases of the newborn, ed 5, Philadelphia, 1983, WB Saunders Co.)

drug equals the elimination of the drug from the body. During this period a constant average plasma concentration (Css) is achieved with some variability around this value, which depends on the dose, dose interval, and drug disposition. As illustrated in Figure 7-3, the minimum effective concentration (MEC) is the concentration (C) at which 50% of patients exhibit the desired response. The maximum safe concentration (MSC) is the C at which 50% of patients exhibit a toxic response. Although concentrations below the MEC are less likely to

result in the desired effect, in some patients they are associated with therapeutic benefit.

The choice of Css is partly determined by the sensitivity at the drug receptor. Developmental differences in number and function of drug receptors may be critical for drug action. An example of the effects of aging on pharmacodynamics is the diminished sensitivity of the cardiovascular system to digitalis, which is associated with a decreased number of receptor sites in the newborn myocardium.

The choice of Css is also determined by the fraction of drug bound to plasma proteins. The goal of drug therapy is to achieve and maintain a free drug concentration at the site of action of the drug that will produce the maximum desired effect with a minimal risk of toxicity. However, the concentration that is measured is usually the total drug concentration in the serum, the sum of bound and free drug. The degree of plasma protein binding (which is often different in pediatric patients, especially newborns) will influence the relationship of total concentration measured to concentration at the active site.

The reported therapeutic range for theophylline in adults is 10 to 20 μg/ml versus a reported therapeutic range in neonates of 4 to 12 μg/ml. Theophylline is reported to be 36% bound to plasma protein at a concentration of 8 μg/ml in newborns as compared with 70% bound in adults. A measured concentration in the serum of 10 μg/ml in an adult would be expected to be 7 μg/ml bound theophylline and 3 μg/ml free theophylline, whereas in the neonate a total concentration of 4.7 μg/ml consists of 1.7 μg/ml bound theophylline and 3 μg/ml free theophylline. When the lower plasma binding is taken into consideration, the unbound effective concentration in neonates and adults is the same. The decreased binding of theophylline to plasma proteins in neonates could be one explanation why therapeutic effect is achieved with lower total serum concentration of theophylline in newborns than in adults. An alternative explanation for the apparent difference in

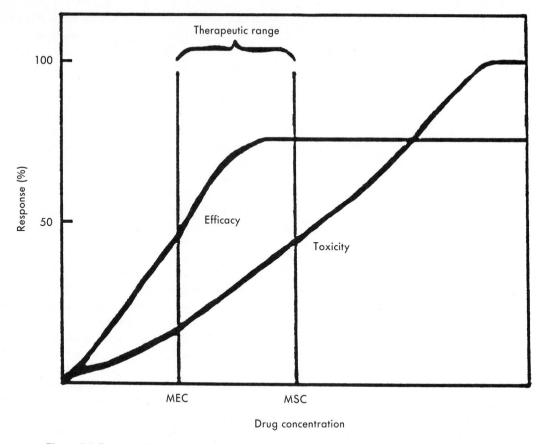

Figure 7-3. Percent of patients with desired and toxic responses as a function of drug concentration. Therapeutic range is bounded by minimum effective and maximum safe concentrations.

theophylline effect is that theophylline is metabolized to an active compound, caffeine, in newborns but not in adults.

With these age-related changes, a new target concentration or a new way of monitoring drug response is required. However, many age-related changes are a result of changes in disposition processes. Stated alternatively, age-related changes are more likely to be the result of different concentrations reaching the site of action. With most pharmacokinetic changes the target plasma concentration remains the same, and the dose or dose interval is adjusted to account for changes in drug disposition. Disposition processes that influence most age-dependent changes in drug response are described in the following paragraphs.

Absorption

The process of absorption determines the rate and the absolute amount of drug entering the bloodstream. The parameter F varies between 0 and 1; $F = 1$ indicates that the extent of availability of that drug to the systemic circulation is 100%.

No systematic studies of absorption of different drugs in sick newborns have been published. Such studies are needed because a variety of differences in absorptive processes are anticipated between newborns and older patients and between well and critically ill newborns. Differences in newborns potentially affecting oral bioavailability include developmental changes in surface area and permeability of gastrointestinal mucosa, age-dependent changes in acid secretion in the stomach, and changes in total gastrointestinal transit time and in gastric emptying time.

Distribution

The volume of distribution of a drug is a useful but theoretical parameter that relates the total amount of drug in the body to the serum or plasma concentration. It may be used to estimate the size of a loading dose or a change in plasma concentration with a given loading dose:

$$\text{Loading dose} \times F = \text{Change in C} \times V$$
$$\text{Change in C} = F \times \text{Loading dose}/V$$

Volume of distribution is usually expressed as a function of body weight, with units of volume per kilogram. Major factors that affect distribution volume are plasma protein binding and body composition. Changes in body composition occur throughout fetal and newborn life. Total body water (TBW) is increased (85% of body weight in preterm infants and 70% in term infants, compared with 55% in adults). Water-soluble drugs (e.g., sulfas, penicillins, aminoglycosides, and cephalosporin) will therefore be distributed in greater volume (i.e., higher TBW of the neonate), thus requiring a larger loading dose on a per kilogram body weight basis.

Premature and term infants have qualitatively and quantitatively different plasma proteins than older infants. Protein binding is decreased in the newborn because of a decreased concentration of albumin and a decreased capacity of fetal albumin to bind to drugs. Certain acidic drugs (e.g., salicylates, ampicillin, phenytoin, phenobarbital, and sulfa drugs) will bind less, thus increasing the free fraction of the drug (with resultant increase in their effect).

Another issue of particular concern in newborn infants is protein binding and increased circulating bilirubin. A number of anionic compounds bind to albumin, thus displacing bilirubin and enhancing neurotoxicity. Binding to plasma proteins by drugs may interfere with the transport of other endogenous substances such as fatty acids. Bilirubin may displace phenytoin from albumin and increase its pharmacologic effect.

Biotransformation (drug metabolism)

Biotransformation (drug metabolism) usually occurs in the liver. Predicting the effect of aging on metabolism is difficult because of the variety of processes that occur in the liver, including oxidation, conjugation, and changing hepatic blood flow. For example, oxidation and glucuronidation are decreased in newborns. Drugs that undergo oxidation (i.e., acetaminophen, phenobarbital, and phenytoin) will have a diminished clearance. Decreased glucuronidation of chloramphenicol has been cited as the cause of "gray baby" syndrome. Furthermore, age-related changes in the pathway of elimination occur. Theophylline is metabolized to an active compound, caffeine, in neonates. In adults theophylline is metabolized to inactive metabolites. A decrease in plasma protein binding may also increase the hepatic clearance of a drug. The clearance of certain drugs through the liver is dependent on the drug's free or unbound fraction.

Clearance (elimination)

Drug clearance (elimination) occurs by excretion or by biotransformation to an inactive metabolite. Most drug elimination pathways become saturated if the dose is high enough. Fortunately, the therapeutic dose for most drugs used in clinical practice is less than that which saturates elimination processes. **When disposition mechanisms are not saturated, then the steady state concentration in the plasma is proportional to the dose rate. Clearance equals the rate of drug elimination divided by the drug concentration. Just as volume of distribution relates to loading dose, clearance relates to maintenance dose at steady state:**

$$(\text{Dose/dose interval}) \times F = Cl \times Css \text{ or}$$
$$Cl = F \times \text{Dose/(interval} \times Css)$$

RENAL EXCRETION

Many common drugs (e.g., aminoglycosides, digoxin, penicillins) have the kidney as their primary route of excretion. Doses of drugs excreted in the urine are modified as a function of age. The glomerular filtration rate (GFR) is low at birth and does not increase significantly until a week of age in term infants. In premature infants the GFR is even less, with a significant increase at a postconceptional age of 34 weeks or more. Aminoglycosides are examples of drugs excreted by glomerular filtration that demonstrate a decreased clearance and a longer half-life in newborns. In adults these drugs might be reduced on the basis of creatinine clearance. However, creatinine is not an ideal marker for glomerular filtration in newborns, since newborn serum creatinine in the first week of life at least partly reflects the mother's creatinine. Complications such as acidosis and anoxia may modify the infant's ability to eliminate a drug and therefore alter the pharmacokinetics of the drug.

HALF-LIFE

The drug elimination half-life is the time required for the drug level to decline by 50%. Half-life is related to both V and Cl, so that

$$t_{1/2} = 0.7 \times V/Cl$$

The half-life is used to predict and interpret the time course of changes in plasma drug concen- trations. **For instance, the time to steady state is 4 to 5 half-lives. The half-life is useful in selecting dose intervals. If the dose interval approximates the half-life, then fluctuation around the average serum concentration will approximate 50%. The importance of considering the effect of various dosing intervals is illustrated in Figure 7-4.**

PREVENTION OF AVOIDABLE THERAPEUTIC MISHAPS

Even after the correct choice of therapeutic agents is made, attention to the following principles is necessary to ensure optimal drug treatment:

1. **Carefully consider predictable factors that may affect the intensity or duration of drug effect with the initial prescription of a given drug.**
2. **Ensure certainty in patient dosing.**
3. **Monitor the effect of therapy and modify the therapeutic plan based on clinical effects and blood concentrations, if warranted.**

Completing the "five rights" of medication administration (Table 7-1) becomes complicated when caring for the newborn because of small dosages and dosage adjustments based on infant weight or surface area. However, without meticulous attention to these issues, potential disasters can and will occur.

Drugs enter the body directly by injection into body fluids, such as the blood, and indirectly by absorption across membrane barriers of the gastrointestinal tract, skin, muscle, and pulmonary alveoli. The rate and extent of drug entry varies with different drug formulations. The administration of drugs to infants is further complicated because dosages are prescribed in amounts not commercially available. Drugs must be diluted from commercially available pediatric or adult dosage forms.

Errors in administration of medications to newborns are not unknown. It has been reported that 8% of all drug doses calculated and

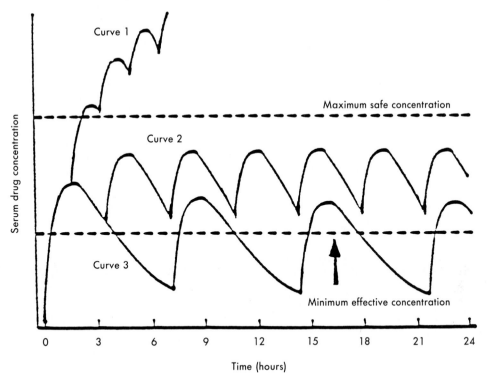

Figure 7-4. Effect of multiple dosing at different time intervals between doses on serum drug concentration. *Curve 1,* Accumulation to toxic levels; *curve 2,* optimal therapeutic levels; *curve 3,* subtherapeutic levels. (From Roberts RJ: Drug therapy in infants, Philadelphia, 1984, WB Saunders Co.)

TABLE 7-1

The "Five Rights" of Drug Administration

Right drug
Right patient
Right route
Right dose
Right time

administered by experienced neonatal intensive care nurses are in fact at least 10 times greater or lesser than the dose ordered. Anecdotal reports exist of infants having digitalis toxicity from receiving 0.09 mg of digoxin when 0.009 mg was ordered. Accuracy of dosage calculation, preparation, and administration of medications is crucial in the care of the neo-

nate. Having two nurses calculate and check the dosage decreases errors.

Although pediatric dosing formulations exist, problems still are reported with such commonly used drugs as digoxin and morphine in 1 to 2 kg babies. The concentration of digoxin preparation available for intravenous (IV) use predisposes to errors in the amount of drug actually administered. A 1 kg newborn given digoxin (5 μg/0.05 ml) every 12 hours receives the dosage by a tuberculin (TB) syringe, which has a dead space sufficient to contain 10 μg of digoxin. In a prospective study, preterm neonates given undiluted preparations of digoxin had an average serum level of digoxin of 4.5 ± 1.1 versus 1.9 ± 1.0 ng/ml (mean ± SD) in preterm infants given a diluted digoxin preparation.

NEONATAL RESUSCITATION MEDICATIONS

Name: _____ Weight: _____ Suction depth: _____

Date of birth: _____ ET tube size: _____

Drug	Strength	Dose	Route	Amount to administer
NaHCO$_3$	0.5 mEq/ml	1-2 mEq/kg	IV	_____
Epinephrine	1:10000	0.1 ml/kg	IV, ET	_____
Atropine	0.1 mg/ml	0.1 ml/kg	IV	_____

Other drugs and dosages could be added (see Table 3-4).

_____
Signature of preparer

Figure 7-5. Calculations for neonatal resuscitation medications.

In emergency situations the prompt and accurate preparation of emergency medications is critical. It is difficult to calculate both quickly and accurately when under the stress of a crisis. A better alternative, in anticipation of emergencies, is the calculation of emergency medications following the infant's admission. Calculations for the most commonly administered medications are posted at the bedside at all times (Figure 7-5).

DATA COLLECTION

Desired effects and potential toxic effects of drug therapy should be recorded, along with the time, to monitor for these effects. The expected dose–effect relationship should be recorded, along with the expected dose–plasma concentration–effect relationship when therapeutic drug monitoring is appropriate.

Dose recommendations and disposition parameters such as distribution volume, clearance, half-life, and bioavailability determined specifically in term or preterm infants should be recorded.

Factors that influence drug response such as chronologic age, maturational age, birth weight, and current weight should also be recorded.

It is important to employ units correctly.

It is important to overcome the problems associated with drug delivery in small infants.

Pharmacokinetics principles may be used to design a dose regimen as follows:

1. In most clinical situations, drugs are administered in such a way as to maintain a steady state of the drug in the body. Therefore the dose input should equal the drug loss from the body. This relationship was previously defined at steady state as dosing rate = $(Cl \times Css)/F$. Thus if the clinician can specify the desired steady state plasma concentration and knows the clearance and bioavailability of that drug in a particular patient, the appropriate dosing rate can be calculated.

Example: Clearance for theophylline in preterm infants is reported as 0.017 L/kg/hr. If the desired average Css = 8 mg/L, then (assuming F = 1):

Dose rate = Css × Cl = 0.136 mg/kg/hr or 1.1 mg every 8 hours

2. When the time to reach steady state is long, as it is with drugs with long half-lives, a loading dose may be desirable. The volume of distribution is the proportionality factor that relates the amount of drug in the body to the plasma concentration. For drugs with one-compartment distribution, the loading dose may be given as a single dose.

Example: Theophylline has a volume of distribution in preterm infants of about 0.7 L/kg. If 8 mg/L is the desired concentration, a loading dose (LD) can be calculated (assuming F = 1):

LD = (Vd × C)/F = 0.7 L/kg × 8 mg/L
   = 5.6 mg/kg of theophylline

Laboratory data

Even when predictable changes are taken into account, other nonpredictable factors may influence a drug's effect. Therefore clinical end points must be followed with the anticipation that dose regimens may require additional modification. For instance the major short-term toxicity of indomethacin for patent ductus arteriosus (PDA) closure is transient, reversible renal dysfunction (i.e., oliguria, reduced GFR, and electrolyte imbalance). When signs of renal dysfunction are observed in infants receiving indomethacin, the next dose is withheld until renal function returns to normal.

Good data collection is essential for accurate timing of dosing and blood sampling. If the drug concentration in the blood has been related to the clinical response, then it is rational to follow blood concentrations in addition to clinical end points. To optimally use measured blood levels, the expected blood concentration must be calculated from the dosing history, measurable patient variables that might affect drug effect, and the timing of blood samples.

TABLE 7-2

Potential Explanations for Discrepancies between Measured and Expected Drug Concentration

Inadequate compliance
Inadequate medication delivery
Inappropriate timing of samples
Laboratory error
Revision in initial estimates of pK required

Comparison of the expected value with the measured value allows rational adjustment of future dosing. This type of comparison can be used to decide if compliance was good, if the timing of samples was appropriate, if a drug measurement error was made in the laboratory, or if a revision in initial pharmacokinetics parameters, such as clearance or volume, is required (Table 7-2).

If a suboptimal clinical response is noted in conjunction with a subtherapeutic target plasma concentration, then revised estimates of clearance may be cautiously made with one or two available plasma concentrations. If a single available concentration is drawn after absorption/distribution is complete and near steady state, then the maintenance dose formula can be rearranged to calculate a revised clearance. The commonsense approach suggests that if a patient has one half the expected concentration of a drug, then perhaps the clearance is twice the initial estimate. On the other hand, if the patient has twice the expected concentration of a drug, one explanation is that the clearance is only half the initial estimate. This technique will be misleading if steady state has not been reached. In response to twice the desired blood concentration, the drug should be discontinued until the blood concentration decays to the target concentration. Then, decreasing the dose rate by one half is anticipated to result in continued achievement of the desired target concentration.

If two concentrations are available after absorption/distribution, then a revised half-life is determined by plotting the concentrations on semilog paper. The revised clearance is then calculated by rearranging the half-life formula as follows:

$$Cl = 0.7 \times V/t_{1/2}$$

PRACTICAL APPLICATION

Following are some examples of simple pharmacokinetics calculations using the principles discussed above. These calculations should not be used unless meticulous attention has been given to the issues of delivery of medication and timing of dosing and blood sampling.

ASSIGNMENT 1: A 0.75 kg, 15-day-old premature infant is receiving an oral theophylline preparation diluted by the pharmacy for apnea of prematurity. He has been given 0.5 mg of theophylline elixir every 12 hours for 5 days. Because his apnea recurs, his theophylline concentration may be subtherapeutic. In addition to other clinical and laboratory evaluation, a theophylline concentration (drawn 6 hours after his last dose) is sent to the laboratory. It will be 4 hours before the theophylline concentrations are run in the laboratory. Estimate what this concentration will be.

ASSIGNMENT 1 ANSWER: The data necessary to address this question include the following:

Total body weight = 0.75 kg
V = 0.69 L/kg = 0.53 L in this patient
Cl = 0.017 L/kg/hr = 0.013 L/hr in this patient
$t_{1/2}$ = 0.7 × V/Cl = 28.5 hr
Time to steady state (Tss) = 4 $t_{1/2}$ = 114 hr
Assume F = 1
MSC = 15 μg/ml
MEC = 5 μg/ml

Therefore:

Css = F × Dose/(Dose interval × Cl)
   = 1 × 0.5 mg/(12 hr × 0.013 L/hr)
   = 3.2 mg/L

ASSIGNMENT 2: Your estimate of the infant's theophylline concentration is subtherapeutic; design a partial IV aminophylline loading dose and an oral theophylline maintenance dose every 8 hours to achieve a steady state concentration of about 10 μg/ml.

ASSIGNMENT 2 ANSWER:
a. Calculate a loading dose to raise concentration 1 (3 mg/L) to concentration 2 (10 mg/L).

Loading dose = (Conc 2 − Conc 1) × V/F
   = (10 − 3) × 0.53 L/1
   = 3.7 mg of theophylline, or since aminophylline is 0.85 theophylline, 4.4 mg of aminophylline

b. Calculate a maintenance dose to achieve a Css of 10 mg/L.

Maintenance dose = (Css × Interval × CL)/F
   = 10 mg/L × 8 hr × 0.013 L/1 = 1 mg of theophylline PO every 8 hours = 1.2 mg of aminophylline every 8 hours

The theophylline concentration submitted in assignment 1 was sent to the laboratory at noon. At 4 PM on the same day (day 1), this concentration was reported by the laboratory to be 3.1 μg/ml.

ASSIGNMENT 3: At 8 AM 5 days later and 4 hours after the patient's last dose of theophylline (1 mg every 8 hours), although apnea has abated, the infant's heart rate is 180 beats/min. Since this infant may be showing signs of theophylline toxicity, the theophylline is discontinued and serum theophylline and caffeine concentrations are sent to the laboratory. At 4 PM the theophylline concentration is reported to be 15 μg/ml (caffeine < 1 μg/ml). Using this concentration, estimate the time at which the concentration will decline to 8 μg/ml and determine an oral theophylline regimen every 12 hours for maintaining that concentration.

The patient's tachycardia resolves.

ASSIGNMENT 3 ANSWER: A revised estimate of clearance can be obtained as follows:

Cl revised = F × Dose/(Interval × Css)
    = 1 × 1 mg/(8 hr × 15 mg/L) = 0.008 L/hr

The revised estimate of $t_{1/2}$ is obtained as follows:

$t_{1/2}$ revised = 0.7 × V/Cl revised
    = 0.7 × 0.53 L/0.008 L/hr = 44.5 hr

Therefore the concentration 40 hours later should be approximately one half the measured 15 mg/L, or about 8 mg/L. To maintain this concentration of 8 mg/L:

Dose = (Interval × Cl revised × Css)/F
    = 12 hr × 0.008 L/hr × 8 mg/L/1
    = 0.8 mg of theophylline PO every 12 hours

ASSIGNMENT 4: Before initiation of the oral regimen, another theophylline concentration is drawn 36 hours after the first concentration and is reported to be 7.5 μg/ml. Since the patient has had no recurrence of apnea, an oral regimen that is based on the last two theophylline concentrations is begun to maintain a theophylline level of 7 μg/ml. Estimate the maintenance dose of theophylline.

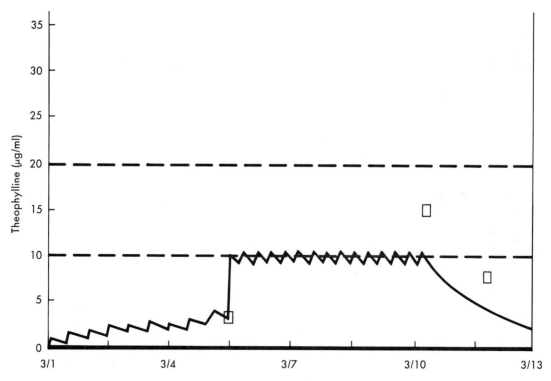

Figure 7-6. Curve represents *expected* concentration versus time curve from published newborn values of clearance and volume. Boxes represent measured plasma concentrations. Points to note are (1) steady state is not achieved until 4 half-lives, or 114 hours; (2) although not expected, clinical symptom of tachycardia and high theophylline concentration suggest toxicity (theophylline was discontinued); (3) third theophylline concentration confirms suspicion of decreased clearance and can be used to estimate individual clearance in this baby as in assignment 4; and (4) dashed lines at 20 and 10 μg/ml represent adult MSC and MEC (not newborn values of 15 and 5 μg/ml).

ASSIGNMENT 4 ANSWER: The theophylline concentration fell 50%, from 15 to 7.5 mg/L, in 36 hours (i.e., the half-life was 36 hours).

The revised clearance can be determined by the formula:

$$Cl \text{ revised} = 0.7 \times V/t_{1/2}$$
$$= 0.7 \times 0.53 \text{ L}/36 \text{ hr}$$
$$= 0.010 \text{ L/hr}$$

Based on this revised clearance, the maintenance dose (MD) is determined as follows:

$$MD = Css \times Interval \times Cl \text{ revised}/F$$
$$= 7 \text{ mg/L} \times 12 \text{ hr} \times 0.010 \text{ L/hr}$$
$$= 0.9 \text{ mg of theophylline PO (every 12 hours)}$$

See Figure 7-6 for a graphic depiction of this problem. The x axis represents days in March.

This practical application section is not intended as a complete approach to the patient but merely as an example of types of calculations useful in therapeutic drug monitoring. The negligible serum caffeine concentration in the example is a simplification for the purpose of illustration of kinetic calculations. The presence of an active metabolite makes theophylline a less than ideal candidate for therapeutic drug monitoring in newborns.

METHODS OF ADMINISTRATION
Oral administration

When oral medications are being administered, the problem of how to get the medication into the infant arises. Oral administration of medication to newborns, especially premature infants, is complicated not only by variations in oral bioavailability, but also by unanticipated loss of the drug. Loss of oral medication occurs when sick infants are unable to take or tolerate their feedings, have frequent and significant regurgitation, or require intermittent oral gastric suctioning and loss of residuals.

If the infant is receiving oral gastric or nasal gastric feedings, the medication is dropped into the center of the barrel of the syringe, which contains a small portion of the feeding. Medication that runs down the side of the barrel may adhere to the plastic and effectively decrease the amount of prescribed medicine delivered to the infant. The administration of the medication is documented on the chart, and any wet burps, emesis, or residual found is noted as to the color and the estimated or measured amount of the feeding lost. For infants receiving oral medications, the documentation of the color of the emesis or residual is important for determining if the color can be attributed to the medication or a pathophysiologic condition.

For infants receiving oral feedings by bottle, putting the medication into the full volume of feedings becomes problematic when the infant refuses to take the full amount of the feeding. If one adds the medication into the bottle, one cannot be assured that the infant will take the entire amount of feeding. The medication can be administered directly into the infant's mouth by gently introducing very small amounts of the medication into the cheek pouch and waiting for the infant to swallow. After this has been repeated several times, the infant will have taken the prescribed amount of medication. A second method is to put 5 to 10 ml of feeding into a Volufeed or bottle and let the infant take the entire amount before continuing with the remainder of the oral feeding. The medication can also be put into a nipple with some formula, and the infant allowed to consume this small volume early in the feeding. For infants who are breastfeeding, the medication can be administered into the mouth as described above, or it can be mixed with a small amount of the mother's breast milk and given to the infant. As with gavage feedings, the medication administration is documented, and the color and amount of any emesis noted.

Intramuscular injection

Unlike the adult who has sufficient muscle mass to receive intramuscular (IM) injections in numerous sites, the infant has relatively little muscle mass to receive injections. When IM injections are required, as with vitamin K, the anterior thigh is the site of choice. The area is cleaned with alcohol, and the medication is injected into the thigh using a 21- to 25-gauge needle. Following injection, the area is massaged. For the infant weighing less than 1500 g, the volume of medication administered IM at one injection should not exceed 0.5 ml. The administration of the medication is documented, as is the site of the injection.

Intravenous administration

IV medication is given to the infant in a newborn unit by a variety of methods, including push injection, antegrade injection, pump infusion, and retrograde injection. Although drugs given IV do not have to cross a membrane barrier to enter the body, the time required to complete drug delivery is a function of dosage (with certain IV methods) volume, IV flow rate, and injection site (Figure 7-7). Failure to recognize potential time lags could easily result in inappropriate timing of expected physiologic responses or presumed peak-and-trough blood concentrations. The use of microbore IV tubing and a distal injection site will partially facilitate the more rapid delivery of the drug, since the volume of the fluid contained in the tubing is greatly reduced.

PUSH INJECTION

The administration of IV push medications consists of preparing both the medication in an appropriate-size syringe and a flush solution (heparin with normal saline [NS], 10% dextrose in water [$D_{10}W$], 5% dextrose in water [D_5W], or sterile water). The IV tubing is inspected for a port that is close to the site of entry, the port is prepared, and the flush is used before and after the injection of the medication. The medication is given over 1 to 2 minutes, depending on the medication and the volume. If postinjection of flush is used, this should be given at the same rate as the medication; if not, then the medica-

tion may be delivered to the infant as a bolus, since it is pushed along by the flush. The use of flush after administering the medication will also remove any of the medication that may be left in the port of the IV tubing.

Certain drugs can safely be given by rapid bolus infusion (IV push)—direct administration of medication into the venous circulation in less than 1 minute. *Slow IV push* is a term common to all nurses, but since interpretation varies widely, a specific rate of injection would be preferable. Many drugs should not be administered by IV push because of the propensity to produce immediate adverse reactions when administered by rapid bolus injection to low birth weight infants.

ANTEGRADE INJECTION

Antegrade injection of medication involves introduction of the medication into an entry port of the IV tubing. The medication is then carried in the tubing with the IV fluid at the same rate of infusion as the fluid. Since infusion rates in newborns are very low, marked delays in drug delivery may result. This method is not recommended for drug delivery to very low birth weight infants.

PUMP INFUSION

To avoid delayed drug delivery times, an IV system employing a mechanical syringe infusion device allows control over the rate of drug delivery to the patient. The major drawback to these small pumps is their cost. The use of pumps for medication delivery has enhanced the consistency of the rate of delivery of the medication to the infant. The pumps vary by manufacturer and the principle by which they deliver fluids to the infant. Generally, pump infusion systems consist of a pump that can be regulated to deliver a specific volume over a specific time period, a syringe or container of medication to be delivered, and connecting tubing/needles to connect the pump to the entry port for drug delivery.

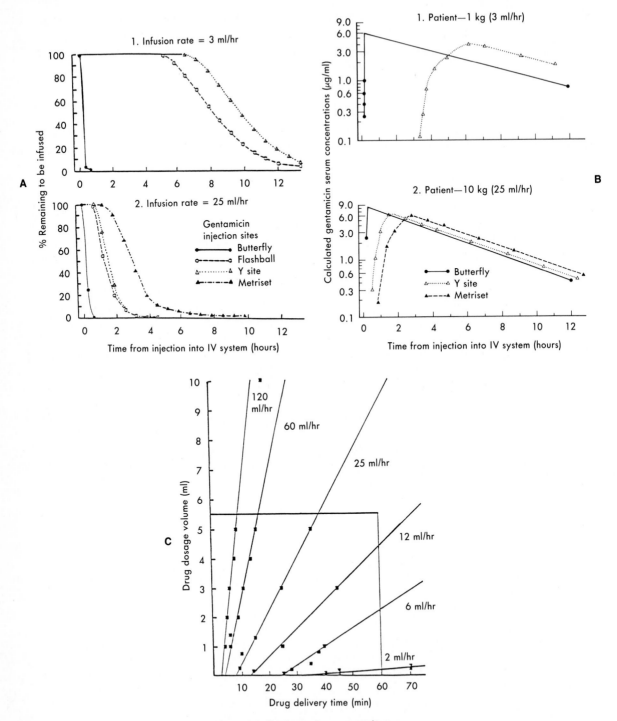

Figure 7-7. For legend see opposite page.

There are two methods of using pumps to deliver medication to ensure that the infant receives the exact amount of medication ordered. Each newborn unit should have a unit policy to ensure that it is uniformly carried out in the same manner by each of the staff.

METHOD 1. The exact amount of medication is drawn into the syringe and diluted, if necessary, to bring the volume to that needed for the operation of the pump. This is then flushed through the connecting tubing/needle, and the syringe is placed in the pump. After the pump has finished the infusion, some of the medication remains in the connecting tubing and hub of the syringe. This medication needs to be flushed into the IV with a flush solution in order for the infant to receive the entire amount ordered.

METHOD 2. The medication is drawn into the syringe through the connecting tubing/needle until the medication volume desired is in the syringe. This is then put on the pump and infused. With this method the connecting tubing/needle is not flushed with a flush solution, since the infant has already received the entire dose ordered. If the medication is flushed through, then the infant receives more than that which was ordered. If the same caretaker who starts the administration of the medication will be there to end it, there should not be a problem.

But if a different caretaker will end it, then the method used needs to be communicated. Setting a unit policy for one method over another would help alleviate any potential medication errors due to lack of communication.

RETROGRADE INJECTION

Retrograde injection is the injection of medication in the opposite direction of the IV fluid flow. This system requires the injection of the medication into the IV tubing, resulting in displacement of a portion of the IV fluid in the tubing. The excess fluid is displaced into an upstream syringe. An alternate method is to use specifically developed retrograde tubing for administration of the medication or retrograde sets that contain a collection bag for the displaced fluid.

Retrograde injection as currently available is not recommended for premature infants. Reported disadvantages are that the amount of fluid injected is limited by the size of the tubing, syringe, or collection bag. There is increased risk of microbial contamination. There is also a total loss of calories, since the displaced fluid is replaced by the medication, which is calorie poor. Since there is no "catch up" on the fluids, the total caloric intake from IV fluids is reduced. In this system the drug delivery rate still depends on the IV infusion rate.

Figure 7-7. **A,** Effects of different IV infusion rates and different injection sites on time required for delivery of drug dose. For example, at 3 ml/hr (*1*), actual infusion of drug begins at 160 minutes after injection into IV system (flashball site) and is completed 6 hours later (i.e., 400 minutes). At more rapid IV infusion rate of 25 ml/hr (*2*), delay in start of actual infusion is less, as is duration required for delivery of dose. Note major difference between injection sites (butterfly versus flashball site). **B,** Effects of IV injection site (butterfly, Y site, or Metriset) on serum gentamicin concentrations. Drug levels were calculated from infusion data shown in **A** for 1 kg patient at 3 ml/hr (*1*) and 10 kg patient at 25 ml/hr (*2*). Note in *view 1* that with use of Y site there is 3-hour delay before drug levels begin to rise in serum. **C,** Influence of dosage volume (*ordinate*) or IV flow rate (*individual data lines*) on time required to complete drug delivery (*abscissa*) with use of manual retrograde injection technique. (**A** modified from Gould T and Roberts RJ: J Pediatr 95:465, 1979. **B** from Roberts RJ: Drug therapy in infants, Philadelphia, 1984, WB Saunders Co. **C** from Leff RD and Roberts RJ: J Pediatr 98:631, 1981.)

OTHER CONSIDERATIONS

The health care provider must be attuned to additional considerations when administering IV medications. The use of filters, protection of certain medications from light sources (especially phototherapy lights), the preservatives used in some medications, and the specific gravity of the medication should be considered before administration of any medication.

A 0.22 μm filter may provide "cold sterilization" (i.e., remove particulate matter and bacterial contamination). There are some medications that cannot be administered using a filter, because the filter removes the active ingredient.

Medications with a lower specific gravity than the IV fluid have a tendency to accumulate at high points in the IV tubing, whereas those medications with higher specific gravity will settle into the low loops of the IV tubing. This can result in delay in the delivery of the medication to the infant.

INSERTING PERIPHERAL IV LINES. Peripheral IV access is often required for medication administration. Needles and catheters used in the neonate are necessarily small (22 to 27 gauge). The most commonly used are the "butterfly" needle and needles with catheter sheaths. Common IV placement sites include the hands, feet, legs, arms, or scalp veins. Extremity vessels that are difficult to visualize may be outlined by diffusing light through the extremity from a transilluminator placed under the extremity. CAUTION: Avoid burning the delicate skin of the premature infant by minimizing or avoiding direct contact of the transilluminator with the skin.

Equipment

Catheters, needles in sizes appropriate for the diameter of the vein
Tape—clear or opaque
Alcohol
Gauze
Syringe with 2 ml of flush solution
Razor (if using head veins)
Tourniquet (rubber band)
Arm/legboard
Infant restraints
Gloves

Procedure. Assemble equipment at the bedside or at a radiant warmer. Provide an adequate heat source throughout this procedure. Tear tape into two short pieces (½ inch by 2 inches) and three longer pieces (½ inch by 6 inches). Select a site for placement of an IV line by determining that the vessel is *not* arterial by palpating for a pulse. Determine the direction of blood flow—in the scalp arteries fill from below, veins from above; in the extremities veins fill distal to central.

Restrain the infant. If using vessels in the extremities, restrain the arm or leg on an armboard. Some care providers prefer to place the armboard after the vessel has been cannulated and the needle/catheter secured in position. If using scalp veins, shave the area and blot with a piece of tape to pick up the hair. Give the hair to the mother for the baby book.

Flush the needle/catheter and remove the syringe. Place the tourniquet around the extremity (optional: many IV lines are placed without a tourniquet). Prepare the site by cleaning with alcohol; allow to dry. After gloving, insert the needle/catheter into the vessel using the hand and fingers to anchor the skin surrounding the vessel. Insert into the vessel at an acute angle and in the direction of blood flow. Observe for blood return or flashback into the tubing or cannula of the catheter. Some vessels will not have a blood return. If there is no return and you feel the needle is in the vessel, a small amount of flush may be injected. If the needle is not in the vessel, a swelling of the tissue at the end of the needle will be obvious. If, with flushing, there is blanching of the skin distal to the insertion site, the vessel is most likely arterial (most common in scalp vein insertion). When there is a blood return, flush is injected to clear the needle and prevent clotting. If using a catheter, remove the needle while gently advancing the catheter.

Secure the IV line by placing a short piece of tape across the needle/catheter. Then cross a longer piece of tape over the needle/catheter, around the back of the catheter, and across the front. Check to see that the IV line is still positioned by disconnecting it from the syringe and watching for a blood return or by infusing a small amount of flush. If necessary, use gauze or a piece of cotton behind the needle for support. Secure this in place by using another long piece of tape. Cover the IV site with half a medicine cup or the clear needle package to protect the site. Infants who are inactive may not need an IV site protective cover. Restrain the extremity if this has not already been done.

If the medication is to be administered intermittently and the line is not needed for fluids and calories, it may be heparin locked and flushed every shift with a heparinized solution (0.2 units of heparin per 1 ml of solution).

TEACHING MODEL. The use of a placenta as a teaching model for insertion of umbilical lines is discussed in Chapter 6. The fetal side of a placenta may also be used for teaching IV insertion of various needles and catheters.

Equipment and supplies
Placenta
Assorted sizes of needles and catheters
Syringes filled with normal saline or flush solution
Gloves
Tape

Procedure. The placenta is placed on drapes with the fetal side up. The fetal membranes are removed, exposing the rich network of vessels. After gloving, insert both butterfly needles and catheters in the larger vessels first and then smaller vessels as the technique is perfected. Any skewering of the vessel is immediately apparent, since blood leaks out through the vessel wall. Tortuous vessels or those with branching patterns are used for various methods of cannulation. Once the catheters are in position, securing the needles/catheters by taping techniques is practiced. Two people may work on one placenta at a time.

COMPLICATIONS
Complications of IV therapy include phlebitis, infiltration, hematomas, chemical burns, and emboli. Frequent (hourly) assessment of the IV site helps prevent complications. Swelling and discoloration of the extremity or of the skin at the needle tip are signs to remove the needle/catheter. In the scalp, infiltration may be difficult to assess, since swelling is not only at the IV site, but also on the dependent side of the head. Scalp edema (on the dependent side) and/or a swollen eye are indicators of scalp vein infiltration. In the extremities, a swollen arm or leg, hand or foot, or fingers or toes indicate an infiltrated IV line.

Footdrop has been associated with positioning a footboard along the lateral aspect of the fibula (caused by pressure on the peroneal division of the sciatic nerve). Use of rolled washcloths as footboards and/or extensive padding of IV boards with cotton, gauze, or washcloths may prevent excessive pressure.

Unnoticed infiltrations may result in skin burns or sloughing and compromised circulation. Warm or hot soaks in an infiltrated site are contraindicated. When warm soaks are used, extravasated fluid is warmed to a temperature that results in burns, maceration, and necrosis. In addition, heat increases the oxygen demand in already compromised tissues.

Elevating the infiltrated area increases venous return and helps decrease edema. Hyaluronidase destroys tissue cement and prevents or minimizes tissue damage by allowing rapid diffusion and absorption of the extravasated fluid. For best results, treat the area within 1 hour of injury. Inject hyaluronidase (15 units/ml) subcutaneously around the periphery of the extravasated area. The effectiveness of hyal-

---

THEOPHYLLINE

Your baby is on a medication called *theophylline.* Other names for this drug include Slo-Phyllin, Theodyl, Theolair, and Aerolate. Theophylline is a very powerful drug that helps your baby breathe by relaxing the small air passages in the lungs.

It is very important that this medication be given on a strict schedule so that the right amount of the drug is in the baby's blood at all times. It is also important to give the right amount of medicine and to give it at the right time. Please be sure to keep all follow-up appointments so that the doctor can adjust the dose of theophylline to meet your baby's needs.

Theophylline can be upsetting to the baby's stomach. To prevent this, please be sure to give the medication with a feeding (formula or breast milk).

THE DOSE OF YOUR BABY'S THEOPHYLLINE IS: _____

THE TIMES TO GIVE THE MEDICATION ARE: _____

Be sure to give the amount of medication ordered by your doctor. Do not change the dose unless the doctor asks you to. Do not give this medication to any other person! Follow your doctor's orders carefully and follow these guidelines when giving this medication.

1. If your baby swallows some of the medicine but not all of it, do not repeat the dose.
2. If your baby vomits after the medication, do not repeat the dose.
3. If you forget to give a dose and it is less than 2 hours late, give the dose and keep the baby on the regular schedule. If the dose is more than 2 hours late when you remember it, give the dose and evenly space the doses over the next 24 hours. Then go back to the regular schedule.
4. If your baby is ill with a cold, flu, or fever; has loss of appetite, diarrhea, vomiting, wheezing, or trouble breathing; or is unusually irritable, CALL THE DOCTOR.
5. Be sure that any doctor seeing your baby knows all of the medicines your baby takes. Do not give other medicines to your baby unless a doctor tells you to.
6. Theophylline should be stored in a safe place. A locked cabinet out of reach of children is best.

IF SOMEONE ACCIDENTALLY TAKES THIS OR ANY OTHER MEDICATION OR POISON, CALL THE POISON CONTROL CENTER IMMEDIATELY!

Figure 7-8. Parent information sheet. (Courtesy University of Colorado Health Sciences Center, Denver, 1987.)

uronidase has not been proved. It may not be effective if diagnoses and administration are delayed.

PARENT TEACHING

The presence of IV lines in newborns is frightening to parents, especially if the IV is in the infant's head. Without information, parents mistakenly believe the fluid is "going into the baby's brain." Reassuring the parents that the fluid is going into large veins in the head (and not into the brain) is important.

Even though their infant has an IV, parents are still encouraged to touch, hold, and feed their infant.

In answer to the question, "Does it hurt?"

parents must be told the truth. "Yes, it hurts to have an IV placed, but once it is in, it doesn't hurt anymore." Parents are usually very cautious when handling their baby and do not want the infant "to get stuck again." The importance of frequent checks in noticing and discontinuing an infiltration should be explained, since some parents mistakenly believe this causes the infiltration. Venous fragility in the newborn, combined with relatively hypertonic solutions, make frequent restarting of IV lines commonplace, and these causes of infiltration should be explained to the parents.

A diagnosis of "rule out sepsis" is often very confusing to families, who do not understand why antibiotics are started before the culture results are known. Explain to the parents that antibiotics can be stopped at 48 to 72 hours if cultures and latex agglutination are negative (in most cases), but that if cultures are positive, delaying the start of antibiotics markedly increases the morbidity and mortality.

Discharge teaching about medications that parents must administer is very important. Parents must know the name of the drug, dosage, frequency of administration, side effects, and any special instructions. Parents must be taught to administer medicines, must demonstrate their ability to do the same, and must receive written instructions (Figure 7-8).

SELECTED READINGS

Aranda JV, Sitar DS, and Parsons, WP: Pharmacokinetics, aspects of theophylline in preterm infants, N Engl J Med 925:413, 1976.

Aranda JV and Turman T: Methylxanthines in apnea of prematurity, Clin Perinatol 6:87, 1979.

Berman W et al: Inadvertent overadministration of digoxin to low birth weight infants, J Pediatr 92:1024, 1978.

Berman W et al: Digoxin therapy in low birth weight infants with patent ductus arteriosus, J Pediatr 93:652, 1978.

Bleyer WA and Koup JR: Medication errors during intensive care, Am J Dis Child 133:366, 1979.

Boerth RC: Decreased sensitivity of the newborn myocardium positive inotropic effects of ouabain. In Marselli PL, Garat-

tine S, and Sereni F, editors: Basic and therapeutic aspects of perinatal pharmacology, New York, 1975, Raven Press.

Burch SM and Chadwick JV: Use of a retroset in the delivery of intravenous medications in the neonate, Neonatal Network 6:51, 1987.

Evans ME, Bhat R, and Vidyasagar D: Factors modulating drug therapy and pharmokinetics. In Yeh TF: Drug therapy in the neonate and small infant, Chicago, 1985, Year Book Medical Publishers, Inc.

Few BJ: Hyaluronidase for treating intravenous extravasations, MCN 12:23, 1987.

Fischer AQ and Strasburger J: Footdrop in the neonate secondary to the use of footboards, J Pediatr 101:1003, 1982.

Giacoia GP and Yaffe SJ: Drugs and the perinatal patient. In Avery G, editor: Neonatology: pathophysiology and management of the newborn, Philadelphia, 1981, JB Lippincott Co.

Glass SM and Giacoia GP: Intravenous drug therapy in premature infants: practical aspects, J Obstet Gynecol Neonatal Nurs 16:310, 1987.

Gould T and Roberts R: Therapeutic problems arising from the use of the intravenous route for drug administration, J Pediatr 95:465, 1979.

Hagedorn MI: Treating intravenous extravasations in the neonate with hyaluronidase objections, Neonatal Network (in press).

Hilligoss D: Neonatal pharmokinetics. In Evans W, editor: Applied pharmokinetics, San Francisco, 1986, Applied Therapeutics.

Holford NHG: Clinical interpretation of drug concentrations. In Katzung BG, editor: Basic and clinical pharmacology, East Norwalk, Conn, 1987, Appleton & Lange.

Holford NHG and Sheiner LB: Understanding the dose effect relationship, Clin Pharmacokinet 6:429, 1981.

Kaufman RE: The clinical interpretation and application of drug concentration data, Pediatric Clin North Am 28:35, 1981.

MacCara ME: Extravasation: a hazard of intravenous therapy, Drug Intell Clin Pharm 17:71, 1983.

Peck CC: Bedside clinical pharmokinetics: simple techniques for individualizing drug therapy, Rockville, Md, 1985, Pharmocometrics Press.

Perlin E, Taylor RE, and Peck CC: Clinical pharmacokinetics: a simplified approach, part I, J Natl Med Assoc 77:475, 1985.

Perlstein PH et al: Errors in drug computation during newborn intensive care, Am J Dis Child 133:376, 1979.

Roberts RJ: Intravenous administration of medication in pediatric patients: problems and solutions, Pediatric Clin North Am 28:23, 1981.

Roberts RJ: Drug therapy in infants, Philadelphia, 1984, WB Saunders Co.

CHAPTER 8

Acid-base homeostasis and oxygenation

WILLIAM H. PARRY • **OLGA R. GUNNELL**

The proper understanding of arterial blood gases and the analyses of acid-base balance are critical to the proper diagnosis, management, and outcome in the neonate. The measurement of arterial blood gases assesses two interrelated but separate processes: oxygenation and acid-base homeostasis. This chapter describes the parameters that reflect oxygenation and acid-base balance, their measurements, and the effects of proposed treatment to maintain homeostasis. Common abbreviations and their meanings are listed in the box at the right.

The assessment of arterial blood gases involves (1) actual measured values (PaO_2, $PaCO_2$, and pH) and (2) calculations from these measurements (oxygen saturation, base excess, and bicarbonate concentration). Some analyzer systems also estimate hemoglobin concentration. To assess acid-

base homeostasis, the results of the pH, PCO_2, base excess, and bicarbonate determinants are examined. The parameters used to assess the adequacy of oxygenation are PaO_2, saturation, and hemoglobin (box, bottom left).

□ The opinions and assertions in this chapter are those of the authors and do not necessarily represent those of the Department of the Army or the Department of Defense.

NORMAL (ARTERIAL) BLOOD GAS VALUES

pH	7.36-7.46
$PaCO_2$	35-45 mm Hg
HCO_3^-	22-26 mEq/L
Base excess	(-4)-$(+4)$
PaO_2	50-80 mm Hg
O_2 saturation	92%-94%

ABBREVIATIONS

pH	Negative log of hydrogen ion concentration
P	Partial pressure (tension, driving force)
a	Arterial
A	Alveolar
v	Venous
c	Capillary
C	Content
S	Saturation
D	Difference
V	Volume
$\dot{V}$	Volume per unit time
V_D	Dead space volume
V_T	Tidal volume
Q	Perfusion (flow)
$\dot{Q}$	Flow per unit time
E	Expiration, expired
I	Inhalation, inspired
F	Fraction

Combined abbreviations

PaO_2	Partial pressure of arterial oxygen
FIO_2	Fraction of inspired oxygen
$PaCO_2$	Partial pressure of arterial carbon dioxide

PHYSIOLOGY
Acid-base homeostasis

An acid is a hydrogen ion donor, and a base is a hydrogen ion receptor. The acid-base balance in the blood is determined by the pH (puissance hydrogen), which refers to the concentration of the hydrogen ion $[H^+]$ in the blood. The hydrogen ion activity actually is minute, amounting to approximately 0.0000001 moles/L. In logarithmic units this is 1×10^{-7} moles/L. The pH is the negative log of the hydrogen ion concentration (pH = 7) (equation 1). A pH of 7 represents a neutral solution, a pH of less than 7 represents increasing acidity, and a pH greater than 7 indicates increasing alkalinity.

(1)

$$pH = -\log[H^+]$$
$$pH = -\log[0.0000001]$$
$$pH = -[-7]$$
$$pH = 7$$

The Henderson-Hasselbalch equation relates the pH to a constant (pK) plus the log of the base to acid concentration ratio (equation 2). Thus if there is too much acid, or an increase in the hydrogen ion reflected in the denominator, the blood pH value decreases. This condition is known as acidemia. Conversely, if there is less acid or more base, the numerator and the pH value increase. This is known as alkalemia.

(2)

$$pH = pK + \log\frac{base}{acid}$$

The pK is the pH at which a substance is half dissociated (cations and anions) and half undissociated (conjugate pair). The pK of whole blood is 6.1, and therefore the pH of blood is:

(3)

$$pH = 6.1 + \log\frac{base}{acid}$$

Assessing the acid-base homeostasis is the first step in determining its status (pH). Physiologic and pathophysiologic processes that tend to change the pH are denoted by the suffix *-osis*.

Thus a process that tends to lower the pH is an acidosis, and the process that tends to raise the pH is an alkalosis. An increase in the hydrogen ion (acid) in the blood causes a decrease in pH and results in acidemia, and a decrease in the hydrogen ion (an increase in the base) results in an elevated pH and alkalemia. The normal human pH is between 7.35 and 7.45; therefore a pH of less than 7.35 is acidemia, and the process that caused it is an acidosis.

Acid-base homeostasis refers to the physiologic mechanisms that maintain the pH in normal range. Pathophysiologic mechanisms result in pH changes that lead to acidemia or alkalemia. A "tendency" to change the pH, not the actual resultant change, connotes a pathophysiologic mechanism.

The arterial carbon dioxide and bicarbonate values in the blood gas analysis evaluate the processes of acidosis and alkalosis that affect the acid status of the body. These parameters assess separate components of acid-base homeostasis: (1) respiratory contribution ($Paco_2$) controlled by alveolar ventilation and (2) nonrespiratory or metabolic contribution (HCO_3^-) controlled primarily by renal excretion, retention, or manufacture of HCO_3^-.

RESPIRATORY CONTRIBUTION

Carbon dioxide, produced by each cell as a waste product of metabolism, is a gas and follows the laws of gas transport. As carbon dioxide is produced, it dissolves in the intracellular fluid and can be measured as the partial pressure (P) of the dissolved gas (Pco_2). As the pressure of the dissolved gas increases in the cell, a gradient develops between this pressure and the extracellular fluid. As the gradient increases, the dissolved carbon dioxide gas moves out of the cell and into the bloodstream (i.e., from the area of greater pressure to the area of lesser pressure). This dissolved carbon dioxide gas is transported by the blood to the lung, where the gradient in the pulmonary capillary is greater than that in the alveoli, and carbon dioxide is excreted in the alveoli in accordance with the direction of the pressure gradient. Ventilation is the only method of excreting carbon dioxide. The amount of carbon dioxide in the blood is balanced by the body's metabolic rate (production) and the alveolar ventilation (excretion). Because metabolism does not change greatly, the measurement of $PaCO_2$ accurately reflects the alveolar ventilation.

Dissolved carbon dioxide is an acidic substance. A minute amount of dissolved carbon dioxide gas combines with water to form carbonic acid, which divides into a hydrogen ion and a bicarbonate ion:

$$H_2O + CO_2 \leftrightarrows H_2CO_3 \leftrightarrows H_+ + HCO_3^-$$

The ratio of the dissolved carbonic acid to the dissociated hydrogen ion and bicarbonate anion is 1000:1.

Elevated $PaCO_2$, resulting in too much "acid" in the blood, causes the pH to fall ($\uparrow PCO_2$, $\downarrow pH$). Hypoventilation causes an increase in carbon dioxide. This process is an acidosis, since the acid in the body increases. Because the amount of carbon dioxide in the body is regulated only by the lung, the process is a respiratory acidosis.

Depressed $PaCO_2$, resulting in less acid in the blood, causes the pH to rise ($\downarrow PCO_2$, $\uparrow pH$). A pathologic or physiologic process, which causes hyperventilation, reduces the dissolved carbon dioxide. Since the result is a decreased amount of acid with a subsequent increase in the pH value, this process is an alkalosis. Because the parameter that is changing is controlled only by the lung, the process is a respiratory alkalosis.

NONRESPIRATORY (METABOLIC) CONTRIBUTION

Nonrespiratory (metabolic) factors involved in acid-base homeostasis are assessed by examining the calculated bicarbonate ion concentration or "base excess." Nonrespiratory parameters are controlled mainly by generating fixed acid by the kidney but are also influenced by pathologic conditions in the gastrointestinal system and other organ systems.

The bicarbonate ion is a hydrogen ion receptor or base. The base excess primarily represents the actual excess or deficit of bicarbonate, but the buffering action of red blood cells also affects the base excess. The base excess is estimated by multiplying the calculated bicarbonate by 1.2, and subtracting the normal bicarbonate value (24 mEq) from the product. A positive value indicates a deficit of fixed acid or an excess of base; a negative value indicates an excess of fixed acid or a deficit of base.

Thus when there is a base excess or the bicarbonate ion increases above normal (normal = 21 to 24 mEq/L), too much base is in the blood, and the pH increases. Any process that raises the pH is an alkalosis, and because the bicarbonate ion or base excess is involved and not carbon dioxide (the respiratory parameter), the process will be a nonrespiratory (metabolic) alkalosis. Conversely, when the bicarbonate ion is below normal, a base deficit or negative base excess is present, and because there is too little base or too much acid, the pH decreases, reflecting an acidosis. Because bicarbonate is a nonrespiratory parameter, this represents a nonrespiratory (metabolic) acidosis.

In the Henderson-Hasselbalch equation discussed previously, the pH was equal to a constant, pK, plus the log of the base/acid ratio. The bicarbonate ion concentration can be substituted for the base, and the dissolved carbon dioxide concentration substituted for the acid.

The Henderson-Hasselbalch equation:

$$pH = pK + \log \frac{base}{acid}$$

Substituting:

$$pH = pK + \log \frac{[HCO_3]}{[PaCO_2]}$$

However, HCO_3^- is in units of milliequivalents per liter, and PCO_2 is in millimeters of mercury. Substituting:

	Respiratory parameter pCO_2	Metabolic parameter HCO_3^-	Cause
Respiratory acidosis	⬆	↑	Hypoventilation
Respiratory alkalosis	⬇	↓	Hyperventilation
Metabolic acidosis	↓	⬇	Add acid or lose base
Metabolic alkalosis	↑	⬆	Add base or lose acid

Figure 8-1. Acid-base derangements. Large arrow indicates primary change that produces change in pH. Small arrow indicates compensatory process.

$$pH = pK + \log \frac{24 \text{ mEq/L}}{40 \text{ mm Hg}}$$

PCO_2 can be converted to milliequivalents per liter by multiplying PCO_2 by its solubility coefficient (0.03 mEq/L).

Converting to common units:

$$pH = pK + \log \frac{24 \text{ mEq/L}}{40 \text{ mm Hg} \times 0.03}$$

The normal bicarbonate concentration is 24 mEq/L. PCO_2 is 40 mm Hg and converts to $40 \times 0.03 = 1.2$ mEq/L. The ratio of base (bicarbonate) to acid (carbon dioxide) is 20:1.

Solving:

$$pH = pK + \log \frac{24 \text{ mEq/L} = 20}{1.2 \text{ mEq/L} = 1}$$

The pK of blood is 6.1. The log of 20 is 1.3. Therefore:

$$pH = 6.1 + 1.3 = 7.4$$

Changes in the 20:1 ratio therefore have profound effects on the pH.

For example, should some process occur causing hypoventilation (respiratory acidosis) of sufficient degree that the $PaCO_2$ is doubled from 40 to 80, the mEq/L of carbon dioxide gas would be 2.4, and the ratio of bicarbonate to carbon dioxide gas becomes 24:2.4, or 10. The logarithm of 10 is 1, and the pH would be 6.1 + 1, or 7.1. Conversely, if a respiratory alkalosis, which results in hyperventilation occurred, lowering the PCO_2 to 20 mm Hg, the resulting ratio would be $\frac{24 \text{ mEq/L}}{0.6 \text{ mEq/L}}$ or 40:1. The log of 40 is 1.6, and the subsequent pH would be 7.70. Similarly, if a metabolic acidosis reduced the bicarbonate ion from 24 mEq/L to 12 mEq/L, the ratio would be 12:1.2 or 10:1, and the pH value would be 7.1. If a metabolic alkalosis acutely raised the bicarbonate ion concentration from 24 mEq/L to 36 mEq/L, the ratio of bicarbonate to carbon dioxide gas would be 30:1, and the subsequent pH would be log 30 = 1.47 + 6.1 = pH 7.57.

Thus far, these derangements (Figure 8-1) have been discussed as if they took place in isolation, but combined respiratory and nonrespiratory problems often occur. These problems occur randomly depending on the pathologic processes occurring in the body. Thus besides the four single acid-base derangements, there are combined acid-base derangements: (1) respiratory acidosis and metabolic acidosis, (2) respiratory acidosis and metabolic alkalosis, (3) respiratory alkalosis and metabolic acidosis, and (4) respiratory alkalosis and metabolic alkalosis. The combined acidoses or combined alkaloses have a cumulative effect on the pH, whereas an acidosis and alkalosis combination tends to negate the effects of each on the pH value.

COMPENSATION

Acid-base homeostasis maintains the pH value near the normal range. Thus if there is a derangement in either the respiratory or nonrespiratory acid-base system, the other system will become "deranged" in the opposite direction in an attempt to balance the primary process. Compensation occurs when the body attempts to balance one pathophysiologic process with a second pathophysiologic process, which opposes the pH effect of the first process.

For example, any respiratory process that leads to retention of carbon dioxide (respiratory acidosis) activates a nonrespiratory system (i.e., the kidney retains bicarbonate) to return the pH to normal range. The nonrespiratory compensation is actually a second pathophysiologic process, and the retention of bicarbonate (metabolic alkalosis) counteracts the primary defect (respiratory acidosis). Thus a neonate with an increased $PaCO_2$ and a compensating elevated bicarbonate is both acidotic and alkalotic but has a pH near the normal range.

Metabolic compensations to respiratory processes can go to remarkable extremes, but respiratory compensations to metabolic processes are limited. For example, hyperventilation cannot lower the $PaCO_2$ much below 8 to 10 mm Hg. Similarly, hypoventilation (in the presence of an intact central nervous system [CNS]) in compensation for a metabolic alkalosis is severely limited by the onset of hypoxemia. Hypoxemia, of course, stimulates the respiratory drive, overriding the compensatory hypoventilation, resulting in the alkalemia continuing unabated.

CORRECTION

Correction of an acid-base disturbance occurs when the pathophysiologic process is detected and the health care provider directs therapy at the primary pathologic process, rather than counterbalancing it with a second pathologic process.

For example, if a respiratory acidosis is present, the clinician assesses the patient to discover the cause for the carbon dioxide retention and directs therapy at improving the ventilatory capacity of the lung, rather than attempting to increase the retention of bicarbonate.

Oxygenation

The remaining components of the blood gas analysis are the PO_2, hemoglobin, and oxygen saturation. Oxygenation is distinct from, although correlated to, ventilation. As previously stated, the $PaCO_2$ correlates inversely to ventilation, whereas other factors besides ventilation influence oxygenation. What is important is the degree of hypoxia at the tissue level. Tissue hypoxia is caused by many factors, including the ability of the lung to oxygenate the blood (arterial hypoxemia).

Another cause of tissue hypoxia is interference with oxygen delivery to the tissue, such as that seen in congestive heart failure (venous hypoxemia). In this situation the PaO_2 may be normal, but because of heart (pump) failure, oxygen is not delivered to the tissue and treatment should be directed toward improving delivery by the pump (Chapter 18).

A third cause of tissue hypoxia may result from a decrease in oxygen content (which occurs with anemia). In this instance the heart and lungs work adequately, so the PaO_2 is normal, but there is insufficient hemoglobin to provide an adequate amount of oxygen.

Finally, tissue hypoxia may result from an abnormal affinity of the oxygen to the hemoglobin molecule. The heart and lungs are performing properly, but inadequate oxygen amounts are at the tissue level because of the abnormal affinity. Fetal hemoglobin has a greater affinity for oxygen than adult hemoglobin and thus requires a lower tissue PO_2 to release comparable amounts of oxygen molecules from the hemoglobin (see Figure 6-1).

Because PaO_2 only measures partial pressure of oxygen in the arterial blood (i.e., measures the amount of dissolved oxygen gas in the blood), it reflects how the lung is working but does not measure tissue oxygenation. Despite oxygenation complexities at the tissue level, the PaO_2 taken with the clinical assessment of tissue perfusion is probably an adequate and accurate reflection of tissue oxygenation. In a few instances hemoglobin determination may be needed for assessing the etiology of tissue hypoxia.

Because respiratory disease is an important aspect of neonatal care, the PaO_2 is frequently measured. Most tissue oxygenation problems are directly related to a respiratory problem rather than to oxygen delivery, oxygen content, or hemoglobin affinity problems. A high PaO_2 can be as dangerous as a low PaO_2. Retrolental fibroplasia has been related to arterial oxygen tensions greater than 100 mm Hg and is directly related to PaO_2 but not to the FIO_2 (see Chapter 17).

Cyanotic congenital heart disease has a fixed shunt that does not allow the PaO_2 to rise when supplemental oxygen is given; thus a low PaO_2 is not related to lung disease. In respiratory distress, hypoxemia because of intrapulmonary shunting or ventilation and perfusion inequality can be overcome by increasing the inspired oxygen tension.

To perform the "shunt test," place a neonate with hypoxemia in 100% oxygen; if the PaO_2 rises to more than 150 mm Hg pressure, cyanotic congenital heart disease is unlikely.

Theoretically, in the normal lung with matched ventilation and perfusion, the alveolar (PAO_2) and the arterial oxygen tension (PaO_2) should be equal. This ideal situation is never obtained, and a difference (gradient) in gas tension exists between the alveolar oxygen tension (PAO_2) and the arterial oxygen tension (PaO_2). The gradient is created by an inequality in ventilation and perfusion, the functional intrapulmonary shunt, and the anatomic shunt. The alveolar-arterial oxygen gradient $D(A\text{-}a)O_2$ is useful to estimate the degree of pulmonary involvement in hypoxemia. The difference between the value of the alveolar oxygen and arterial oxygen tensions should be less than 20. The $D(A\text{-}a)O_2$ will be greater than 20 in pulmonary disease.

To calculate the alveolar-arterial oxygen difference:

(1)

$$D(A\text{-}a)O_2 = PAO_2 - PaO_2$$

Substitute the calculation of alveolar oxygen tension:

(2)

$$D(A\text{-}a)O_2 = \left(PIO_2 - \frac{PaCO_2}{RQ} \right) - PaO_2$$

Substitute the calculation of inspired oxygen tension:

(3)

$$D(A\text{-}a)O_2 = \left[(PB - 47)\, FIO_2 - \frac{PaCO_2}{RQ} \right] - PaO_2$$

The arterial PaO_2 is measured by blood gas analysis. The alveolar PAO_2 is calculated by first determining the inspiratory PO_2, which is the barometric pressure minus the water vapor pressure multiplied by the fraction of the inspired oxygen.

To calculate the inspired oxygen tension:

(4)

$$PIO_2 = (PB - PH_2O)\, FIO_2$$

BUT

$$PH_2O = 47$$

THUS

$$PIO_2 = (PB - 47)\, FIO_2$$

Thus the inspired oxygen pressure when one is breathing room air at sea level is $760 - 47(0.21) = 150$ mm Hg. The alveolar oxygen is equal to the inspired oxygen minus the alveolar carbon dioxide divided by the respiratory quotient (RQ). Clinically, the alveolar carbon dioxide is equal to the arterial carbon dioxide, and RQ is 0.8.

To calculate the alveolar oxygen tension:

(5)

$$PAO_2 = PIO_2 - \frac{PACO_2}{RQ}$$

BUT

$$PACO_2 = PaCO_2$$

AND

$$RQ = 0.8$$

THUS

$$PAO_2 = PIO_2 - \frac{PaCO_2}{0.8}$$

Therefore when one is breathing room air at sea level with a $PaCO_2$ of 40 mm Hg, the alveolar oxygen pressure is equal to the PIO_2 (150 mm Hg) minus 40 divided by 0.8 (which is 50), or 100 mm Hg. The alveolar-arterial oxygen gradient in an infant with a PaO_2 of 160 mm Hg and a $PaCO_2$ of 40 mm Hg in an atmosphere of 40% oxygen at sea level is 75 mm Hg.

$$D(A\text{-}a)O_2 = \left[(760 - 47)\, 0.4 - \frac{40}{0.8} \right] - 160 = 75$$

The alveolar-arterial oxygen gradient is useful in predicting the FIO_2 required to result in a desired PaO_2. Working from a known $D(A\text{-}a)O_2$ and rearranging equation 3:

(6)

$$FIO_2 = \frac{D(A\text{-}a)O_2 + PaCO_2 + PaO_2}{(PB - 47)}$$

For example, to obtain a PaO_2 of 90 mm Hg in an infant with an alveolar-arterial gradient of 75 mm Hg and a $PaCO_2$ of 40 mm Hg at sea level, an atmosphere of 30% oxygen ($FIO_2 = 0.3$) is required.

$$FIO_2 = \frac{75 + \dfrac{40}{0.8} + 90}{(760 - 47)} = 0.3$$

Knowledge of the $D(A\text{-}a)O_2$ can help the clinician adjust the arterial oxygen concentration by working the equation backward (equation 6). Thus if the alveolar-arterial gradient is known, an FIO_2 on the ventilator can be determined that will predict a desired PaO_2.

Equation 6 can be simplified. The rule of seven states: the estimated percentage change in inspired oxygen is equal to the desired change in PaO_2 divided by 7.

(7)

$$\%O_2 \text{ change} = \frac{\text{New } PaO_2 - \text{Old } PaO_2}{7}$$

For example, to obtain a PaO_2 of 90 mm Hg in an infant with a PaO_2 of 160 mm hg, a reduction of 10% inspired oxygen is required.

$$\%O_2 \text{ change} = \frac{90 - 160}{7} = \frac{-70}{7} = -10\%$$

SATURATION

Saturation is defined as the percentage of hemoglobin that combines with oxygen. Oxygen binding with hemoglobin increases as the partial pressure of oxygen increases but not linearly. The oxygen dissociation curve is a measure of the affinity that hemoglobin has for oxygen (Figure 8-2).

The "30-60-90" rule is useful in remembering percent saturation and reconstructing the hemoglobin dissociation curve if required (Figure 8-2). At a PaO_2 of 30 mm Hg, the oxygen saturation is 60%; at a PaO_2 of 60 mm Hg, saturation is 90%; and at 90 mm Hg, PaO_2 is 95% saturated. At a normal venous oxygen tension of 40 mm Hg, the oxygen saturation is 75%.

Factors that affect this affinity include temperature, pH, and hemoglobin structure. Hypothermia, alkalemia, hypocapnea, and fetal hemoglobin increase the affinity of hemoglobin for oxygen (shift the curve to the left), whereas

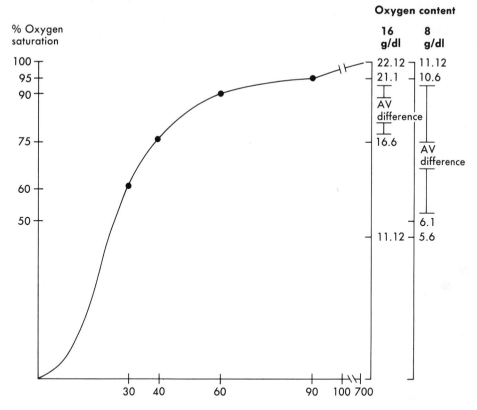

Figure 8-2. Oxygen hemoglobin dissociation curve; 30-60-90 rule is demonstrated. *Right,* Oxygen content for hemoglobin concentration of 16 and 8 g/dl is given, demonstrating effect of anemia on venous saturation and tissue Po_2.

fever, acidemia, and hypercapnea decrease the affinity of hemoglobin for oxygen (shift the curve to the right). At a given tissue Po_2, an increased affinity for oxygen releases less oxygen at the tissue level, whereas a decreased affinity releases more oxygen to the tissue. Alternately, the Po_2 at which the hemoglobin is 50% saturated (the P_{50}) is low when the hemoglobin affinity is great and higher when the hemoglobin affinity is low.

CONTENT

Oxygen content is calculated from the hemoglobin saturation and hemoglobin concentration. One gram of hemoglobin binds 1.39 cc of oxygen. The oxygen content in cubic centimeters per deciliter is the product of the saturation percentage and the hemoglobin in grams per deciliter plus the amount of dissolved oxygen. For clinical purposes the amount of dissolved oxygen in plasma can be neglected because it is only 0.003 cc/dl/mm Hg.

Oxygen content becomes critical in anemia, which can cause a significant derangement in tissue oxygenation. An infant with a hemoglobin of 8 g/dl will have one half the oxygen content of an infant with a hemoglobin of 16 g/dl at an equivalent percentage saturation. In

Figure 8-2, an infant with 16 g hemoglobin that is 95% saturated (PaO_2 = 90 mm Hg) carries 21.1 cc/dl oxygen, whereas the infant with 8 g hemoglobin carries 10.6 cc/dl oxygen. Approximately 4 to 5 cc/dl oxygen is required by the tissues for metabolism. Therefore venous blood contains 4 to 5 cc/dl oxygen less than the arterial blood. The venous oxygen content in an infant with 16 g hemoglobin would be between 16 and 17 (21.1 − 4.5 = 16.6), which corresponds to approximately 75% saturation (16.6/22.24 = 74.6%) or a PvO_2 of 40 mm Hg. However, the venous oxygen content in the infant with 8 g hemoglobin would be 6.1 cc/dl oxygen (10.6 − 4.5 = 6.1). The 55% saturation corresponds to PO_2 of less than 30, indicating tissue hypoxia, as compared with the infant with 16 g/dl hemoglobin.

BLOOD FLOW

The total amount of oxygen in arterial blood is determined by the product of oxygen content (CaO_2) and the blood flow. The total blood flow (Qt) can be divided into the amount of blood in the pulmonary capillaries (Qc) and in the shunt (Qs). The degree of shunting can be calculated by knowing the venous oxygen content, arterial oxygen content, and oxygen content in the pulmonary capillaries exposed to ventilated alveoli:

(8)

$$\frac{Qs}{Qt} = \frac{CcO_2 - CaO_2}{CcO_2 - CvO_2}$$

A shunt occurs when blood passes from the systemic venous to the systemic arterial circulation without receiving oxygen, because of anatomic defects in the heart (such as cyanotic congenital heart disease) or because of blood perfusing alveoli that are not ventilated (such as intrapulmonary shunts). Shunts lower the final arterial oxygen saturation. The usual degree of shunt in the newborn is 15% to 20% of the cardiac output.

The oxygen saturation can determine the percentage of the shunt. (The equation is usually derived in terms of oxygen content, but for clinical purposes dealing with the saturation is adequate.)

(9)

$$\frac{Qs}{Qt} = \frac{ScO_2 - SaO_2}{ScO_2 - SvO_2} \times 100$$

Venous and arterial saturation can be calculated from venous and arterial blood gases, and the pulmonary capillary saturation can be estimated from the calculated alveolar oxygen tension (see equation 5). Calculation of the shunt helps distinguish lung disease from congenital heart disease or helps document changes in the severity of lung disease.

ETIOLOGY
Acid-base homeostasis

Ventilation is usually defined as the amount of gas leaving the mouth per units of time (e.g., minute ventilation, $\dot{V}E$). Minute ventilation is equal to the product of the tidal volume (VT) and the respiratory frequency in breaths per minute:

$$\dot{V}E = VT \times f$$

The tidal volume can be divided into (1) the gas in the airway plus the gas in nonperfused alveoli (physiologic dead space, VD), and (2) the gas in the alveolar space, which is involved in gas exchange (alveolar volume, VA). Therefore:

(1)

$$\dot{V}E = (VD + VA)f$$

OR

(2)

$$\dot{V}E = \dot{V}D + \dot{V}A$$

Alveolar ventilation ($\dot{V}A = \dot{V}E - \dot{V}D$) is measured by collecting the volume of expired gas ($\dot{V}E$) and measuring the concentration of carbon dioxide gas in the expired volume ($FECO_2$) and the arterial carbon dioxide tension ($PaCO_2$) and a constant:

$$\dot{V}A = \frac{\dot{V}E(FECO_2)}{PaCO_2} \times K = \frac{VCO_2(k)}{PaCO_2}$$

Thus the $PaCO_2$ is inversely related to alveolar ventilation.

An acid-base disturbance in the respiratory system (a change in PCO_2) is caused by a derangement in alveolar ventilation. In a respiratory acidosis when carbon dioxide excretion is below normal, several conditions must be considered. The most common cause of carbon dioxide retention is obstructive lung disease. Meconium aspiration is a common cause of obstructive lung disease in the neonate, and transient tachypnea of the newborn is an obstructive lung disease. Obstructive lung disease is found in the recovery phase of uncomplicated respiratory distress syndrome and in bronchopulmonary dysplasia. Alveolar ventilation is decreased in these conditions by increasing physiologic dead space that occurs with (1) debris in the large and small airways, (2) inflammation in the large and small airways, and (3) ventilation and perfusion mismatch. An increase in dead space leads to carbon dioxide retention.

Another major cause of carbon dioxide retention is poor respiratory effort from (1) narcosis because of maternal anesthesia before delivery, (2) depressed respiratory drive because of sepsis, (3) severe intracranial hemorrhage, including intraventricular hemorrhage, or (4) metabolic disturbances, such as hypoglycemia, affecting the respiratory center.

The third cause involves injuries or changes in the thoracic cage, such as diaphragmatic hernia, phrenic nerve paralysis, or pneumothorax, and results in a derangement in alveolar ventilation, which decreases in phrenic nerve paralysis and pneumothorax because of a decline in tidal volume, respiratory rate, or a combination of these.

In respiratory alkalosis the carbon dioxide excretion is greater than normal. The mechanism for this increased excretion is hyperventilation. Respiratory alkalosis because of hyperventilation may be (1) iatrogenic, resulting from vigorous ventilator therapy in a neonate with respiratory disease, (2) a result of restrictive lung disease, such as early respiratory distress syndrome, (3) caused by central nervous system stimulation of the respiratory drive (i.e., high altitude and encephalitis), and (4) present in hypoxemia, which stimulates the respiratory centers through chemoreceptors.

In nonrespiratory (metabolic) acidosis the metabolic component either results from adding nonvolatile acid (an acid other than carbon dioxide) or losing base bicarbonate. Abnormal acids that are associated with diseases are lactic acid in hypoxia, organic acids in renal failure, and ketoacids in diabetic acidosis. Loss of base occurs in renal tubular acidosis (a defect in the ability of the renal tubules to reabsorb bicarbonate), diarrhea with loss of bicarbonate in the feces, or through urinary excretion resulting from the effects of certain drugs, such as acetazolamide (Diamox).

Nonrespiratory (metabolic) alkalosis is due to either a loss of acid or adding base, principally bicarbonate. Adding bicarbonate is most likely iatrogenic. Loss of acid occurs with nasogastric suctioning or severe vomiting, which may occur in pyloric stenosis. Acid loss also occurs from the kidney through the influence of certain drugs such as diuretics, digitalis therapy, and corticosteroids, which preferentially excrete sodium and potassium, causing depletion. Thus a hydrogen ion is substituted in the urine to conserve sodium or potassium. Acid is lost because of the hydrogen ion excretion, the base remains, and the body fluids become alkaline.

Oxygenation

Although tissue hypoxia may be caused by delivery system failure (heart failure), anemia, abnormal hemoglobin affinity for oxygen, and a decreased PaO_2, hypoxemia results from only lung disease or cyanotic congenital heart disease. The most common abnormality of the lung leading to hypoxemia is mismatched ventilation and perfusion. Perfect matching of ventilation and perfusion takes place when an adequate amount of blood flows past oxygenated and ventilated alveoli, but this ideal situation rarely occurs, and there is always some degree of ventilation and perfusion mismatch. Two extreme examples of mismatch are (1) ventilated and oxygenated alveoli without perfusion (e.g., pulmonary emboli) and (2) the well-perfused but nonventilated alveoli (atelectasis). The former is an example of wasted ventilation (V/Q = infinity), and the latter is an example of a shunt (V/Q = O). Either extreme of ventilation and perfusion abnormality is incompatible with life if it is extensive, and thus the degree of ventilation and perfusion mismatch is somewhere between the ends of the spectrum.

Hypoxemia because of ventilation and perfusion mismatch can be overcome by administering supplemental inspired oxygen. In spite of poorly ventilated alveoli, raising the inspired oxygen tension will wash nitrogen from the alveoli, resulting in a higher alveolar oxygen tension, which increases artery oxygen tension. In a shunt, however, no oxygen is exposed to any of the shunted blood, and the PaO_2 cannot increase.

Central hypoventilation from narcosis may cause hypoxemia. As the alveolar carbon dioxide rises, the PAO_2 falls, and subsequently PaO_2 decreases. However, this condition should be clinically evident and should not be confused with lung or congenital heart disease. Other causes of hypoxemia are sufficiently rare in the infant that they need only be mentioned: decreased inspired oxygen tension, which may occur at high altitude, and oxygen diffusion limitations.

Most conditions that were thought to be diffusion limited actually are caused by ventilation and perfusion mismatch. The oxygen molecule must diffuse from the alveolus across the alveolar cell, an interstitial space, the capillary endothelial cell, and the plasma to the red blood cell. A pathologic condition may occur that interferes with the diffusion process (e.g., thickening of the interstitial space). These processes, however, do not affect oxygen diffusion as much as they alter ventilation

and perfusion relationships. Consequently, the hypoxemia is caused by the abnormal ventilation and perfusion relationship rather than diffusion limitation.

PREVENTION

Perinatal asphyxia has profound effects on neonatal oxygenation, involving the following factors: (1) decreased inspired oxygen tension, (2) aggravated ventilation and perfusion mismatch (increased intrapulmonary shunt) and anatomic shunt through the ductus arteriosus and foramen ovale, (3) decreased cardiac output through asphyxic cardiomyopathy, and (4) decreased oxygen affinity by shifting the oxygen dissociation curve to the right during asphyxic acidemia that resulted from combined metabolic and respiratory acidosis.

Prevention of acid-base and oxygenation disturbances and maintenance of acid-base homeostasis require attention to detail. Prevention of premature births or transport of pregnant women who may deliver a high-risk infant to tertiary care centers can minimize perinatal asphyxia. Prompt and efficient resuscitation measures can also significantly improve the survival rate of premature infants with acid-base and oxygenation problems.

With respiratory disturbances, immediate assessment and prompt therapy, including supplemental inspired oxygen and assisted ventilation when indicated, minimize the respiratory component of acid-base and oxygenation disturbances (see Chapter 17). Careful monitoring of fluid intake and output, minimizing blood loss, observing for sepsis, and monitoring urine electrolytes for potential abnormalities will enable the clinician to control the continuous nonrespiratory conditions and ideally prevent development of nonrespiratory acid-base disturbances.

Monitoring inspired oxygen tensions and arterial oxygen tensions and supplying appropriate concentrations of additional inspired oxygen will prevent low arterial oxygen tensions

(see Chapter 17). The monitoring may be accomplished intermittently through indwelling arterial catheters or continuously through transcutaneous oxygen monitors (see Chapter 6). Monitoring the hemoglobin concentration and blood loss with replacement to an adequate hemoglobin concentration ensures a potentially adequate oxygen content. Careful attention to fluids, electrolytes, and acid-base homeostasis minimizes adverse effects of asphyxic cardiomyopathy by reducing the strain of the heart.

DATA COLLECTION

History, physical examination, and laboratory data augment each other in assessing disturbances in acid-base homeostasis and oxygenation (see outline below).

Evaluation of acid-base disturbances and oxygenation problems in the neonate

I. History
   A. Obstetric and perinatal
   B. Neonatal
   C. Family
II. Physical examination
   A. Vital signs
   B. General appearance
   C. Respiratory effort
   D. Pulmonary examination
   E. Cardiac examination
   F. Abdominal examination
   G. Neurologic examination
III. Laboratory
   A. Chest x-ray film
   B. Arterial blood gases
   C. Urinalysis
   D. In selected cases: sepsis evaluation, urine electrolytes, and serum electrolytes

History

An adequate obstetric and perinatal history may warn of potential acid-base and oxygenation disturbances:

- Premature delivery predisposes the infant to shock and respiratory distress.
- Meconium staining may indicate respiratory difficulties.
- Prolonged rupture of membranes, infants of diabetic mothers, or abnormal maternal bleeding may be associated with either metabolic or respiratory acid-base disturbances and hypoxemia.
- A neonatal history of vomiting, diarrhea, or other gastrointestinal disturbances can cause acid-base disturbances.
- The infant's general appearance, feeding habits, and activity level may indicate sepsis or CNS injury, both of which promote acid-base disturbances and hypoxemia.
- Nosocomial infections and pneumonia may significantly influence acid-base and oxygen disturbances.
- A family history of inherited renal problems such as tubular acidosis may suggest an acid-base disturbance.
- A family history of salt-losing endocrinopathies may produce an acid-base disturbance.

Signs and symptoms

Signs of acid-base disturbance vary widely and are often undetected. Vital signs that show hypothermia and low blood pressure reflect metabolic derangements in acid-base homeostasis. Respiratory rate and pattern, grunting, flaring, and retracting indicate respiratory derangements of acid-base homeostasis and oxygenation. Abnormal auscultation of the chest or heart may suggest present or future acid-base or oxygenation disturbances, including possible congenital heart disease. Examining the abdomen, particularly for the proper number and size of kidneys, is important in assessing potential acid-base disturbances. Lethargy, seizures, generalized neurologic signs, or focal neurologic signs increase concern about either potential respiratory or metabolic acid-base disturbances or hypoxemia.

Laboratory data

A chest x-ray examination may demonstrate a respiratory cause for acid-base disturbance and hypoxemia.

URINALYSIS

The routine urinalysis records urine specific gravity and demonstrates that urine is being produced.

ARTERIAL BLOOD GASES

The assessment of the arterial blood gas will point to the primary acid-base derangement, and may reveal a secondary compensation and define the degree of hypoxemia. Although the pathophysiologic condition of the acid-base disturbance is determined through the analysis of arterial blood gases, further assessment of the infant is required:

1. Respiratory alkalosis or acidosis should be evident from the physical examination, arterial blood gas analysis, and chest x-ray examination.
2. Consider shock and sepsis in metabolic acidosis. Urine electrolytes may provide additional information to delineate causes. Blood pressure measurement, a complete blood cell count, serum and urine electrolyte and glucose determinations, and assessment of intake and output of fluids are necessary to assess a metabolic disturbance.
3. Oxygenation disturbances may be analyzed from the preceding laboratory tests, and when indicated, electrocardiogram and arterial blood gas responses to increased inspired oxygen concentration are used to evaluate the possibility of cyanotic congenital heart disease.

TREATMENT

In respiratory acidosis, the pathophysiologic condition is hypoventilation, which is associated with hypoxemia. Treatment is directed at the underlying cause. Where primary lung disease exists, ventilatory assistance must be provided. Hypoxemia, because of ventilation and perfusion mismatch in respiratory disease, is treated with increased inspired oxygen concentration or ventilatory support including constant positive airway pressure (see Chapter 17).

Asphyxia often leads to a combined respiratory and metabolic acidosis. Ventilation will resolve the respiratory acidosis, and the improved oxygenation may allow the lactic acidosis to resolve without bicarbonate therapy. In narcosis, temporary ventilatory support may be required. The narcosis may be reversed with naloxone (Narcan) at a dose of 0.01 mg/kg. (Repeated doses may be required; see Chapter 3.)

The other acidoses and alkaloses must have a careful search for the causes, with therapy directed toward them. This may require drug therapy, replacement of losses, or surgical correction of abnormalities.

COMPLICATIONS

The outcome of unrecognized and untreated acid-base or oxygenation disturbances may be an increased mortality or an increased morbidity in the survivors. Complications of the correction of the acid-base and oxygenation disturbance vary according to the disturbance and treatment provided.

The major effect of acidosis on the body is CNS depression. In metabolic acidosis the rate and depth of respiration are increased, whereas in respiratory acidosis respiration is depressed. The major effect of alkalosis on the body is increased excitability of the CNS and tetany (often of the respiratory muscles).

Respiratory acidosis with treatment by assisted ventilation can produce all of the complications of assisted ventilation, including infection, trauma, oxygen toxicity, sepsis, air leak, subglottic stenosis, and others (see Chapter 17).

Complications of oxygen therapy include the risks of hypoxemia and hyperoxemia. Immediate effects of hypoxia include pulmonary vasoconstriction, a change from aerobic to anaerobic metabolism (with eventual metabolic acidosis), cyanosis, bradycardia, hypotonia, and decreases in CNS and cardiac functions. Prolonged high inspired oxygen concentrations increase pulmonary morbidity through pulmonary oxygen toxicity and contribute to retrolental fibroplasia. If ventilatory support is required to attain adequate oxygenation, the complications are those of ventilator therapy (see Chapter 17).

•   •   •

Maintenance of acid-base homeostasis and oxygenation significantly improves the survival of a critically ill neonate. Understanding arterial blood gases and the acid-base balance provides the clinician with the foundation for prevention, early identification, and prompt treatment of acid-base and oxygenation problems.

SELECTED READINGS

Avery ME, Fletcher BD, and Williams RG: The lung and its disorders in the newborn infant, ed 4, vol 1, Major problems in clinical pediatrics, Philadelphia, 1981, WB Saunders Co.

Duc G: Assessment of hypoxia, Pediatrics 48:469, 1971.

Shapiro BA: Clinical application of blood gases, ed 2, Chicago, 1980, Year Book Medical Publishers, Inc.

Spearman C and Sheldon R: Fundamentals of respiratory therapy, ed 4, St Louis, 1982, The CV Mosby Co.

Thebault DW and Gregory GA: Neonatal pulmonary care, Menlo Park, Calif, 1979, Addison-Wesley Publishing Co.

Tisi GM: Pulmonary physiology in clinical medicine, Baltimore, 1980, Williams & Wilkins.

West JB: Respiratory physiology: the essentials, ed 2, Baltimore, 1979, Williams & Wilkins.

PART II

Nutritional and Metabolic Care of the Neonate

CHAPTER 9

Neonatal nutrition

JOSEPH W. KAEMPF · CORALIE BONNABEL · WILLIAM W. HAY, JR.

Nutrition can be defined as the taking in of materials necessary for the body's metabolic requirements of growth, replacement, and energy production. Good nutrition in the neonate implies a diet that provides for normal growth, development, and body composition—one that not only promotes a state of good health, but may actively inhibit disease. Neonatal nutrition also has a unique qualitative aspect—the powerful psychologic interplay between mother and infant during feeding that constitutes nurturing.

The focus of this chapter is twofold: first, to present an overview of the physiology of growth, gastrointestinal function, and nutritional requirements in preterm infants and, second, to discuss various feeding regimens with special emphasis on the unique problems that challenge the clinician trying to provide good nutrition to the preterm or sick newborn.

PHYSIOLOGY
Growth

Growth is the fundamental characteristic of fetal and neonatal life. Growth is not simply the accumulation of mass, but also consists of the development of function. The determinants of growth are not completely understood. Genetic, placental, environmental, and nutritional factors all play important roles. From a nutritional standpoint, maternal weight gain during pregnancy is well correlated with fetal growth rate.[22,31] The quality of the maternal diet in terms of the intake of protein, calories, and other nutrients directly affects fetal growth.[22,27] The pregnant woman subjected to significant dietary deprivation does not adapt to sustain fetal growth, but rather to protect her own nutrient stores.[29] In most circumstances, however, there is a large maternal reserve of nutrients available to the fetus, and maternal diet is not the rate-limiting factor in growth.

Placental size is a major determinant of fetal growth. However, at a given placental size (as measured by weight), small, average, and large fetal weight groups are quite discrete, suggesting that factors other than placental size influence fetal growth[26] (Figure 9-1). Both morphologic and transport studies of the placenta show an increasing capacity for diffusion of nutrients through term. Thus the decrease in fetal growth rate toward term (36 to 42 weeks) appears to be a biologic phenomenon mediated by developmental factors within the fetus. The major factor is probably endocrine, but the mechanisms are not known. The most influential fetal growth–promoting hormone is insulin.[14] Apancreatic infants are among the most growth retarded of all babies (Figure 9-2), whereas anencephalic infants and panhypopituitary dwarfs are near normal in age-specific size at birth. In contrast, infants of diabetic mothers, responding with high insulin secretion to elevated glucose concentrations, are among the largest of human newborns (Figure 9-3).

Most clinicians agree that the postnatal growth of premature infants should approximate normal intrauterine growth rates, of which we have several standards (Figure 9-4; see also Figure 4-13). However, it may be inappropriate to apply these intrauterine standards to extrauterine life, given that the premature

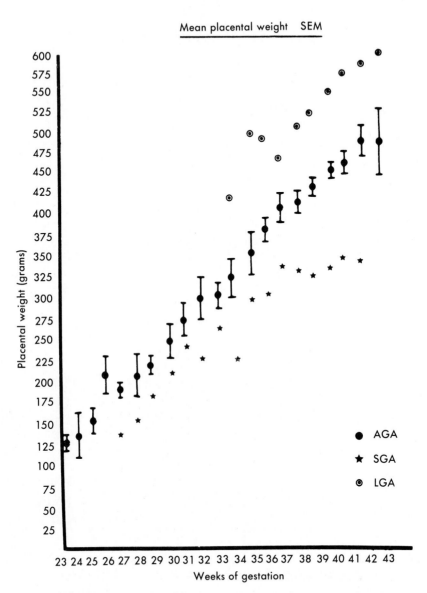

Figure 9-1. Mean placental weights for appropriate-for-gestational-age (AGA), small-for-gestational-age (SGA), and large-for-gestational-age (LGA) infants at each gestational age (±SEM given for AGA infants only). (From Molteni RA et al: J Reprod Med 21:327, 1978.)

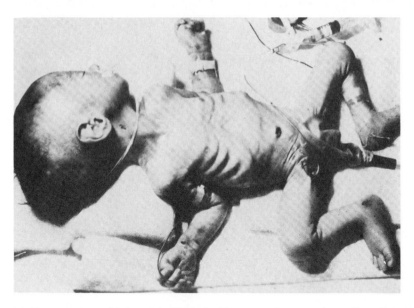

Figure 9-2. Term newborn (birth weight 1280 g) with pancreatic agenesis confirmed at autopsy. Plasma insulin was absent. Note marked deficiency of adipose tissue and muscle development. (Reproduced by permission from Hill D: Semin Perinatol 2:319-328, 1978.)

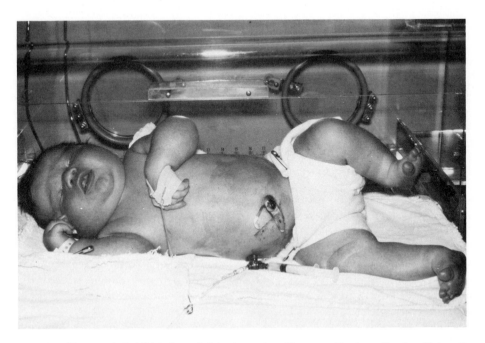

Figure 9-3. Characteristic LGA infant of diabetic mother. (Courtesy Newborn Service, University of Colorado Health Sciences Center, Denver.)

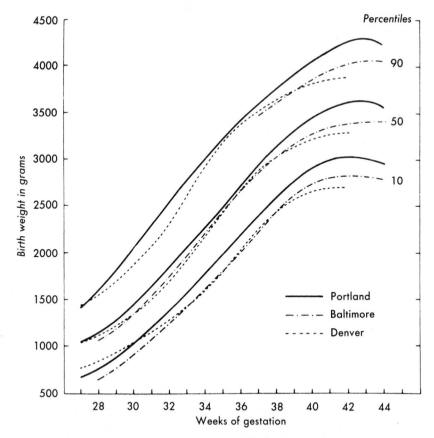

Figure 9-4. Comparisons of fetal weight curves for different populations in United States. These growth curves suggest that maternal socioeconomic status and race may influence fetal growth rate as much as altitude. (From Babson SG et al: Pediatrics 45:937, 1970. Reproduced by permission of Pediatrics.)

infant must use his or her own metabolic and gastrointestinal functions to process the diet and must face multiple energy-consuming challenges from which the fetus is protected (temperature maintenance, resistance to gravity, breathing). It is more important to assess and evaluate the infant's growth combining several parameters. Daily weight and weekly head circumference and length should be plotted on a graph similar to Figure 9-5. Caloric and water intake can be recorded in a similar fashion

using this chart. This information combined with biochemical parameters (serum electrolytes, hemoglobin, total protein, albumin) and the physical examination provide the best overall picture of an infant's growth.

Clinical measurements of growth and adequate nutrition include:

1. Measure weight daily.
   a. Use the same scale, amount of clothing, and "equipment."
   b. Keep a nursery catalog of average

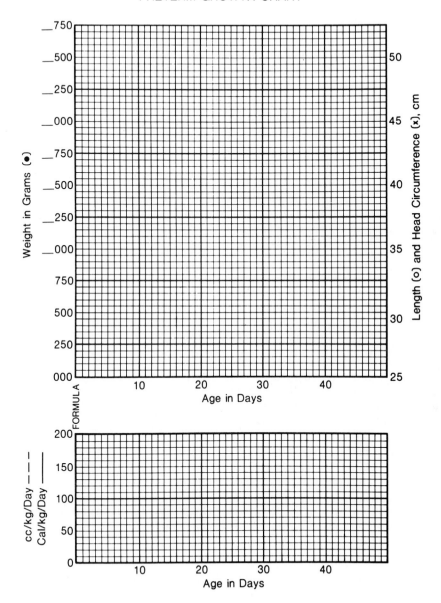

PRETERM GROWTH CHART

Figure 9-5. Preterm infant growth chart allowing simultaneous comparison of diet, fluid intake, total caloric intake, weight, length, and head circumference.

weights of "equipment" such as diapers, IV boards, tubing, syringes, and articles of clothing.

c. Weigh at the same time each day, preferably before a feeding.

d. Many scales are accurate to only ±10 g, which may be the weight of a stool, a urine-soaked diaper, or the average daily weight gain.

2. Measure the length and head circumference weekly and plot with weight on intrauterine growth curves (see Figure 4-13).

a. With the baby lying flat, measure length from the top of the head to the bottom of the heel (foot flexed 90 degrees at the ankle) with the legs held extended.

b. The head circumference is the largest measurement around the frontal parietooccipital axis.

c. The ponderal (weight-length) index should be followed weekly to assess the quality of growth. Weight gain without an increase in length or head circumference is usually edema or excessive fat deposition. True organ growth is related to length increase, not just weight gain. Ponderal index = (100 × weight in grams) divided by (length in centimeters cubed).

d. The triceps skinfold thickness and midarm or midthigh circumference are poorly defined for growing preterm infants, but sequential measurements on a given infant may be useful for trending.

3. Weekly serum electrolytes, calcium, phosphorus, total protein, albumin, and hemoglobin should be monitored to prevent specific deficiencies in the diet. Biweekly alkaline phosphatase should be checked in the very low birth weight (VLBW) infant at risk for osteopenia. Hypoproteinemia in premature infants must be assessed against the low protein concentra-

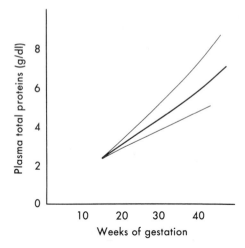

Figure 9-6. Approximate regression line for 95% confidence limits for plasma total proteins in human cord blood of infants appropriately sized for gestational age but delivered at different gestational ages. (Data from Baum D et al: Biol Neonate 18:311, 1971; S Karger AG, Basel.)

tions during fetal life that normally increase gradually with advancing gestation[2] (Figure 9-6).

Normal in utero growth averages 20 to 30 g per day in the last 12 weeks of gestation. It is unrealistic to expect the premature infant, especially the sick VLBW infant, to achieve these growth rates in the first 1 to 2 weeks of life. Respiratory disease, cold stress, inability to use the gastrointestinal tract, fluid and electrolyte imbalances, etc., all make it difficult to provide optimal calories and nutrients to the sick premature infant.

Gastrointestinal development and function

The gastrointestinal tract of the premature infant has the remarkable ability to adapt and grow to suit the nutritional and metabolic demands of extrauterine life. Because of the enormity of the respiratory and neurologic problems that beset the VLBW infant, there is a tendency to forget that the gastrointestinal tract is also immature and has several anatomic and functional limitations.

TABLE 9-1

Development of the Gastrointestinal Tract in the Human Fetus: First Appearance of Developmental Markers

Anatomic part	DEVELOPMENTAL MARKER	WEEKS OF GESTATION
Esophagus	Superficial glands develop	20
	Squamous cells appear	28
Stomach	Gastric glands form	14
	Pylorus and fundus defined	14
Pancreas	Differentiation of endocrine and exocrine tissue	14
Liver	Lobules form	11
Small intestine	Crypt and villi develop	14
	Lymph nodes appear	14
Colon	Diameter increases	20
	Villi appear	20
Functional ability		
Suckling and swallowing	Mouthing only	28
	Immature suck-swallow	33-36
Stomach	Gastric motility and secretion	20
Pancreas	Zymogen granules	20
Liver	Bile metabolism	11
	Bile secretion	22
Small intestine	Active transport of amino acids	14
	Glucose transport	18
	Fatty acid absorption	24
Enzymes	Alpha-glucosidases	10
	Dipeptidases	10
	Lactase	10
	Enterokinase	26

From Lebenthal E: Pediatr Ann 16:211, 1987.

Table 9-1 summarizes some important developmental milestones in the fetal gastrointestinal tract.

Protein digestion and absorption are remarkably efficient in the premature infant despite the fact that enterokinase, the rate-limiting enzyme in the activation of pancreatic proteases, has only 10% of the adult activity. Carbohydrate absorption is limited by a relative deficiency of lactase, which splits lactose to glucose and galactose. Lactase in the infant of less than 34 weeks gestation is present at only about 30% of the activity found in the normal term infant. Premature infants may malabsorb 10% to 30% of dietary fat because of a small bile acid pool size and relative lack of pancreatic lipase. An effective suck and swallow do not develop until approximately 34 weeks postconception.[19]

Despite these anatomic and functional shortcomings, there is much to be gained by slow, careful feeding of the premature infant. There is very good evidence to suggest that enteral feeding, above and beyond providing calories and nutrients, may be a trigger for intestinal growth, maturity, and metabolic adaptation. Recent reviews of this subject emphasize the positive, trophic effects of feeding that may be mediated by various gut hormones such as gastrin and enteroglucagon.[15,23] It is probably unwise to deprive the sick premature infant of any enteral feeding for prolonged periods of time unless there is a specific contraindication for feeding, such as necrotizing enterocolitis.

Nutritional requirements
WATER

During the latter half of gestation, the human fetus accumulates water at the rate of about 20 ml/day. Total body water decreases from about 90% to 70% of weight, and its distribution shifts from extracellular to intracellular spaces[4] (Figure 9-7). After birth the extrauterine environment adds several new sources of water loss for the neonate, including skin and respiratory epithelium evaporation, low humidity, increased respiratory rate, and urine and stool losses. Water requirements for the first day of life in healthy term infants are approximately 60 to 70 ml/kg and may increase to 140 to 150 ml/kg/day by the end of the first week. Higher values are occasionally necessary in smaller, preterm infants. **Fluid administration must be individualized according to changes in the infant's weight, urine output, urine specific gravity, serum electrolytes, blood urea nitrogen (BUN), and physical examination.**

CALORIES

The caloric requirements of the human fetus have been calculated from the reported values of fetal oxygen consumption and the composition of new tissue deposited during growth[32]:

Human fetal caloric requirements*

Oxidation	55 kcal/kg/day
Growth	40 kcal/kg/day
TOTAL	95 kcal/kg/day

Human fetal oxygen consumption (8 ml/kg/min) has been estimated from comparative animal physiology studies under nonstressed conditions. The caloric requirements represented by this oxygen consumption would be 56 kcal/kg/day. The

*Modified from Sparks JW et al: Biol Neonate 38:113, 1980.

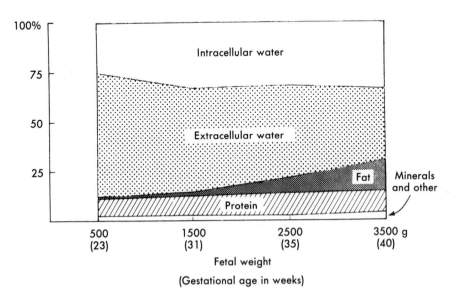

Figure 9-7. Body water, mineral, and nutrient composition of human fetuses in relation to fetal weight and gestational age. (From Dweck HS: Clin Perinatol 2:183, 1975.)

TABLE 9-2

Daily Caloric Requirements for Preterm Infants

CALORIC REQUIREMENT	KCAL/KG/DAY
Basic metabolic rate	35-50
(Day 1)	(35)
(Day 2)	(45)
(Day 28)	(50)
Intermittent activity (highly variable)	15
Occasional cold stress	10
Fecal loss	8
Specific dynamic action (energy cost of digestion and metabolism)	12
Growth	25
TOTAL	105-120

Modified from Sinclair JC et al: Pediatr Clin North Am 17:863, 1970.

TABLE 9-3

Caloric Calculations

A. For growth (120 cal/kg/day)
   1. Baby's weight in kilograms × 120 = calories needed per day.
   2. Ounces needed per day = calories needed per day ÷ number of calories per ounce.
   3. Ounces needed per day × 30 ml/oz = milliliters needed per day.
   4. Number of milliliters per feeding = milliliters per day ÷ number of feedings per day.
B. Twenty-four-hour intake is known. Calculate the number of calories per kilogram per day the baby received:
   1. Milliliter intake over 24 hours × 1 oz/30 ml = number of ounces in 24 hours.
   2. Number of ounces of intake × number of calories per ounce = number of calories taken.
   3. Calories per kilogram per 24 hours = number of calories ÷ weight in kilograms.

caloric requirement for tissue accretion increases from 10 kcal/kg/day at 20 weeks gestation to 40 kcal/kg/day at term, largely because of the deposition of white fat.

The total caloric requirement at birth of 90 to 100 kcal/kg/day decreases during the first day of life to about 50 kcal/kg/day because of the cessation of growth. This requirement progressively increases over several days to 100 to 120 kcal/kg/day with the addition of physical activity, cold stress, specific dynamic action, fecal loss, and growth (Tables 9-2 and 9-3). As with water needs, caloric requirements need to be individualized according to the patient's age, weight, and specific disease processes.

PROTEIN

Protein accretion is critical for optimal growth. It is the net result of two opposing processes: synthesis and degradation. The amount and type of protein necessary for optimal growth in premature infants have been difficult to establish. In fact, an almost trial-and-error series of clinical studies have been performed that have compared the effects of varying quantities of bovine and human milk protein on neonatal growth. Prior to the 1940s human milk was considered the diet of choice for premature infants. Subsequent studies, however, have shown greater growth rates in premature infants fed high-protein, cow's milk formulas as compared with those fed human milk.[3,10] The metabolic cost of this greater growth rate achieved with a high-protein, cow's milk diet has been called into serious question. Studies have shown decreased blood pH, increased BUN, and markedly variable plasma amino acid levels in infants fed high-protein, cow's milk diets. These values were quite different from those on human milk diets.[16,28] Furthermore, lower intellectual functioning has been found in infants fed high-protein, casein-predominant cow's milk formulas.[9,25]

Human milk is a whey-predominant food (whey/casein ratio of 80:20), whereas cow's milk is casein predominant (whey/casein ratio of 18:82). Whey protein is particularly rich in essential amino acids and contains more cystine than cow's milk, an essential amino acid for the newborn. Also, human milk protein is relatively low in tyrosine and phenylalanine, thereby decreasing the chance of hypertyrosinemia and hyperphenyl-alaninemia, which have been associated with lower IQ scores. Taurine is an amino acid that is found in relatively high concentration in human milk but is almost absent from cow's milk. Although taurine is a constituent of bile salts, a specific deficiency state has not been described in humans. However, animal data suggest that taurine plays an important role in neural transmission and retinal development, and it may be important in brain development and growth modulation in humans.[8] Taurine should be included in the diet of the newborn infant.

There are legitimate concerns that mature breast milk may not provide adequate protein for the growing preterm infant. However, there is evidence that milk expressed from mothers of preterm infants is higher in protein ("preterm milk") than milk from mothers of term infants ("mature milk").[20] Furthermore, several studies have shown that premature infants grow at acceptable rates when fed preterm human milk only.[11,12]

In summary, breast milk from an infant's own mother is the preferred source of protein for the premature infant. An intake of 3 to 3.5 g/kg/day (whether the infant receives human milk or formula) should provide for optimal growth. Supplemental protein (e.g., from Human Milk Fortifier*) may need to be added in certain circumstances if there is poor growth and biochemical indicators of inadequate protein intake.

FAT

Human neonates are unique among animals in having a white fat content of 16% to 18% of body weight at term.[32] This fat deposition occurs during the last 12 to 14 weeks of gestation. Brown fat is present in all mammals at birth and serves to maintain body temperature by exothermic triglyceride turnover in response to cold-induced norepinephrine release by sympathetic nerve endings in the brown fat.

*Mead Johnson.

Newborn infants, particularly premature ones, absorb fat less efficiently than older children. Pancreatic lipase and bile acids are less available for fat digestion and absorption.[19] Fat digestion is augmented in the newborn by lingual lipase and mammary lipase (if the infant is receiving breast milk), which considerably improve fat digestion and absorption.[17] Most neonatologists recommend that 40% to 45% of the infant's total caloric intake should be fat, with 3% of the total calories as linoleic acid. Human breast milk contains considerable quantities of linolenic acid, another fatty acid that may be important for the newborn.[12]

Medium-chain triglycerides do not require bile salts for absorption and can be directly absorbed into the portal venous circulation. Although this offers theoretical advantages for the premature infant, there is little evidence that the inclusion of medium-chain triglycerides improves growth in the healthy, feeding premature infant,[35] and their routine use is not recommended. Medium-chain triglycerides can improve fat absorption and energy intake in those infants with hepatic dysfunction or short gut syndrome.

Carnitine is an amine that facilitates the transport of long-chain fatty acids into the mitochondria, where beta-oxidation occurs. The newborn infant has a limited ability to synthesize carnitine, and fatty acid oxidation may be impaired if an exogenous source is not provided. Carnitine deficiency may lead to impaired fat utilization in sick premature infants, particularly those who are maintained on intravenous (IV) fluids and nutrients alone.[13] Human milk and cow's milk formulas contain sufficient carnitine to restore plasma carnitine levels after birth.

CARBOHYDRATE

From as early as the start of the second trimester in many of the organs of the developing fetus, carbohydrate reserves accumulate as glycogen.[30] This glycogen serves local glucose needs (e.g., the heart), and hepatic glycogen is used by other glucose-dependent tissues, primarily the brain. Immediately after birth the neonate relies heavily

TABLE 9-4

Minerals and Trace Elements in Neonatal Nutrition

MINERAL OR ELEMENT	BIOLOGIC ROLE	DEFICIENCY STATE	RECOMMENDED ORAL INTAKE FOR RAPIDLY GROWING PRETERM INFANTS
Sodium	General growth and tissue accretion, body fluid equilibrium, cellular energy and electrical charge balance	Poor growth, fluid imbalance, neurologic dysfunction, lethargy, seizures	3-5 mEq/kg/day
Potassium	General growth and tissue accretion, acid-base balance, cellular energy and electrical charge balance	Myocardial damage, arrhythmia, hypotonia, muscle weakness	2-3 mEq/kg/day
Chloride	General growth and tissue accretion, cellular energy and electrical charge balance	Failure to thrive, muscle weakness, vomiting	3-5 mEq/kg/day
Calcium	Bone and tooth formation, fat absorption, nerve conduction, muscle contraction	Bone demineralization, tetany, arrhythmias, seizures	185-200 mg/kg/day
Phosphorus	Bone and tooth formation, energy transfer compounds	Bone demineralization, weakness	100-140 mg/kg/day
Magnesium	Metalloenzymes, cellular electrical charge balance	Neurologic dysfunction, anorexia, diarrhea, renal disease	5-10 mg/kg/day
Iron	Hemoglobin formation, metalloenzymes	Anemia, pallor, apathy, intellectual dysfunction	2 mg/kg/day after 1-2 months of age
Zinc	Metalloenzymes, DNA-RNA synthesis, wound healing, host defenses	Growth retardation, dermatitis, alopecia, diarrhea, delayed wound healing	1-1.5 mg/kg/day
Copper	Metalloenzymes, protein metabolism	Neurologic dysfunction, anemia, neutropenia, bone demineralization	100-200 μg/kg/day
Manganese	Metalloenzymes, carbohydrate metabolism, antioxidants, hemostasis	Neurologic dysfunction, defects in lipid metabolism, reduced coagulants, animals—growth retardation	10-20 μg/kg/day
Chromium	Carbohydrate metabolism, component of nucleic acids	Impaired glucose tolerance, impaired growth	2-4 μg/kg/day
Selenium	Metalloenzymes, antioxidant	Cardiomyopathy	1.5-2.5 μg/kg/day
Iodine	Thyroid hormone synthesis	Hypothyroidism	1 μg/kg/day
Fluoride	Bone and tooth formation	Dental caries	No need to supplement preterm infants
Molybdenum	Metalloenzymes, purine metabolism	Neurologic and visual dysfunction, animals—growth retardation	2-3 μg/kg/day

Modified from Forbes GB: Pediatric nutrition handbook, Elk Grove Village, Ill, 1985, American Academy of Pediatrics; and Tsang RC, editor: Vitamin and mineral requirements of preterm infants, New York, 1985, Marcel Dekker, Inc.

TABLE 9-5

Vitamins in Neonatal Nutrition

VITAMIN	BIOLOGIC ROLE	DEFICIENCY STATE	RECOMMENDED ORAL REQUIREMENT
Vitamin A (1 IU = 0.3 μg retinol)	Component of visual purple; integrity of epithelial tissues, bone cell function	Night blindness, xerophthalmia, keratomalacia, poor growth, impaired resistance to infection	1400 IU/day
Vitamin D (D_2-activated calciferol; D_3-activated dehydrocholesterol; 1 IU = 0.025 μg)	Formation of calcium transport protein in duodenal mucosa; facilitates bone resorption, phosphorus absorption	Rickets, osteomalacia	400 IU/day
Vitamin E (1 IU = 1 mg of alpha-tocopherol acetate)	Antioxidant, role in red blood cell membrane fragility	Hemolytic anemia in premature infants; associated with edema (?), increased red blood cell osmotic fragility, and thrombocytosis	25 IU/day for first 2-4 weeks, then 5 IU/day
Vitamin K	Blood coagulation: factors II, VII, IX, X	Hemorrhagic manifestations	1 mg at birth (0.5 mg for infants weighing less than 1500 g), then 5 μg/kg/day
Vitamin C (ascorbic acid)	Exact mechanism unknown; functions in folacin metabolism, collagen biosynthesis, iron absorption and transport, tyrosine metabolism	Scurvy	30 mg/100 kcal
Vitamin B_1 (thiamine)	Coenzyme for decarboxylation, other reactions	Beriberi, neuritis, edema, cardiac failure, hoarseness, anorexia, restlessness, aphonia	250 μg/100 kcal

Modified from Forbes GB: Pediatric nutrition handbook, Elk Grove Village, Ill, 1985, American Academy of Pediatrics; and Tsang RC, editor: Vitamin and mineral requirements of preterm infants, New York, 1985, Marcel Dekker, Inc.

on this stored glycogen for energy and can exhaust this supply within 12 hours if food or IV glucose is not provided.

Lactose, a disaccharide composed of glucose and galactose, is the predominant carbohydrate in breast milk. Although premature infants have only 30% of the lactase activity of term infants, they tolerate lactose quite well in most circumstances.[24] Galactose is of major interest in neonatal metabolism, since it makes up 50% of the carbohydrate calories. However, neither a specific role for dietary galactose nor a typical deficiency state have been identified in human infants. Galactose may play a key role in energy storage, since in the newborn it is more readily taken up by the liver to form liver glycogen than is glucose.[18]

Forty percent to 45% of the newborn's caloric intake should be provided as carbohydrate, pre-

TABLE 9-5—cont'd

Vitamins in Neonatal Nutrition

VITAMIN	BIOLOGIC ROLE	DEFICIENCY STATE	RECOMMENDED ORAL REQUIREMENT
Vitamin B_2 (riboflavin)	Cofactor for many enzymes	Photophobia, cheilosis, glossitis, corneal vascularization, poor growth	335 μg/100 kcal
Vitamin B_6 (pyridoxine)	Cofactor for many enzymes	Dermatitis, glossitis, cheilosis, peripheral neuritis; infants—irritability, convulsions, anemia	250 μg/100 kcal
Vitamin B_{12} (cobalamin)	Coenzyme component, red blood cell maturation, CNS metabolism	Pernicious anemia, neurologic deterioration	0.15 μg/100 kcal
Niacin	Component of coenzymes I and II (NAD, NADP), many enzymatic reactions	Pellagra, dermatitis, diarrhea, dementia	4 mg/100 kcal
Pantothenic acid	Component of coenzyme A, many enzymatic reactions	Observed only with use of antagonists; depression, hypotension, muscle weakness, abdominal pain	1.0-1.4 mg/kg/day
Folacin (group of compounds containing pteridine ring, p-aminobenzoic and glutamic acids)	Tetrahydrofolic acid (the active form); synthesis of purines, pyrimidines, methylation reactions	Megaloblastic anemia	15 μg/kg/day
Biotin	Coenzyme	Dermatitis, anorexia, muscle pain, pallor	0.6-2.3 mg/kg/day
Choline	Neurotransmission, cell membrane structure, phospholipids, lipoproteins	Unknown	5-9 mg/kg/day

ferably lactose. If the infant shows signs of lactose intolerance (frequent, loose stools, abdominal distention, cramping, positive stool Clinitest), then a portion of the carbohydrate can be given as glucose polymers. Glucose polymers have the added advantage of keeping formula osmolality low.

MINERALS AND TRACE ELEMENTS

Mineral requirements for the premature infant have been largely estimated from in utero accretion rates. Recently the American Academy of Pediatrics Committee on Nutrition[1] and Tsang[33]

have published recommended daily intakes for minerals and trace elements for the healthy, feeding, premature infant. Table 9-4 describes the biologic role of these minerals and trace elements, as well as their deficiency states and recommended daily oral requirements.

VITAMINS

Table 9-5 is a summary of the recommended vitamin intakes for orally fed preterm infants, as well as a brief description of the biologic role and deficiency state of each vitamin.[33]

FEEDING TREATMENTS AND STRATEGIES
Human milk

Human milk is the preferred food for the term newborn. With milk, nature has provided the ideal means for giving the term infant sufficient stores of calories, fat, carbohydrate, protein, micronutrients, and water to ensure proper growth and nutrition. The premature infant, however, has special nutritional needs. Recommended daily requirements for macronutrients and micronutrients are greater for the preterm infant, yet such infants have a less developed gastrointestinal tract with which to satisfy these requirements. There are neonatologists who believe human milk may not be the ideal food for premature infants, primarily because of its relatively low contents of protein, calcium, and phosphorus.[6,7] Table 9-6 compares the macronutrient and micronutrient contents of term human milk with standard and "premature" formulas. It should be remembered there is good evidence that milk from mothers of premature infants has a greater protein, sodium, and chloride content than term milk, particularly in the first 4 weeks postpartum[20] (Table 9-7). Furthermore, there are several studies that demonstrate excellent growth in premature infants fed their own mother's milk.[11,12]

The advantages of breast milk are legion. The protein and fat are easily digestible. Selected nutrients in milk, such as epidermal growth factor, nerve growth factor, and taurine, appear to be important modulators of infant metabolism. Other components of breast milk, including secretory IgA, lactobacillus growth factor, complement, lactoferrin, lactoperoxidase, lysozyme, and leukocytes, are important antimicrobial agents that probably contribute to the lower rate of certain infections in breastfed infants.[34] The psychologic benefits of a mother providing milk for her premature infant are great and often unappreciated. Parents are separated, both physically and emotionally, from their infant when the infant is cared for in an intensive care setting. These parents are often frightened and frustrated about not being the baby's primary caretaker. Providing milk is a tangible and important contribution the mother can make to the infant's good health and reasserts the primary importance of the mother-infant bond.

Milk from the premature infant's own mother is the food of choice in the intensive care nursery. The VLBW infant should also receive a daily multivitamin preparation, and supplements of protein, calcium, phosphorus, and/or sodium chloride may need to be added in certain circumstances as the individual situation dictates (poor growth, decreased serum proteins, osteopenia, elevated alkaline phosphatase, decreased serum phosphorus, hyponatremia). Nutrient fortifiers for human milk are available to make breast milk supplementation practical and accurate (Table 9-8).

Formulas

Many mothers elect not to provide milk for their infant in the intensive care setting. Fortunately, there are excellent cow's milk formulas designed for term and preterm infants. Infants weighing more than 1800 g can be adequately nourished with one of the formulas designed for term infants (Table 9-6). More immature infants, particularly those weighing 1500 g or less, should be fed one of the "premature" formulas (Table 9-6). The manufacturers have done an admirable job of "humanizing" these formulas. Higher-quality whey protein has been provided in a 60:40 ratio with casein. Easily digested, lower-osmolality glucose polymers provide approximately half the carbohydrate calories (lactose provides the other half), and medium-chain triglycerides are added to ensure fat absorption. The concentrations of minerals, vitamins, and trace elements have been adjusted to meet the special needs of the premature infant.

Soy protein formulas should be reserved for formula-fed babies who are clearly allergic to cow's milk protein and should not be used for prolonged periods in the VLBW infant. Pregestimil° is an elemental formula designed for infants with compromised gastrointestinal tracts or malabsorptive problems. It should not be used routinely in the nursery in VLBW infants without a specific indication.

Occasionally, because of fluid, respiratory, or cardiac problems it is necessary to restrict free water intake to the infant. This can be safely done without compromising caloric intake by adding glucose polymers, corn oil, medium-chain triglycerides, casein powder, powdered formula, or milk fortifier to the formula. Alternatively, the formula base can be mixed to a 24 kcal/oz or 27 kcal/oz ratio instead of the usual 20 kcal/oz preparation.

Feeding regimens

One of the greatest challenges in the intensive care nursery is to provide enteral nutrition to a baby too immature or too sick for well-coordinated sucking, swallowing, esophageal motility, and appropriate gastric emptying. Tube feeding can be used successfully in these infants. Tubes can be passed from the nares or mouth into the stomach, duodenum, or jejunum. Feedings can be given by continuous, interrupted, or bolus infusion. No one method of feeding has been shown to be clearly superior in all situations. Gut growth and development have been shown to be augmented by enteral feeding, and it is unwise to keep the premature infant without food for prolonged periods (>1 week) unless there is a specific contraindication to feeding, such as necrotizing enterocolitis.

Intermittent or bolus feedings have the theoretical advantage of promoting the intestinal endocrine and metabolic responses observed after normal neonatal fast-feed patterns of nutrition. Reflux and regurgitation may be a problem, and milk may be put into the lung by inadvertent tracheal intubation. Continuous feeding can

°Mead Johnson.

prove to be beneficial in those cases in which intermittent or bolus infusions are associated with reflux, aspiration, or hypoxia. This method, however, has been associated with lactobezoar formation and gastrointestinal perforation. Transpyloric tubes are helpful if there is a marked delay in gastric emptying time or severe reflux. This method has the disadvantage of more difficult tube placement, and food bypasses gastric and duodenal digestive processes, which is particularly important in fat absorption.

Gavage feeding
PURPOSE

The purpose of gavage feeding is to provide a means of feeding an infant who is too immature to allow for safe nipple feeding or who is too sick to take adequate nourishment.

PRECAUTIONS

Aspiration of feeding into the lungs is of major concern in any infant less than 34 weeks of gestational age who does not have a neurologically mature swallow, gag, or cough reflex and will not cough adequately, if at all, in the event of aspiration. Any debilitated infant with rapid, labored respirations or an infant with an endotracheal tube has a high chance of aspirating, since the vocal cords are forced open and the seal around the tube may not be tight. The gavage tube position must be checked very carefully. These infants must not be overfed. Feedings must run slowly to prevent overfilling or too rapid filling of the stomach and subsequent emesis. *Gavage feeding should never be pushed.*

Passage of the gavage tube should be done gently, since it can cause trauma.

Passage of the gavage tube may stimulate the vagus nerve, causing the infant to become apneic or bradycardic. Tactile stimulation usually will cause the infant to breathe. However, the tube may have to be withdrawn if the symptoms do not subside.

Aspiration of the stomach contents via the

TABLE 9-6

Formula Comparison (Amounts per Deciliter)

		COW'S MILK			
	MATURE HUMAN MILK	SIMILAC 20	ENFAMIL 20	SMA 20	SIMILAC LBW 24
Protein source					
Whey/casein	80:20	18:82	60:40	60:40	18:82
Amount (g)	1	1.56	1.5	1.5	2.2
Calories (%)	6	9	9	9	11
Fat source (%)					
Medium-chain triglycerides	—	—	8.1	—	50
Polyunsaturated (linoleate [olive])	16	37	29	15	18
Saturated (coconut)	38	45	47.3	44	75
Monounsaturated (oleate [safflower])	42	18	15.5	41	7
Amount (g)	4.5	3.6	3.8	3.6	4.5
Calories (%)	55	48	50	48	47
Cholesterol (mg)	14.5	1.1	1.1	3.3	1.4
Vitamin E/PUFA (mg/g)	0.4	1.1	1.9	1.3	2.3
Carbohydrate source (%)					
Lactose	100	100	100	100	50
Glucose polymers	—	—	—	—	50
Amount (g)	7.1	7.2	6.9	7.2	8.5
Calories (%)	39	43	41	43	42
Calories	73	68	68	68	81
Calories/fl oz	22	20	20	20	24
Minerals					
Calcium (mg)	33	51	46	42	73
Phosphorus (mg)	15	39	32	28	57
Ca/P ratio	2.2:1	1.3:1	1.47:1	1.5:1	1.3:1
Sodium, mg (mEq)	16 (0.7)	22 (1.0)	18.1 (0.8)	15 (0.7)	36 (1.6)
Potassium, mg (mEq)	51 (1.3)	81 (2.1)	72 (1.84)	56 (1.4)	122 (3.1)
Chloride, mg (mEq)	39 (1.1)	51 (1.5)	42 (1.19)	38 (1.1)	89 (2.5)
Magnesium (mg)	4	4.1	5.2	4.5	8.1
Zinc (mg)	0.16	0.5	0.52	0.5	0.8
Iron (mg)	0.021	0.12	0.11	1.2	0.3
Iodine (μg)	30	10	6.8	6	12
Copper (μg)	25-40	61	63	47	81
Manganese (μg)	7-15	3.4	10.5	15	4.1
Osmolality (mOsm/kg)	300	290	300	300	290
Estimated renal solute load (mOsm/L)	71	105	97	91	160

| | COW'S MILK | | | CASEIN HYDROLYSATE | SOY | | |
SIMILAC SPECIAL CARE 24	ENFAMIL PREMATURE 20	PREMIE SMA 24	PREGESTIMIL 20	PROSOBEE 20	ISOMIL 20	NURSOY 20
60:40	60:40	60:40				
2.2	2.4	2	1.9	2	1.8	2.1
11	12	10	11	12	11	12
50	40	11	37.6	8.1	–	–
21	23	15.4	36.2	29.1	37	15
66	25.7	48	9.1	47.3	46	44
13	11.7	35	17.1	15.5	17	41
4.4	4.1	4.4	2.7	3.6	3.6	3.6
47	44	48	35	48	49	48
2.5	–	2-4	–	0	0	0
2.7	3.9	1.6	1.6	0.5	1.1	1.3
50	40	50	–	Sucrose	Sucrose	Sucrose
50	60	50	100	Corn syrup	Corn syrup	–
8.6	8.9	8.6	9.1	6.8	6.83	6.9
42	44	42	54	40	40	40
81	81	81	68	68	68	68
24	24	24	20	20	20	20
146	95	75	63	63	71	60
73	48	40	42	50	51	42
2.0:1	2.0:1	1.9:1	1.5:1	1.3:1	1.4:1	1.43:1
41 (1.8)	32 (1.4)	32 (1.4)	32 (1.4)	24 (1.04)	32 (1.4)	20 (0.9)
114 (2.9)	90 (2.3)	75 (1.9)	74 (1.9)	82 (2.1)	95 (2.4)	70 (1.8)
73 (2.1)	69 (1.9)	53 (1.5)	58 (1.6)	56 (1.58)	44 (1.3)	38 (1.1)
10	4	7	7.4	7.4	5.1	6.7
1.2	0.8	0.8	0.4	0.5	0.5	0.5
0.3	0.2	0.3	1.3	1.3	1.2	1.15
5	6.4	8.3	4.8	6.9	10	6
203	130	70	63	63	51	47
10	10.6	20	21	16.9	20	20
300	300	280	350	200	250	296
156	152	128	125	127	123	122

Continued.

TABLE 9-6—cont'd

Formula Comparison (Amounts per Deciliter)

	MATURE HUMAN MILK	COW'S MILK			
		SIMILAC 20	ENFAMIL 20	SMA 20	SIMILAC LBW 24
Vitamins and essential nutrients					
A IU	190-240	203	210	200	244
D IU	2.2	41	42	40	49
E IU	0.2-0.7	20	2.1	1	2.4
K (μg)	2	2	5.8	5.5	6.5
C (mg)	4.3-5	5.4	5.4	5.5	10
B_1 (thiamine) (μg)	14	6	52	67	102
B_2 (riboflavin) (μg)	37	101	105	100	122
B_6 (pyridoxine) (μg)	11	41	42	42	49
B_{12} (μg)	0.05	1.7	0.15	0.13	0.2
Niacin (mg)	0.15-0.18	0.7	0.84	0.5	0.85
Folic acid (μg)	5.2	10	10.5	5	12
Pantothenic acid (μg)	180-230	304	310	210	365
Biotin (μg)	0.7	3	1.5	1.5	3.6
Choline (mg)	9	10.8	10.5	10	13
Inositol (mg)	14	3.2	3.1	3.2	3.8

gavage tube assists in checking for placement and residual amounts from previous feedings. This should be done gently, because the tube may lodge against the wall of the stomach and because the suction during aspiration may cause trauma and bleeding. Injecting a small amount of air into the tube while listening with a stethoscope over the stomach helps confirm placement.

Intolerance of feeding may be the first symptom of illness in an infant. Serious conditions that cause feeding intolerance are hypoxia, dyspnea, congestive heart failure, sepsis, and necrotizing enterocolitis. Symptoms at first may be very subtle, so the caretaker should be constantly aware of any change in the infant's overall condition and feeding intolerance.

EQUIPMENT

1. Prepackaged gavage set with no. 8 Fr catheter, 20 ml syringe, and medicine cup
2. One no. 5 or 3.5 Fr catheter for very immature infant for indwelling gavage tube
3. Stethoscope

PROCEDURE

I. Intermittent gavage feeding
  A. Before starting a feeding, make sure the infant tolerated the previous feeding.
    1. Before the feeding, determine the amount of formula according to the infant's size, gestational age, physical condition, amount of previous feeding, and feeding regimen.
    2. Alter the amount of formula depending on how the infant tolerated the last feeding. In the following conditions, it may be necessary to decrease the amount of formula given:
      a. Vomiting between feedings
      b. Unusual abdominal distention
      c. Residuals of previous feeding in the stomach

COW'S MILK			CASEIN HYDROLYSATE	SOY		
SIMILAC SPECIAL CARE 24	ENFAMIL PREMATURE 20	PREMIE SMA 24	PREGESTIMIL 20	PROSOBEE 20	ISOMIL 20	NURSOY 20
550	970	240	210	210	203	200
122	260	48	42	42	41	40
3.2	3.7	1.5	1.6	2.1	2	0.95
10	10.6	7	10.6	10.6	10	10
30	29	7	5.5	5.5	6	5.5
203	200	80	53	53	41	67
503	290	130	63	63	61	100
203	200	50	42	42	41	42
0.45	0.24	0.2	0.21	0.21	0.3	0.2
4.1	3.3	0.6	0.85	0.85	0.9	0.5
30	29	10	10.6	10.6	10	5
1543	970	360	320	320	507	300
30	1.63	1.8	5.3	5.3	3	3.5
8.1	6.1	12.7	9	5.3	5.4	8.5
4.5	3.8	3.2	3.2	3.2	3.4	2.7

(1) Gently aspirate the entire amount of stomach contents into the syringe. Note amount, color, and appearance of contents. Immediately report bloody or "coffee grounds" (heme positive), green or yellow (test these for bile), or fecal-appearing aspirates. Withhold feeding pending a decision about the feeding plan.

(2) Unless residuals are mostly mucous, return them to the stomach to prevent loss of electrolytes. Subtract this amount from the total given. For example, if a baby is to receive 30 ml and 5 ml of residual is aspirated, return the 5 ml and give only 25 ml of additional formula. (Large aspirates may indicate that the baby is being overfed and may necessitate decreasing the amount of formula. Large aspirates may often indicate partial ileus or early signs of sepsis, necrotizing enterocolitis, or obstruction).

3. Increase the amount of feeding with great care. Following orders for advancing feeds without constantly evaluating the baby is dangerous.

B. Insert the feeding tube (oral placement).

1. Oral tube placement is preferred to nasal tube placement for infants because infants are obligatory nose breathers. However, because of less stimulation of the gag reflex, nasal tube passage may be chosen in certain situations (e.g., older preterm infant who needs supplementation

TABLE 9-7

Nutritional Composition of Preterm and Term Breast Milk

NUTRIENT	7 DAYS		14 DAYS		28 DAYS		>56 DAYS	
	PRETERM	TERM	PRETERM	TERM	PRETERM	TERM	PRETERM	TERM
Calories (kcal/dl)	73.86	73.62	74.59	71.81	73.33	72.71	70.10	76.33
	±1.81	±3.32	±1.96	±3.57	±2.14	±1.88	±1.424	±2.34
Protein nitrogen (g/L)	2.76	2.55	2.39	1.97	1.90	1.76	1.99	1.96
	±0.18	±0.18	±0.16	±0.14	±0.09	±0.08	±0.10	±0.10
Sodium (mEq/L)	17.23	9.54	12.36	9.37	9.56	7.04	8.85	7.14
	±1.88	±1.30	±1.42	±1.95	±0.70	±0.96	±0.80	±0.51
Calcium (mg/L)	293	293	266	274	282	267	310	314
	±16	±8	±15	±13	±12	±13	±16	±12
Fat (g/dl)	3.1	2.98	3.42	3	3.24	3.07	3.43	3.46
	±0.71	±0.28	±0.18	±0.26	±0.16	±0.21	±0.16	±0.32
Lactose (g/dl)	6.38	6.43	6.86	6.63	6.79	6.92	7.21	6.68
	±0.22	±0.13	±0.16	±0.23	±0.17	±0.36	±0.11	±0.22

Modified from Lemons JA et al: Pediatr Res 16:113, 1982.

after nippling but who fights, gags, and vomits with oral tube passage). Small (3.5 or 5 Fr) indwelling nasogastric tubes can be placed for gavage feedings, and the infant can learn to nipple with the tube in place.

2. Measure for approximate tube length by holding one end of the tube at the back of the earlobe and drawing the tubing to the mouth and down to the tip of the xiphoid process. Observe this point in relation to the black marking on the tube.

3. Use the natural bend of the tube to follow the natural curves of the mouth and throat for easier insertion.

4. Insert the tube in the mouth and toward the back of the throat, gently pushing it down the esophagus until reaching the premeasured mark on the tubing.

C. Check tube position.
   1. Verify the exact position of the gavage tube on insertion and before every feeding. During insertion, the tube may go into the trachea instead of the esophagus. If this occurs, the infant may respond instantly by fighting, coughing, and becoming cyanotic. The gavage tube may also enter only the esophagus and not actually go into the stomach.

   2. Attach the syringe to the gavage tube. Aspirate gently on the tube while rotating the tube between the thumb and index finger. This helps prevent aspirating stomach mucosa. Usually a few curds of formula or mucus are in the stomach. Pull stomach contents back into the tube to verify that the gavage tube is in the stomach.

   3. If the infant is very active or vigorous, wrap the infant in a blanket to prevent the infant from pulling on the tube.

   4. Tape the tube in place or always keep one hand on the tube at the premeasured mark to prevent the tube from slipping.

TABLE 9-8

Nutrient Composition of Human Milk Fortifier and Natural Care*

	HUMAN MILK FORTIFIER† (AMOUNT PER FOUR PACKETS)	NATURAL CARE‡ (AMOUNT PER 124 ML)
Calories (kcal)	14	100
Protein (g)	0.7	2.7
Fat (g)	0.05	5.4
Carbohydrate (g)	2.73	10.6
Calcium (mg)	60	210
Phosphorus (mg)	33	105
Sodium (mg)	7	50
Chloride (mg)	17.7	90
Vitamin A (IU)	780	680
Vitamin D (IU)	260	150
Vitamin C (mg)	24	37

*This table lists the major constituents; refer to product for complete listing of vitamins, minerals, and trace elements.
†Mead Johnson, Evansville, Ind.
‡Ross Laboratories, Columbus, Ohio.

D. Begin feeding.
1. After determining that the tube is in position and it is safe to feed the infant, begin feeding by removing the plunger from the syringe and affixing the syringe to the gavage tube. Pour the predetermined amount of formula into the syringe. (Flow down the tube may begin spontaneously or require a gentle nudge with the plunger.) *Allow feedings to be run by gravity.* (The higher the tube is held, the faster the milk will flow.) Let the formula run at a slow, steady pace to prevent the infant from vomiting.
2. When all the formula has run in, pinch the gavage tube to prevent drops on the end from falling into the infant's throat and being aspirated. Withdraw the tube.
II. Continuous gavage feeding
A. An indwelling gavage tube should be used for infants who need maximal total intake but cannot tolerate a bolus of formula at any one feeding; for example:
1. Very small immature infants
2. Infants of diabetic mothers—to stabilize blood glucose
3. Some bowel surgery patients with short gut or dumping syndrome
B. Normally, use the oral route. The nasal route may be chosen for greater stability of the tube and if the infant has increased gagging, apnea, and bradycardia with an oral tube. To pass a tube into the duodenum or jejunum, pass it into the stomach first. Then, hourly advance the tube a small distance. (Once the pH is greater than 7, the tube is probably past the pylorus.) Transpyloric mercury-tipped tubes may be left in place for 3 to 7 days. Ascertain the correct position of the tube. Once in position, secure the tubing with tape.
C. Run continuous gavage feedings into a sterile, measured container such as a large syringe or a Buretol (Travenol, in-line burette) *without* a membrane. To control the rate of flow appropriately, attach the container to a volumetric or syringe pump.
D. Because of the danger of infection, change continuous drip feeding (syringe, tubing, and milk) at 4-hour intervals.[21]
E. Carefully watch the infant for emesis or abdominal distention. Check stomach residuals every 2 to 4 hours. Every hour check the amount of formula infused and record it in the same manner as an
IV.
Position the infant after any feeding to prevent aspiration in case regurgitation occurs:
1. Elevate the infant's head to prevent regurgitation.
2. Place the infant on the right side or prone to prevent aspiration.

Nippling

In general, healthy babies (>34 to 36 weeks gestation) can be fed human milk or 20 kcal/oz formula ad libitum starting as soon after birth as adequate breathing, circulation, swallowing, and temperature control are established.

For the premature infant, the ability to nipple feed develops as the neurologic system matures. Criteria for initiating nipple feeding must be individualized and include the following:

1. Adequate neurologic development. The coordination of sucking, swallowing, and breathing develops at around 34 weeks, and the gag reflex develops at around 36 weeks gestational age.

   Nonnutritive suckling on a pacifier during gavage feedings quiets, comforts, and teaches the baby that sucking and satiety are related. The ability to suck on a pacifier, fingers, or a gavage tube *does not* ensure the baby's ability to perform nutritive suckling.

   Since the expression and swallowing phases of nutritive suckling (see Chapter 12) are missing in nonnutritive suckling, the presence of a gag reflex is *absolutely essential* before the preterm baby attempts to nipple. A preterm infant without a gag who attempts to nipple is at increased risk for aspiration.

2. Adequate respiratory function. Respirations are unlabored, less than 60 breaths/min, and the oxygen requirement is less than 30% to 40%. The premature infant with bronchopulmonary dysplasia may be very tachypneic, thus complicating attempts at nipple feeding, since the infant must coordinate sucking and swallowing with rapid respirations. Extreme care and caution is warranted in oral feeding—much time and patience, correct positioning, and an unhurried care provider are essential.

3. Consistent weight gain.

Nipple feedings should begin slowly at one feeding per day, then increase as tolerated to once every 8 hours, then once every third feeding, then every other feeding, and finally all feedings should be nipple feedings. Scheduling nipple feedings for parent visits enables them to actively participate in their baby's care. A too-rapid change to nipple feeding results in weight loss; the baby tires with feedings and is unable to take in caloric requirements or needs gavage supplementation after nippling to meet caloric needs (with inherent danger of vomiting the nippled feeding and aspiration). Diligent attention is warranted, and a decrease in nipple feedings is necessary to prevent dehydration, malnutrition, and a worsening of the infant's condition.

Charting

Chart the following on a flowsheet:

1. Type of feeding
2. Method of feeding
3. Amount of feeding
4. Time of feeding
5. Amount of aspiration
6. Infant's toleration of feeding

Feeding protocols should not be rigid or blindly followed. Each feeding plan should be individualized with careful attention to the infant's physical examination, previous feeding tolerance, and overall status. After a period of stabilization and recovery from any birth stress, most premature infants can accept slow, enteral feeding at a time when the cardiorespiratory status begins to improve. Table 9-9 is a suggested guideline for feeding the premature infant.

PROBLEMS
Underfeeding

Underfeeding can lead to total undernutrition (growth failure and marasmus) or to selected nutritional deficiencies (vitamin, mineral, trace element, essential fatty or amino acid). Severe protein undernutrition is called kwashiorkor. Ma-

TABLE 9-9

Suggested Guidelines for Feeding the Preterm Infant

WEIGHT	DAY OF FEEDING	TYPE OF FOOD	VOLUME	FREQUENCY
<1000 g	1	Breast milk or 20 kcal/oz formula	2 ml	q 2 hours
	3-4	Breast milk or 20 kcal/oz formula	4 ml	q 2 hours
	7-8	Breast milk or 20 kcal/oz formula	8 ml	q 2 hours
	10-12	Breast milk or 20-24 kcal/oz formula (± supplements)	10-15 ml	q 2 hours
1000-1500 g	1	Breast milk or 20 kcal/oz formula	2 ml	q 2 hours
	3-4	Breast milk or 20 kcal/oz formula	6 ml	q 2 hours
	7-8	Breast milk or 20 kcal/oz formula	10-12 ml	q 2 hours
	10-12	Breast milk or 20-24 kcal/oz formula (± supplements)	15-30 ml	q 2-3 hours
1500-2000 g	1	Breast milk or 20 kcal/oz formula	4-5 ml	q 2-3 hours
	3-4	Breast milk or 20 kcal/oz formula	10-15 ml	q 2-3 hours
	5-7	Breast milk or 20-24 kcal/oz formula (± supplements)	25-40 ml	q 2-3 hours

rasmus and kwashiorkor are seldom if ever seen in advanced form in neonatal intensive care units, but many of their manifestations can be found in milder degrees (Table 9-10).

The major causes of underfeeding in neonatal intensive care units are severe illness and extreme prematurity. Neurologic injury (e.g., intracerebral hemorrhage or facial palsy) may lead to functional feeding inabilities. Respiratory disease with chronic endotracheal intubation may promote gastric reflux and pulmonary aspiration. Gastritis, strictures, and short gut secondary to necrotizing enterocolitis are common gastrointestinal problems. Babies with omphalocoeles or gastroschises are particularly difficult to manage because of gut malrotation and poor peristaltic development.

A major concern with chronic undernutrition is the potential neurologic injury it may inflict. During development, significant undernutrition can adversely affect cell division, cell migration, and cell maturation. In the brain, reduced cell number primarily involves the glial cells. Brain lipid and myelin membrane content may be reduced, and enzyme levels are altered. The severity of these changes, the precise developmental stage at which they occur, and the length of time they persist interact to determine the degree, nature, and reversibility of neurologic injury in the pre-

TABLE 9-10

Manifestations of Marasmus and Kwashiorkor

	MARASMUS	KWASHIORKOR
Growth failure	++	++
"Wasting" (loss of subcutaneous tissue, primarily fat)	++++	++
Malabsorption	++	++
Vomiting	+	±
Infections	++	++
Edema	−	+++
Abdominal distention	+	++
Hypoproteinemia	+	+++
Decreased BUN	±	++
Extracellular water/ intracellular water	+	+++
Ketonuria	+	+
Hypoglycemia	+	?

mature infant. It is unlikely that neurologic injury in the premature infant is caused by fetal nutritional deficiencies unless postnatal underfeeding is prolonged and severe.

In the presence of vomiting, excessive residual, or feeding intolerance, withhold feedings until stomach and intestinal emptying is

effective. Add an indwelling gastric gavage tube to low, intermittent suctioning when a functional or anatomic obstruction is suspected. Give subsequent feedings in smaller amounts and less frequently, and advance more cautiously. Elevate the head and thorax. The prone position may minimize reflux. Keep a bulb syringe at the head of the bed for quick suctioning of vomited material. Take abdominal girth measurements every 4 to 8 hours.

To measure abdominal girth, place cloth or paper tape underneath the baby's back and bring the ends of the tape around the abdomen over the umbilicus. Do not pull the tape too tightly. Mark the tape measurement location on the abdomen for consistency of subsequent measurements.

Signs of intestinal obstruction include gastric content retention (increased residual), emesis (may be bilious), abdominal distention, and a persistent air-fluid pattern shown by abdominal x-ray examination.

In most cases of diarrhea the following treatment is successful:

1. Restriction of enteral feedings
2. IV feeding
3. Correction of water and electrolyte imbalances
4. Cautious resumption of feedings
5. Smaller volumes per feeding
6. Low-osmolality solution that emphasizes materials that are readily absorbed (glucose polymers, sucrose, medium-chain triglycerides)

In late metabolic acidosis, a brief period of bicarbonate supplementation and lower protein intake usually corrects the problem. It seldom is so severe or protracted as to lead to further metabolic consequences or growth failure.

Overfeeding

Overfeeding involves giving the infant too much food too fast. This simple problem is one of the

most frequent feeding problems in preterm infants. The guidelines for feeding in Table 9-9 emphasize slow, careful advancement of the feeding with constant reassessment of the baby's physical examination and clinical status. The clinician must continually be alert for signs of overfeeding and intolerance.

Regurgitation and vomiting

The most common causes of regurgitation and vomiting are as follows:

1. Overfeeding (too much, too fast)
2. Physiologic "spitting up" (? mechanism)
3. Chalasia/poor lower esophageal sphincter tone
4. Ileus (immaturity, injury, infection, aganglionosis)
5. Infection (gastroenteritis)
6. Tachypnea/respiratory distress
7. Intestinal obstruction
8. Pyloric stenosis
9. Hiatal hernia
10. Metabolic disorders (galactosemia, amino acidurias, electrolyte imbalance, etc.)
11. Increased intracranial pressure
12. Drug withdrawal

The first three causes listed above are the most common reasons for regurgitation and vomiting. The chief danger is aspiration and pneumonitis.

Abdominal distention

Abdominal distention may result from overfeeding or delayed passage of intestinal contents (ileus, immature gut motility, meconium plug, meconium ileus, microcolon, aganglionosis). A distended abdomen may also represent air swallowing, tracheoesophageal fistula, pneumoperitoneum, peritonitis, necrotizing enterocolitis, or abdominal visceromegaly (enlarged bladder, hydronephrosis, hepatosplenomegaly).

Diarrhea

Frequent, loose stools are a common finding in premature infants who are milk-fed. The usual cause is overly rapid advancement of the amount of the baby's feeding. Secondary causes may include hyperosmolality and a disproportionate amount of lactose for the baby's digestive capacity. Transient disaccharidase deficiencies such as lactase deficiency following gastrointestinal infections and with phototherapy are also associated with diarrhea in the premature infant. Several other causes of diarrhea include:

1. Congenital, developmental, or secondary lactase deficiency
2. Sucrase-isomaltase deficiency
3. Primary immune defects
4. Pancreatic insufficiency/cystic fibrosis
5. Viral, bacterial, or parasitic infections
6. Cow or soy protein intolerance
7. Short gut syndrome
8. Primary hepatobiliary disease
9. Endocrine disorders (thyroid, adrenal)

Lactobezoars

Lactobezoars are concretions of milk substances that form in the stomach and small intestine. Several years ago an increasing number of premature infants, usually fed concentrated "premature" formulas by continuous nasogastric infusion, acquired lactobezoars.[5] They are quite unusual in the breast milk–fed baby. The presentation is variable but usually includes abdominal distention and regurgitation. Diagnosis is confirmed by x-ray examination of the stomach showing a mass containing radiodense calcium deposits. Withdrawal of feeds for a short period of time is usually sufficient therapy, but persistent signs of obstruction may indicate the need for surgical removal.

Late metabolic acidosis

Late metabolic acidosis is a condition occurring during the early phase of "full" feeding in preterm infants. Acid balance is positive for several reasons: (1) an excessive cation and acid load from relatively high protein intake, (2) relatively low hydrogen ion excretion, and (3) bicarbonaturia.

Neurologic injury

Neurologic injury occurs with certain hyperaminoacidemias (e.g., with hyperphenylalaninemia and hypermethioninemia). Follow-up studies of babies fed very large amounts of protein (>4 g/kg/day) suggested an inverse correlation between protein intake and IQ.[9] These studies have not been repeated, and the possible influences of protein quality and associate or incidental neurologic derangements were not rigorously excluded.

PARENT TEACHING

Holding and feeding an infant are two of the most important and enjoyable aspects of parenting. Unfortunately, such practices are often denied parents of sick, premature infants in intensive care nurseries. The babies are literally isolated from their parents, and the feelings of helplessness and frustration that such conditions induce in parents must be devastating, especially when added to the already overwhelming burden of guilt and fear. It is absolutely essential that physicians and nurses involve parents in the care and especially the nourishment of their baby.

Feeding is one of the best ways parents can be involved with their baby's care. Of course, the mother who provides her own milk is at an advantage. This simple process provides extraordinary support for these mothers. But the nonnursing mother (and father) can also be involved with the baby's feeding:

1. **Explain the developmental aspects of enteral food processing in premature infants.**
2. **Talk about the infant's specific illnesses that may affect feeding.**
3. **Discuss formula or breast milk composition in a straightforward fashion.**
4. **Discuss all types of feeding, but be supportive of each parent's choice and continue to focus on the advantages of the selected feeding.**

5. **Teach parents to follow the daily weight and caloric charts.**

6. **Emphasize the slow progress and routine "ups-and-downs" of feeding premature infants.**

Finally, most parents are eager and capable of feeding their babies and can safely nipple or gavage feed with assistance from the nurses. Nothing encourages "bonding" quite so well as holding, feeding, and watching the baby grow.

REFERENCES

1. American Academy of Pediatrics Committee on Nutrition: Nutritional needs of low-birth-weight infants, Pediatrics 75:976, 1985.
2. Baum D et al: Studies on colloid osmotic pressure in the fetus and newborn infant, Biol Neonate 18:311, 1971.
3. Davidson M et al: Feeding studies in low birth weight infants, J Pediatr 70:695, 1967.
4. Dweck HS: Feeding the prematurely born infant, Clin Perinatol 2:183, 1975.
5. Erenberg A, Shaw RD, and Yousefzadeh D: Lactobezoar in the low-birth-weight infant, Pediatrics 63:642, 1979.
6. Fomon SJ, Ziegler EE, and Vazquez HD: Human milk and the small premature infant, Am J Dis Child 131:463, 1977.
7. Forbes GB: Fetal growth and body composition: implications for the premature infant, J Pediatr Gastroenterol Nutr 2(suppl 1):552, 1983.
8. Gaull GE: Taurine in milk: growth modulator or conditionally essential amino acid? J Pediatr Gastroenterol Nutr 2(suppl 1):266, 1983.
9. Goldman HI et al: Late effects of early dietary protein intake on low-birth-weight infants, J Pediatr 85:764, 1974.
10. Gordon H, Levine SZ, and McNamara H: Feeding of premature infants: a comparison of human and cow's milk, Am J Dis Child 73:442, 1947.
11. Gross SJ: Growth and biochemical responses of preterm infants fed human milk or modified infant formula, N Engl J Med 308:237, 1983.
12. Heim T: Energy and lipid requirements of the fetus and the preterm infant, J Pediatr Gastroenterol Nutr 2(suppl 1):516, 1983.
13. Helms RA et al: Enhanced lipid utilization in infants receiving oral L-carnitine during long-term parenteral nutrition, J Pediatr 109:984, 1986.
14. Hill D: Effect of insulin on fetal growth, Semin Perinatol 2:319, 1978.
15. Hughes CA: Intestinal adaptation. In Tanner MS and Stocks RJ, editors: Neonatal gastroenterology contemporary issues, Newcastle upon Tyne, Eng, 1984, Intercept.
16. Janas LM, Picciano MF, and Hatch TF: Indices of protein metabolism in term infants fed human milk, whey-predominant formula, or cow's milk formula, Pediatrics 75:775, 1985.
17. Jensen RG et al: The lipolytic triad: human lingual, breast milk, and pancreatic lipases: physiological implication of their characteristics in digestion of dietary fats, J Pediatr Gastroenterol Nutr 1:243, 1982.
18. Kliegman RM et al: The effect of enteric galactose on neonatal canine carbohydrate metabolism, Metabolism 30:1109, 1981.
19. Lebenthal E and Leung YK: The impact of development of the gut on infant nutrition, Pediatr Ann 16:211, 1987.
20. Lemons JA et al: Differences in the composition of preterm and term human milk during early lactation, Pediatr Res 16:113, 1982.
21. Lemons PM et al: Bacterial growth in human milk during continuous feeding, Am J Perinatol 1:76, 1983.
22. Lin CC and Evand MI: Intrauterine growth retardation: pathophysiology and clinical management, New York, 1984, McGraw Hill Book Co.
23. Lucas A: Hormones, nutrition and the gut. In Tanner MS and Stocks RJ, editors: Neonatal gastroenterology contemporary issues, Newcastle upon Tyne, Eng, 1984, Intercept.
24. MacLean WC and Fink BB: Lactose malabsorption by premature infants: magnitude and clinical significance, J Pediatr 97:383, 1980.
25. Menkes JH: Early feeding history of children with learning disorders, Dev Med Child Neurol 19:169, 1977.
26. Molteni RA, Stys SJ, and Battaglia FC: Relationship of fetal and placental weight in human beings: fetal/placental weight ratios at various gestational ages and birth weight distributions, J Reprod Med 21:327, 1978.
27. Philipps C and Johnson NE: The impact of quality of diet and other factors on birth weight of infants, Am J Clin Nutr 30:215, 1977.
28. Raiha NC et al: Milk protein quantity and quality in low-birth-weight infants. I. Metabolic responses and effects on growth, Pediatrics 57:659, 1976.
29. Rosso P: Nutrition and maternal-fetal exchange, Am J Clin Nutr 34:744, 1981.
30. Shelley H: Glycogen reserves and their changes at birth and in anoxia, Br Med Bull 17:137, 1961.
31. Simpson JW, Lawless RW, and Mitchell AC: Responsibility of the obstetrician to the fetus. II. Influence of prepregnancy weight gain on birth weight, Obstet Gynecol 45:481, 1975.

32. Sparks JW, Girard J, and Battaglia FC: An estimate of the caloric requirements of the human fetus, Biol Neonate 38:113, 1980.

33. Tsang RC, editor: Vitamin and mineral requirements of preterm infants, New York, 1985, Marcel Dekker, Inc.

34. Welsh JK and May JT: Anti-infective properties of breast milk, J Pediatr 94:1, 1979.

35. Whyte RK et al: Energy balance in low birth weight infants fed formula of high or low medium-chain triglyceride content, J Pediatr 108:964, 1986.

CHAPTER 10

Fluid and electrolyte management

EUGENE W. ADCOCK III · CAROL ANN CONSOLVO

Although advances in management of specific neonatal disorders have contributed to a remarkable decline in morbidity and mortality, fluid and electrolyte therapy, thermal regulation, and maintenance of oxygenation remain the central features of modern, supportive neonatal intensive care. It is assumed, therefore, that all infants requiring tertiary care (and most infants requiring so-called intermediate, level II, or secondary care) will receive parenteral fluid and electrolytes. Much useful information has accumulated about full-term infants, but some crucial information is still missing, especially about very low birth weight (VLBW) infants. At best, approximations for therapy are necessary in many clinical situations. This chapter is based on the following fundamental principles: (1) rapidly assessing the infant's initial condition, (2) developing a short-term, time-oriented, management plan, (3) initiating therapy, and (4) monitoring the infant and modifying the plan based on clinical and biochemical data.

PHYSIOLOGY

Neonates show dramatic physiologic differences when compared on a per kilogram basis with older children and adults: (1) their basic metabolic rate is at least double; (2) their water requirements are four or five times greater; and (3) their sodium excretion is only 10% of that in older children and adults. The subdivisions of total body mass (TBM) are illustrated in Figure 10-1. Total body weight as a percentage of TBM demonstrates a curvilinear decline with increasing age (Figure 10-2). Intracellular fluid (ICF) and extracellular fluid (ECF) as percentages of TBM change in opposite directions as gestation advances.

These physiologic and body composition phenomena result in a narrow margin of safety in calculating fluids and electrolytes for small infants, especially those weighing less than 1250 g. Caretakers should calculate independently all requirements and compare calculations with each other. Intravenous (IV) fluid should be administered by a special infusion pump, which can regulate fluid at rates of 1 ml/hr or less. The intake should be measured hourly, and the output should be quantitated as soon as it occurs. The balance of intake and output should be made at least every 8 to 12 hours using a standard form (Figure 10-3). Once clinical signs of fluid overload or deficit occur, it may be extremely difficult to regain balance. Fluid balance should be viewed prospectively. A similar procedure should be a part of every initial care plan.

The effect of gestational age on body composition is striking (Figure 10-4). Because gestational age is an important determinant of the percentage and distribution of total body water (TBW), accurate assessment is important. Changes in distribution and percent of body water may also depend on intrauterine growth, maternal fluid balance, postnatal age, diet, daily water intake, and changing metabolism.

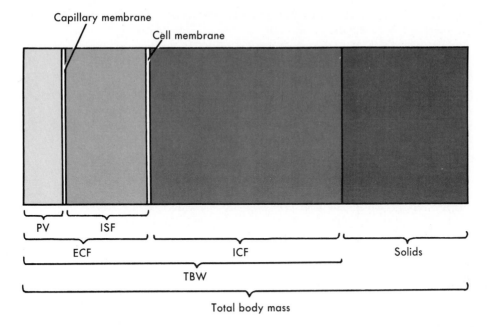

Figure 10-1. Major subdivisions of total body mass. *PV,* Plasma volume; *ISF,* interstitial fluid; *ECF,* extracellular fluid; *ICF,* intracellular fluid; *TBW,* total body water. (From Winters RW, editor: The body fluids in pediatrics, Boston, 1973, Little, Brown & Co.)

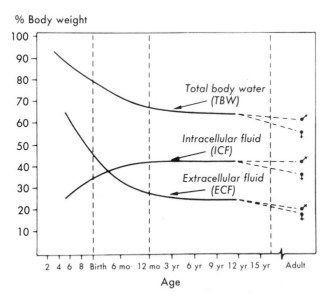

Figure 10-2. Effects of age on TBW, ICF, and ECF. Note curvilinear changes that are maximal during perinatal period. (From Winters RW, editor: The body fluids in pediatrics, Boston, 1973, Little, Brown & Co.)

The maternal history and the intrapartum course are helpful in calculating the infant's fluid and electrolyte requirements. For example, if the mother received large amounts of electrolyte-free fluids in the intrapartum period, the neonate may be hyponatremic and have expanded ECF at birth. Because small-for-gestational-age (SGA) infants have reduced amounts of fat, body water (as a percentage of TBM) increases. Conversely, large-for-gestational-age (LGA) infants have a smaller percentage of TBW because of an increased amount of body fat.

Electrolyte composition of interstitial fluid (ISF) and plasma is similar but strikingly different from ICF (Figure 10-5).

Sodium is the major cation in ECF (both ISF

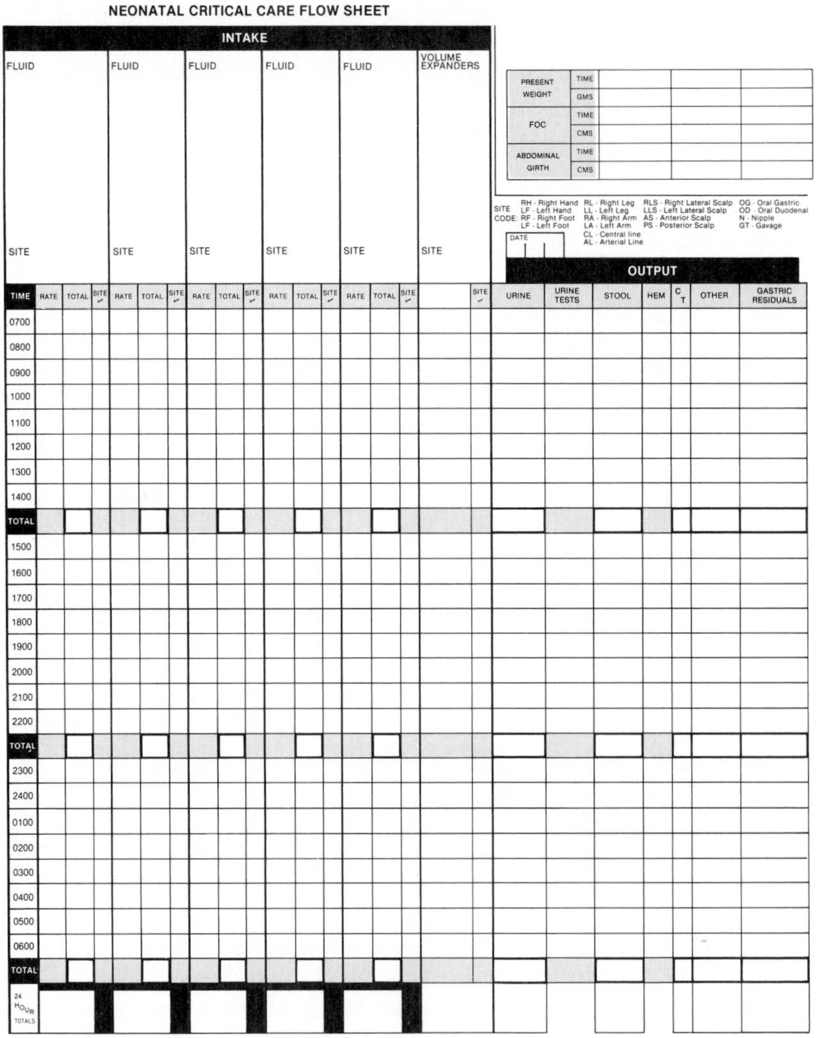

Figure 10-3. Model intake and output sheet. (Courtesy University Children's Hospital at Hermann, Houston, Tex.)

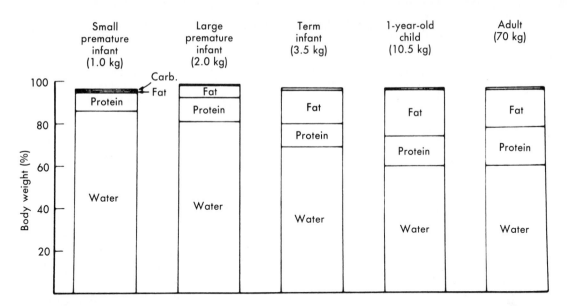

Figure 10-4. Effects of gestational age on body composition compared with older children and adults. (From Heird WC et al: J Pediatr 80:352, 1972.)

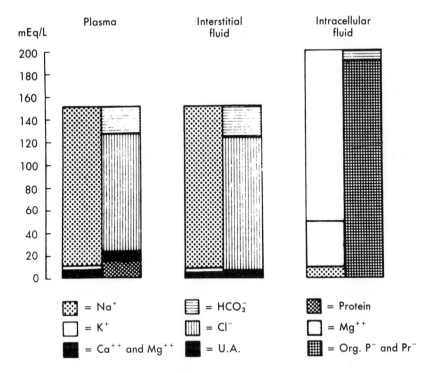

Figure 10-5. "Gamblegram" of plasma ISF and ICF. (From Winters RW, editor: The body fluids in pediatrics, Boston, 1973, Little, Brown & Co.)

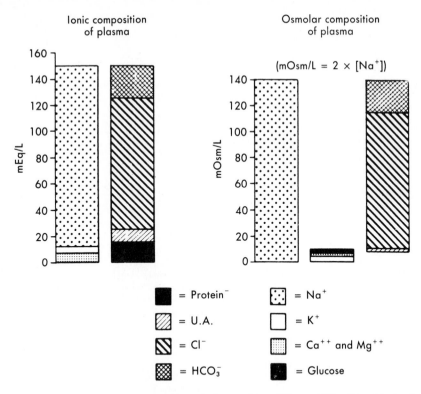

Figure 10-6. Ionic and osmolar composition of plasma. (From Winters RW, editor: The body fluids in pediatrics, Boston, 1973, Little, Brown & Co.)

and plasma) and is easily measured. Potassium, the major cation in ICF, cannot be measured readily, because ICF is not clinically accessible. Since 90% of the total body potassium is intracellular, when plasma potassium is low, it is assumed that the total body potassium is invariably low.

Osmotic force or pressure is a phenomenon that is a colligative property of any solution. Osmotic phenomena are dependent on the number (N) of particles (regardless of size or charge) in a solution and are measured in milliosmoles, according to the equation:

$$mOsm = (mM) \times (N)$$

Following are three examples:

	mM	N	mOsm
NaCl	1	2	2
Glucose	1	1	1
$CaCl_2$	1	3	3

Unfortunately, two physical chemistry terms are used interchangeably in clinical medicine: (1) osmolality (milliosmole per kilogram of water) and (2) osmolarity (milliosmole per liter of solution). In most laboratories osmotic forces are determined by the technique of freezing point depression, so osmolality is the correct term (normally 280 to 300 mOsm/kg water). The difference in terms is usually unimportant, since the total solid content per liter of plasma is small.

Osmotic forces can be satisfactorily estimated (Figure 10-6) in many clinical settings by the formula:

Plasma mOsm/kg water = 2(Na⁺) +

$$\frac{BUN\ (mg/dl) \times 10}{28} + \frac{Glucose\ (mg/dl) \times 10}{180}$$

The molecular weight of two nitrogen atoms and glucose are 28 and 180, respectively, and BUN is blood urea nitrogen.

Osmotic forces are responsible for apparently low plasma electrolyte concentrations in some common clinical settings.

In hyperglycemia, the plasma sodium concentrate reported by the laboratory is usually low, but the total effective osmolality may be normal, as seen in this example:

$$Glucose = 720\ mg/dl$$
$$(Na^+) = 120\ mEq/L$$
$$mOsm/L = 280$$

$$\frac{720 \times 10}{180} + 120 \times 2 = 280$$

Although hyperlipidemia is less frequent, an analogous situation exists (Figure 10-7). Low laboratory values for plasma sodium occur because the increase in plasma solids (lipids) causes a lower plasma water content and hence a lower sodium concentration per liter of whole plasma. In this case the plasma water sodium concentration may be normal.

Osmotic forces largely determine shifts in the internal redistribution of water in hydration disturbances.

Four pure disturbances of hydration exist: (1) too much electrolyte, (2) too little electrolyte, (3) too much water, and (4) too little water. Combinations of these disturbances may also occur.

Neonatal renal "immaturity" influences fluid and electrolyte needs. Various renal functions do not develop at the same rate.

Glomerular filtration rate (GFR) is low at birth and, despite the initial gestational age, characteristically rises rapidly during the first 6 weeks of life. A VLBW infant in satisfactory condition at 6 weeks may have an adequate GFR.

Urinary sodium excretion increases slowly during the first 2 years of life.

Measuring the urine sodium concentration should be considered part of the routine assessment of fluid and electrolyte balance. All neonates tend to retain sodium if it is given in large amounts.

Urine sodium losses are influenced by sodium intake and gestational age.

Urine sodium may rise when moderately increased amounts of sodium are given to more mature infants. VLBW infants, however, tend to lose urine sodium, which may be greater per kilogram than that of term infants, when receiving the normal (1 to 4 mEq/kg) sodium intake.

The capacity to dilute and concentrate the urine appears limited but can be influenced by nutrient intake.

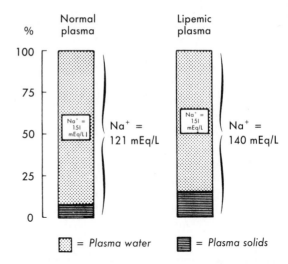

Figure 10-7. Effects of hyperlipemia on plasma water and plasma sodium concentration. (From Winters RW, editor: The body fluids in pediatrics, Boston, 1973, Little, Brown & Co.)

Urea is usually the major component of urine osmolality (and hence specific gravity), whereas electrolytes quantitatively contribute less. When parenteral nutrition is being provided, urine specific gravity may rise because of the low renal threshold for glucose and amino acids. When specific gravity rises, therefore, the cause must be ascertained before altering the fluid infusion rate. A diagnostic test (Bili-Labstix) can screen for glucose and protein but misses amino acids, which must be detected by amino acid chromatography when necessary.

Neonatal urinary acidification is limited, and the bicarbonate threshold is reduced.

Both physiologic and pathophysiologic factors can contribute to an alkaline urine. For example, VLBW infants have a limited capacity for hydrogen ion excretion, whereas other infants may have acute illnesses such as bicarbonate-losing tubular necrosis or urinary tract infection.

The roles of hormones, such as antidiuretic hormone, aldosterone, atrial natriuretic factor, and parathormone, in regulating neonatal fluid and electrolyte balance are not well defined.

Hormonal influences can be primary, such as in the syndrome of inappropriate secretion of antidiuretic hormone and in some cases of hypocalcemia. Secondary hormonal influences can be caused by certain drugs, such as spironolactones, which are aldosterone antagonists.

Insensible water loss (IWL) occurs via both pulmonary and cutaneous routes and is influenced by the factors listed below. Because clinical states and environmental factors influence water needs, there is normally a wide range (30 to 60 ml/kg/24 hr) of IWL in healthy term infants.

Factors that decrease IWL may do so by as much as one third in VLBW infants and should be given consideration in each patient. When operative concomitantly, several of these factors can increase IWL by as much as 200%, such as when phototherapy is used and a VLBW infant is under a radiant warmer. For every 1° C rise in body temperature, metabolism and fluid needs increase approximately 10% ("Q-10 effect"). These expected increases must be recognized in calculating fluid requirements.

Factors that influence IWL

Decrease IWL	Increase IWL
Heat shield or double-walled incubators	Inversely related to gestational age and weight
Plastic blankets	Respiratory distress
Clothes	Ambient temperature above thermoneutrality
High relative humidity (ambient or ventilator gas)	Fever
	Radiant warmer
	Phototherapy
	Activity

ETIOLOGY

The causes of common electrolyte problems and common clinical syndromes are discussed in the section on treatment.

PREVENTION

Prevention of fluid and electrolyte imbalance in the neonate begins with knowing the proper calculation of fluid and electrolyte requirements. The estimated metabolic rate forms the reference base for all calculations. The metabolic rate (and hence oxygen consumption) normally increases steadily over the first weeks of life, so increases in water and probably electrolyte needs should be anticipated.

If the caloric requirement is approximately 100 cal/kg/day, the physiologic basis of metabolic rate may be used in calculating needs; however, in most settings use the 100 ml/kg basis, which will be modified by factors that influence IWL and adjusted depending on body weight, clinical composition, and urine volume and composition (Figure 10-8 and Table 10-1).

Preterm infants usually have slightly lower metabolic rates per kilogram than term infants. SGA infants may have higher metabolic rates than preterm infants of similar weight, which is thought to be related to their relatively large brain/body mass ratio. Both SGA and preterm

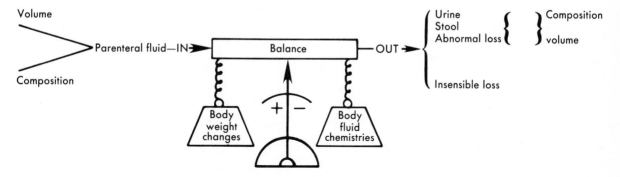

Figure 10-8. Basic scheme for monitoring and modifying therapy.

TABLE 10-1

Guidelines for Fluid (ml/kg/day) and Solute Provision by Patient Weight and Days of Age

WEIGHT	RANGES OF WATER LOSS		DAY 1*	DAY 2-3*	DAY 4-7*
<1250 g	IWL†	40-130			
	Urine	50-100			
	Stool	5-10			
	TOTAL	95-230	120	150	175-200
1250-1750 g	IWL†	20-50			
	Urine	50-100			
	Stool	5-10			
	TOTAL	75-160	90	110	130-140
>1750 g	IWL†	15-40			
	Urine	50-100			
	Stool	5-10			
	TOTAL	70-150	80	90	100-120

Increment for phototherapy: 20-30 ml/kg/day
Increment for radiant warmer: 20-30 ml/kg/day
Maintenance solutes: Glucose: 7-12 g/kg (4-8 g/kg in VLBW infants)
                                 Na: 1-4 mEq/kg (2-8 mEq/kg in VLBW infants)
                                  K: 1-4 mEq/kg
                                 CL: 1-4 mEq/kg
                                 Ca: 1 mEq/kg

*Adjustment based on a urine flow rate of 2 to 7 ml/kg/hr with a specific gravity of 1.003 to 1.010 and stable weight.
†May be reduced by 30% if the infant is on a ventilator.

infants, especially VLBW infants, are expected to require more frequent modification of requirements.

Preterm infants, however, often are subject to other problems that may make this physiologic fact less crucial in calculating needs. SGA infants often require more water per kilogram than either preterm or term, normally grown infants. Input should be recorded every hour and output recorded as it occurs. VLBW infants require frequent monitoring of fluid balance, so that if output is unusually large, intake must be adjusted immediately. If fluid intake decreases, critically ill infants may not tolerate "catching up." Continuous monitoring is necessary to ensure that fluid is infusing in appropriate amounts. Infusion pumps that accurately register 1 ml/hr or less must be used.

Requirements for fluid and electrolytes can be divided into maintenance and deficit needs. Maintenance needs keep the organism in a zero balance state and can be subdivided into (1) normal loss, which consists of water and electrolyte loss through sweat, stool, urine, and insensible (lung and skin) routes, and (2) abnormal or ongoing losses, such as diarrhea, ostomy, or chest tube drainage.

All diapers should be preweighed on a gram scale and marked with dry weight. After each stool or void, the diaper is reweighed, and the difference equals the amount of loss. For example, if the dry weight is 20.7 g and the "wet" weight is 26.4 g, the difference is 5.7 g or 5.7 ml of stool or urine. All losses should be calculated to the nearest milliliter. IV volumetric chambers or small urine collection cups can be used for collection chambers for tube drainage.

Deficit needs refer to previously incurred losses. These should be extremely rare in the newborn but are common in older neonates with disorders that have an insidious or delayed onset, such as renal tubular dysfunction or nonvirilizing congenital adrenal hyperplasia.

Deficits are best estimated by body weight

comparisons. A weight loss greater than 10% to 15% in 1 week should be considered dehydration. VLBW infants are particularly difficult to maintain within 10% to 15% of birth weight during the first week of life.

The initial choice of parenteral solutions is dependent on the weight and age of the infant (Table 10-1). Maintenance of water needs in larger infants on the first day of life can usually be met by a 7.5% to 10% glucose solution infused at 80 ml/kg/day. The infusion rate should be increased gradually to 100 to 120 ml/kg/day using principles of monitoring discussed later.

All sick infants require IV access for fluid administration. The IV equipment should include (1) a needle or catheter, (2) connecting tubing, (3) a volumetric chamber to measure small volumes, and (4) an infusion pump. IV infusions should never be given without a volumetric chamber and infusion pump.

Electrolytes such as sodium and potassium are usually omitted the first day and then added as chloride salts in amounts of 1 to 4 mEq/kg. Mildly acidotic and VLBW infants may be given their sodium requirements as sodium bicarbonate or acetate. Hypocalcemia also may be frequent in tertiary care patients.

Potassium should never be added to IV fluid until urine flow and renal function have been assessed. On the first day, the maintenance requirement for calcium is 0.5 to 1 mEq (100 to 200 mg)/kg given as calcium gluconate. This maintenance is most important in VLBW infants and those who are severely ill.

Factors that influence IWL must be identified early and maintenance needs adjusted appropriately to prevent problems with water and electrolyte balance.

VLBW infants present special problems because data on their management are incomplete. Our recent experience with 30 infants weighing 1250 g or less can be summarized as follows:

1. Water requirements should start at 110 to

120 ml/kg at birth and often need to be increased by 20 to 40 ml/kg/day over days 2 to 4 of life, at which time they plateau at 175 to 200 ml/kg/day.

2. Sodium requirements (including medications) were 2 to 3 mEq/kg/day after 12 hours of age and reached a maximum of 7 mEq/kg/day on days 5 and 6, which was required to prevent hyponatremia.

3. Cumulative weight loss plateaued at 10.8% to 12.7% of birth weight (95% confidence limits) by day 3.

4. Maintenance of normal serum glucose concentrations (<150 mg/dl) required relatively less glucose than in term infants (4 to 8g/kg/day). As anticipated, infants weighing 900 g or less were the most difficult to manage without causing either excessive weight loss or hyponatremia.

VLBW infants, especially those under radiant warmers, may have greatly increased IWL. They also commonly receive phototherapy. Hence their fluid requirements may be 175 to 200 mg/kg/day. After the first week of life, as the epithelium becomes more cornified, the requirements decrease toward 120 to 150 ml/kg/day.

Neonates requiring maintenance fluids when significant oral caloric intake is low (<50 kcal/kg/day) for more than 3 to 5 days should be given parenteral nutritional support with increased glucose, amino acids, lipids, vitamins, and micronutrients (see Chapter 13).

DATA COLLECTION

All parenteral therapy should be based on the following principles: (1) assessing the patient, including maintenance needs, factors that modify IWL, and specific medical or surgical disorders; (2) calculating short-term (12 to 24 hours) fluid and electrolyte needs; (3) initiating therapy at the proper site and rate; and (4) monitoring and modifying based on clinical and biochemical data.

History

A history of factors that influence IWL (see list on p. 210) includes gestational age, birth weight, and postnatal age.

Signs and symptoms

Weight and urine output are the best overall clinical guide to assessing the adequacy of therapy. Weight is the most sensitive index of IWL and must be accurately determined at least every 24 hours. Accurate daily weights in VLBW infants require special nursing efforts and often the use of electronic bed scales.

Urine output should be 1 to 3 ml/kg/hr with a specific gravity of 1.002 to 1.010 (60 to 300 mOsm) (Figures 10-9 and 10-10). Blood pressure and peripheral perfusion may reflect changes in vascular volume and cardiac output. Normal capillary refill occurs within 3 seconds, but hypothermia may falsely delay capillary refill.

Loss of skin turgor is a late and variable sign and is usually not helpful in assessing the therapy, but vital signs (heart and respiratory rate and skin and core temperature) provide helpful clues about the metabolic rate and stress. Drainage from ostomy sites, chest tubes, and nasogastric or other tubes must be quantitated accurately. These types of drainage represent abnormal or ongoing maintenance requirements that must be added to the calculation of abnormal maintenance needs (abnormal + normal = total maintenance).

Laboratory data

Plasma, serum, and whole blood concentrations of electrolytes (Na^+, K^+, Cl^-, Ca^{++}), red blood cells (hematocrit), glucose, BUN or creatinine, and acid-base status should be performed serially. Occasionally serum osmolality and protein concentrations are helpful in assessing the neonate's condition.

Urine specific gravity and volume must be measured as soon as voiding occurs. Urine os-

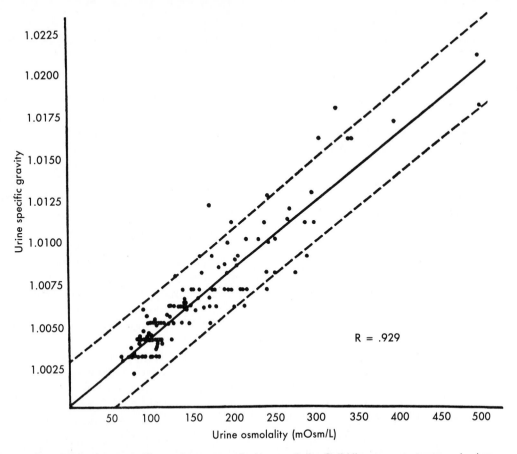

Figure 10-9. Urine specific gravity compared with osmolality. Solid line represents mean; broken line represents 95% confidence limits. (From Jones MD, Gresham EL, and Battaglia FC: Biol Neonate 21:322, 1972.)

molality and electrolyte concentration help clarify fluid and electrolyte balance when glucose, protein, or unusual solutes appear in the urine.

The water content of urine evaporates rapidly under a radiant warmer. Glucosuria and proteinuria (>2+) cause modest elevations in specific gravity, whereas radiographic dyes excreted in the urine cause extreme increases in the specific gravity. All urine samples should be screened with a diagnostic test (BiliLabstix).

All drainage must be collected and mea-

sured, so that the concentration of solutes can be determined. Collections every 4 to 6 hours are preferable to a single "spot" urine, which is commonly misleading. Occasionally determining trace elements, hematocrit, and protein content of urine or drainage can be crucial to management.

TREATMENT
Techniques of IV therapy

Peripheral veins are the most easily accessible and have the least adverse effects for paren-

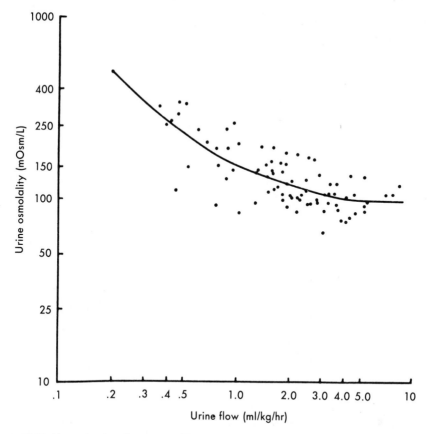

Figure 10-10. Normal urine flow rates. (From Jones MD, Gresham EL, and Battaglia FC: Biol Neonate 21:324, 1972.)

teral therapy. Scalp vein infusion sets are most commonly used in the foot, hand, or scalp veins. However, the advent of extremely small catheter and introducer sets (Quick-Cath, Angiocath, and others) has permitted prolonged (5 to 7 days) use of a single peripheral infusion site.

Often, a rubber band is the most effective tourniquet for the extremity of a small infant. The area of skin should be cleaned with an antiseptic, and efforts should be made to avoid shaving the head, because parents often find this upsetting. Before puncturing the skin, have the "setup" (as described previously) and the appropriate fluid ready.

It is important to recognize the high potential of infiltration and skin sloughs with peripheral IVs. The risk is greatest in the foot, less with the hand, and the least on the scalp. Calcium-containing solutions present an added risk. Although the needle or catheter must be taped in place, the tape must not obscure adequate visualization. At least every hour record the fluid administered, and observe the site for any sign of infiltration. The arm or leg can be positioned on a padded tongue blade (armboard or footboard) to prevent needle displacement. A "flap" of tape can be made at the end of the board, which can be pinned or tied to the bed for further immobilization. Padded sandbags can be used to hold an infant's head or extremity still for a period of time but must be removed regularly to allow some movement. The need for immobilization is less with catheters than with scalp vein sets. However, the board may need to be removed after several hours for additional assurance of no infiltration, as well as mobilization of the limb.

Deep and central veins can be approached by two techniques. Percutaneous insertion using Silastic catheters can be accomplished readily only after much experience. Saphenous or antecubital insertion with advancing the catheter to a deep vein is a relatively simple technique (long lines), and even subclavian cannulation of VLBW infants can be accomplished with relative ease. The risk of infection and thrombosis is probably no greater than with peripheral infusion, but the consequences may be much more serious (see Chapter 13).

The second technique, venesection or cutdowns, can be performed readily with modest training. Catheterization for total parenteral nutrition requires special consideration (see Chapter 13). The catheter is also advantageous because patient mobility is greater, but the risks of infection and thrombosis may be greater than those with percutaneous techniques.

Umbilical vessel catheterization should not be performed for only fluid infusion, except in emergencies (see Chapter 6).

Common problems

In neonatal intensive care units virtually all patients receive IV fluid therapy, so that conventional rules of pediatric fluid therapy, which estimate losses and project deficit replacement, are not completely satisfactory. Weight, urine output and concentration, and the concentration of various solutes in serum and other body fluids are usually known. The correct diagnosis usually rests on clinical and laboratory measurements (not estimates), which are supported by the clinical setting. A pure disorder of hydration is rarely encountered, but mixed disorders or syndromes usually are.

For example, one can compute the amount of sodium required to correct a deficit by the following formula:

$$\text{Sodium required} = (\text{Sodium desired} - \text{Sodium observed}) \times \text{TBW}$$

This calculation considers that the sodium will be given as a "dry salt." The total amount and the rate given is a matter of clinical judgment. In practice, the caretaker usually begins sodium deficit therapy, measures serum (and perhaps urine) sodium, and modifies the IV solution. The cause of the deficit must be identified while these conditions are being corrected, or it is likely to recur.

Common electrolyte disorders
HYPOCALCEMIA
(INFANTS WITH <7 mg/dl)

Clinical findings may correlate poorly with biochemical data (total or ionized calcium). Jitteriness and twitching are nonspecific, and serum calcium (and probably glucose) should be measured.

Hypocalcemia is strongly associated with infants of diabetic mothers, asphyxia, and prematurity (especially the VLBW infant). "Early" (<72 hours) hypocalcemia can be prevented by the inclusion of 18 mg/kg of elemental calcium as 200 mg/kg of calcium gluconate in maintenance IV solution (1 mEq = 2 ml of 10% calcium gluconate).

Bolus infusion (also associated with arrhythmias) and slow infusion for 2 to 3 minutes are not as successful as more gradual attempts to correct hypocalcemia. Either repeated (every 6 hours), slow infusion or continuous infusion is best. Additional elemental calcium should be given intravenously at 18 to 75 mg/kg for 4 to 6 hours if seizures or biochemical abnormality persists. "Late" (>7 days) hypocalcemia usually has a specific cause, such as high phosphate intake, malabsorption and postdiarrhea state, hypomagnesemia, hypoparathyroidism, or rickets, and should be evaluated in detail.

Care should be taken in administering the IV calcium: (1) place the baby on a cardiac monitor to detect bradycardia, (2) immediately discontinue calcium administration if bradycardia occurs, and (3) check the peripheral IV site for patency before and during administration because of sloughing, calcification, and necrosis caused by infiltrated calcium.

HYPERNATREMIA
(INFANTS WITH >150 mEq/L)

Clinical signs of hypernatremia are rare, except for seizures that occur late. The most common causes of hypernatremia are: (1) dehydration, (2) injudicious use of sodium-containing solution (sodium bicarbonate bolus infusion and sodium-containing medications can be overlooked), and (3) congenital reduction in antidiuretic hormone. Both nephrogenic and central diabetes insipidus are uncommon. Cerebral palsy and intracranial bleeding correlate strongly with hypernatremia. Management is directed toward the causes, and serum sodium should be reduced slowly to prevent seizures.

HYPONATREMIA
(INFANTS WITH <130 mEq/L)

Hyponatremia is usually asymptomatic because of chronic rather than acute development of imbalance, but a late clinical sign is seizures. Most common causes include (1) overhydration as a result of maternal or neonatal administration of electrolyte-free solutions, (2) renal loss of sodium commonly in VLBW infants and in any neonate receiving diuretic therapy, and (3) a syndrome of inappropriate antidiuretic hormone secretion that is suspected clinically when decreased serum sodium and increased urine specific gravity occur. This syndrome is associated with central nervous system (CNS) and lung pathologic conditions. Criteria include (1) low serum sodium, (2) continued urine

sodium loss, (3) urine osmolality greater than plasma, and (4) normal adrenal and renal function. Management is by water restriction until diuresis follows and is directed toward the etiology.

HYPERKALEMIA
(INFANTS WITH >6 mEq/L)

Clinical signs	Electrocardiographic changes
Muscular weakness	Short QT interval
Cardiac arrhythmias	Widening QRS
Ileus	Sine wave QRS/T

Causes of hyperkalemia include (1) acidosis with or without tissue destruction, (2) renal failure (water overload may limit management), and (3) adrenal insufficiency (relatively uncommon).

Management is directed toward the causes and nonspecific treatment, depending on the severity of hyperkalemia:

1. **Stop all potassium administration.**
2. **Infuse 100 to 200 mg of calcium gluconate to lower the cell membrane threshold (this is transient but may be lifesaving).**
3. **Infuse sodium bicarbonate, 1 to 2 mEq/ kg, diluted at a 1:2 ratio with water, which is another transient therapy aimed at enhancing intracellular sodium and hydrogen exchange for potassium.**
4. **Administer 1 g/kg cation exchange resin (sodium polystyrene-sulfonate [Kayexalate]) as an oral or rectal solution. Little experience has been reported in neonates, and technical problems of retention can be substantial.**
5. **Perform peritoneal dialysis, but frequently sodium bicarbonate must be added to dialysate to prevent acidosis.**

HYPOKALEMIA
(INFANTS WITH <3.5 mEq/L)

Clinical signs of hypokalemia are related to muscular weakness and cardiac arrhythmias.

Ileus may occur also. Electrocardiographic changes include a decreased T wave and ST depression. The most common causes of hypokalemia are (1) increased gastrointestinal losses from an ostomy and a nasogastric tube and (2) renal losses common in diuretic therapy.

About 90% of total potassium is intracellular. Management is directed toward the causes: (1) low serum potassium always implies significant intracellular depletion, (2) intracellular potassium can be low with normal serum potassium, and (3) IV solutions should not exceed 40 mEq/L potassium.

Common clinical syndromes

Acute renal failure is most often caused by (1) extrinsic factors such as asphyxia, shock, and heart failure; (2) intrinsic factors, such as congenital or acquired lesions; and (3) obstructive uropathy, including urethral or extragenitourinary mass. Oliguria or anuria usually occurs initially. Electrolyte-free glucose infusion should be limited to IWL and urine output. Elevations of BUN often do not occur, because protein intake is commonly low. Recovery is usually associated with natriuresis and osmotic diuresis. This may develop rapidly, and sodium loss as high as 20 mEq/kg/day may occur. Body weight and fluid losses must be carefully and frequently measured, at least every 12 hours. Nonrenal losses, such as gastrointestinal drainage, must be measured also. Ideally, balance treatment is directed toward no weight gain or 1%/day weight loss until recovery is nearly complete. Any weight gain demands careful reevaluation of the fluid plan.

Asphyxia is frequently associated with:
1. Hypotension
2. Renal failure (Tubular necrosis is suggested by proteinuria and hematuria.)
3. Respiratory failure (Ventilators reduce IWL from lungs.)
4. Myocardial ischemia (Echocardiography can often assess ventricular function.)
5. Syndrome of inappropriate antidiuretic hormone secretion (early or late in the clinical course)
6. Cerebral edema (usually after 24 hours)

The asphyxiated neonate should be managed by prospectively reducing the initial fluid estimates by 30% to 60%. IWL and urine output may be the best initial plan, although volume expansion to treat hypotension may be a greater priority.

Major surgery

Surgical trauma is superimposed on the normal metabolic responses of the neonate, determined by both gestational and postnatal age. In healthy term infants, negative balance of water, electrolytes, nitrogen, and calories with associated weight loss occurs during the first 3 to 5 days, with transition to positive balance and weight gain by 7 to 10 days. Similar transition times for preterm infants vary enormously. Deficits may exist as a result of delayed diagnosis, with external loss or internal loss. "Third-space" (especially peritoneal) loss is a notorious source of deficit underestimation.

The exactness of the metabolic response to surgery is not resolved and varies widely among individual patients, even with similar lesions. Perhaps too many uncontrollable variables exist to define a normal postoperative physiologic response of neonates, especially those weighing less than 2 kg. Negative nitrogen balance always occurs postoperatively but is considerably less than in adults. The control of this tendency to minimize nitrogen loss is unknown. Thermal regulation is almost never controlled as well in the operating room as in the intensive care unit, but transport incubators, warmed operating rooms, radiant warmers, and prewarmed solutions should be used in an attempt to achieve thermoneutrality. Intraoperative fluid balance is rarely precise despite the best efforts. Blood loss on sponges, drapes, and other objects should be measured, but IWL from open body cavities is difficult to estimate.

The principles of postoperative management

are (1) serial monitoring of clinical and chemical variables, and meticulously and frequently (every 4 to 6 hours) watching fluid balance, including drainage; (2) providing 30 to 40 kcal/kg as glucose and planning a zero balance of water and electrolytes for 1 to 3 days; and (3) using total parenteral nutrition if significant enteral feedings (>50 kcal/kg) cannot be achieved by 3 to 5 days. Gastrointestinal motility returns rapidly in term infants as compared with adults. Almost all VLBW infants require total parenteral nutrition following surgery.

Water intoxication (hypotonicity) is common in neonates because of small volumes of urine and infusates. A high index of suspicion and meticulous attention to the details of IV therapy prevent hypotonicity. Increased antidiuretic hormone secretion commonly occurs and may progress to a syndrome of inappropriate antidiuretic hormone. Water intoxication may be hard to distinguish from hypotonic dehydration. Water restriction and continued sodium administration should be instituted only after the diagnosis is established. Fresh frozen plasma (10-20 ml/kg) given with a diuretic (1-2 mg/kg furosemide [Lasix]) may be used in the diagnosis, since a good diuresis suggests dehydration or decreased plasma volume.

COMPLICATIONS

Increased fluid administration (>180 ml/kg) has been associated with (1) bronchopulmonary dysplasia, (2) necrotizing enterocolitis, and (3) patent ductus arteriosus. Reduced fluid administration (to prevent increased fluid administration) has been associated with (1) hypertonicity; (2) CNS damage, including bleeding and cerebral palsy; and (3) renal failure and tubular damage.

PARENT TEACHING

The need for and presence of an IV line in the newborn may be frightening for parents. Clear, physiologically sound explanations of the need for fluid and electrolyte support in the sick neonate allay their fears. Scalp vein IVs are particularly of concern (1) if the hair must be shaved and (2) because a common fantasy is that the needle is in the baby's brain. Explain to parents that scalp vein IVs are in the large veins of the head and not the brain and that an IV in the head stays in longer, thus decreasing the need for multiple vein puncture and allowing more mobility. In answer to the question: "Does it hurt?" a truthful answer, "Yes, when it is put in" or "No, not after it is in the vein," relates to peripheral venipuncture.

Infiltrates at peripheral IV sites should be addressed prospectively with parents. Erythema and edema are expected. Sloughing of the skin is not infrequent in VLBW infants and is more common on the feet and hands than on the scalp. Topical therapy similar to thermal burn management is indicated, whereas skin grafting is rarely needed.

Including parents in the care of their sick neonate requires an explanation about the importance of measuring intake and output. Inadvertent disposal of diapers and giving fluids that are not recorded are prevented by emphasizing the importance of saving them for the baby's nurse. "A little spitting up" after feeding may seem insignificant if parents are not instructed in the importance of telling the nurse and saving it for inspection or testing.

• • •

Continuous assessment of renal status and water and electrolyte balance can be achieved through meticulous attention to detail. Proper care requires that the management team repeatedly assess, monitor, and modify, because the first estimates are often prone to error.

SELECTED READINGS

Heird WC et al: Intravenous alimentation in pediatric patients, J Pediatr 80:351, 1972.

Jones MD, Gresham EL, and Battaglia FC: Urinary flow rate and urea excretion rates in newborn infants, Biol Neonate 21:322, 1972.

Winters RW: The body fluids in pediatrics, Boston, 1973, Little, Brown & Co.

CHAPTER 11

Glucose homeostasis

JANE E. DiGIACOMO · MARY I. HAGEDORN · WILLIAM W. HAY, JR.

During intrauterine life the fetus depends on the constant transfer of glucose across the placenta to meet its glucose requirements. After birth neonates must maintain glucose homeostasis by producing and regulating their own glucose supply. This requires activation of a number of metabolic processes, including gluconeogenesis and glycogenolysis, as well as intact regulatory mechanisms and an adequate supply of metabolic substrates.

PHYSIOLOGY

Throughout gestation maternal glucose provides the major source of energy for the fetus via facilitated diffusion across the placenta. Fetal glucose concentration varies directly with maternal concentration and is usually approximately 70% of the maternal value. Changes in maternal metabolism, including increased caloric intake and decreased sensitivity of the maternal tissues to insulin, provide the additional substrate necessary to meet fetal energy demands. During maternal normoglycemia the fetus produces little, if any, glucose, although the enzymes for gluconeogenesis are present by the third month of gestation.[24] If fetal energy demands cannot be met, however, as is the case in maternal starvation with resultant maternal hypoglycemia, the fetus is capable of adapting both by using alternate substrates, such as ketone bodies, and by "turning on" its endogenous glucose production. There is additional evidence that even in the basal state, the fetus relies on fuels other than glucose to meet some of its energy demands. These include both lactate and amino acids.

Fetal glycogen synthesis begins as early as the ninth week of gestation. Most fetal glycogen is synthesized from glucose; this may occur indirectly via three-carbon intermediates such as lactate. The major sites of glycogen deposition are liver, lung, heart, and skeletal muscle. Rates of hepatic glycogen deposition vary with different species depending on the length of gestation; in the human, with a relatively long gestation, hepatic glycogen increases slowly throughout the first two trimesters of pregnancy, with a more rapid rate of deposition during the third trimester[30] (Figure 11-1). By 40 weeks gestation, hepatic glycogen stores are two to three times adult levels. Skeletal muscle glycogen content also increases during the third trimester to as much as five times adult levels. In contrast, lung and cardiac muscle glycogen stores decrease as the fetus approaches term, although they are still of physiologic significance. Survival after asphyxia, for example, has been shown to be directly related to cardiac glycogen content. The decrease in lung glycogen, which begins at 34 to 36 weeks, may be related to ongoing developmental processes that require utilization of stored energy. An example would be the dramatic increase in the rate of surfactant synthesis seen at the same gestational age.

Several factors can affect rates of glycogen accumulation. Decreased availability of substrate, as in maternal malnutrition, placental insufficiency, or multiple gestations, has been associated with a decreased rate of glycogen synthesis. Acute intrauterine hypoxia does not appear to produce a measurable change in glycogen content, but chronic hypoxia, as seen in maternal preeclamp-

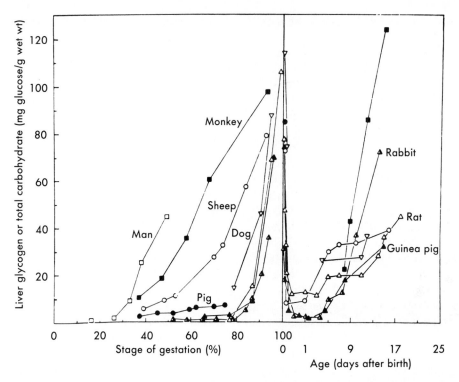

Figure 11-1. Liver glycogen content: changes with gestational and postnatal age. (From Shelley HJ: Br Med Bull 17:137, 1961.)

sia, does result in lower tissue glycogen content as compared with normoxic controls.

In addition to glycogen, the human fetus also stores energy as adipose tissue. Most triglyceride synthesis occurs during the third trimester. By 40 weeks the human fetus has a fat content of about 16%, making it the fattest of all terrestrial newborn mammals. The human placenta transports some free fatty acids, although the amount transported has not been well quantified. Preliminary studies suggest that the maternal fatty acids transported to the fetus are not sufficient to account for the amount of adipose tissue present; therefore the fetus must also synthesize triglycerides directly from glucose. Again, conditions in which fetal glucose supply is reduced will result in less adipose tissue accumulation.

Insulin, considered a major stimulus for fetal

growth, is present in the fetal pancreas by 8 to 10 weeks. Pancreatic insulin content increases in late gestation, exceeding adult levels by the time the infant reaches term.[17] However, the fetal pancreas seems to be less sensitive than the adult pancreas to the insulin secretion–stimulating effects of increased glucose concentration. Nevertheless, insulin secretion is augmented by higher glucose concentrations; increasing amino acid concentration adds to this effect. The elevated insulin concentration increases both fetal glucose utilization and glucose oxidation rates without increasing total fetal oxygen consumption.[12,31] This implies that other substrates (e.g., amino acids) become available for nonoxidative metabolism, which may promote tissue accretion and growth. Animal studies have demonstrated increased rates of protein synthesis and glucose uptake with increased insulin concentration and, conversely, decreased cell numbers and DNA content with insulin deficiency, supporting insulin's role as a growth-promoting factor. The fetuses of diabetic mothers have an increased islet cell response to hyperglycemia compared with controls, releasing more insulin than normal fetuses at any given blood glucose concentration.[17] The higher insulin levels, in turn, lead to increased growth, producing the macrosomia typically seen in infants of diabetic mothers (IDMs).

The related pancreatic hormone glucagon, which, like insulin, does not cross the placenta, has been detected as early as 15 weeks gestation. The role of glucagon in regulating fetal glucose metabolism remains unclear. The concentration of glucagon in fetal blood is relatively low, even though pancreatic content is higher than in the adult. The high insulin-to-glucagon ratio in the fetus may be important in preferentially maintaining glycogen synthesis and suppressing gluconeogenesis, since glucagon is a potent inducer of gluconeogenic enzymes.[24]

At birth the infant is removed abruptly from its glucose supply, and blood glucose concentration falls. Several hormonal and metabolic changes occur at birth that facilitate the adaptation necessary to maintain glucose homeostasis. Catecholamine levels increase markedly at birth, possibly as a response to cooling in the delivery room, with a subsequent increase in glucagon levels and a reversal of the fetal insulin/glucagon ratio.[34] The elevated glucagon and norepinephrine levels activate hepatic glycogen phosphorylase, which induces glycogenolysis; simultaneously the falling glucose concentration stimulates hepatic glucose-6-phosphatase activity, which leads to an increase in hepatic glucose release.[5] Increased catecholamines also stimulate lipolysis, providing substrate for gluconeogenesis. The reversal of the insulin/glucagon ratio, such that the glucagon concentration is greater than the insulin concentration, induces synthesis of phosphoenolpyruvate carboxykinase (PEPCK), which is considered the rate-limiting enzyme in hepatic gluco-

neogenesis. The concentrations of PEPCK and other gluconeogenic enzymes continue to increase with postnatal age during the first 2 weeks of life regardless of gestational age[5,24] (Figure 11-2). These changes act in concert to provide glucose to replace the supply previously received via the placenta.

Studies in normal infants using several different methods have determined that the steady state glucose production/utilization rate in the term neonate is 3.5 to 5.5 mg/min/kg,[6] approximately twice the weight-specific rate measured in adults. As in the fetus, it appears that approximately half of this glucose is oxidized to CO_2 during normal metabolic processes, whereas the remainder is used in nonoxidative pathways such as glycogen and fat synthesis.

Maintenance of glucose homeostasis depends on the balance between hepatic glucose output and peripheral glucose utilization. Hepatic glucose output is a function of rates of glycogenolysis and gluconeogenesis, which are regulated by the factors discussed above. Peripheral glucose utilization varies with the metabolic demands placed on the neonate. Some circumstances in which peripheral utilization is increased include hypoxia, since anaerobic metabolism of glucose is less efficient than aerobic glycolysis; hyperinsulinemia, which increases glucose uptake by the insulin-sensitive tissues, including muscle and liver; and cold stress, under which the infant must increase the metabolic rate to maintain body temperature. If rates of glycogenolysis and gluconeogenesis do not match the rate of glucose utilization, because of failure of the hormonal control mechanisms or variability of substrate supply, then disturbances of glucose homeostasis occur. These disturbances are recognized clinically by the presence of hypoglycemia or hyperglycemia.

ETIOLOGY
Hypoglycemia

Hypoglycemia during the first 72 hours of life was defined previously as a whole blood glucose concentration of less than 35 mg/dl in the term

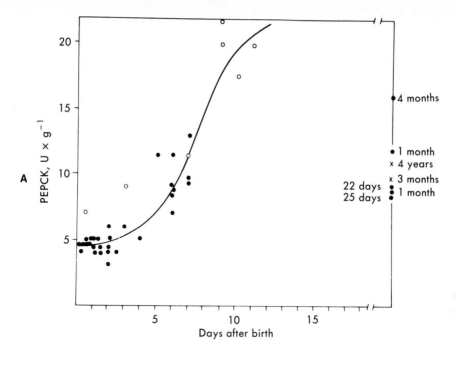

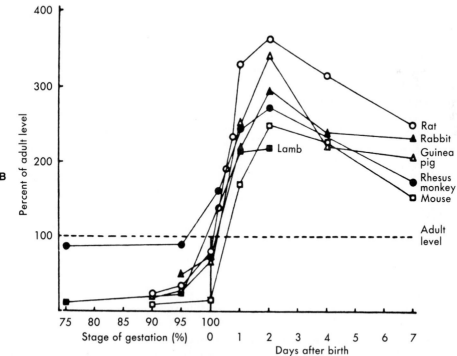

Figure 11-2. Changes in representative hepatic enzymes before and after birth. **A,** Phospho-enolpyruvate carboxykinase. **B,** Glucose-6-phosphatase. (**A** from Marsac C et al: Biol Neonate 28:317, 1976. Reproduced by permission of S Karger AG, Basel. **B** from Dawkins MJR: Br Med Bull 22:27, 1961.)

infant or less than 25 mg/dl in the preterm infant, or alternatively as a plasma concentration of less than 40 mg/dl or less than 30 mg/dl, respectively. These definitions were based on statistical analyses of glucose concentrations measured in large groups of neonates. The definition of hypoglycemia was based on the glucose concentration two standard deviations (2 SD) below the mean for the group. The overall incidence of hypoglycemia has been estimated at 1.3 to 4.4/1000 live births; differences in incidence figures probably reflect the difference between those studies that reported only symptomatic infants and those that evaluated data from screening measurements on all infants, thus including those with asymptomatic hypoglycemia. In premature infants the incidence of hypoglycemia is increased, with estimates ranging from 1.5% to 5.5%[22] (Figure 11-3).

More recently with changes in nursery care, including earlier feeding and the liberal use of intravenous (IV) dextrose infusions, average glucose concentrations in newborns appear to be increased. As a result, several authors have suggested redefining hypoglycemia based on current data. For example, a recent study[14] of blood glucose levels in 65 normal term neonates found that 95% had values greater than 30 mg/dl in the first 24 hours of life and greater than 45 mg/dl after 24 hours of life. Similarly, Srinivasan et al[36] found that in infants who received the first feeding by 3 hours of age, subsequent plasma glucose values were higher than previously reported "normal" values; in addition, several infants with plasma glucose concentrations within 2 SD of the study mean had symptomatic hypoglycemia. These data suggest that the definition of hypoglycemia may need to be revised to reflect both changes in newborn care and the higher "normal" glucose concentrations that have now been documented on the second and third days of life.

A further consideration when evaluating blood glucose concentrations is that significant metabolic derangements, including decreases

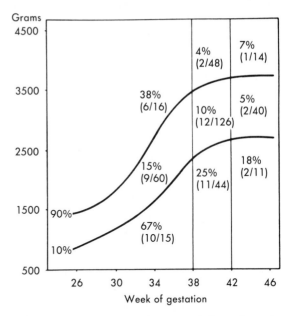

Figure 11-3. Incidence of neonatal hypoglycemia (blood glucose <30 mg/dl) by birth weight and gestational age. (From Lubchenco LO and Bard H: Pediatrics 47:831, 1971. Reproduced by permission of Pediatrics.)

in cerebral glucose supply, may occur at glucose concentrations above the "hypoglycemic" level as defined by large population studies. The infant with polycythemia, for example, may have a normal blood glucose concentration but may have decreased cerebral delivery of glucose because of reduced plasma flow. Therefore in the infant at risk for continued hypoglycemia, there may be some benefit to maintaining glucose concentrations in the "average normal" rather than the "low normal" range.

The causes of hypoglycemia can be divided into several broad categories based on the mechanism(s) producing the hypoglycemia. These include inadequate substrate supply, abnormal endocrine regulation of glucose metabolism, and increased rate of glucose utilization. There are also a number of etiologies whose mechanisms are not well defined.

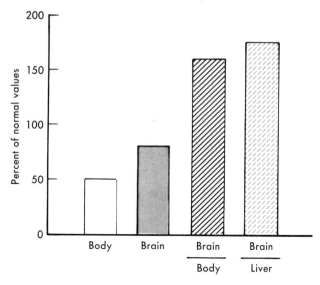

Figure 11-4. Differences in organ/body weight ratios in SGA infant compared with appropriate-for-gestational-age (AGA) counterpart. (From Lafeber HN, Jones CT, and Rolph TP: Some of the consequences of intrauterine growth retardation. In Visser HKA, editor: Nutrition and metabolism of the fetus and infant, Boston, 1979, Martinus Nijhoff, Publishers.)

INADEQUATE SUBSTRATE SUPPLY

If the substrate supply to the liver is inadequate, the hepatic glucose output will not meet metabolic demands. Most often this is due to subnormal fat and glycogen stores, which therefore do not provide enough energy to maintain glucose homeostasis until gluconeogenesis reaches adequate levels. Since most hepatic glycogen is accumulated during the third trimester, infants born prematurely will have diminished glycogen stores. The infant with intrauterine growth retardation secondary to placental insufficiency is also at risk for decreased glycogen production, presumably because of diminished transfer of precursors across the placenta. The limited supply is then used for oxidative metabolism and tissue growth, rather than fat or glycogen accretion. Postnatally catecholamine- and glucagon-stimulated lipolysis and glycogenolysis rapidly deplete the already less than adequate supplies at a time when gluconeogenesis is still impaired because of low levels of PEPCK and other gluconeogenic enzymes. Hypoglycemia then results. These infants may be asymptomatic with the initial episode of hypoglycemia, but they can become symptomatic if the hypoglycemia persists.

Although inadequate stores of glycogen and lipid have been cited as the major etiology of hypoglycemia in the premature and small-for-gestational-age (SGA) infant, a number of other factors may also play a role. The preterm infant with respiratory distress syndrome, for example, has increased metabolic demands because of the increased work of breathing. Infants with intrauterine growth retardation and hypoglycemia have been shown to have an increased rate of glucose disappearance when receiving an IV glucose infusion, as well as reduced fat mobilization in response to hypoglycemia, when compared with normoglycemic SGA newborns. Because of the increased brain weight/liver weight ratio in the infant with asymmetric growth retardation, cerebral glucose requirements are high relative to the liver's capacity to respond, even if glycogen stores are normal for size[18] (Figure 11-4). Inappropriately elevated insulin/glucose ratios have also been observed in some SGA infants. These findings suggest that other disturbances in glucose metabolism in addition to lower than normal energy stores may be present in some growth-retarded infants.

A much rarer, but related, problem occurs in several types of glycogen storage disease. In these inherited disorders hypoglycemia is due, not to inadequate glycogen stores, but rather to the inability to utilize stored glycogen as a result of one of several enzyme deficiencies.[22] Hypoglycemia has also been reported in children with severe congenital heart disease and congestive heart failure; in these cases inadequate uptake of substrate by the liver, secondary to either hepatic congestion or poor cardiac output with resultant poor hepatic perfusion, leads to decreased rates of gluconeogenesis and glycogenolysis.[13]

ABNORMALITIES OF ENDOCRINE REGULATION

Hyperinsulinemia is the most common endocrinologic disturbance resulting in neonatal hypoglycemia and may be the most common cause of persistent hypoglycemia in the first year of life. Excessive insulin secretion in the newborn produces an increased rate of glycogen synthesis and intracellular glucose uptake. In addition, high circulating insulin levels inhibit lipolysis, ketogenesis, and glycogenolysis, impairing the infant's response to the increased glucose demand.

The most common clinical situation in which hyperinsulinemia occurs is in the IDM. In utero the fetus becomes hyperglycemic because of increased transfer of glucose across the placenta from the hyperglycemic mother. The fetal pancreatic beta cells are stimulated by the increased fetal glucose concentration to produce abnormally increased quantities of insulin. As mentioned previously, the islet cells seem to be abnormally sensitive to this stimulus. Prior to delivery, the increase in cellular glucose uptake in response to the increased insulin secretion is matched by the increased availability of glucose from the mother. After delivery, however, the source of glucose is abruptly removed while the hyperinsulinemia persists, producing hypoglycemia. The decrease in glucose concentration postpartum is a result of insulin-stimulated peripheral glucose uptake, as well as inhibition of gluconeogenesis and glycogenolysis by the high insulin concentrations. While some studies have reported other abnormalities in glucose kinetics in the IDM, Cowett et al[4] found no difference in glucose kinetics in IDMs versus controls. This may reflect the fact that maternal diabetic control was maintained during pregnancy in the group studied, although a large review of pregnancies in diabetic mothers found no association between the incidence of neonatal hypoglycemia and the number of episodes of maternal hyperglycemia (a reflection of the degree of control) late in pregnancy.[10] The incidence of hypoglycemia in IDMs ranges from 15% to 75%; these infants are frequently asymptomatic. The incidence of a number of other complications is increased in these infants as well, including polycythemia, which may add to disturbances of glucose homeostasis, hypocalcemia, dystocia secondary to macrosomia, and congenital anomalies. Although typically macrosomic, the infants of mothers with severe diabetic vasculopathy may have intrauterine growth retardation due to decreased placental blood flow.

Like the IDM, infants with Beckwith-Wiedemann syndrome are also macrosomic and hyperinsulinemic; in addition, they have other associated anomalies, including macroglossia, which may cause airway obstruction, and omphalocele. Up to 50% have symptomatic hypoglycemia in the first few days of life. As in the IDM, the hyperinsulinemia is due to pancreatic beta-cell hyperplasia; however, in these infants maternal or fetal hyperglycemia has not been documented, and the etiology of the islet cell hyperplasia is unknown.

Islet cell hyperplasia is also seen in some infants with severe erythroblastosis fetalis. The mechanism responsible for the hyperplasia is unknown, but glutathiones released from erythrocytes during hemolysis may indirectly stimulate islet cell hyperplasia by inactivating circulating insulin. Regardless of the etiology, infants with erythroblastosis may exhibit symptomatic or asymptomatic hypoglycemia. The incidence ranges from 2% to 20%, increasing with decreasing umbilical cord hemoglobin concentrations. Exchange transfusion, often required to treat severe anemia or hyperbilirubinemia, may further contribute to hyperinsulinemia.[29] The high dextrose content of the CPD blood used for the exchange transfusion stimulates insulin release from the hyperplastic beta cells. When the transfusion is completed, glucose entry rates return to baseline but insulin levels remain high, causing "rebound" hypoglycemia.

A number of infants have been described as having persistent hyperinsulinemia due to islet cell dysplasias such as nesidioblastosis (diffuse increase in beta-cell number) or discrete islet cell adenomas. Seventy percent of infants with these disorders manifest refractory hypoglycemia in the first 3 days of life. Because the hyperinsulinemia begins in utero, these infants, like the others described above, are also usually macrosomic at birth.

Hypoglycemia has also been noted following the use of beta-agonist agents for tocolysis. Both animal[37] and human[28] studies have documented increased insulin concentrations in infants whose mothers received such drugs prior to delivery; the risk of developing hypoglycemia may be inversely related to the length of time between the last dose received by the mother and delivery.

Finally, several cases of iatrogenic hyperinsulinemia have been reported in infants whose umbilical artery catheters were inadvertently positioned with the tip near the origin of the pancreatic artery.[23] The islet cells were then exposed to the high glucose concentration of the solution being infused through the catheter and responded with an increased rate of insulin release, producing hypoglycemia, which resolved when the catheter was repositioned.

In addition to hyperinsulinemia, global endocrine disturbances can also result in hypoglycemia. These disturbances include abnormalities of the hypothalamic-pituitary axis, with the most severe being panhypopituitarism. Such infants frequently have growth hormone deficiency and hypothyroidism in addition to severe hypoglycemia. If pituitary dysfunction is due to a structural central nervous system (CNS) lesion, other neurologic problems, including abnormal muscle tone and neonatal seizures, may be present. Adrenal failure and hypoglycemia can occur as a result of adrenal hemorrhage, often in association with neonatal sepsis. Isolated defects, including primary hypothyroidism and cortisol deficiency, may also be associated with hypoglycemia.

INCREASED GLUCOSE UTILIZATION

Some term infants may have normal energy stores at birth and intact regulating mechanisms, but may be stressed by one of several conditions so that the available supplies do not meet the neonate's energy requirements. The asphyxiated newborn is one common example. Following asphyxia and subsequent tissue ischemia, the neonate relies largely on anaerobic metabolism for energy production. Since this process is relatively inefficient, more glucose is metabolized to produce the amount of energy required than would be used under aerobic conditions. As a result, glucose from lipolysis and glycogenolysis is rapidly consumed. Hypoxic-ischemic damage to the liver may further impair synthesis of gluconeogenic enzymes and thus delay the normal postnatal onset of gluconeogenesis. Elevated insulin levels may also be present, providing an additional etiology for the hypoglycemia.

Hypothermia, often due to inappropriate management of the infant after delivery, may result in hypoglycemia due to rapid depletion of brown fat stores for nonshivering thermogenesis. Hypoglycemia also has been observed in some infants with sepsis. A study done in several such infants found that they had an increased rate of glucose disappearance in response to an IV glucose infusion, suggesting an increased rate of glucose utilization.[19] Stimulation of glucose utilization may be a result of circulating endotoxins, which increase the rate of glycolysis. In addition, increased catecholamine levels in response to the stress of acute infection may play a role.

Hyperglycemia

Hyperglycemia in the newborn is usually defined as a blood glucose concentration of greater than 125 mg/dl in the term infant or greater than 150 mg/dl in the premature infant. Incidence is difficult to determine; estimates range from 5.5% of all infants receiving IV infusions of 10% dextrose in water ($D_{10}W$) to as high as 40% in infants weighing less than 1000 g.

Most often the neonate with hyperglycemia is a low birth weight (LBW) infant (<32 weeks gestation and <1200 g birth weight) who cannot tolerate an IV glucose infusion at the usual rate of 4 to 8 mg/kg/min (i.e., $D_{10}W$ at 60 to 100 ml/kg/day). This relative glucose intolerance is probably due to general immaturity of the usual regulatory mechanisms, including a decreased insulin response to glucose. Some investigators have also reported that unlike fetuses and adults, preterm as well as some term infants fail to suppress endogenous glucose production despite the administration of an adequate exogenous supply (e.g., IV infusion)[3]; however, other investigators did not measure any glucose production in premature infants receiving IV glucose at a rate of more than 2 mg/kg/min.[40] The risk of developing hyperglycemia is significantly increased with decreasing birth weight, as well as with an increasing rate of glucose infusion, even within the accepted range of glucose infusion rates.[21] Delay in initiating enteral feedings may be an additional risk factor, since the incidence of hyperglycemia is higher in LBW infants receiving all of their nutrition parenterally than in those who receive at least a part of their nutrition enterally. The rate at which the glucose concentration is increased in the hyperalimentation solution may also play a role. The presence of respiratory distress syndrome with its requirement for mechanical ventilation is also associated with an increased risk of developing hyperglycemia. This may be due to increased circulating catecholamines, leading to increased lipolysis and glycogenolysis.

Although SGA infants are more likely to be hypoglycemic, a few cases of what has been termed *transient diabetes mellitus* have been reported in growth-retarded infants.[32] In these cases hyperglycemia is thought to be a result of partial insulin insensitivity, but increased levels of catecholamines and other stress-related hormones may play an important role. Unlike true diabetes mellitus, ketosis does not develop. Most cases are self-resolved or respond to decreasing the glucose administration rate; occasionally insulin therapy may be required.

There are several other etiologies that must be considered in infants with hyperglycemia. Increased blood glucose concentrations have been reported in association with gram-negative sepsis.[16] IV lipid infusions may also produce hyperglycemia if given rapidly at rates of more than 0.25 g/kg/hr; however, this exceeds the rate at which lipids are usually given.[38] Methyl xanthines are frequently used to treat apnea in the preterm infant and may be a cause of hyperglycemia. This problem has been well documented after theophylline overdose; one study also measured increased blood glucose concentrations in infants with therapeutic theophylline levels, including concentrations in the hyperglycemic range in two infants.[35] Neonates undergoing surgical procedures are also at increased risk for hyperglycemia, probably because of a combination of the large quantities of glucose-containing fluids and blood products that may be administered during the procedure and the effects of stress-related hormones.

PREVENTION

Recognition of those infants at risk for disturbances in glucose homeostasis is the most important step in preventing both hypoglycemia and hyperglycemia. In infants with conditions

predisposing to hypoglycemia, such as the SGA infant or the IDM, early feeding and hourly monitoring of blood glucose concentrations until the infant is stable may prevent a decrease in blood glucose or at least reduce the severity of the hypoglycemia. Maintenance of a neutral thermal environment is especially critical to minimize energy expenditure in those infants at risk for hypoglycemia. Other conditions associated with hypoglycemia, such as asphyxia and hypothermia, may be avoidable through appropriate obstetric and neonatal intervention.

Hyperglycemia occurs most often in premature infants receiving IV glucose. In the very low birth weight (VLBW) infant, hyperglycemia may be avoided by starting IV glucose infusions at rates of 2 to 3 mg/kg/min and following blood glucose concentrations frequently (as often as every 3 to 4 hours) while these infants continue to receive IV glucose. However, hyperglycemia

may be unavoidable in the very immature infant.

DATA COLLECTION
History

The history of any neonate must include a detailed prenatal and family history, including a history of any abnormal maternal glucose tolerance test, previous macrosomic infants, unexplained stillbirth or neonatal demise, or any history of diabetes, preeclampsia, hypertension, Rh incompatibility, or other risk factors discussed earlier. Other important data include a history of family members with hypoglycemia or metabolic disease and a history of maternal drug exposure, especially to beta-agonist tocolytic agents.

The most important information to be obtained from the infant's history are gestational age, Apgar scores, and details of events in the

TABLE 11-1

Neonatal Hypoglycemia: Etiologies and Time Course

MECHANISM	CLINICAL SETTING	EXPECTED DURATION
Decreased substrate availability	Intrauterine growth retardation	Transient
	Prematurity	Transient
	Glycogen storage disease	Prolonged
	Inborn errors (e.g., fructose intolerance)	Prolonged
Endocrine disturbances		
Hyperinsulinemia	IDM	Transient
	Beckwith-Wiedemann syndrome	Prolonged
	Erythroblastosis fetalis	Transient
	Exchange transfusion	Transient
	Islet cell dysplasias	Prolonged
	Maternal beta-sympathomimetics	Transient
	Improperly placed umbilical artery catheter	Transient
Other endocrine disorders	Hypopituitarism	Prolonged
	Hypothyroidism	Prolonged
	Adrenal insufficiency	Prolonged
Increased utilization	Perinatal asphyxia	Transient
	Hypothermia	Transient
Miscellaneous/multiple mechanisms	Sepsis	Transient
	Congenital heart disease	Transient
	CNS abnormalities	Prolonged

TABLE 11-2 _____

Etiologies of Neonatal Hyperglycemia

Iatrogenic (e.g., during IV glucose infusion)
Decreased insulin sensitivity (e.g., VLBW infant or transient diabetes mellitus)
Sepsis
Methyl xanthine side effect

_____

delivery room, especially any findings that would suggest the presence of significant perinatal asphyxia. An infant with a history of any of the conditions listed in Tables 11-1 and 11-2 should be considered at high risk for developing a problem with glucose homeostasis.

Physical examination

Careful measurement of birth weight and head circumference in combination with accurate gestational age assessment will establish whether the infant is premature, LBW, SGA, or large-for-gestational-age (LGA) and thus at increased risk for hypoglycemia. IDMs frequently have small heads relative to their general macrosomia and have been described as having "tomato facies" because of plethora and increased buccal fat. The physical findings associated with Beckwith-Wiedemann syndrome have already been listed.

SIGNS AND SYMPTOMS

Signs of neonatal hypoglycemia are nonspecific and extremely variable. They include general findings, such as abnormal cry, poor feeding, hypothermia, and diaphoresis; neurologic signs, including tremors and jitteriness, hypotonia, irritability, lethargy, and seizures; and cardiorespiratory disturbances, including cyanosis, pallor, tachypnea, periodic breathing, apnea, and cardiac arrest. These findings may also be seen in prematurity, sepsis, intraventricular hemorrhage, asphyxia, hypocalcemia, congenital heart disease, and structural CNS lesions, among other etiologies. In the pres-

ence of any of the above signs, however, hypoglycemia should always be considered, since the diagnosis can be made relatively easily and prompt treatment is essential in the symptomatic infant.

Hyperglycemia is usually asymptomatic and is most often diagnosed on routine screening of the infant at risk.

Laboratory data

When the diagnosis of hypoglycemia is suspected, the plasma glucose concentration must be determined. Ideally, this determination should be made using one of the preferred enzymatic methods, such as the glucose oxidase method. The sample should be obtained from a warmed heel or by venipuncture and transported in a sample tube containing a glycolytic inhibitor. If a standard serum chemistry tube is to be used (i.e., one without a glycolytic inhibitor), the sample must be processed promptly, since the erythrocytes in the sample will continue to metabolize glucose and may falsely reduce the value obtained.

In the usual clinical setting, more rapid determination of the glucose concentration is frequently desirable. Several different enzyme/chromogen test strips are available for this purpose; the two most often encountered are Dextrostix and Chemstrips bG. These produce a color change that varies with the glucose concentration present in a drop of blood applied to the surface. The specimen can be obtained from a heelstick specimen. The glucose concentration present is determined either by comparison of the test strip with a set of colorimetric standards provided on the package or by placing the strip in a reflectance colorimeter.

These methods can be quite useful in screening infants in whom abnormal glucose concentrations are suspected, provided that the user is aware of their limitations. Accuracy depends in part on the technique used. An adequate drop of blood must remain in contact with the enzyme-impregnated test strip for the designated length of time. Isopropyl alcohol remaining on the heel after it is prepped can falsely elevate the value.[9] Outdated strips may yield falsely low results. Even with proper technique, test strip methods have an associated wide variance, whether or not a reflectance colorimeter is used to obtain results. They may either overestimate or underestimate the glucose concentration present, depending on the range of concentrations tested and the specific product used.[11,26]

Because of the associated problems, the diagnosis of hypoglycemia or hyperglycemia should never be made solely by test strip results. Borderline or suspicious values should be confirmed by a specimen sent to the chemistry laboratory. However, treatment for suspected hypoglycemia should not be withheld until the confirmatory report has been obtained, since this may mean a delay of several hours. Similarly, if hypoglycemia is suspected on the basis of clinical symptoms, initial treatment should be instituted even if the test strip result is "normal." If the actual value is abnormal, a delay in therapy could be harmful; if the actual value is within the normal range, therapy can be stopped without serious side effects.

Most cases of neonatal hypoglycemia will have an identifiable etiology (e.g., the IDM, the SGA infant, etc.). Those infants with idiopathic hypoglycemia, whether symptomatic or asymptomatic, generally improve spontaneously within 2 to 5 days, and no further evaluation is needed. However, in rare cases hypoglycemia will persist beyond the first week of life with no obvious cause detected. The diagnostic evaluation of these children should include simultaneous determination of glucose and insulin concentrations; evaluation of pituitary function, including measurement of thyroid-stimulating hormone (TSH), thyroxine (T_4), adrenocorticotropic hormone (ACTH), cortisol, and growth hormone levels; pancreatic ultrasound (if hyperinsulinemia is present); and appropriate studies to diagnose inborn errors of metabolism, such as lactate and pyruvate concentrations.

TREATMENT
Hypoglycemia

Early identification of the infant at risk for developing hypoglycemia and institution of prophylactic measures to prevent its occurrence constitute the best treatment for this disorder. In those infants in whom hypoglycemia does occur, the treatment goals are twofold: to return the glucose concentration to normal levels and, once normalized, to maintain it within the normal range.

In the asymptomatic, otherwise well infant with hypoglycemia, an attempt may be made to normalize blood glucose concentrations by immediately feeding the infant formula or a solution of $D_{10}W$ and following glucose concentrations hourly until the infant is stable. In most cases, however, including all cases of symptomatic neonates, IV therapy should be used. The usefulness of a bolus of 200 mg/kg given as $D_{10}W$ (i.e., 2 ml/kg of $D_{10}W$) given over 1 to 3 minutes has been established.[20] This schedule has several advantages; there is a lower incidence of hyperglycemia immediately following the bolus, and the slower rate of administration decreases the insulin response to glucose infusion, thus lowering the risk of rebound hypoglycemia after the bolus. Following the bolus, a continuous IV infusion of glucose should be started at a rate of 4 to 8 mg/kg/min[20] (Figure 11-5). These rates cover the range of hepatic glucose production in normal term newborns; rates at the lower end of the range are suggested for IDMs to avoid enhancing insulin stimulation, whereas higher rates may be necessary in SGA infants, given their high brain/body weight ratio. When glucose infusion rates are being calculated, it is important to remember that commercially prepared glucose solutions actually contain glucose in its hydrated form (MW 198 versus MW 180 for anhydrous glucose), which lowers the actual glucose content of the solution by approximately 8%. Thus $D_{10}W$ contains approximately 9.2 g of glucose per deciliter.

The infant's blood glucose should be moni-

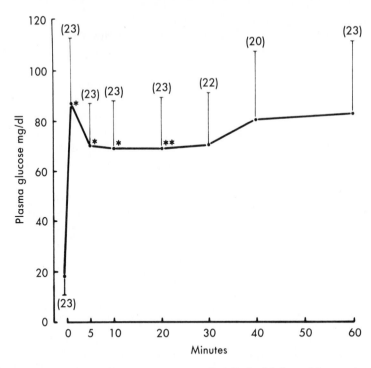

Figure 11-5. Plasma glucose response to glucose "minibolus" followed by continuous glucose infusion (8 mg/min/kg) as therapy for neonatal hypoglycemia. (From Lilien LD et al: J Pediatr 97:295, 1980.)

tored frequently until the infant is stable, using one of the methods discussed above. Usually glucose infusion at "maintenance" rates will be sufficient to preserve normoglycemia, but in some infants, especially those with hyperinsulinemia, much higher rates of glucose infusion may be required. In such infants the infusion rate can be increased by 1 to 2 mg/kg/min every 30 to 60 minutes until the blood glucose concentration stabilizes in the low normal range. The minimum rate adequate to maintain normoglycemia should be used to avoid continued stimulation of excessive insulin secretion. If necessary, additional bolus infusions of 10% glucose can be administered to treat recurrent hypoglycemia; each bolus should be followed by an increase in the IV glucose infusion rate until the glucose concentration remains stable.

Once the infant's requirement has been determined, the infusion usually should be maintained at that level for a minimum of 2 to 4 days. Feedings can be instituted when clinically indicated. When feedings are well tolerated, the IV infusion generally can be slowly tapered, provided the glucose concentration and clinical status remain stable.

ADJUNCTIVE THERAPY

STEROIDS. Steroids may ameliorate hypoglycemia by decreasing peripheral glucose utilization, increasing gluconeogenesis, and enhancing the response to glucagon. Use of steroids should be limited to those neonates who require more than 15 to 18 mg/kg/min of glucose to maintain normoglycemia. They can be given as hydrocortisone, 5 to 10 mg/kg/day divided into two to four doses, or as prednisone, 2 mg/kg/day in one or two doses. If effective, the steroids are continued until the blood glucose concentration has been stable for 24 to 48 hours and the infant is tolerating tapering of the IV glucose infusion.

GLUCAGON. Glucagon, 30 μg/kg IV or intramuscularly (IM), will release glycogen from hepatic stores. Its administration may be useful diagnostically, since failure to respond to glycogen administration with an increase in serum glucose concentration suggests depletion of hepatic glycogen stores. IDMs may require much larger doses, up to 300 μg/kg, to produce a response. Glucagon is most useful in infants with hypoglycemia secondary to increased circulating insulin levels, since hyperinsulinemia stimulates glycogen formation and inhibits glycogenolysis even in the presence of hypoglycemia. Glucose infusion should be maintained following glucagon administration, since there is a risk of increased insulin secretion in response to the glucagon-produced surge in glucose production. In addition, the rapid, but transient, increase in glucose concentration immediately following glucagon injection may produce a false sense that the hypoglycemia has resolved, even though the underlying etiology still exists.

SOMATOSTATIN. Somatostatin, which inhibits release of both insulin and glucagon from the pancreas, has been used successfully to treat refractory hypoglycemia in some infants with islet cell dysplasias. It is administered as a continuous infusion at rates of 3 to 10 μg/hr in combination with replacement glucagon administration. It should not be considered definitive therapy but rather a means of stabilization of these infants prior to surgical treatment, usually subtotal or total pancreatectomy, or as adjunctive therapy following surgery.

DIAZOXIDE. Because it also suppresses pancreatic insulin release, diazoxide has been suggested as a treatment for hypoglycemia due to hyperinsulinemia. Experience in neonates has been limited, and its effectiveness is not well documented[2]; however, in infants beyond the neo-

natal period it has been useful in controlling persistent hyperinsulinemia due to islet cell dysplasias when surgery has not achieved complete remission.

MISCELLANEOUS. In those infants with hypoglycemia due to a specific medical problem, therapy should be directed toward alleviating the underlying illness. This includes administration of antibiotics to treat sepsis, partial exchange transfusion to relieve hyperviscosity, hormone replacement in cases of hypopituitarism, and dietary intervention in infants with metabolic disorders. Surgery is usually required in cases of nesidioblastosis and islet cell adenomas, since these are relatively unresponsive to medical therapy alone.

Hyperglycemia

GLUCOSE. Most cases of hyperglycemia can be treated by reducing the neonate's glucose intake. Many LBW infants will tolerate glucose infusions at rates of up to 4 mg/kg/min, although Zarif et al[39] reported that more than 40% of infants weighing less than 1000 g had a blood glucose concentration higher than 125 mg/dl while receiving glucose at an average rate of 4.4 mg/kg/min. In addition, the VLBW infant, with high fluid requirements due to large insensible water losses through the skin, may require a combination of water and glucose intake that could only be administered by using a hypotonic solution such as $D_{2.5}W$. The use of a low glucose concentration necessitates the addition of sodium (e.g., $D_{2.5}W$ has approximately 130 mOsm/L, requiring the addition of sodium chloride to produce an isotonic solution with 280 mOsm/L), which may further complicate management of fluids and electrolytes. Further, the VLBW infant needs adequate caloric intake (50-60 kcal/kg/day) to avoid a negative nitrogen balance and tissue catabolism. These needs often cannot be met without resultant hyperglycemia. If the glucose is only mildly elevated (e.g., concentrations of 150 to 200 mg/dl) and the infant has no evidence of adverse

effects such as osmotic diuresis, there may be no indication for reducing the rate of IV glucose administration.

INSULIN INFUSION. Because of the above considerations, some authors have suggested the use of a continuous insulin infusion in the infant who cannot tolerate infusion of glucose solutions with concentrations greater than 5 g/dl (i.e., D_5W). Infusion of insulin at rates of 0.2 to 0.8 mU/kg/min (0.01 to 0.05 units/kg/hr) for 12 to 24 hours will result in improved glucose tolerance, although some infants may require supplemental insulin at higher rates or for a longer time.[25] Hypoglycemia can be avoided by starting with a low infusion rate and increasing the rate by 10% to 20% every 60 to 90 minutes until the glucose concentration is less than 150 mg/dl. Blood glucose concentrations should be monitored every 15 to 20 minutes during initiation of the insulin infusion, and an IV glucose infusion should be maintained to avoid any abrupt changes in blood glucose. Despite some promising results, there have also been reports of resistance to insulin infusion developing after 1 to 3 days of use, leading to a recurrence of hyperglycemia.[8] Insulin infusion may also be useful in the treatment of more mature infants with transient diabetes mellitus, although these infants will frequently respond to an adjustment of the glucose infusion rate.

MISCELLANEOUS. Galactose was administered IV to a group of glucose-intolerant VLBW infants by Sparks et al,[33] resulting in a 65% to 80% increase in total carbohydrate intake, with resolution of hyperglycemia and improvement in glycosuria. Whole-blood galactose levels reached a plateau of 14.8 ± 2 mg/dl in the treated infants, a value significantly higher than the highest value measured in normal milk-fed infants (4.2 mg/dl). However, the peak in treated infants was still well below the range seen in infants with galactosemia, and no adverse effects were detected clinically. With further clinical trials, galactose may emerge as an alternative source of carbohydrate for the glucose-intolerant infant.

In addition to specific measures to lower the blood glucose concentration, close attention must be paid to fluid balance in the hyperglycemic infant, since hyperglycemia can induce an osmotic diuresis. The VLBW infant is at increased risk for this problem because of generally increased fluid requirements and a low renal threshold for tubular glucose excretion as compared with the term infant. Finally, as in hypoglycemia, efforts should be made to treat any underlying etiology, such as sepsis.

PROGNOSIS
Hypoglycemia

The outcome for infants with neonatal hypoglycemia appears to be related to the duration and severity of the hypoglycemia, as well as the underlying etiology. Those with asymptomatic hypoglycemia usually have a normal neurodevelopmental outcome, although minor abnormalities such as learning disabilities and abnormal electroencephalograms (EEGs) without seizure disorder occasionally have been reported at long-term follow-up. Symptomatic infants have a poorer diagnosis, with abnormalities ranging from learning disabilities to cerebral palsy and seizure disorders, as well as mental retardation of varying degree.[7] Computed tomography (CT) scans performed in a small group of infants who had severe neonatal hypoglycemia (blood glucose concentrations of 10 to 20 mg/dl) were abnormal in 50% of the infants, with most showing cortical or cerebral atrophy; however, these infants did not represent a randomly selected population.[15] Prompt initiation of treatment is thought to be associated with better outcome, although this has not been well documented.

The incidence of neurodevelopmental abnormalities in IDMs ranges from 0% to 35%; the lower figures are from more recent studies and may represent improvement in obstetric and neonatal care. None of the long-term follow-up studies has shown an association between the presence of neonatal hypoglycemia and later neurodevelopmental impairment.[10,27] Instead, outcome has been related to such factors as prematurity, presence of congenital anomalies, and degree of control of maternal disease.

Infants with islet cell dysplasias, who are more likely to have recurrent and prolonged episodes of hypoglycemia, generally have poor outcomes,[1] possibly because these infants do not generate ketone bodies, which could serve as an alternative source of energy for cerebral metabolism during periods of hypoglycemia. Hypoglycemia secondary to hypopituitarism is also associated with a poor outcome; often this is due to other CNS or endocrine dysfunction rather than the hypoglycemia itself.

Hyperglycemia

Although there is little direct evidence, it has been postulated that hyperglycemia in the premature infant may increase the risk of intraventricular hemorrhage by causing rapid changes in osmolarity with resultant rapid fluid shifts within the brain and germinal matrix. One study did report an increased mortality in hyperglycemic premature infants as compared with their normoglycemic counterparts, although hyperglycemia may have been a marker for those infants with more severe illness rather than a direct cause of the increased mortality. Increased morbidity may be seen in the form of greater difficulty with fluid and electrolyte management, as well as problems establishing adequate nutrition.

Infants with transient diabetes mellitus usually recover spontaneously within the first week; persistent insulin resistance is extremely rare. No neurologic sequelae have been directly attributed to the presence of transient hyperglycemia in these neonates.

PARENT TEACHING

Parent teaching should begin prior to delivery, with emphasis placed on good nutrition and early and regular prenatal care. The goal of teaching during pregnancy should be to provide the fetus with an environment that is optimal for normal growth. This includes the prevention of some of the clinical conditions known to increase the risk of neonatal hypoglycemia, such as intrauterine growth retardation associated with maternal cigarette smoking and poor maternal nutrition. In addition, regular prenatal care assures the early detection of potentially serious problems, including preeclampsia and gestational diabetes.

Prenatal teaching is especially important in the woman with known diabetes mellitus, since overall outcome (although not necessarily the incidence of hypoglycemia) is directly related to the degree of control during pregnancy. In addition, the possibility of neonatal hypoglycemia and requirement for IV therapy can be discussed with the parents before delivery so that they will be aware that the infant may require a longer hospital stay even if delivered at term.

If IV therapy is selected to treat neonatal hypoglycemia, regardless of etiology, a thorough explanation of the treatment plan must be given to the parents at the time therapy is instituted. Frequent progress reports should be provided to resolve unanswered (and often unasked) questions and relieve parental anxiety. Since the majority of cases of neonatal hypoglycemia resolve quickly without permanent sequelae, little teaching is required about problems to expect after discharge. The exceptions to this are those children with islet cell dysplasias who may have recurrent episodes of hypoglycemia; their parents need to be aware of the symptoms of hypoglycemia and emergency treatment measures that can be instituted prior to the child's being seen by a physician. Parents of infants with inborn errors of metabolism also need counseling with regard to prognosis, as well as genetic counseling about risks of recurrence in future pregnancies.

•　　•　　•

Hypoglycemia is a frequently encountered problem in the newborn; with the increasing survival of very premature infants, hyperglycemia will become increasingly common. A favorable prognosis in both of these conditions requires prompt identification of infants at risk and early institution of appropriate therapy. As we develop a better understanding of the control of glucose homeostasis in the fetus and newborn, better information on prevention and optimal treatment of these problems will become available.

ACKNOWLEDGMENTS

Supported by NIH grants DK35836, HD00781, and HD20761. Dr. DiGiacomo is supported by NIH Training Grant HD07186.

REFERENCES

1. Aynsley-Green A: Nesidioblastosis of the pancreas in infancy, Dev Med Child Neurol 23:372, 1981.
2. Barrett CT and Oliver TK: Hypoglycemia and hyperinsulinism in infants with erythroblastosis fetalis, N Engl J Med 278:1260, 1968.
3. Cowett RM, Oh W, and Schwartz R: Persistent glucose production during glucose infusion in the neonate, J Clin Invest 71:467, 1983.
4. Cowett RM et al: Glucose kinetics in infants of diabetic mothers, Am J Obstet Gynecol 146:781, 1983.
5. Dawkins MJR: Biochemical aspects of developing function in newborn mammalian liver, Br Med Bull 22:27, 1961.
6. Denne SC and Kalhan SC: Glucose carbon recycling and oxidation in human newborns, Am J Physiol 251:E71, 1986.
7. Fluge G: Neurological findings at follow-up in neonatal hypoglycemia, Acta Paed Scand 64:629, 1975.
8. Goldman S and Hirata T: Attenuated response to insulin in VLBW infants, Pediatr Res 14:50, 1980.
9. Grazaitis DM and Sexson NR: Erroneously high Dextrostix values caused by isopropyl alcohol, Pediatrics 66:221, 1980.
10. Haworth JC, McRae KN, and Dilling LA: Prognosis of infants of diabetic mothers in relation to neonatal hypoglycemia, Dev Med Child Neurol 18:471, 1976.
11. Hay WW Jr and Osberg IM: The "Eyetone" blood glucose reflectance colorimeter evaluated for in vitro and in vivo accuracy and clinical efficacy, Clin Chem 29:558, 1983.
12. Hay WW Jr et al: Effect of insulin on glucose uptake in the near-term fetal lamb, Proc Soc Exp Biol Med 178:557, 1985.
13. Haymond MW et al: Glucose homeostasis in children with severe congenital heart disease, J Pediatr 95:220, 1979.
14. Heck LF and Erenberg A: Serum glucose levels during the first 48 hours of life in the healthy full-term neonate, Pediatr Res 17:317A, 1983.
15. Hirabayashi S, Kitakara O, and Hishidi T: Computed tomography in perinatal hypoxic and hypoglycemic encephalopathy with emphasis on follow-up studies, J Comput Assist Tomogr 4:451, 1980.
16. James T III, Blessa M, and Boggs TR Jr: Recurrent hyperglycemia associated with sepsis in a neonate, Am J Dis Child 133:645, 1979.
17. Ktorza et al: Insulin and glucagon during the perinatal period: secretion and metabolic effects in the liver, Biol Neonate 48:204, 1985.
18. Lafeber HN, Jones CT, and Rolph TP: Some of the consequences of intrauterine growth retardation. In Visser KHA, editor: Nutrition and metabolism of the fetus and infant, Boston, 1979, Martinus Nijhoff Publishers.
19. Leake RD, Fiser RH, and Oh W: Rapid glucose disappearance in infants with infection, Clin Pediatr 20:397, 1981.
20. Lilien LD et al: Treatment of neonatal hypoglycemia with minibolus and intravenous glucose infusion, J Pediatr 97:295, 1980.
21. Louik C et al: Risk factors for neonatal hyperglycemia associated with 10% dextrose infusion, Am J Dis Child 139:783, 1985.
22. Lubchenco LO and Bard H: Incidence of hypoglycemia in newborn infants classified by birth weight and gestational age, Pediatrics 47:831, 1971.
23. Malik M and Wilson DP: Umbilical artery catheterization: a potential cause of refractory hypoglycemia, Clin Pediatr 26:181, 1987.
24. Marsac C et al: Development of gluconeogenic enzymes in the liver of human newborns, Biol Neonate 28:317, 1976.
25. Ostertag SG et al: Insulin pump therapy in the very low birth weight infant, Pediatrics 78:625, 1986.
26. Perelman RH et al: Comparative analysis of four methods for rapid glucose determination in neonates, Am J Dis Child 136:1051, 1982.
27. Persson B and Gentz J: Follow-up of children of insulin-dependent and gestational diabetic mothers, Acta Paediatr Scand 73:349, 1984.
28. Procianoy RS and Pinheiro CEA: Neonatal hyperinsulinemia after short-term maternal beta-sympathomimetic therapy, J Pediatr 101:612, 1982.
29. Schiff D et al: Metabolic effects of exchange transfusions. II. Delayed hypoglycemia following exchange transfusion with citrated blood, J Pediatr 79:589, 1971.
30. Shelley HJ: Glycogen reserves and their changes at birth and in anoxia, Br Med Bull 17:137, 1961.
31. Simmons MA et al: Insulin effect on fetal glucose utilization, Pediatr Res 12:90, 1978.
32. Sodoyez-Goffant F and Sodoyez JC: Transient diabetes mellitus in a neonate, J Pediatr 91:395, 1977.
33. Sparks JW et al: Parenteral galactose therapy in the glucose-intolerant premature infant, J Pediatr 100:255, 1982.
34. Sperling MA et al: Fetal-perinatal catecholamine secretion: role in perinatal glucose homeostasis, Am J Physiol 247:E69, 1984.

35. Srinivasan G et al: Plasma glucose changes in preterm infants during oral theophylline therapy, J Pediatr 103:473, 1983.

36. Srinivasan G et al: Plasma glucose values in normal neonates: a new look, J Pediatr 109:114, 1986.

37. Tenenbaum D and Cowett RM: Mechanisms of beta-sympathomimetic action on neonatal glucose homeostasis in the lamb, J Pediatr 107:588, 1985.

38. Vileisis RA, Cowett RA, and Oh W: Glycemic response to lipid infusion in the premature neonate, J Pediatr 100:108, 1982.

39. Zarif M, Pildes S, and Vidyasagar D: Insulin and growth-hormone responses in neonatal hyperglycemia, Diabetes 25:428, 1976.

40. Zarlengo KM et al: Relationship between glucose utilization rate and glucose concentration in preterm infants, Biol Neonate 49:181, 1986.

SELECTED READINGS

Cowett RM and Schwartz R: The infant of the diabetic mother, Pediatr Clin North Am 29:1213, 1982.

Fisher DA: Endocrine physiology (I). In Smith CA and Nelson NM, editors: The physiology of the newborn infant, ed 4, Springfield, Ill, 1976, Charles C Thomas, Publisher.

Gutberlet RL and Cornblath HM: Neonatal hypoglycemia revisited, 1975, Pediatrics 58:10, 1976.

Hay WW Jr: Fetal and neonatal glucose homeostasis and their relation to the small for gestational age infant, Semin Perinatol 8:101, 1984.

Hill DE: Effect of insulin on fetal growth, Semin Perinatol 2:319, 1978.

Ogata ES: Carbohydrate metabolism in the fetus and neonate and altered neonatal glucoregulation, Pediatr Clin North Am 33:25, 1986.

Pildes RS and Pyati SP: Hypoglycemia and hyperglycemia in tiny infants, Clin Perinatol 13:35, 1986.

CHAPTER 12

Breastfeeding the sick neonate

SANDRA L. GARDNER · JAYNE P. O'DONNELL · LEONARD E. WEISMAN

It has long been recognized that breast milk has many advantages over homemade and commercial formulas. Posters dating from 1918 show the difference in the mortality of breastfed and bottle-fed infants. Research has identified specific anti-infective properties of breast milk. These properties provide protection against gastrointestinal infections and respiratory infections. Although breastfeeding can be a struggle for the mother of a healthy newborn, and even more difficult for the mother of a sick or premature newborn, more mothers are choosing to breastfeed their infants because of the benefits it offers. The goal of this chapter is to give the health care provider the skill and knowledge to support the breastfeeding dyad, particularly when it involves the sick neonate. Methodology and resource material for successful clinical management of this situation are provided. Recommendations are based on reasonable available data wherever possible and on many years of experience.

PHYSIOLOGY[6,9,11,17]
Nutritional value of breast milk

When evaluating the components of breast milk, one should realize that the composition varies with the (1) stage of lactation, (2) time of day, (3) sampling time during a feeding, (4) maternal nutrition, and (5) variation among individuals.

Colostrum is produced during the first week after birth. It contains a higher ash content and higher concentrations of sodium, potassium, chloride, protein, fat-soluble vitamins, and minerals than mature milk. Colostrum has a lower fat content, especially of lauric and myristic acids, than mature milk. This milk is yellowish, thick, rich in antibodies, has a specific gravity between 1040 and 1060, and contains 67 kcal/dl. Multipara and women who have previously breastfed have more colostrum during the first few days than women who have not.

Transitional milk is produced between 1 and 2 weeks postpartum, and mature milk is produced 2 weeks postpartum and usually contains 75 kcal/dl. During a feeding, the relative content of protein and the absolute content of fat increase. The morning feeds have a higher fat content than the afternoon and evening feeds. Malnourished mothers produce less milk. Water-soluble vitamins in breast milk may be affected by deficient diets.

Cow's milk versus human milk

Cow's milk has significant differences from human milk. Cow's milk has 18 parts whey to 82 parts casein, whereas human milk has 60 parts whey to 40 parts casein. Casein is composed of proteins with esther-bound phosphate, high proline content, and low solubility at a pH of 4 to 5. Casein forms curd by combining with calcium

□ The opinions and assertions in this chapter are those of the authors and do not necessarily represent those of the Department of the Army or the Department of Defense.

caseinate and calcium phosphate. The cysteine and taurine content is low in cow's milk but high in human milk, whereas the methionine content is high in cow's milk and low in human milk. Human milk also has lower aromatic amino acids, phenylalanine, and tyrosine. Human milk contains 6.8 g of lactose/dl, and cow's milk contains 4.9 g of lactose/dl. Sodium, phosphorus, calcium, magnesium, citrate, and total ash content are higher in cow's milk, but potassium and the calcium/phosphorus ratio are higher in human milk. Human milk contains more iron than unsupplemented cow's milk but less iron than supplemented cow's milk. Cow's milk has a mean pH of 6.8, osmolality of 350 mOsm, and 221 mOsm renal osmolar load. Human milk has a mean pH of 7.1, osmolality of 286 mOsm, and 79 mOsm renal osmolar load.

Cow's milk forms curd much easier and thus delays gastric emptying. The newborn cannot handle certain proteins well because of lack of specific enzymes required for metabolism. Iron is more bioavailable in human milk and iron absorption from human milk is more efficient, but cow's milk has a higher concentration of zinc and contains more fluorine than human milk.

Preterm versus term breast milk

A great deal of information, some conflicting, recently has been published about the contents of preterm breast milk. Most authors agree that preterm breast milk has a higher protein, sodium, and possibly calcium content than term breast milk.[12]

Immunologic value of breast milk[13,15]

The protective properties of human milk can be divided into cellular and humoral factors. Investigations about allergy, necrotizing enterocolitis, tuberculosis, and neonatal meningitis suggest that breast milk provides a protective function.

Cellular components

About 10^6 leukocytes/ml are present in colostrum, but this number decreases significantly about the third to fifth day postpartum. Mature milk contains about 4000 cells/ml. Macrophages, which make up 90% of the cells present in breast milk, are large complex phagocytes and are laden with lipids. Macrophages are inhibited by the lympho kine migration inhibitory factor (MIF) and are functionally active in colostrum and when evaluated in vitro.

Macrophages phagocytize microorganisms and kill bacteria. They produce lysozyme, lactoferrin, and complement, and when removed from animal stomachs have retained the ability to phagocytize. Animal studies have shown that macrophages add a protective quality to breast milk. Specifically, macrophages have been shown to decrease the risk of necrotizing enterocolitis in at-risk rats. Efforts to confirm this in humans have been inconclusive, but current storage and handling techniques could adversely affect the properties involved in this protection.

Lymphocytes, which make up 10% of breast milk cells, produce MIF. Both T and B lymphocytes are present in breast milk, although two thirds appear to be T cells. The B cells synthesize IgA. The T and B cells respond to mitogens and antigens by proliferation. Intact lymphoid cells have been found in the stomach, intestines, and traversing the mucosal wall. Suggested immunologic significance includes sensitization, graph versus host phenomenon, and immunologic tolerance. Lymphocytes may also be incorporated in the tissue and adoptively immunize the neonate.

Humoral components

Immunoglobulins (IgA, IgM, IgG) are present in breast milk in greater amounts during the first 4 to 6 days and then decrease significantly with time. IgA is the predominant immunoglobulin in both colostrum and mature milk. These previously mentioned immunoglobulins provide local intestinal protection against gastrointestinal viruses and bacteria, such as poliomyelitis and *Escherichia coli.*

Lactobacillus bifidus is a gram-positive nonmotile anaerobic bacillus that is the predominant bacteria in breastfed infants (instead of gram-negative organisms). The bifidus factor appears to be a dialyzable nitrogen-containing carbohydrate without amino acids.

Lactobacillus produces large amounts of acetic acid and lactic acid. This acidic environment is more conducive to the growth of lactobacillus than to gram-negative organisms.

The antistaphylococcal factor may protect the neonate against staphylococcal infections. This factor is stable at extreme temperatures and part of the free fatty acid component, yet separate from linoleic acid.

Lysozyme is a thermostable, acid-stable enzyme that increases with lactation and is 300 times greater in human milk than in cow's milk. Lysozyme is bacteriostatic against gram-negative and gram-positive bacteria in vitro.

Lactoferrin, an iron-binding protein stable in stomach pH, is normally saturated 50% with iron. It is highly concentrated in milk but gradually decreases with time. Lactoferrin is bacteriostatic against staphylococci, *E. coli,* and *Candida albicans* by depriving the organism of iron but may be disrupted by oral iron therapy that interferes with saturation.

An interferon-like substance was produced and secreted in colostral cells in vitro but is not present in the supernatant fluid of colostrum. No clinical evidence of this function has been documented in the neonate.

Several factors of complement are found in small amounts in milk but decrease with time and may aid lysis of this bacteria. Unsaturated B_{12}-binding protein is present in milk in large amounts. The B_{12}-binding protein makes B_{12} unavailable for bacterial growth of *E. coli* and other organisms. Nonimmunoglobulin macromolecules and fatty acids in milk appear to have some immunologic value also.

Antiallergic properties

The small intestine in the neonate has increased permeability to macromolecular antigens. Production of secretory IgA in the intestine is delayed until about 2 months of age. Secretory IgA in breast milk appears to inhibit absorption of these antigens.

Normal lactation

Breast development during pregnancy is stimulated by luteal and placental hormones, lactogen, prolactin, and chorionic gonadotropin. Estrogen stimulates growth of the milk collection (ductal) system, whereas progesterone stimulates growth of the milk production system.

If women should abort as early as 16 weeks, their breasts will secrete colostrum. Therefore mothers are capable of breastfeeding any viable infant.

The estrogen and progesterone function as inhibitors to actual milk production. Therefore stimulation of the breast before delivery will not create milk. Once the infant and placenta are delivered, stimulation of the nipple becomes effective in producing milk.

Stimulating the nipple by the infant's sucking action causes an increase in the prolactin released in the bloodstream and induces the synthesis and release of oxytocin. The amount of prolactin is directly related to the quantity and possibly quality of nipple stimulation; since prolactin stimulates the synthesis and secretion of milk, the quantity of prolactin is related to the quantity of milk. A decrease in the quality of stimulation causes a decrease in prolactin production and thus a decrease in milk production.

Adequate prolactin secretions control the supply-and-demand quality of breastfeeding. The sooner the infant nurses, the sooner milk comes in. More milk is produced, not by the length of the infant's nursing, but by the quality (nutritive versus nonnutritive) of the infant's suckle. **As the infant becomes larger, he or she will want to nurse longer but will be able to empty most of the breast in 4 to 7 minutes after letdown has taken place.**

Oxytocin brings about the letdown reflex and

uterine contractions. Eventually, oxytocin is released by only a thought of breastfeeding or the sound of an infant crying, in addition to the infant's nursing.

Natural weaning through adding solids can be unnoticed by the mother. Early weaning by introducing a bottle can cause temporary engorgement, which resolves in a few days. Weaning should be performed by adding one bottle or cup feeding every 2 or 3 days. Sudden weaning will cause increased engorgement and discomfort for the mother. A breast binder and ice may help to relieve the mother's discomfort.

Psychologic values of breastfeeding

In animal studies, the lactating female appears to be protected from large changes in response to certain situations.

The short-term advantage of breastfeeding is early mother and infant contact. The "en-face" position of breastfeeding enhances this contact. In the sick neonate, early contact, whether it is breastfeeding or another physical means, sometimes must be delayed or modified.

The long-term psychologic effect of unrestricted nursing appears to be a more even mood cycle as a result of elevated prolactin levels, which enhance coping mechanisms associated with caring for a new family member.

All referring physicians and nursing personnel who admit infants to the intensive care unit should support and assist mothers who wish to breastfeed their infant.

Lactation and reproduction

Lactation is not a form of birth control, although some women have no menses for as long as 12 months while breastfeeding. Since ovulation may occur in the absence of menses, it is possible to become pregnant while lactating. Contraceptive methods other than birth control pills should be discussed with the lactating woman (see section on establishing breastfeeding and drugs).

ETIOLOGY

Although breastfeeding is a normal, natural function, it is not simple, but rather a highly complex interaction and interdependence between mother and baby. To be successful, the breastfeeding dyad must synchronize their behavior and physiology and receive support from their environment. In the past, breastfeeding sick or preterm babies was thought to be impossible, but now breast milk may be the preferred nutrition for premature infants, even though feeding at the breast may be necessarily delayed. Delayed breastfeeding may be as successful as immediate feeding when (1) problems are prevented, (2) mothers receive support and encouragement in maintaining their milk supply, and (3) everyone is patient and knowledgeable about teaching the baby to suckle.

PREVENTION

Problems with breastfeeding may be a maternal problem, a neonatal problem, or a combination of these. Breastfeeding problems should be prevented. To solve a breastfeeding problem, the mother must be observed feeding the infant.

Maternal problems

Maternal problems include engorgement, painful nipples, and cracked nipples.[10] A primipara is at high risk for developing engorgement. Frequent emptying of the breast is the best prevention.

Engorgement occurring in the early postpartum period is characterized by general discomfort, usually in both breasts in a well, afebrile woman. Areolar engorgement blocks the nipple and makes grasping the areola difficult for the infant. Gentle breast massage and manual expression of a small amount of milk softens the areola so the infant is able to "latch on." When the body of the breast(s) and the areola are affected, the goal of management is to make the mother comfortable so that nursing may continue. Supporting the breasts is crucial, and the mother should wear a well-fitting but adjustable brassiere 24 hours a day.[11] Applying cold packs decreases pain, and pain relievers may be prescribed. Applying heat (packs or a warm shower) and expressing some milk is good preparation for feeding. A nursing baby, manual expression, or an effective pump helps initiate and maintain milk flow.

Preparation may prevent sore, cracked, and painful nipples, although many mothers do not prepare their breasts and have no problems. Fair-skinned women (especially redheads) usually have more problems. Prenatally, stimulation of the nipple by gently pulling and twisting or rubbing with a towel helps condition the nipple and makes it pliable. Massaging the entire breast helps maintain patency of the milk ducts and can also be performed during pregnancy. When the infant begins to suck, or if the nipples are becoming sore from breast pumps, nipple conditioning should cease.

The initial grasp of the nipple by the infant often causes discomfort because of the negative pressure on the empty ductules.[11] Hand expression of a few drops of milk starts the flow and immediately rewards the hungry baby so that tugging and pulling at the nipples are unnecessary at the beginning of the feeding. Poor positioning of the infant causes painful and eventually cracked nipples. Prevention and treatment involve careful positioning of the infant close to the mother (Figure 12-1). Compression of the areola behind the nipple extracts milk from the storage sinuses[16] (Figure 12-2). Changing the infant's position on the nipple several times during the feeding may also be helpful. Figure 12-3 shows the "football hold" position.

Nursing the least painful or unaffected breast first initiates milk flow in the affected side and provides initial relief from hunger, so that the baby does not suck too vigorously when nursed on the painful nipple. Keeping nipples clean and dry promotes healing. Clear water (no soap or alcohol) is all that is necessary to

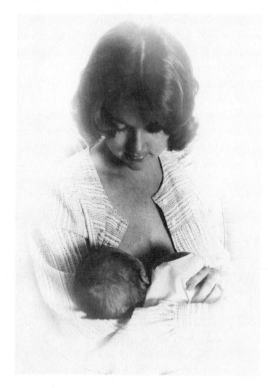

Figure 12-1. Proper positioning of breastfeeding infant. (© Lact-Aid International, Inc. Reprinted by permission.)

keep the nipples clean. Drying nipples well, not using plastic nursing pads, and exposing nipples to air and dry heat (sunlight, light bulb sauna, or a low setting on a hair dryer) is comforting. Using medications may affect the infant and the maternal letdown reflex. Using ointments may not be helpful, since they prevent exposure to air and drying, but if used, a small amount (i.e., one drop) should be gently massaged into the nipple. Lanolin (if there is no allergy to wool) or A and D ointment may be used safely. Nipple shields are not recommended, because they are awkward for the mother and confusing for the infant.

Flat or inverted nipples may be difficult for

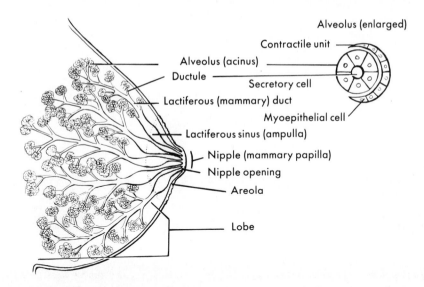

Figure 12-2. Structure of human breast during lactation. (From Riordan J: A practical guide to breastfeeding, St Louis, 1983, The CV Mosby Co.)

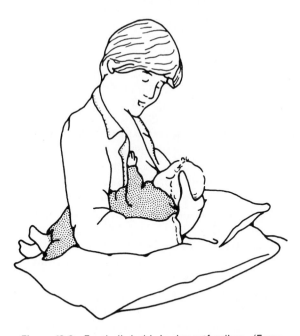

Figure 12-3. Football hold in breastfeeding. (From Bowman J and Hill R: Pediatrics 35:815, 1965; and Breastfeeding, Evanston, Ill, 1981, American Academy of Pediatrics. Copyright American Academy of Pediatrics, 1965 and 1981. Reproduced by permission of Pediatrics.)

the infant to grasp and result in maternal engorgement and infant frustration (Figure 12-4). Inverted nipples may be treated by wearing plastic breast cups or shields (Figure 12-5).

Neonatal problems

Neonatal problems include nipple confusion, sucking defects, choking, and multiple births. Because increased stimulation creates an increased milk supply, it is possible to breastfeed multiple infants. In the early weeks it will be difficult and time consuming, but eventually it can become faster and more convenient than bottle feeding. Two infants can be fed at the same time, in the cradle position or in the football hold position (Figure 12-6). The babies should change breasts with each feeding, because one may have a stronger suck than the other and each breast should receive an equal amount of stimulation.

Normal sucking on the breast differs greatly from sucking on an artificial nipple. Understanding the mechanisms of suckling is essential to preventing, assessing, and intervening in

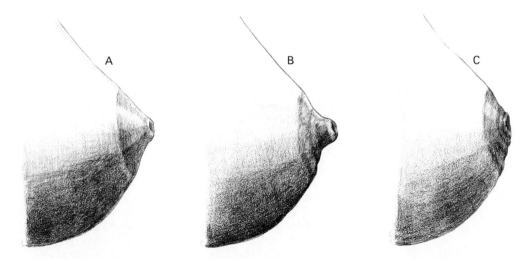

Figure 12-4. Inverted nipples. **A,** Normal and inverted nipples may look similar when nipple is not stimulated. **B,** Normal nipple protrudes when stimulated. **C,** Inverted nipple retracts when stimulated. (© Jimmy Lynne Scholl Avery. Reprinted by permission.)

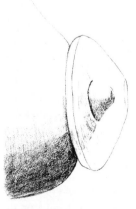

Figure 12-5. Breast shield. Special breast shields may be worn under bra during last 3 to 4 months of pregnancy. Gentle pressure at edge of areola gradually forces nipple through center opening of shield to help increase nipple protractility. It can be used after childbirth if needed. NOTE: Milk can leak from breasts into shields. Since maternal body warmth can foster rapid bacterial contamination, such milk should be discarded. (© Jimmy Lynne Scholl Avery. Reprinted by permission.)

neonatal suckling problems. Human nutritive suckling is composed of five separate yet interrelated processes: (1) rooting, (2) orienting, (3) suction, (4) expression, and (5) swallowing[5,11] (Figure 12-7). Rooting, the tactile stimulating of the baby's face and lips, elicits the head to turn toward the stimulus and enables the infant to find the mother's nipple. Orienting, or latching on, consists of the initial suction and jaw and tongue movements used to draw the mother's nipple high in the palate. The lactiferous sinuses, located behind the nipple and areola, must be stimulated by the infant's mouth for milk to be extracted (see Figure 12-2).

Suction, the application of negative pressure in the infant's mouth, holds the nipple and areola in place and extracts milk. At the beginning of breastfeeding, a strong suction stretches and shapes the nipple, but only moderate suction is required to maintain adequate grasp of the nipple. During the feeding, occasional burst of suction assist the milk flow. Ex-

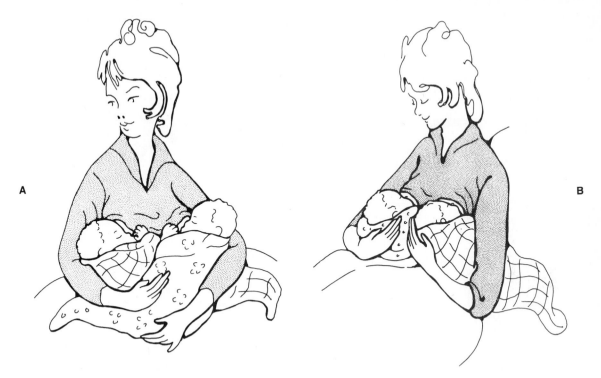

Figure 12-6. Breastfeeding twins. **A,** Cradle position. **B,** Football hold position. (From The womanly art of breast feeding, Franklin Park, Ill, 1976, La Leche League International.)

pression, or squeezing milk out by using pressure, is performed through a series of jaw and tongue movements. The infant thrusts the lower jaw upward, while simultaneously moving the tongue upward and stroking back toward the palate. With this chewinglike motion, milk is expressed from the lactiferous sinuses. Swallowing the milk also reflexively initiates the expression cycle of jaw and tongue movements. Therefore nutritive suckling is primarily expression and swallowing of milk. During nursing, just enough suction to keep the nipple in proper position is used, even during the expressive phase of suckling.

Suckling an artificial nipple requires different behaviors than suckling the breast. When an artificial nipple is being used, fluid flows into the posterior oropharynx (Figure 12-8). In an attempt to regulate the milk flow and prevent choking and gagging, infants may curl their tongue up behind the nipple, clench their gums, or obstruct the nipple's holes with their tongue.

"Nipple confusion," a learned and correctable suckling defect, describes the difficulty of babies who have been fed with artificial nipples before learning to breastfeed. The infant who has learned to obstruct fast flow from a bottle nipple often sucks so strongly on the breast that milk flow is blocked. Tongue thrusting (used in bottle feeding) results in (breast) nipple extrusion and prevents the infant from obtaining milk from the breast. Flutter sucking, caused by inefficient fluttering movements of the

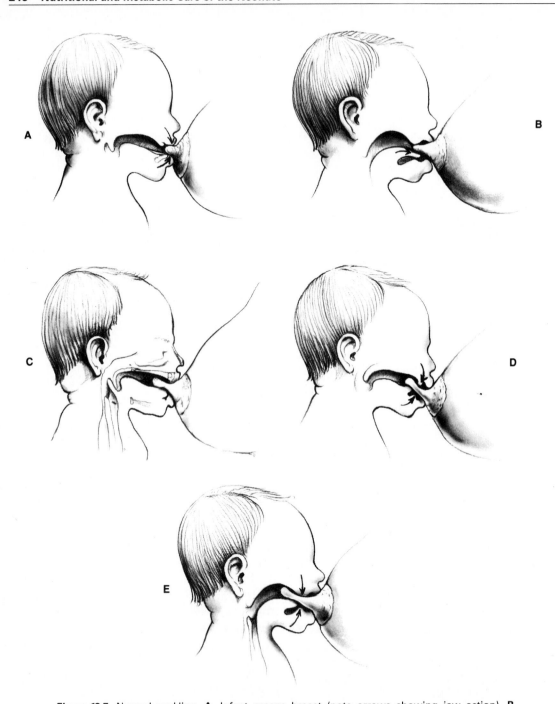

Figure 12-7. Normal suckling. **A,** Infant grasps breast (note arrows showing jaw action). **B,** Tongue moves forward to draw nipple in. **C,** Nipple and areola move toward palate as glottis still permits breathing. **D,** Tongue moves along nipple, pressing it against hard palate, creating pressure. **E,** Ductules under areola are milked, and flow begins. Glottis closes. (From Lawrence RA: Breastfeeding: a guide for the medical profession, ed 2, St Louis, 1985, The CV Mosby Co.)

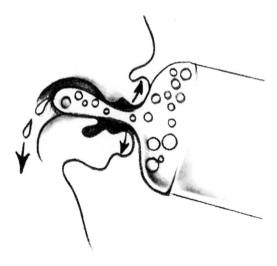

Figure 12-8. Artificial nipple. (From Lawrence RA: Breastfeeding: a guide for the medical profession, ed 2, St Louis, 1985, The CV Mosby Co.)

tongue, does not produce adequate stimulation for milk ejection. The common receding jaw of the infant may make it difficult for the nipple to stay in place, and support at the angle of the jaw often helps.

If the infant cannot coordinate sucking and swallowing, choking occurs. Assessment of the problem includes evaluation of the method of feeding and possibly using alternative nutritional methods until the cause is determined. If the infant is bottle-fed, choking may be a result of a soft nipple, a fast flow that the infant cannot control, or a nipple that is too long for the infant's (particularly the preterm infant's) mouth. If the mother is breastfeeding and the ejection is strong, the first rush of milk could cause choking, which may be prevented by manual expression of a small amount (several spurts) of milk before offering the nipple to the baby. Stopping and restarting the feeding may also resolve sucking problems.

Some suckling problems are not preventable, since they are the sequelae of perinatal events or of physical disorders and represent develop-

mental delays. These sucking difficulties require diagnostic evaluation and appropriate intervention into the underlying cause.

Ideally, no term or preterm infant who will be breastfed should ever be fed with an artificial nipple, but this is not always possible, especially for the sick premature infant who requires prolonged hospitalization. Knowledgeable choice of artificial nipples for an infant who eventually will be breastfed prevents later nipple confusion. Use of the NUK orthodontic nipple is recommended, since the process used to suck this artificial nipple is the same process used to suckle the human breast. Using a NUK nipple or pacifier, rather than other types, teaches the proper sequence for suckling the breast and prevents nipple confusion. However, teaching the premature infant to suck often starts long before nutrition is obtained from a nipple. When the premature infant is gavage fed, giving a pacifier teaches the infant to equate satiety with sucking. Using a pacifier provides nonnutritive sucking that calms and soothes the preterm infant, as well as providing the opportunity to develop a sucking skill. When the mother is present for gavage feeding, placing the baby in direct skin contact with her breast enables nuzzling and licking behaviors and teaches that relief from hunger and the breastfeeding position are associated.

The Lact-Aid Nursing Trainer system assists a variety of breastfeeding problems, including suckling defects (Figure 12-9). Formula or expressed breast milk is contained in a presterilized, disposable bag suspended between the mother's breasts by a cord, and the liquid is delivered by a thin, flexible tube attached to the bag. The end of the tube is placed against the mother's nipple to enable the infant to suckle the tube and nipple at the same time. This device provides the correct rate of flow and volume of liquid that elicits the reflexes of swallowing and expression. The Lact-Aid trainer provides oral therapy and nutritional supplement for the infant and mammary therapy that enhances the mother's lactation.[4] It is effective in

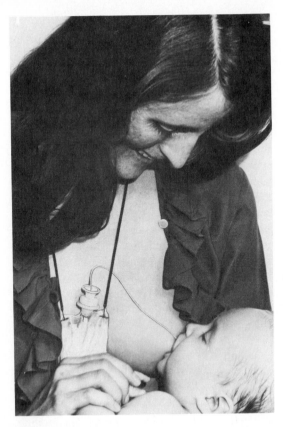

Figure 12-9. Lact-Aid Nursing Trainer. (Courtesy Lact-Aid International, Inc.)

managing low milk production in the mother caused by separation, delayed breastfeeding, poor technique, or other correctable problems and in giving nutritional and oral therapy to the infant who is slow in gaining weight or has a suckling dysfunction. CAUTION: To prevent the spread of serious infections, Lact-Aid should never be borrowed, rented, or loaned from another mother.[7]

Problems with the letdown reflex may be maternal, neonatal, or a combination of these. The mother's emotional state may interfere with letdown. A tense mother will not have a letdown reflex. Often, especially in breastfeeding a pre-

mature infant, this is because of fear of failure or lack of privacy. Knowledge of the mechanisms of lactation can help avoid a fear of failing. It is important to give the mother as much privacy and the least stressful environment as possible when pumping her breasts and while breastfeeding. If a mother experiences a weak or delayed letdown, she should massage the colostrum or milk down to the nipple before putting the infant to the breast. Infants with a poor suck (i.e., preterm infants or infants with Down's syndrome or a neurologic deficit) understimulate the breast and do not trigger the letdown reflex. Use of the Lact-Aid Nursing Trainer provides oral therapy, improves these infants' suckling ability, and enables a successful nursing relationship.

DATA COLLECTION AND INTERVENTION
Establishment of breastfeeding
AVAILABLE FEEDING AND SUCKLING NEONATE

If the infant is premature or ill but can be held near the breast, several methods and devices can help the infant in learning to take the breast.

The low birth weight infant may have a weak suck, but as soon as the infant is strong enough to breastfeed, he or she may be placed at the breast. Although the suck is weak, the infant is usually able to get some nutrition. Breast massage may assist in bringing down the milk, thus making it easier to obtain.

Infants who have been admitted to a level II or level III nursery often present a dilemma to care providers regarding the most favorable time to begin putting the infant to the breast. The infant's present physical status coupled with considerations regarding nutrition and energy expenditure provide data for arriving at such decisions. Recent studies show that the preterm infant may be able to breastfeed far earlier (<1500 g; 33 to 36 weeks) than is customary.[13,14] Although including a small sample size (five preterm infants) these studies showed[13]:

1. Fluctuations and a sharper decrease in transcutaneous Po_2 ($TcPo_2$) occurred with bottle feeding but not with breastfeeding.
2. Skin temperature elevated during breastfeeding because of bodily contact with the mother.
3. Bradycardia occurred with bottle feeding but not with breastfeeding—possibly related to faster milk flow from the bottle (no infant had difficulty with letdown) and interference with breathing.
4. Breastfeeding sessions lasted longer than bottle feeding (done by nurses).
5. There was a differential pattern of sucking bursts and better coordination of sucking and breathing with breastfeeding.

The infant's respiratory status should be reviewed. Infants requiring supplemental oxygen can breastfeed. If the infant requires 35% oxygen or less, oxygen may be delivered via a nasal cannula to ensure adequate and consistent oxygenation. This will eliminate another source of concern for the mother (i.e., having to worry about juggling the blow-by oxygen line). If the infant has not previously been placed on a nasal cannula, the nurse should initiate the cannula and then assess oxygenation using a pulse oximeter. Once oxygenation has been documented, the pulse oximeter may be discontinued, and the breastfeeding experience may begin. If the infant requires more than 35% oxygen, the oxygen line should be attached to a blender. The infant should be assessed by using a pulse oximeter before the feeding begins. The line should be anchored securely near the infant's nose or held in place by the nurse or the father.

The infant's suck-swallow-breathe coordination should be assessed before initiation of breastfeeding for infants of less than 36 weeks gestation. The nurse should be available during the initial breastfeeding to provide support to the mother, to assure that the infant exhibits no signs of distress (i.e., color changes), and to provide guidance for the mother if the infant chokes with letdown. The nurse also needs to reinforce to the mother that the infant's sucking pattern will be a pattern of bursts and pauses. The pauses are present in all infants and provide rest periods for the infant.

The infant's temperature status requires review. Attention should be directed toward preventing hypothermia with infants who require significant thermal support. The infant should be swaddled, and a hat should be placed on the infant's head to prevent heat loss.

Families and staff often fear that the infant will not get enough during a breastfeeding. This concern is especially predominant when infants have been hospitalized for prematurity, and fluids and calories have been scrutinized closely. Health professionals need to be sensitive to such concerns and refrain from employing methods such as weighing infants before and after feedings or using gavage tubes to attempt to determine the exact amount of breast milk ingested during the feeding. These methods are inaccurate and only serve to heighten the mother's anxiety. Health professionals need to focus on cues that can be used during and after hospitalization by both caretakers and the family. These cues include the infant's satisfaction after the feeding, the frequency of feedings, and the voiding pattern (minimum of six to eight wet diapers per day). Trends in weight gain can also demonstrate the success of the mother and infant in breastfeeding.

The small infant may have difficulty taking a large nipple into the mouth. The mother should shape her nipple by pinching behind the areola to allow more of the nipple to be placed in the infant's mouth. The thumb and index finger or the first two fingers should be parallel to the infant's nose and chin. The breast must be soft enough to be pinched down in this manner. It is important that the mother hold the infant closely for the comfort of both with the infant's entire body, not just the head, turned toward the mother's body (see Figure 12-1).

A breast shield allows the infant to get a nipple in the mouth but increases the amount of sucking required to obtain milk and decreases the amount of stimulation received at the nipple. Therefore using a nipple shield is not recommended and does not provide a rewarding experience for the mother or the infant. Preventing maternal and neonatal problems associated with breastfeeding is essential in making this a successful experience for both mother and baby (see section on prevention).

Since nonnutritive suckling does not stimulate prolactin secretion and milk production, infants should not be placed on an empty breast to feed. Without positive reinforcement (i.e., milk) for their efforts, babies soon learn that the breast does not give milk, become frustrated, and refuse to feed. The Lact-Aid Nursing Trainer may be used to initiate proper suckle and supplement intake in the small premature infant able to nurse (see section on prevention).

If the nurse has worked with the mother and assessed that she readily "lets-down" after the infant begins suckling, breastfeeding may actually be an easier mode of feeding for the infant. Once letdown is established, the infant expends little energy in sucking. He or she only needs to coordinate swallowing and breathing with an occasional burst of sucking to assist the mother. Supplementing breast feedings with bottle-fed formula is energy and calorically inefficient, since the baby expends energy, thus calories, to feed twice. More energy and calorically efficient methods of initiating breastfeeding include feeding more often (i.e., smaller, more frequent feeds), supplementing by gavage feeding, or use of a Lact-Aid Nursing Trainer.

On some occasions, the infant will be able to nurse but the mother is not available. The infant should use the NUK orthodontic nipple, and the mother should pump her breasts to maintain her milk supply.

NONAVAILABILITY OF A FEEDING OR SUCKLING NEONATE

If premature birth or neonatal or maternal illness delays the onset of breastfeeding, the mother experiences a decrease in her milk production. Depending on how long breastfeeding has been delayed, mammary involution and the return of menstrual hormonal cycles may inhibit breastfeeding. The ill or preterm infant may be weak and tire easily, so that adequate lactation is not established. A mother may be so concerned about the welfare of her infant that she spends most of her time at the hospital and receives inadequate rest, which is a common cause of milk production problems. The care plan includes encouraging, educating, and giving a mother permission to go home and rest, which may require someone to assist with the care of siblings. The stress of having a sick infant and the time spent at the hospital may preclude adequate maternal nutrition.

It is necessary to add about 600 kcal to the nonpregnant diet and to replace elements, such as calcium, minerals, and fat-soluble vitamins, used in producing milk. The recommended dietary increases are similar to those during pregnancy. Adequate fluid intake, 6 to 8 glasses of water, skim milk, or other noncaffeine liquids, should be consumed every day. Certain components of breast milk, such as quantity, protein, and calcium content, do not vary with maternal diet, whereas others (i.e., fatty and amino acids, lysine, methionine, and water-soluble vitamins) vary with maternal intake.

A mother's diet does not have much effect on the quality of the breast milk (unless malnutrition intervenes) but affects the mother's overall health. She should be reminded to eat a balanced diet. Vegetarian diets should be supplemented with about 4 mg of cyanocobalamin per day.

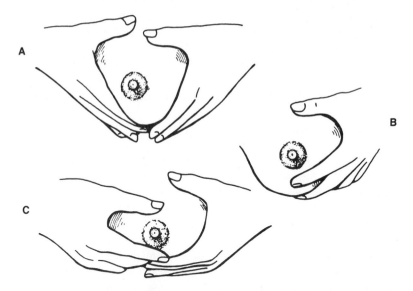

Figure 12-10. Breast massage. **A,** Place hands with palms toward chest at breast. Encircle breast with fingers and thumbs. **B** and **C,** Applying pressure, move hands forward, overlapping as they near nipple. Stop posterior to areola. Continue for 1 to 2 minutes or until milk is on nipple. Repeat on opposite breast. (From Bowman J and Hill R: Pediatrics 35:815, 1965; and Breastfeeding, Evanston, Ill, 1981, American Academy of Pediatrics. Copyright American Academy of Pediatrics, 1965 and 1981. Reproduced by permission of Pediatrics.)

It is important that the mother and infant be comfortable while breastfeeding. A comfortable chair with armrests or a pillow often helps, and the mother should be assured of privacy during breastfeeding and breast pumping.

If a neonate is unable to feed at the breast, breast milk can be produced through artificial stimulation of the breast. The mother should establish a regular routine of breast massage and pumping soon after the baby's birth. It is often necessary for the care provider to help the mother start her routine. Each breast should be pumped every 2 to 4 hours for 10 to 15 minutes. Mothers who have not prepared their nipples should begin pumping each breast for 4 to 5 minutes and increase as tolerated to 10 to 15 minutes. Mothers should use a breast pump during waking hours only; undisturbed sleep at night is more important than pumping. CAUTION: Mothers should be counseled regard-ing the potential risks of using breast shields or manual breast pumps that have been used by other women. Breast shields, pumps, and lactation aids are intimate care items and are meant for one mother–one baby use.

INDUCTION AIDS. Various induction aids using tactile, mechanical, and biochemical principles are available to assist the mother in lactating and relactating. Knowledge of the different systems and their advantages and disadvantages enables the health care provider to help the mother choose the most helpful aid.

Breast massage before breastfeeding or pumping may help unplug breast ducts and allow milk to flow more easily. Breast massage during pumping provides the important tactile stimulation that is missing without the baby's nursing and facilitates prolactin synthesis. Figure 12-10 shows a breast massage technique.

HAND EXPRESSION. Once breast milk supply

has been established, hand expression is the simplest and most cost-effective way to collect milk. However, some mothers find this method aesthetically unsatisfactory, and they should use other methods.

Technique

1. Place the forefinger and thumb on either side of the nipple at the back of the areola.
2. Press fingers back toward the ribs, pinch fingers together, and pull forward.
3. Continuously repeat this maneuver for 10 to 15 minutes every 2 to 4 hours.
4. Collect the milk in a plastic bag or container.

MECHANICAL DEVICES. There are many different breast pumps costing from a few dollars to more than $1000. Two classes of breast pumps are available: (1) the continuous sucking device and (2) the intermittent sucking device. The continuous sucking device's (Marshall Breast Pump Infant Nurser) major advantages are that it is relatively inexpensive, portable, and sanitary. The major problem with the continuous sucking device is discomfort and soreness. The intermittent sucking device (Egnell Electric Breast Pump) is used when there is a problem with or a problem anticipated with another device. The disadvantages are cost and lack of portability.

Breast pumps provide stimulation to initiate and maintain a milk supply until the baby is able to suckle. Beginning on the low or normal pump setting and carefully breaking the suction at the breast with a finger helps to prevent sore nipples. Painful maternal engorgement is relieved by pumping each breast just enough to obtain relief. Nipple/areolar engorgement must be relieved so that the infant is able to grasp and suckle the nipple.

To increase milk supply, the pump should be used every 2 to 4 hours. Because the breast pump is not so efficient as the suckling infant, tactile stimulation and breast massage may help increase the milk supply. Looking at the baby's picture or listening to a tape recording of the baby's cry stimulates milk production with a pump. To decrease engorgement, the pump should be used only as necessary to relieve discomfort, and only enough milk to make the breast more comfortable should be removed.

DRUGS

HORMONES. Estrogen and progesterone stimulate the proliferation of the alveolar and ductal systems while prolactin production increases. Milk secretion is inhibited during pregnancy by the presence of estrogen and progesterone, even though the prolactin level is high.[11] After delivery, estrogen and progesterone decrease greatly, and prolactin initiates milk production.

Estrogen and progesterone therapy is not recommended for lactating women because of the possible effect on the infant via the milk. Although these hormones may enhance proliferation, they may inhibit lactation.[11]

OXYTOCIN. Oxytocin is critical in the milk ejection reflex and may help in initiating this ejection.[11] Stimulation of the nipple in the lactating woman releases oxytocin by the hypothalamus. Oxytocin then triggers the release of milk by stimulating the contraction of the myoepithelial cells and ejection of the milk.[11] Administering oxytocin nasal spray (Syntocinon) to enhance letdown without necessarily changing the volume produced has met with some success. Its greatest application is in the mother who wishes to relactate, but it is not effective during the first few weeks. Oral administration by tablet has not been as effective as the nasal spray.[11] Diminished effect and even lactation suppression may occur with prolonged use of oxytocin. A rebound effect is avoided by a 3-day use cycle.

Theophylline increases pituitary prolactin secretions. Theoretically, tea and coffee should then enhance lactation, yet excessive amounts may inhibit letdown.[11]

ALCOHOL. Experimentally, the milk-ejection

reflex can be at least partly blocked by alcohol by a central effect preventing the release of oxytocin. The alcohol dosage used in laboratory animals to obtain this effect is equivalent to moderate to heavy drinking in humans. Small amounts of alcohol (a cocktail, glass of beer or wine), especially in the early evening when the milk supply is at its lowest and fatigue and tension are at their highest, relax the mother and enhance letdown.

Emotional support during breastfeeding of a normal or sick infant facilitates a successful experience for both the mother and the infant. Support groups with mothers who have had similar experiences are helpful in supplement-

ing support obtained from significant others and professionals.

COMPLICATIONS

Information on perinatal complications and breastfeeding is contained in Table 12-1.[1,8]

Drugs in breast milk

Information about specific drugs excreted in breast milk is provided in Table 12-2.[2,11] Protein binding, degree of ionization, molecular weight, and solubility of drugs influence the passage of drugs into milk. Protein-bound drugs and drugs of large (>200 molecular weight) molecular weight are less likely to pass

TABLE 12-1

Perinatal Complications and Breastfeeding

	BREASTFEED		
COMPLICATIONS	YES	NO	COMMENTS
Maternal complications			
Cesarean section	x		Regional anesthesia enables contact and feeding in recovery room. Pain medication is best given after feeding so levels peak before next feeding.
Pregnancy-induced hypertension	x		Preterm or SGA infants may be delivered, making delayed breastfeeding and pumping necessary. Maternal drugs may affect infant; see Table 12-2.
Venous thrombosis and pulmonary embolism	x		Depending on mother's ability; radioactive materials may be used for diagnosis, and anticoagulants may be used for therapy; see Table 12-2.
Bacterial infections			
Urinary tract	x		Choice of antibiotics is important; see Table 12-2.
Mastitis	x		Continued emptying of breast (i.e., nursing baby or breast pump), bed rest, antibiotic therapy that is safe for infant, application of heat and cold, and use of analgesics are therapeutic.
Sexually transmitted diseases	x		No contraindication once mother is treated appropriately.
Tuberculosis		x	Culture-positive mothers must be separated from their infants.
	x		After therapy, when it is safe for mother to contact infant, then it is safe to breastfeed.
Diarrhea	x		Proper hand washing should be done and breastfeeding continued.

Modified from American Academy of Pediatrics: Report of the Committee on Infectious Disease, ed 19, Evanston, Ill, 1982, American Academy of Pediatrics; and Hill R: Breastfeeding, Evanston, Ill, 1981, American Academy of Pediatrics.

Continued.

TABLE 12-1—cont'd

Perinatal Complications and Breastfeeding

	BREASTFEED		
COMPLICATIONS	YES	NO	**COMMENTS**
Viral infections			
Rubella	x		Isolate infected infant from other infants and susceptible personnel. Mother is not contagious postpartum and need not be isolated from infant. Rooming-in may be considered.
Rubella immunization	x		There is no known adverse effect on infant.
Herpes simplex (HSV)	x	x	May breastfeed if there is no active lesion on breast. Strict hand washing, as well as covering of genital lesions, is necessary. Rooming-in supports breast-feeding while isolating infant from others in nursery.
Varicella (chickenpox)	x	x	If mother has chickenpox within 6 days of delivery, isolate mother and do not allow her to breastfeed until she is no longer contagious.
Measles (rubeola)	x	x	If infant has measles, may isolate mother and infant together and allow breastfeeding. Mothers with measles postpartum have breastfed, and neonates have acquired mild disease. Secretory antibodies are probably present in milk in 48 hr. Mother exposed before delivery without active disease should be isolated from infant, because 50% of infants contract disease.
Hepatitis	x	x	Hepatitis B antigen has been found in breast milk, but transmission by this route is not well documented. Both infants of chronic HBsAg carriers and those with acute hepatitis should receive high titer hepatitis B immunoglobulin and hepatitis vaccine.
HIV (AIDS; human immunodeficiency virus)		x	Breastfeeding is absolutely contraindicated in mothers who are HIV positive.
Parasitic infections			
Toxoplasmosis	x		No transmission of toxoplasmosis has been demonstrated in humans. Antibodies are present in breast milk.
Other infections			
Trichomoniasis		x	Metronidazole is contraindicated for infant; milk may be pumped and discarded until therapy is completed.
Other maternal complications			
Diabetes	x		Lactation is antidiabetogenic. Lactosuria must be differentiated from glycosuria.
Thyroid disease	x	x	Radioisotopes and propylthiouracil are found in breast milk and may adversely affect infant. Neither hypothyroidism nor hyperthyroidism is contraindication alone.
Cystic fibrosis	x	x	May cause nutritional drain on mother and excessive electrolyte intake for infant.
Smoking	x	x	Nicotine interferes with letdown and is excreted in milk.

TABLE 12-1—cont'd

Perinatal Complications and Breastfeeding

COMPLICATIONS	BREASTFEED		COMMENTS
	YES	NO	
Neonatal complications			
Medical			
Diarrhea	x	x	Maintain breastfeeding in infectious diarrhea unless milk is source of infection. Congenital lactase deficiency is rare but requires lactose-free formula.
Respiratory disease	x	x	Breast milk by gavage may be used if infant's condition permits.
Galactosemia		x	Galactose (lactose) free diet is required.
Inborn errors of metabolism	x	x	Combination of breast milk and special formula may sometimes be used. Careful monitoring of blood and urine levels of the amino acid is required.
Acrodermatitis enteropathica	x		Low plasma zinc levels are corrected by human milk and zinc sulfate supplementation.
Down's syndrome	x		Hypotonia and poor suck reflex contribute to poor let-down and inadequate supply. Proper positioning, manual expression to begin feeding, and supporting the breast so infant does not lose nipple are helpful. Support from mother with Down's syndrome infant is helpful.
Hypothyroidism	x		Enough T_3 may be ingested to mask symptoms.
Hyperbilirubinemia	x		May have slightly higher bilirubin than bottle-fed infant. There is no evidence that supplements are beneficial (see Chapter 15).
Breast milk jaundice	x	x	Uncommon occurrence ($\frac{1}{200}$ breastfed infants); diagnosis of exclusion; if all other causes are excluded, a temporary cessation of breast milk may be indicated; see Chapter 15.
Cystic fibrosis	x		Increased losses of and lower electrolyte content of breast milk may cause electrolyte imbalance.
Surgical			
Cleft lip and/or palate size	x		Associated lesions, size, and position of defect influence successful feeding. Positioning and stabilizing breast in infant's mouth may help seal defect. Cleft lip nipple, breast shield, or expressed milk in bottle with special nipple may be used.
Gastrostomy	x		If gastrostomy feedings are used, expressed breast milk is appropriate.
Partial obstruction (meconium plug, ileus, Hirschsprung's disease)	x		If oral feedings are indicated, breast milk is feeding of choice because of digestibility and mild cathartic effect.
Necrotizing enterocolitis	x		Breastfeeding may be partially protective and may be used when feedings resume.
Gastrointestinal bleeding	x		Most common cause is maternal bleeding nipple. Perform Apt test to differentiate fetal from adult hemoglobin.
CNS malformations	x		Weak suck and uncoordinated suck and swallow may be problems.

TABLE 12-2

Drugs Excreted in Breast Milk

DRUGS	BREAST MILK	INFANT
Analgesics	Heroin, codeine, meperidine, pentazocine, dextropropoxyphene, and diazepam appear in variable amounts.	Symptoms of depression and floppiness have been associated with these drugs.
Antibiotics and sulfa drugs		
Sulfa drugs	These appear in breast milk and may interfere with bilirubin binding in neonate; infants with G-6-PD deficiency may develop hemolysis.	Should not be used for breastfeeding mother in the first month or if infant has G-6-PD deficiency.
Chloramphenicol	Appears in breast milk.	Contraindicated in nursing mother because infant may accumulate it and develop gray baby syndrome.
Tetracycline	Appears in breast milk at 50% of serum level; may cause staining of teeth and growth abnormalities.	May develop these problems, especially when therapy exceeds 10 days; nursing mothers should avoid this drug if possible.
Metronidazole	Appears in breast milk in levels equal to serum levels.	Side effects include decreased appetite, vomiting, blood dyscrasia, and animal evidence of tumorigenicity.
Cephalexin, cephalothin, oxacillin, chloroquine, and para-amino-salicylic acid	Very small amounts appear in breast milk.	Rash and sensitization are possible. May also affect bacterial flora.
Anticholinergics	Atropine appears, but quaternary ammonium derivatives do not appear in breast milk.	The neonate of a nursing mother receiving atropine should be observed for tachycardia, constipation, and urinary retention.
Anticoagulants	Heparin and warfarin (Coumadin) do not appear in breast milk.	
Antithyroidal drugs		
Iodide	Passes into milk.	May cause goiters and is contraindicated during breastfeeding.
Thiouracil	Higher concentration in maternal milk than in blood.	Neonatal problems include suppression of thyroid activity and agranulocytosis. If breastfed, infant should be given thyroid supplement and thyroid function should be followed.
Anticonvulsants		
Phenobarbital, phenytoin, carbamazepine (Tegretol), and valproic acid (Depakene)	All appear in small amounts.	Sedation is possible, but rarely are clinical symptoms significant enough to cause adverse effects.

Modified from Lawrence RA: Breastfeeding: a guide for the medical profession, ed 2, St Louis, 1985, The CV Mosby Co; and American Academy of Pediatrics, Committee on Drugs: Pediatrics 72:375, 1983.

TABLE 12-2—cont'd

Drugs Excreted in Breast Milk

DRUGS	BREAST MILK	INFANT
Cardiovascular drugs		
Digitalis and propranolol	Appears only in small amounts.	Digitalis and propranolol appear to be safe.
Reserpine	Appears in breast milk.	Symptoms include diarrhea, lethargy, nasal stuffiness, bradycardia, and respiratory difficulties; contraindicated in breastfeeding.
Cathartics		
Aloin, cascara sagrada, and anthraquine preparations	Appear in breast milk.	Colic and diarrhea are possible side effects.
Diagnostic radioactive compounds		
^{67}Ga, ^{125}I, and ^{131}I	Appear for 24-48 hr.	Discontinue breastfeeding for 48 hr.
Diuretics	May suppress lactation.	Inadequate milk; no significant risks are present.
Psychotherapeutics		
Lithium	Appears in breast milk; inhibits lactation.	Contraindicated in pregnancy and lactation. Inhibits cyclic 3'-5' AMP, a substance significant to brain growth.
Phenothiazines	Appear in small amounts.	No contraindications.
Diazepam (Valium)	Appear in breast milk and may accumulate in infant, since it is detoxified in liver.	Poor feeding, weight loss, hypoventilation, and drowsiness may be seen.
Tricyclic antidepressants	Appear in minimal amounts.	Apparently safe for infant.
Stimulants		
Caffeine	Appears in small amounts but may accumulate in infant.	Symptoms include jitteriness, wakefulness, and irritability.
Theophylline	Appears in moderate amounts.	Irritability, jitteriness, and wakefulness may be seen in infant.

into milk. Conversely, lipid-soluble drugs pass more easily into the milk. Since breast milk is slightly acidic as compared with plasma, weakly alkaline compounds are equal or greater in breast milk than in plasma. Weakly acidic compounds have a higher concentration in plasma than in breast milk.

Several factors influence the drug effect on the infant. Most drugs appear in milk, but drug levels usually do not exceed 1% of the ingested dose and are not dependent on the milk volume.[11] Many variables, such as gastric empty-ing, pH, and effects of intestinal enzymes affect absorption. Finally, the chronologic and gestational ages of the infant affect the maturity of the systems involved in excretion and detoxification.

PARENT TEACHING

Parent teaching has been discussed throughout this chapter, since it is so essential to a successful breastfeeding experience for both mother and baby.

Before a premature or sick baby is actually

TREATMENT AND STORAGE OF BREAST MILK

Treatment

1. Heat—Significant loss of lysozyme, lactoferrin, immunoglobulins, lactoperoxidase, lymphocyte function, complement, phagocytosis, and macromolecules may occur.
2. Lyophilization—Effects are similar to those of heat treatment.
3. Freezing—Limited information; cells are not viable, but there is no effect on IgA content.

Storage

1. Use sterile plastic bags (amount for one feeding/bag); glass may change immunologic properties of breast milk.
2. Label with name, date, and time of collection.
3. Store in refrigerator for 24 hours or freeze for longer periods.

---

nursed at the breast, the colostrum and breast milk are pumped and fed to the infant. If the mother's production is adequate, no supplement is necessary. Before collecting the mother's milk, perform the following:

1. Screen (by history) mother for disease.
2. Screen (by history) mother for maternal drugs.
3. Instruct mother in sterile technique.
4. Perform a culture for bacterial contamination (<10,000 organisms/ml).

Proper collection and storage must be discussed with each family so that stored milk does not cause infections. Often the mother pumps and collects the milk, and the father transports it to the neonatal intensive care unit (NICU) (see Chapter 22). Methods of treatment and storage are listed in the boxed material above. Rewarming techniques include placing frozen milk in (1) a room temperature water bath, (2) a hot water bath, (3) a microwave oven, or (4) under cold running water and then tepid water. Slow room temperature rewarming is a concern because of bacterial overgrowth, especially if

thawing is prolonged. Most nurseries use room temperature water bath rewarming to avoid exposure to the high temperatures of the hot water bath and the microwave. Fresh breast milk is preferable for feedings because of its immunologic properties. If the mother visits the infant at feeding time, she may pump her breasts and the breast milk is immediately fed to the baby.

Human milk banks that collect, store, and distribute milk to infants other than those of the donating mother exist around the world. This support is not available to some NICUs; others intentionally choose not to store donor milk. The reservations about storing donor milk generally involve questions concerning adequate nutrition and immunologic benefit versus harm to the high-risk infant. Adequate screening of human milk donors (for cytomegalovirus [CMV], human immunodeficiency virus [HIV], etc.) is essential, as is informed consent. Many nurseries do not give human milk other than the mother's.

Anticipatory guidance for the mother breastfeeding a preterm infant is essential. The mother must be informed in the beginning that her milk supply may dwindle, even though she closely adheres to the pumping schedule. This is normal, since no pump stimulates the breast as efficiently and physiologically as the suckling baby. When the pumping regimen begins, explaining and drawing the mother a picture (Figure 12-11) of what is commonly experienced helps alleviate guilt due to a dwindling milk supply. A rather sparse supply of milk does not mean she cannot nurse the baby, since the milk supply will build in response to the baby's nutritive suckle. The parent should be taught that there is no correlation between the amount of breast milk expressed and the amount of milk a mother actually lets down when the infant is at the breast.

Establishing realistic parental expectations for the first time the infant breastfeeds decreases disappointment from unattainable

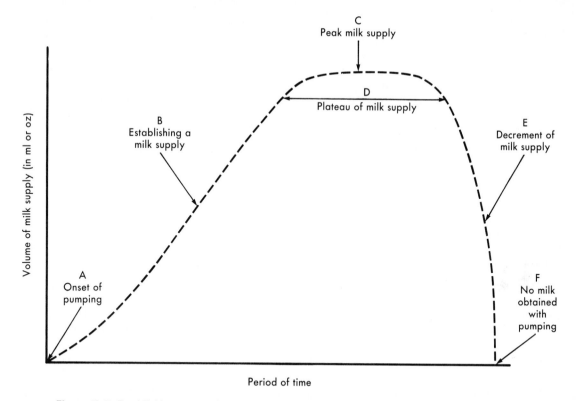

Figure 12-11. Establishing and maintaining milk supply by pumping. *A,* Pumping begins. *B,* Milk supply is established and increases. *C,* Peak or maximum volume of milk is established and plateaus. *D,* Gradually, supply begins to dwindle and, *E,* may totally cease. *F,* Volume of milk and time period for decline in supply to begin and end in no milk production is an individual process. Some women begin and end cycle in days or weeks; others are able to pump for months. Even if supply dwindles to no milk, nutritive suckle of baby with Lact-Aid Nursing Trainer in place will reestablish supply.

goals. Breastfeeding, like parenting, is not instinctual but is a learned behavior for both the mother and the infant. No one, including the health care provider, should expect immediate latch-on and vigorous sucking. The first several attempts at breastfeeding may consist only of direct skin contact, nuzzling, and licking behaviors by the baby, and cuddling and positioning by the mother. Any actual sucking is an "extra" reward but should not be anticipated.

• • •

Medical and nursing staff need to receive education and training regarding the many facets of the breastfeeding experience.[3] Staff attitudes and behaviors are important to breastfeeding families and provide input into the breastfeeding experience. A multidimensional approach to such education includes having manuals, guides, and other educational materials available for staff as well as scheduling routine classes, in-services, and workshops. Moreover, professionals with clinical expertise should be identified. These reliable resource personnel can increase the staff's competency in counseling and assisting breastfeeding families.

Protocols addressing breastfeeding can outline a consistent approach for staff, as well as provide resource material that addresses successful strategies for handling common problems. Protocols can also serve to diminish the amount of incorrect information that is disseminated.

Breast milk is the best milk, even for the sick or premature infant. By understanding normal lactation, the health care provider can support the breastfeeding dyad when breastfeeding is delayed or disrupted.

REFERENCES

1. American Academy of Pediatrics: Report of the Committee on Infectious Disease, ed 19, Evanston, Ill, 1982, American Academy of Pediatrics.
2. American Academy of Pediatrics, Committee on Drugs: The transfer of drugs and other chemicals into human breast milk, Pediatrics 72:375, 1983.
3. American Academy of Pediatrics, Task force on the promotion of breastfeeding: The promotion of breastfeeding, Pediatrics 69:654, 1982.
4. Avery JL: Relactation and induced lactation. In Riordan J: A practical guide to breastfeeding, St Louis, 1983, The CV Mosby Co.
5. Bosma JF, editor: Oral sensation and perception, Department of Health, Education and Welfare Pub No (NIH)73-546, Bethesda, Md, 1973, US Department of Health, Education and Welfare.
6. Freier S and Eidelman AI: Human milk, its biological and social value, Excerpta Medica, International Congress Series 518, 1980.
7. Gardner SL and Avery JL: Hazardous breastfeeding practices: a white paper, Athens, Tenn, 1989, Lact-Aid International.
8. Hill R: Breastfeeding, Evanston, Ill, 1981, American Academy of Pediatrics.
9. Jelliffe DM and Jelliffe EFP: Human milk in the modern world, London, 1978, Oxford University Press.
10. LaLeche League International: The womanly art of breastfeeding, Danville, Ill, 1987, The Interstate Printers & Publishers, Inc.
11. Lawrence RA: Breastfeeding: a guide for the medical professional, ed 2, St Louis, 1985, The CV Mosby Co.
12. Lemons JA et al: Differences in the composition of preterm and term human milk during early lactation, Pediatr Res 16:113, 1982.
13. Meier P and Anderson GC: Responses of small preterm infants to bottle and breastfeeding, Matern Child Nurs J 12:97, 1987.
14. Meier P and Pugh EJ: Breastfeeding behavior of small preterm infants, Matern Child Nurs J 10:396, 1985.
15. National Institute of Child Health and Human Development: Immunology of breast milk (monograph), New York, 1979, Raven Press.
16. Riordan, J: A practical guide to breastfeeding, St Louis, 1983, The CV Mosby Co.
17. Vorherr H: Human lactation, Semin Perinatol 3(3):191, 1979.

SELECTED READINGS

Auerbach K and Avery JL: Relactation after an untimely weaning: report from a survey, Resources in Human Nurturing (monograph 2), 1979.

Auerbach K and Avery JL: Relactation and the premature infant: report from a survey, Resources in Human Nurturing (monograph 3), 1979.

Auerbach K and Avery JL: Relactation after a hospital induced separation: report from a survey, Resources in Human Nurturing (monograph 4), 1979.

Auerbach K et al: Breastfeeding the premature infant: a symposium, Keeping Abreast J 2(2):98, 1977.

Avery GB: Breastfeeding, Pub No 017-026-00084-4, Washington, DC, 1979, US Government Printing Office.

Eiger M and Olds S: The complete book of breastfeeding, New York, 1972, Workman Publishing Co, Inc.

Eleventh Round Table: Counseling the mother on breastfeeding, Columbus, Ohio, 1980, Ross Laboratories.

Larson B: Lactation: a comprehensive treatise, ed 4, New York, 1978, Academic Press, Inc.

Lawrence RA: Medications and breast milk, Childbirth Educator, p 47, spring 1987.

Lawrence RA: Breastfeeding, Clin Perinatol 14:1, 1987.

Meier P: A program to support breast feeding in the high-risk nursery, Perinatol Neonatol 5:43, 1980.

Patient Care Panel: Drugs excreted in mother's milk, Pract Primary Physicians, p 2, June 30, 1980.

Pryor KD: Nursing your baby, New York, 1973, Harper & Row Publishers, Inc.

CHAPTER 13

Total parenteral nutrition

HOWARD W. KILBRIDE · LORETTA FORLAW

Only since the mid 1960s have intravenous (IV) carbohydrates been administered routinely to very low birth weight (VLBW) infants. In 1966 Auld et al[3] showed that early provision of carbohydrates in this way could avoid catabolism and hypoglycemia, and Cornblath et al[4] demonstrated that its early administration decreased mortality in VLBW infants. Two years later Dudrick et al[5] demonstrated that nutrition adequate for growth could be supplied by continuous infusion of nutrients through a deep venous catheter. Since that time, total parenteral nutrition (TPN) has been used in many critically ill neonates and infants with great success and undoubtedly has been partly responsible for the improved survival reported in these infants. This chapter will familiarize the reader with indications for TPN, the nutritional needs of the critically ill newborn, and parenteral methods of meeting these needs. Mechanical, infectious, and metabolic complications are discussed with special emphasis on prevention or early identification.

PHYSIOLOGY
Fuel stores

During periods of fasting, tissue stores of energy provide the major source of fuel for the body. Carbohydrate is stored in the liver and muscle as glycogen. The formation of glycogen (glycogenesis) and its breakdown to form glucose (glycogenolysis) are balanced by hormonal regulation to maintain stable blood sugar levels. Newborns, particularly those who are growth retarded or preterm, have low glycogen stores.

The greatest body energy stores are in the form of fat, which provides an energy yield of 9 kcal/g. In addition to normal deposits of adipose tissue, newborns (and hibernating adult animals) have unique stores termed *brown fat*. These stores, which are anatomically located between the scapulae, in the axillae, mediastinum, and around the adrenals, protect the body from hypothermia through nonshivering thermogenesis (see Chapter 5).

Protein makes up lean body mass. Although protein is not used as an energy store, it may be oxidized for this purpose during periods of starvation. Catabolism usually leads to some bodily dysfunction as noted below.

Effects of starvation

During and after the last trimester of pregnancy, the fetal and neonatal brain is rapidly growing, including increases in glial and neuronal cell numbers, myelinization, synaptic connections, and dendritic arborization. An infant who receives inadequate nutrition prenatally or postnatally may have an interruption of brain growth and will be at risk for permanent brain injury. Autopsy studies of brains of malnourished infants have shown diminished cell numbers and deficiencies in the lipid and phospholipid content. Additionally, investigators have related postnatal microcephaly or decreased head growth velocity in preterm infants with later detrimental outcome.[10]

Malnutrition may cause more immediate clinical problems. These include muscle wasting, hypotonia, loss of ventilatory drive, apnea, and difficulty in weaning from the ventilator. Immune responses may be depressed with increased susceptibility to infection.

Nutritional requirements of the neonate
CALORIC

Caloric requirements for the growing preterm infant are°:

Basal	40-50	kcal/kg/day
Activity	5-15	kcal/kg/day
Cold stress	0-10	kcal/kg/day
Fecal loss	10-15	kcal/kg/day
Specific dynamic action	10	kcal/kg/day
Growth	20-30	kcal/kg/day
TOTAL	85-130	kcal/kg/day

These estimates are based on enteral intake. Parenteral requirements are about 20% less or about 85 to 90 kcal/kg/day.

Basal values of caloric requirements must be adjusted according to the patient's activity, body temperature, and degree of stress. An elevation of body temperature increases the caloric expenditure by approximately 12% for each degree centigrade above 37.8° C (100.2° F). Activity and catabolic states can cause a 25% to 75% increase in metabolic demands.

WATER

Water requirements vary with gestational and postnatal age (conceptual age) and environmental conditions such as incubator versus radiant heat source and phototherapy (see Chapter 15).

MINERAL

Sodium requirements are minimal for the first days of life. After 1 week the average requirement is 2 to 3 mEq/kg/day. Large renal losses (>5 mEq/kg/day) may occur in very immature infants (<28 weeks gestation) in the first weeks of life.

Potassium and chloride requirements are approximately 2 mEq/kg/day and 3 to 4 mEq/kg/

°From Sinclair JC et al: Pediatr Clin North Am 17:863, 1970.

day, respectively (see Chapter 10). Glucosuria may cause increased sodium and potassium urinary losses.

Initial calcium requirements to avoid hypocalcemia are 0.5 to 1 mEq/kg/day for VLBW infants. During rapid growth the requirement may be 4 mEq/kg/day or greater. Low levels of ionized calcium may result in irritability or tetany.

Phosphorus requirements are 20 to 60 mg/day. Since it is a major constituent of cellular activity (as adenosine triphosphate, 2,3-diphosphoglycerate, creatine phosphate), important cellular functions such as hemoglobin-oxygen dissociation curve and leukocyte functions may be disturbed.

Magnesium requirements are 0.25 to 0.5 mEq/kg/day.

Since body calcium is mainly present in the bone as calcium phosphate, depletion of either of these minerals may result in osteomalacia, rickets, and bone fractures. Excess calcium ion may depress the central nervous system (CNS). A patient receiving parenteral calcium as a bolus infusion should have his or her cardiorespiratory status monitored. Bolus calcium administration may cause bradycardia in any infant and may cause asystole in infants with underlying cardiac disease.

Features of phosphorus deficiency include weakness, convulsions, and other neurologic abnormalities. The amount of these minerals to be administered is limited by their solubility product (see section on solutions).

Magnesium deficiency states mimic hypocalcemia manifesting as irritability, tremulousness, tetany, and cardiac arrhythmias.

CARBOHYDRATE

In parenteral nutrition caloric requirements are met by carbohydrate given as dextrose, which has 3.4 cal/g in the hydrated state. The minimum dextrose requirement is that which avoids hypoglycemia, usually 6 to 8 mg/kg/min. Requirements are greater for infants who are stressed (e.g., because of sepsis or hypothermia) or hyperinsulinemic (i.e., infants of diabetic mothers or with Beckwith-Wiedemann syndrome).

PROTEIN

The quantity of daily protein required by a term newborn infant based on estimates from breast milk intake is approximately 325 mg/kg/day (approximately 2 g/kg/day). Requirements for preterm infants are much higher, as indicated by in-utero accretion rates during the latter half of pregnancy. At 28 weeks gestation the fetus requires 350 mg/kg/day of nitrogen, this figure declining to 150 mg/kg/day by term gestation.[24] When this estimated accretion rate is added to the obligatory postnatal nitrogen excretion, the requirement for a 28-week gestation preterm infant in the neonatal intensive care unit (NICU) may be calculated to be approximately 495 mg/kg/day (3.1 g/kg/day of protein).

Despite these estimates, protein requirements for optimal growth of preterm infants remain controversial. Finnish investigators demonstrated that adequate growth may be achieved with a protein intake of 2.25 g/kg/day.[18] However, a recent controlled trial of protein quantity in which caloric intake was held constant concluded that weight gain and linear growth were greater when protein intake was 3.5 g/kg/day as compared with 2.24 g/kg/day.[15]

Excessive quantities of protein may be associated with hyperaminoacidemia, hyperaminoaciduria, azotemia, and hyperaminemia. Indeed, these metabolic abnormalities may contribute to detrimental long-term outcome. In one study infants with a birth weight of less than 1300 g who received 6 g/kg/day of protein in the neonatal period had, on the average, lower IQ scores at 5- to 7-year follow-up than infants who had had a lower protein intake.[12]

Provision of specific amino acid requirements for the growing preterm infant is perhaps more important than the total protein quantity made available. An essential amino acid is one that cannot be synthesized in adequate quantity to meet the requirements for normal growth and develop-

ment. The differentiation between essential and nonessential amino acids is not clear in newborn infants, since the ability to synthesize some amino acids may vary with the clinical situation or stage of maturity. Lysine and threonine are essential in their entirety. The requirements for other amino acids may be met by providing ketoanalogs, which may accept a nitrogen group during transamination. There is a high requirement for branched amino acids (leucine, isoleucine, and valine) in the growing newborn. These are primarily metabolized in skeletal muscle. Their administration during parenteral nutrition may be advantageous, since protein is not preferentially directed to the liver, as it would be during enteral feedings.

Methionine is an essential sulfur-containing amino acid that is metabolized to cysteine, cystine, and taurine. Cysteine has been thought to be an essential amino acid to the newborn because of decreased activity of hepatic cystathionase. However, recent studies have indicated that cystathionase activity is present in extrahepatic tissues in the fetus and preterm infant.[25] Thus the neonatal requirement for this amino acid is unsubstantiated. Phenylalanine is an essential amino acid for protein synthesis. However, if given in excess, it may be neurotoxic (as evidenced in classic phenylketonuria). Taurine and histidine may be essential amino acids only for the preterm newborn. Early investigations suggest that taurine may be important for retinal development.

Nonessential amino acids make up the largest percentage of the amino acid pool in the fetal body. Although, as with essential amino acids, the desired quantities of these amino acids are not known, it is thought that they should be provided in parenteral solutions in a balanced formulation rather than overrepresentation by one amino acid.

FAT

Long-chain fatty acids are essential in the newborn for brain development. Essential fatty acids (EFAs) include linoleic and arachidonic acids. Biochemical evidence of EFA deficiency may be seen in less than a week in low birth weight

TABLE 13-1

Vitamins: Suggested Intake and Signs and Symptoms of Deficiency and Toxicity

ADVISABLE INTAKE		SIGNS AND SYMPTOMS	
		DEFICIENCY	TOXICITY
Vitamin A	500-2000 IU	Failure to thrive; apathy; mental retardation; dry, scaly skin; corneal ulceration; night blindness	Anorexia; irritability; increased cerebrospinal fluid pressure; desquamation of skin; bone abnormalities
Vitamin D	400 IU	Biochemical and roentgenographic signs of rickets; decreased bone mineralization	? Infantile hypercalcemia; failure to thrive; vomiting; mental retardation; aortic stenosis; nephrocalcinosis
Vitamin E	1-3 mg	Hemolytic anemia; edema; thrombocytosis; deficiency symptoms may be accentuated if receiving iron therapy	Increased incidence of sepsis; necrotizing enterocolitis; possible intracranial hemorrhage following pharmacologic doses in preterm infants
Vitamin C	50-75 mg	Scurvy; anorexia; weight loss; irritability; hemorrhage; bone changes; elevated tyrosine and phenylalanine levels in premature infants	Renal stones; acidosis
Vitamin B_1 (thiamine)	0.2 mg	Beriberi; cardiac failure; aphonia; vomiting; edema	? Shock
Vitamin B_2 (riboflavin)	0.4 mg	Seborrhea; glossitis; cheilosis; corneal vascularization	None
Niacin	5 mg	Pellagra; dermatitis; diarrhea; dementia	Flushing; abnormal liver function test
Vitamin B_6 (pyridoxine)	0.4 mg	Vomiting; anemia; weight loss; irritability; seizures	None
Vitamin B_{12}	1.5 μg	Megaloblastic anemia	None
Pantothenic acid	2 mg	Headache; fatigue; muscle cramps; decreased motor coordination; vomiting and diarrhea	None
Biotin	12 μg	Seborrhea; alopecia; vomiting; muscle pain; diarrhea	None
Vitamin K_1	150 μg	Deficiency of vitamin K–dependent coagulation factors; hemorrhagic disease of the newborn	Hemolysis and increased bilirubin if water-soluble analog used
Folate	50-100 μg	Megaloblastic anemia; hypersegmented neutrophils	Mask vitamin B_{12} deficiency

Modified from Anderson TA and Fomon SJ: Vitamins. In Fomon SJ, editor: Infant nutrition, Philadelphia, 1974, WB Saunders Co; and Barness L: Pediatric nutrition handbook, Evanston, Ill, 1979, American Academy of Pediatrics.

TABLE 13-2

Trace Elements: Recommendations and Signs and Symptoms of Deficiency

ELEMENT	RECOMMENDATIONS*	DEFICIENCY SIGNS AND SYMPTOMS
Zinc	300 μg/kg/day (preterm) 100 μg/kg/day (term)	Acrodermatitis enterohepatica; alopecia; rash; growth disturbance; diarrhea; increased susceptibility to infection
Copper	30-50 μg/kg/day	Anemia; neutropenia; hypothermia; psychomotor retardation; hypotonia; osseous changes including cupping and flaring of long bones and metaphyses, flaring of ribs, and submetaphyseal fractures; pallor, hypopigmentation
Manganese*	2-10 μg/kg/day	Deficiency not recognized in humans; in animals growth retardation, ataxia, bony abnormalities
Chromium*	0.2 μg/kg/day	Impaired glucose tolerance; in animals hypercholesterolemia, impaired growth, and corneal opacities
Selenium*	1-3 μg/kg/day	Protects cell components from oxidative damage due to peroxides; in adults cardiac and skeletal myopathies have been described; in children four cases of macrocytosis and pseudoalbinism have been described in association with low levels
Iodide*	5-15 μg/kg/day	? Hypothyroidism

Modified from Hambidge KM: Pediatr Clin North Am 24:95, 1977; and Shaw JCL: Am J Dis Child 133:1260, 1979, and 134:74, 1980.
*Neonatal requirements unknown; deficiency not yet recognized.

(LBW) infants receiving a deficient diet, and the administration of parenteral glucose and amino acids may accelerate these abnormalities. EFA deficiency results in an imbalance in fatty acid production, with an overproduction of nonessential fatty acids. These biochemical changes are measured as an elevated triene/tetraene ratio (>0.4). Clinical manifestations appearing at variable times after biochemical changes of EFA deficiency include scaly dermatitis, poor hair growth, thrombocytopenia, failure to thrive, poor wound healing, and increased susceptibility to bacterial infection. Early studies suggested that clinical manifestations of EFA deficiency would be avoided if 3% to 4% of caloric intake were supplied as linoleic acid. Recent animal studies, however, indicate that 7% of total calories must be provided as linoleic acid to correct EFA deficiency.[2]

In addition to preventing EFA deficiency, lipid emulsions are a rich source of nonprotein calories. Recent studies have demonstrated that lipid may be more effective than dextrose in promoting nitrogen retention.

Preterm infants appear to have limited capability to oxidize fatty acids. This limitation may be related to a deficiency of carnitine, which in the form of acyl-carnitine promotes transfer of fatty acids into mitochondria where oxidative metabolism occurs.

VITAMIN

Vitamin requirements, and signs and symptoms of deficiencies and toxicities are listed in Table 13-1.

In addition to the classical signs and symptoms of vitamin A deficiency, lower levels of this vitamin are found in infants with bronchopulmonary dysplasia (BPD) than in those without chronic lung disease.[14] In a controlled, blind trial, Shenai et al[20] were able to decrease morbidity from chronic lung disease in high-risk neonates by injection of high-dose (2000 IU) retinyl palmitate. Current investigations are under way to better define the role of vitamin A in healing processes in the preterm infant.

Because of antioxidant properties of vitamin E, it also has been suggested for treatment and/or prevention of BPD and retrolental fibroplasia.

Studies have demonstrated no role in BPD amelioration and conflicting results regarding prevention of retinopathy. Although the final word on this therapy is not in, recent reports of high mortality among parenterally treated infants and the ill-defined risk of intracranial hemorrhage suggest that this drug should be used with caution in the newborn infant until more data are available.[1]

TRACE MINERAL

Although trace minerals are relatively scarce (less than 0.01% of the weight of the human body by definition), they play an important role in normal growth and development. Deficiencies of both zinc and copper have been identified in infants receiving long-term TPN. Manifestations of deficiency and recommendations for parenteral intake are given in Table 13-2. The recommendations for manganese, chromium, selenium, and iodide are included because parenteral solutions are now available for these trace elements. Deficiency states have not yet been identified in newborns, and requirements are not yet firmly established for these or lesser known trace elements such as molybdenum, nickel, vanadium, tin, silicon, and fluorine.

ETIOLOGY

Clinical indications for parenteral nutrition include any situation in which there will be a delay in establishing adequate oral nutrition. When parenteral nutrition is administered through a peripheral vein (PPN), caloric intake is limited by the concentration of carbohydrate (usually <12.5% dextrose) and fluid volume that can be delivered. Using lipid emulsions, a caloric intake of 60 to 90 kcal/kg/day and a protein intake of 2 g/kg/day can be achieved. This intake may prevent catabolism and in some cases effect moderate growth. This is usually adequate for term newborns with transient bowel disease (such as may be seen following the repair of a small omphalocele) or for preterm infants whose oral feedings are delayed for 1 to 2 weeks. PPN is commonly used to supplement nutrition in newborns who are able to receive only part of their requirements orally. When caloric needs can be met by peripherally administered TPN, this route is preferred to the central route because the catheter insertion risks are avoided and generally the risk of infection is less. The placement of a central line for parenteral nutrition allows a higher carbohydrate load to be used, giving more calories in less fluid. In preterm infants at risk for a patent ductus arteriosus and pulmonary edema, diminishing fluid intake and improving nutritional status may be important in management. TPN by a central catheter should be considered in:

1. VLBW infants (<1000 g) who do not tolerate oral feedings after a week of age and who cannot receive adequate caloric intake by PPN
2. Infants who have had gastrointestinal surgery and will have a significant delay in enteral nutrition because of complications such as a large gastroschisis, extensive bowel resection following necrotizing enterocolitis, or meconium peritonitis
3. Infants with chronic dysfunction such as intractable diarrhea

DATA COLLECTION
Monitoring growth

Weight loss or inadequate weight gain is the initial effect of inadequate caloric intake. Linear growth, although less affected, will be diminished after longer periods of poor nutrition. Because of "brain sparing," head circumference growth is the least affected.

Fetal weight gain in utero at each week of gestation is currently used as the standard to assess adequacy of potential growth. Weight acquisition in utero is approximately 20 g/day at 28 weeks gestation and 30 g/day at 33 weeks gestation according to the "reference fetus" model of Ziegler et al.[24] However, it may not be appropriate for the preterm infant to grow at the same rate as the fetus in utero.

Adequate nutrition is probably better defined by evidence of adequate fat and muscle

acquisition in the neonate. Triceps skin fold thickness has been used to measure fat. The upper arm circumference minus the triceps skin folds has been used for muscle acquisition determinations in term infants and older children.[9] Standards are not yet available for preterm infants. In older children arm radiography devised by Behnke[3a] (available as part of the standard chest x-ray examination) has been used to assess fat acquisition and bone development.

This information is available on most chest x-ray films taken of preterm infants, but standards need to be established.

Minimum monitoring of growth should consist of:

1. Weight monitored daily b.i.d. or t.i.d. in LBW infants with marked fluid shifts
2. Length monitored weekly
3. Head circumference monitored weekly

These measurements should be recorded at least weekly on an appropriate growth curve for premature infants to assure adequate growth assessment.

Biochemical monitoring

In addition to anthropometric measurements, biochemical parameters may be monitored to assess nutritional adequacy. Tests for protein malnutrition have included serum total protein, albumin, transferrin, retinol-binding protein, and prealbumin; the latter two have been most promising in preterm infants. Routine clinical use of these measures awaits greater definition of normal variation and independent effects of systemic illness.

Biochemical monitoring of the infant's physiologic status is necessary to avoid complications of TPN (see section on metabolic complications and Table 13-6).

TREATMENT
Central catheter placement

Although many materials have been used, silicone elastomer catheters (Silastic) are preferred for central venous placement because of their pliability and low incidence of thromboembolic complications. Placement of a small (0.635 mm outside diameter) catheter has been successfully accomplished by both cutdown and percutaneous techniques using limb and scalp veins.[6,11]

It is best that veins that may be used for percutaneous central line placement not be sites for routine venipuncture. Therefore these veins should be marked to be reserved for this technique in an infant who is identified as potentially requiring TPN. The procedure involves stabilization of the vein and skin preparation with povidone-iodine solution. A needle (19-gauge butterfly needle with tubing cut off) is used to puncture the skin and create a subcutaneous tunnel before entering the vein. Once the needle is within the vein, the catheter is passed through it and advanced a premeasured distance to the approximate location of the right atrium (if the basilic vein is used, turn the infant's head to face the insertion site to minimize the risk of the catheter's entering neck vessels). The catheter tip position should be documented radiographically. The sharp needle is carefully removed from the skin and threaded off the catheter. A blunt-end needle is reattached to the catheter. Once the catheter is appropriately located in position, heparinized flush solution should be periodically instilled to prevent stasis and thrombosis.

The length of tubing outside of the infant's body should be measured and recorded. Excess may be carefully curled at the site of insertion and covered with a transparent, adhesive, nonocclusive polyurethane dressing. If an armboard was used for stabilization, it may be removed. Arm restraints should not be necessary.

Large-bore Silastic catheters (Broviac) are placed surgically in infants in whom the percutaneous method is not technically possible or for home (long-term) TPN. Generally, the catheters are placed in the internal or external jugular veins or common facial vein by cutdown and threaded to a central venous site. The distal end is tunneled subcutaneously and exited through the anterior chest wall or skin incision in the scalp to decrease the risk of wound contamination. The catheter must be secured and dressed using sterile technique. A small piece of Elastoplast to which the catheter is sutured may be placed near the catheter site.

Composition of infusate
CARBOHYDRATE

The prime source of calories is usually dextrose given peripherally as a 10% to 12% solution. Centrally a 15% to 30% solution may be used. The glucose load will be increased if either the infusion rate or glucose concentration of the infusate is increased. Too rapid an increase in glucose load may exceed an infant's carbohydrate tolerance and result in hyperglycemia. A rapid decrease in the infusion rate or the glucose concentration of the infusate may result in hypoglycemia.

When calculating caloric intake:

$$1 \text{ g dextrose} = 3.4 \text{ kcal}$$

OR

$$100 \text{ ml/kg of } D_{10}W = 34 \text{ kcal/kg}$$

OR

$$100 \text{ ml/kg of } D_{30}W = 102 \text{ kcal/kg}$$

Administered glucose load can be calculated:

Glucose load =

$$\text{Glucose (mg/kg/ml)} \times \frac{\text{Volume (ml)}}{\text{Time}}$$

Generally, a neonate will initially tolerate a 10% dextrose in water ($D_{10}W$) solution at an infusion rate to yield a load of 6 to 8 mg/kg/min. Some advocate the use of insulin added to the infusate to facilitate carbohydrate conversion, decrease glycosuria, and improve caloric intake. Generally, this is unnecessary. When there is glucose intolerance, it is usually preferable to add additional forms of calories such as fat emulsions.

TABLE 13-3

Composition of Fat Emulsions (10%)

	INTRALIPID	LIPOSYN II
Fatty acid distribution (%)		
Linoleic acid	50	66
Oleic acid	26	18
Palmitic acid	10	9
Linolenic acid	9	4
Stearic acid	4	3
Components (g/dl)		
Soybean oil	10	5
Safflower oil	—	5
Egg phosphatides	1.2	1.2
Glycerol	2.25	2.5
Caloric content (kcal/dl)	110	110

Blood sugar determinations and screening for glycosuria should be performed several times each day when glucose delivery is altered.

LIPIDS

To treat or prevent EFA deficiency, 0.8 to 1 g/day of fat emulsion per 100 calories administered is sufficient. In those cases in which there is inadequate caloric intake from carbohydrates, fat emulsions are used as an additional source of nonprotein calories. Fat emulsions should be given cautiously, beginning with 0.5 g/kg/day every 1 to 2 days as tolerated and increasing to 4 g/kg/day maximum. The composition of two available fat emulsions is presented in Table 13-3. Daily requirements for linoleic acid may be obtained with either emulsion. The emulsified fat particles are similar in size and metabolic rate to naturally occurring chylomicrons. Most are cleared through passage in the adipose and muscle tissue. The capillary endothelial lipoprotein lipase hydrolyzes triglycerides and phospholipids, generating free fatty acids (FFAs), glycerol, and other glycerides. Most of the fatty acids diffuse into

TABLE 13-4

Concentrations of Amino Acids Adjusted to 3% Solutions and Compared with Recommendations for Amino Acid Requirements

AMINO ACID	RECOMMENDATIONS		SOLUTIONS			
	SNYDERMAN (MG/KG/DAY)	GHADIMI (MG/KG/DAY)	TRAVASOL (MG/DL)	FREAMINE III (MG/DL)	AMINOSYN-PF (MG/DL)	TROPHAMINE (MG/DL)
Essential						
L-Leucine	240	400	185	272	356	420
L-Phenylalanine	144	100	184	168	128	144
L-Methionine	72	15	176	160	54	101
L-Lysine	168	120	174	219	204	246
L-Isoleucine	180	200	143	208	228	244
L-Valine	168	200	137	198	194	235
L-Histidine	58	50	133	85	95	146
L-Threonine	144	60	126	121	155	126
L-Tryptophan	36	30	53	45	52	59
Nonessential						
L-Alanine	444	100	624	212	211	161
L-Arginine	122	250	310	285	368	364
L-Proline	192	50	127	339	247	207
L-Tyrosine	144	12.5	12	—	19	69
L-Cysteine	72	85	—	—	*	<10*
L-Serine	166	100	150	177	142	165
L-Glycine	396	100	623	421	116	110
L-Glutamine	48	12.5	—	—	—	—
L-Taurine	—	—	—	—	196	70

Modified from Kerner JA and Sunshine P: Parenteral alimentation, Semin Perinatol 3:417-430, 1979. By permission.
*Cysteine hydrochloride supplement may be added.

the adipose tissue for reesterification and storage. A small portion circulates to be used by other tissues for fuel or for conversion by the liver into very low density lipoprotein. Extremely immature and small-for-gestational-age (SGA) infants with decreased adipose tissue have demonstrated delayed clearance of fat emulsion. Rates of administration should be slowest in these infants. The rate-limiting step for lipid clearance is the metabolism by lipoprotein lipase. The use of heparin stimulates the release of this enzyme and will result in an increase in serum FFA; therefore heparin must be used with caution. Carbohydrate must be administered with fat to provide the necessary substrates for fatty acid oxidation. Increased infusion of dextrose with the fat emulsion promotes fatty acid clearance.

AMINO ACID SOLUTION

The composition of four crystalline amino acid solutions available for parenteral use are presented in Table 13-4 and compared with recommendations for amino acid requirements. For neonatal use, the amino acid solution is usually administered in a 1.5% to 2.5% concentration. Each solution supplies an excess of nonessential amino acids, although more recently available solutions have sought to balance the nonessential amino acid profile.

L-Cysteine, which may be an essential amino acid in preterm infants, is not stable in solution.

With the use of Trophamine and Aminosyn-PF, this amino acid may be added immediately before the solution is administered.

Trophamine and Aminosyn-PF also include taurine, which is not available in other solutions. An additional theoretical advantage of Trophamine is the greater calcium/phosphorus solubility.[7]

To allow for safe and effective use of parenteral nitrogen, the maximal quantity provided should be guided by the nonprotein calories infused. A calorie/nitrogen ratio of approximately 200 to 300 calories to 1 g nitrogen (1 g nitrogen = 6.4 g protein of Aminosyn-PF or 5.9 g protein of Travasol) is a general guideline. If 50 cal/kg/day were infused, based on 300 cal/1 g nitrogen, the maximum nitrogen that could safely be administered would be 0.17 g, or 1.1 g protein/kg/day (0.17 × 6.4).

ELECTROLYTES

Sodium is given in the maintenance quantity (2 to 3 mEq/kg/day) as long as the serum sodium is 135 to 140 mEq/L and there are no excessive losses.

Potassium is given in maintenance amounts (2 mEq/kg/day) unless there is excessive loss or renal disease. Potassium needs may increase with anabolism.

As long as the patient does not have renal tubular dysfunction, sodium and potassium requirements may be evaluated by monitoring urinary electrolyte levels (i.e., if sodium were depleted, low urine concentration would be expected).

Sodium and potassium may be supplied as chloride, acetate, or phosphate salts. The daily chloride requirement is approximately 3 mEq/kg/day and should be balanced with acetate to avoid alkalosis or acidosis (acetate is converted to bicarbonate). Amino acid preparations also supply anions that must be recognized to calculate a balanced anion solution. For example, Aminosyn-PF supplies 10 mEq of acetate per gram of nitrogen.

MINERALS

Phosphorus may be provided as sodium or potassium phosphate. Calcium is supplied as 10% calcium gluconate (9.7 mg of elemental calcium/100 mg of salt). In preparing a solution with both calcium and phosphate, care must be taken to avoid calcium phosphate precipitation. Magnesium is supplied as magnesium sulfate.

When a potassium phosphate solution at pH 7.4 is used, 4.4 mEq of potassium supplies 93 mg of elemental phosphorus. When a solution of sodium phosphate is used at pH 7.4, 4 mEq of sodium is given with each 93 mg of elemental phosphorus.

CALCIUM

1. Because of the increased risk of precipitation, calcium chloride should not be used.
2. An elevation in temperature, increased storage time, rise in pH, and decrease in protein or glucose concentration may increase the likelihood of precipitation.
3. In preparing the solution, phosphate salts should be added before the calcium salts, and thorough mixing should occur throughout the entire addition.
4. With appropriate precautions, it should be safe to mix 20 mEq of calcium and 20 mm of potassium phosphate in a liter of solution.

VITAMINS

A preparation containing the American Medical Association's recommended formulation of IV vitamins has recently become available for general use.° Requirements may be approximated by providing 1 vial per day for term newborns. It is recommended that preterm infants with a birth weight of less than 1500 g receive 65% and infants with a birth weight of less than 1000 g receive 30% of a vial, although these guidelines are still under investigation.[13,17]

°MVI Pediatric, Armour Pharmaceutical Co., Kankakee, Ill.

TRACE ELEMENTS

Commercially available amino acid solutions contain trace elements as contaminants, but variability even in the same brand means they cannot be relied on for delivering maintenance trace elements.

Zinc may be supplied as zinc sulfate. Serum zinc levels usually approximate the maternal levels and decline over the first week of life. By the second week of life, neonates not receiving dietary zinc should have supplementation. It may be necessary to initiate zinc intake earlier in neonates with intestinal loss such as following gastrointestinal surgery.

Copper is supplied as cupric sulfate.

Some centers also provide manganese, chromium, and selenium salts for long-term parenteral nutrition, although requirements and deficiency states have been less well defined.

Table 13-5 outlines a suggested composition for a TPN solution (guideline only).

The following case example serves to illustrate the above points regarding writing orders for TPN:

History: A male infant born at 29 weeks gestation at 1300 g is now 14 days old and unable to be fed because of bowel resection (status post) necrotizing enterocolitis. Because there will be a prolonged delay in oral alimentation, a central vein catheter is placed for TPN. He is currently receiving $D_{10}W$ at 120 ml/kg with maintenance electrolytes. He appears cachectic and weighs 1100 g. His serum electrolytes and blood glucose are normal.

The approach to calculating TPN requirements is as follows:

Caloric requirements: Since this patient has already had a significant postpartum period without adequate nutrition, achieving the necessary caloric intake for growth is a very important part of his care at this time to assure survival without excessive morbidity. The infant will probably require 120 cal/kg or more for growth. We will begin with 55 to 60 kcal/kg and advance daily to reach this level.

Carbohydrate: Initially a dextrose load just above

TABLE 13-5

Suggested Composition for Intravenous Nutrition Regimen

	DAILY AMOUNT
Calories	
Dextrose, 3.4 kcal/g	10-20 g/kg
Lipids, 1.1 kcal/ml (10% solution)	1-4 g/kg
Nitrogen*	0.315 g/kg
Protein (6.4 g protein = 1 g N_2)	2 g/kg
Electrolytes	
Sodium	3 mEq/kg
Potassium	2-3 mEq/kg
Chloride	3-4 mEq/kg
Phosphate	2 mM/kg
Calcium	1 mEq (20 mg)/kg
Calcium gluconate, 10%	200 mg/kg
Magnesium	0.8 mEq (20 mg)/kg
Vitamins	
MVI-Ped	1 packet
Vitamin A	700 μg
Thiamine (B_1)	1.2 mg
Riboflavin (B_2)	1.4 mg
Niacin	17 mg
Pyridoxine (B_6)	1 mg
Ascorbic acid (C)	80 mg
Ergocalciferol (D)	400 IU
Vitamin E	7 IU
Pantothenic acid	5 mg
Cyanocobalamin	1 μg
Folate	140 μg
Vitamin K	200 μg
Trace elements	
Zinc (zinc sulfate)	300 g/kg
Copper (cupric sulfate)	20-30 μg/kg
Manganese sulfate	2-10 μg/kg
Chromium chloride	0.2 μg/kg
Selenium	1-2 μg/kg

*L-Cysteine, 50 mEq/kg, should be added before administration.

what has been previously tolerated should be used. Thus the patient should receive $D_{12.5}W$ at perhaps 130 ml/kg/day, depending on the fluid requirements of the infant. Overhydration with its risks of cardiovascular and pulmonary complications should be avoided. This represents:

12.5 g glucose/dl × 130 ml/kg = 16.2 g glucose

16.2 g glucose/kg × 3.4 kcal/g glucose =
$$55.1 \text{ kcal/kg}$$

Lipid emulsion may be added to increase the caloric intake, starting with 0.5 g/kg/day.

5 ml/kg (0.5 g) 10% fat emulsion × 1.1 kcal/ml = 5.5 kcal/kg/day (or 2.5 ml/kg of 20% fat emulsion)

Thus the total nonnitrogen calories on the first day of TPN will be 60.6 (55.1 + 5.5).

Protein: In calculating the quantity of protein to be given using the ratio 200 kcal/1 g nitrogen, 0.3 g of nitrogen/kg may be given with 60.6 calories: $\left(\dfrac{60.6}{200} \times 1 \text{ g} \right)$. This quantity of nitrogen (as Aminosyn-PF) represents 1.9 g protein/kg (0.3 g/nitrogen × 6.4 g protein/g nitrogen).

Electrolytes: The patient should receive maintenance sodium ion (3 mEq/kg) and potassium ion (2.5 mEq/kg) unless there are excessive renal or gastrointestinal losses.

Anions: Balancing anions is the next consideration. The 0.3 g of nitrogen if given as Aminosyn-PF will add 3 mEq of acetate/kg to the solution (10 mEq acetate/1 g nitrogen). If potassium is administered as potassium chloride, 2.5 mEq/kg of chloride will be given. If 0.5 mEq of sodium/kg is given as sodium chloride, the solution will provide 3 mEq/kg of chloride. This will approximate maintenance requirements of this anion and will balance the 3 mEq/kg of acetate. The additional 2.5 mEq/kg of sodium can be given as sodium phosphate, which will provide approximately 58 mg/kg of elemental phosphorus.

$$(2.5 \text{ mEq Na}^+/\text{kg}) \times \left(\frac{93 \text{ mg (P)}}{4 \text{ mEq Na}^+} \right)$$

Minerals, vitamins, and trace elements: Calcium, magnesium, vitamins, and trace elements should be ordered at this point. Calcium initially should be started at 1 mEq/kg but should be increased as the infant begins to grow.

Volume: Calculating the concentration of each ingredient in a 250 ml bottle of TPN solution is the next step. Since the per kilogram figure of each additive is to be delivered in 130 ml, the amount of each to be put in the 250 ml bottle

should be calculated by multiplying by 1.92 (250/130).

TPN orders: Thus the TPN orders would be written for this patient as follows:

1. $D_{12.5}W$ with the following per 250 ml to run 6 ml/hr:

   0.58 g nitrogen (3.7 g protein)
   1.0 mEq sodium as sodium chloride
   4.8 mEq sodium as sodium phosphate
   4.8 mEq potassium as potassium chloride
   111.6 mg phosphorus as sodium phosphate
   5.8 mEq acetate (in 0.58 g Aminosyn-PF)
   1.9 mEq calcium
   1.5 mEq magnesium
   1.25 vials MVI-Ped
   576 μg zinc
   58 mg copper
   12 μg manganese
   0.5 μg chromium
   2.1 μg selenium
   96 mEq L-cysteine

2. 5.5 ml of 10% fat emulsion through a peripheral IV to run 1 ml/hr.

   Then discontinue fat emulsion infusion and IV. Progression: On subsequent days the dextrose concentration and lipids would be advanced slowly to increase the caloric intake to requirements as tolerated. The quantity of protein would also be increased to about 2.5 g/kg.

Solution preparation

Solutions should be prepared in the hospital pharmacy under a laminar flow hood in a work area isolated from traffic and contaminated supplies. There should be quality control checks to monitor for breaks in sterility in equipment, personnel, environment, and solutions.

Since many additives potentially may be incompatible, a mixing sequence should be established that separates the most incompatible ingredients. Calcium and phosphate should be separated as far as possible in the mixing sequence. Both single- or multiple-bottle sequences have been advocated.

Although the TPN solution may be stored for

weeks in dark, refrigerated conditions, certain additives such as vitamins C and A may lose activity over time. Storage also increases the risk of microbial contaminations; therefore TPN solutions should be prepared on the day they are needed.

Administration of the TPN solution

Proper administration of the TPN solution is as important as its preparation in preventing complications. The solution label should always be checked for proper identification of the patient and the current formula order.

Routine procedures must be established to avoid infectious complications from solution contamination. A standardized schedule should be maintained. Bottles should be changed and initiated at the same time each day.

A parenteral nutrition solution container should arrive from the pharmacy "spiked" with an IV set.

Solutions on the nursing units may be returned to the pharmacy for additives before hanging, but no additives can be placed in the solution once it is hanging.

Infections may occur from contamination of the solution bottle or by breathing or touching during tubing changes. Parenteral nutrition solution is infused via a 0.22 μm bacterial particulate and air–eliminating filter.

Mask and gloves must be worn when changing bottles, filters, and other support equipment. Extension tubing must be fastened down with a rubber-shod clamp before changing bottles, filters, and other equipment to avoid "bleeding back" into the catheter. When "bleeding back" occurs, the interior of the catheter becomes coated with blood, increasing the risk of complications from a fibrin sleeve and clot formation.

Changes in TPN infusion rates result in changes in glucose delivery to the newborn and may lead to hypoglycemia or hyperglycemia if the glucose homeostatic mechanisms do not adjust fast enough. Reactive hypoglycemia may

occur if the glucose load is abruptly discontinued. Parenteral nutrition solutions must infuse at a constant rate via an infusion pump. Attempts to rush or slow down solutions should not occur.

If the parenteral nutrition infusion is suddenly discontinued because of a clotted catheter or accidental removal, $D_{10}W$ should be infused via a peripheral vein and blood glucose monitored.

Use of parenteral nutrition may increase an infant's risk of developing hyperglycemia during surgery. Since rapid fluid infusions may be necessary during operative procedures, the TPN solution should be discontinued and replaced with a physiologic infusate during the perioperative period. After surgery TPN should be resumed when the patient is euglycemic.

Discontinuation of the TPN solution may begin by tapering as the infant begins to tolerate oral feedings. When the patient is taking approximately two thirds of the required calories orally, the central line should be aseptically removed by the surgical team that placed it. Percutaneously placed catheters may be removed as a routine IV line once parenteral access is no longer necessary. The length of the indwelling portion of the catheter should be measured and compared with that stated in the original procedure note. Careful attention to this detail will alert the clinician to the unlikely occurrence of catheter fragmentation, in which a portion is left in the tissue or vessel.

Administration of fat solution

Since fat emulsions support bacterial growth and improper administration may lead to contamination of the central venous line, fat emulsions should be administered alone via a peripheral vein. If this is not possible, a Y-tube may be used to bypass the filter.

Fat emulsions are never given via a filter, since they will disrupt and clog it.

Rapid infusion of the fat emulsion may exceed its clearance rate from the body and accentuate complications; therefore fat emulsions should not be infused faster than 0.15 g/kg/hr.

To minimize the risk of metabolic imbalances and administrative error, many clinicians provide lipid emulsion in small quantities continuously, as with dextrose solutions.

General care of the central line

Avoiding frequent breaks in the line minimizes infectious complications and prolongs catheter life. General care of the central venous line should include:

1. Only parenteral nutrition solution or dextrose and water should be infused, no medications
2. No blood drawing
3. No stopcocks
4. Daily change of tubing

If the line is malfunctioning, it must be properly checked to avoid the possibility of complications from a release of clot into the bloodstream. If a clotted line is suspected, the line may be aspirated using strict sterile technique. If a good blood return occurs or a clot is aspirated and removed, the catheter may be irrigated with sterile, dilute heparin solution (250 units heparin/5 ml normal saline). The catheter must not be irrigated without blood return.

Some clinicians will flush a partially occluded line with urokinase. This practice is not yet generally accepted in most neonatal centers.

Specific management protocols for long-term Silastic catheter complications are discussed later in the section on home care.

COMPLICATIONS
Mechanical complications

Potential complications include pneumothorax, hemothorax, hydrothorax, subclavian hematoma, air embolism, thromboembolism, catheter misplacement, or cardiac perforation. Chest x-ray examination and documentation of catheter placement are necessary before instill-

ing a hypertonic solution.

The preceding complications may occur at any time as long as the catheter is present. The risk is greatest if the catheter is moved following initial placement. The chest x-ray examination should be repeated if there is any history of pulling or tension on the catheter or any apparent change in its external position.

A pleural effusion may be blood or chyle or may signal that the catheter has eroded into the pleural space. The effusion may be the infusate.

Superior vena cava syndrome and thrombophlebitis may occur with continued use of a catheter.

Complications are unusual with percutaneously placed small-bore, Silastic catheters. However, because of their narrow diameter the catheters may occasionally need to be removed because of occlusion, particularly secondary to lipids or calcium phosphate crystals.

Infectious complications
CONTAMINATED SOLUTION PREPARATION

Rigid criteria for sterile preparation of the solutions are mandatory (see previous section on solution preparation).

An in-line 0.22 μm membrane filter is capable of trapping bacteria and fungi (although not endotoxin) and should be helpful in minimizing the risk of septicemia from a contaminated IV bottle. However, a filter provides a break in the line and another potential place for contamination. Additionally, filters minimize the risk of an air embolism.

There should be no additives to the TPN bottle after it leaves the pharmacy.

CONTAMINATION OF THE IV LINE FROM MISUSE

General guidelines to avoid IV contamination are as follows:

1. Blood should not be drawn or given through the catheter, because this increases the formation of a fibrin sleeve and clots.

2. Stopcocks should never be used.
3. Medicines should not be injected or "piggy backs" given through the central venous line.
4. When changing IV fluid bottles, extension tubing should be changed with a rubber-shod clamp to avoid bleeding back through the catheter.

Infections usually result from contamination with an organism that has colonized on the skin.

The procedure for a dressing change is as follows:

1. Organize supplies at the bedside (see boxed material at right).
2. Wash hands thoroughly for at least 2 minutes.
3. Don a sterile gown, hat, and mask.
4. Remove the old dressing and place in a paper bag.
5. Inspect the catheter site and surrounding skin for signs of irritation, leakage, edema, and erythema.
6. Put on sterile gloves and thoroughly cleanse a 2- by 3-inch area with sterile alcohol-acetone–saturated gauze pads. Using a circular motion from center to periphery, cleanse with friction. Use sterile applicators to cleanse the sutures and catheter sites.
7. Repeat cleansing with povidone-iodine scrub three times.
8. Remove the povidone-iodine scrub with a sterile alcohol gauze pad.
9. Change the extension tubing and filters. Fill the new extension tubing and filter with fluid.
10. Drape the area with a fenestrated drape.
11. Change gloves.
12. Prepare the area from center to periphery with povidone-iodine solution on sterile gauze or a swabstick. Blot pooled solution and allow to dry.
13. Apply povidone-iodine ointment to sterile 2- by 2-inch gauze cut to fit around the catheter at the insertion site.

EQUIPMENT FOR CENTRAL VENOUS CATHETER CARE

Masks (2)
Clean gown
Examination gloves (2 pairs)
Paper bag
TPN tray containing 2- by 2-inch gauze sponges, 4- by 4-inch gauze sponges
Medicine glasses (4)
Scissors
Sterile applicators
Sterile fenestrated drape (1)
Acetone, 10%; isopropyl alcohol, 70%
Povidone-iodine scrub
Povidone-iodine solution
Isopropyl alcohol, 70%
Telfa pad
Povidone-iodine ointment
Extension tubing
Micropore tape, 2-inch roll
Transpore tape, ½-inch roll
Elastoplast, 3-inch roll
Tincture of benzoin

From Forlaw L: Reprinted from Critical Care Nursing Quarterly (formerly Critical Care Quarterly), Vol. 3, No. 4, pp. 12-13, with permission of Aspen Publishers, Inc., © March 1981.

---

14. Cover the 2- by 2-inch gauze and catheter sheath with a Telfa pad.
15. Paint the skin with benzoin and allow to dry.
16. Apply Elastoplast to include the junction of the catheter and extension tubing.
17. Tape the extension tubing to the Elastoplast with a "butterfly" crossing of tape. Do not tape the filter to the dressing.
18. Label the dressing, including the date of change and the initials of the person performing the dressing change.
19. Chart the dressing change, appearance of the site, and problems encountered.

With appropriate care, catheter-related sepsis should occur in less than 1% of patients.

With the development of sterile, occlusive, transparent dressings, equally good results may be achieved with less frequent dressing changes, and the surgical site may be examined through the dressing material. If this dressing is used, it is placed over the insertion site and along the catheter to secure it to the skin. Therefore steps 14 to 17 are eliminated.

EVALUATING THE INFANT FOR AN INFECTIOUS DISEASE COMPLICATION

Generally, patients receiving parenteral nutrition who develop catheter-induced sepsis demonstrate persistent fever spikes, but this sign may be less dramatic in a newborn than in an older child. Sepsis must be suspected when nonspecific findings such as lethargy or apnea occur.

Of the catheters removed on suspicion of catheter sepsis, 75% are removed unnecessarily.[23] Other sources of infection must be investigated. Routine catheter removal is not required unless the infant is extremely ill.

Some guidelines for management of an infant on TPN with temperature instability or other signs of suspected sepsis are:

1. The bottle of parenteral nutrition should be aseptically discontinued and an appropriate dextrose and water solution with electrolytes substituted. The parenteral nutrition bottle with tubing should be sent to the laboratory for culturing.
2. The infant should be evaluated for potential sources of infection, including a general physical examination looking for non-TPN–related sources and inspection of peripheral and central venous sites for erythema.
3. Laboratory aids should include screening tests such as (a) a complete blood count including platelet count, (b) acute-phase reactants, (c) aerobic and anaerobic bacterial cultures of blood (drawn from a peripheral site), (d) urine culture, (e) cerebrospinal fluid culture, and (f) wound and/or stool culture if indicated.
4. Radiologic evaluation should be considered for an abscess if fever persists.
5. If another infection source is found, it should be treated appropriately. If the infection responds to treatment but a positive blood culture was present, there is a risk that the catheter may be the focus for continued seeding of the blood. Follow-up blood cultures obtained through the catheter and close clinical monitoring are important if the catheter is to be left in place.
6. If no source for the fever is found and it persists for 8 to 12 hours, septicemia should be suspected. If the infant is stable, this may be treated using appropriate antibiotics through the catheter, thus prolonging the life of the TPN line.[23] Quantitative blood cultures may be helpful to determine if catheter-related sepsis is being adequately treated.[16] If the patient appears critically ill, the catheter should be removed immediately and appropriate antibiotic therapy initiated.

Catheter removal should be performed according to the following steps:

1. Prepare the skin site as for surgery.
2. Obtain a blood culture specimen through the catheter.
3. Remove the catheter sutures and culture if there is evidence of infection.
4. Remove the catheter and place the tip in an anaerobic culture medium.
5. Obtain a peripheral blood culture.

Metabolic complications
GLUCOSE METABOLISM

Hyperglycemia may occur with an increased carbohydrate load, especially in very premature infants who may have inadequate endogenous insulin production or decreased sensitivity to insulin. Elevated blood glucose may lead to hyperosmolality and osmotic diuresis, resulting in hyperosmolar dehydration. Manifestations include polyuria, glucosuria, and dry, hot, flushed skin. Serum sodium is not a reliable measure of serum osmolality if there is hyperglycemia. Direct measurement or an estimate using the following formula is necessary:

Serum osmolality = 1.86 Na +
    Blood urea nitrogen (BUN)/2.8 + Glucose/18

Transient glucose intolerance may be seen with stress. If hyperglycemia occurs without an apparent change in glucose infusion, the possibility of sepsis, hypoxemia (i.e., as a result of apnea or pneumothorax), intraventricular hemorrhage (especially if the infant is <34 weeks gestation), or an inadvertent increase in carbohydrate administration (mistake in preparation or rate of infusion) should be considered.

Glucose intolerance may also be accentuated during infusions of lipid emulsion, especially in the VLBW infant. Discontinuation of the lipid infusion without alteration of the carbohydrate load will often eliminate hypoglycemia in this situation.

Hypoglycemia may result from an abrupt interruption of glucose infusion or excessive exogenous insulin administration. Manifestations of hypoglycemia include tachycardia, lethargy, jitteriness, and seizures. If these occur immediately following an interruption of the TPN infusion, an IV glucose infusion must be initiated at once, followed by close monitoring of the blood glucose to allow appropriate glucose administration. The glucose concentration of the infusate can usually be safely decreased by 5 mg/dl every 12 hours. Blood glucose values should be monitored hourly for 3 hours after each change.

AMINO ACID METABOLISM

Hyperammonemia may be seen in preterm infants given excessive protein loads. Hyperammonemia will also occur in neonates with urea cycle defects who are challenged with an amino acid load. Hyperammonemia may be manifested as somnolence, lethargy, seizures, and coma. Biochemical screening is necessary to avoid these complications before there are symptoms.

Azotemia may occur before hyperammonemia, depending on the liver's ability to convert ammonia to urea. Azotemia may also be a sign of dehydration.

Initially BUN should be monitored daily, then three times a week. If an elevation of BUN is the only abnormal finding, the patient should be evaluated for evidence of dehydration such as decreased urine output, increased urine specific gravity, or weight loss.

Approximately 30% of infants receiving TPN for more than 2 weeks will develop cholestatic jaundice (direct bilirubin >2 mg/dl). The risk appears greatest for the least mature infants and those receiving the longest period of TPN without enteral feeding. It occurs earliest and is most severe in those infants with the highest protein intakes and is possibly accentuated by hypertonic dextrose loads. The etiology appears to be multifactorial, including lack of bile flow stimulation, malnutrition, and amino acid toxicity or deficiency. Fat emulsions have been associated with cholestasis, but objective evidence of an etiologic role has not been provided. An increase in serum bile acid concentration usually precedes elevated conjugated bilirubin levels. Serum amino transferases are often normal early in the clinical course. Serum albumin and prealbumin levels usually remain normal. An abnormality in hepatic synthetic function or early rise in isoenzyme levels should lead the clinician to investigate other forms of liver disease. The differential of cholestatic jaundice would include:

1. Bacterial sepsis
2. Congenital viral infection
3. Postpartum acquisition of cytomegalovirus
4. Neonatal hepatitis

5. Bile duct obstruction such as biliary atresia or choledocal cyst
6. Galactosemia
7. Cystic fibrosis
8. Alpha-I-antitrypsin deficiency

Management of cholestatic jaundice should include:

1. Reduction of parenteral protein to 1g/kg/day
2. Reduction of dextrose to 20%
3. Enteral feedings if possible

LIPID METABOLISM

Infants with decreased adipose tissue may demonstrate intolerance to fat emulsions. Lipids may be poorly tolerated by extremely premature and SGA infants in the first week of life. Parenteral fats should be used cautiously in these infants. Hyperlipidemia may result, causing elevated triglycerides, FFAs, and increased lipoprotein levels. Serum may be checked daily for evidence of visible lactescence (increased plasma turbidity) by observation of plasma in a hematocrit that has been spun in a centrifuge. Some laboratories can measure fat emulsion levels by nephelometry (light-scanning index). A level greater than 100 mg/day is associated with hyperpre-beta-lipoproteinemia, hypertriglyceridemia, hypercholesterolemia, and hyperphospholipidemia. Since visual inspection of the plasma and nephelometry may give false-negative results, intermittent triglyceride and fatty acid levels should be obtained to monitor the lipid therapy.

Hyperlipidemia is responsible for the known and theoretical complications of fat emulsions.

Competitive displacement of bilirubin by FFAs may increase the risk of kernicterus in infants with hyperbilirubinemia, particularly those of less than 30 weeks gestation. Hyperbilirubinemia requiring therapy is a theoretical contraindication to lipid infusion, although the risks appear to be minimal when concentrations are low and infused slowly.[21]

TABLE 13-6

Metabolic Variables to Be Monitored during Intravenous Nutrition

VARIABLE TO BE MONITORED	INITIAL PERIOD*	LATER
Plasma electrolytes	Daily	2× weekly
BUN	3× weekly	2× weekly
Plasma calcium	3× weekly	2× weekly
Plasma magnesium phosphorus	Weekly	Weekly
Dextrostix†	q.8h.	Daily
Urine glucose	q. void	Daily
Serum albumin	2× weekly	Weekly
Liver function studies		
Transaminases	2× weekly	Weekly
Blood NH₃	Weekly	Weekly
Blood acid-base status	Daily	2× weekly
Hemoglobin	Daily	2× weekly
Serum turbidity‡	Daily	Daily
Serum triglyceride, cholesterol, FFA‡	Weekly	Weekly
Clinical observations (activity, vital signs, weight)	Daily	Daily

Modified from Kerner JA and Sunshine P: Parenteral alimentation, Semin Perinatol 3:417-430, 1979. By permission.
*While patient is metabolically unstable.
†Blood glucose to verify as needed.
‡While receiving fat emulsions.

Severe pulmonary disease or hypoxemia and/or altered pulmonary function are relative contraindications to the use of lipid emulsions.

Fat accumulation in alveolar macrophages and pulmonary capillaries has been identified in postmortem lung evaluations from infants who had received parenteral Intralipid.[8] However, more recent studies have found lipid-stained macrophages and alveolar cells in infants who had not received fats. These studies question the validity of the previous postmortem investigations.[19] In vivo hypoxemia has been noted with high-dose lipid infusion. In human studies, however, no effect on oxygenation has been seen with low-dose infusions.[22]

SEPSIS. The altered immune function by lipid deposition in macrophages and the reticuloendothelial system must be considered in infants with sepsis.

COAGULATION ABNORMALITIES. Evaluation of the effects of lipids on platelet count and function and hypercoagulability have not demonstrated consistent abnormalities in newborns.

Risk of accelerating atherosclerosis. Pathologic studies of babies receiving long-term parenteral fat emulsions have shown deposition in the intima of major vessels, accelerating atherosclerosis.

An additional concern of using plant fatty acid infusion is the risk of phytosterol substitution for cholesterol in the developing CNS. Long-term studies are needed to evaluate this theoretical risk.

Infants receiving TPN without fat emulsions or another fat source may develop biochemical evidence of EFA deficiency as early as 1 week of age. EFA deficiency should be suspected in infants with:

1. Scaly dermatitis
2. Poor wound healing
3. Elevated aspartate aminotransferase
4. Elevated triene/tetraene (>0.4)

A summary of metabolic screening is given in Table 13-6.

PARENT TEACHING
In hospital

Clinicians caring for an ill newborn must be attentive to the involvement and emotional state of the parents (see Chapter 22). There is a higher incidence of child abuse, foster placement, and relinquishment among infants who have been cared for in an NICU as compared with healthy "normally treated" newborns.

Bonding problems may be made worse by early separations that may occur in the NICU. When a newborn infant cannot be fed orally, an important normal part of the infant's care is no longer available for the parents. The placement of a central line with bandages around the head and neck can be frightening to parents and result in less handling and caretaking on their part.

Infants requiring chronic care such as TPN should have primary nursing (one regular nurse) and one physician who communicates regularly with the parents. Attempts should be made to keep the parents involved in other parts of the infant's care, since they are not able to feed the baby. They should be fully informed regarding the purpose of and appropriate care of the infant's central line so they will feel comfortable handling their infant with the line in place.

At home

Home parenteral nutrition has been used in neonates with congenital intestinal anomalies or following massive bowel resection for necrotizing enterocolitis.

TPN is initiated in the hospital. If growing and otherwise well, the infant may be a candidate for TPN at home. **The parents should be fully informed and cooperative, since they will be involved with assessment and management of the catheter and TPN administration. Since many professionals are involved, it is important to have a "team" approach with one person who communicates with the family. Physicians must be available to provide follow-up for the infant at least weekly in the clinic.**

The infant or young child will usually be receiving TPN intermittently (10 to 16 hours per day). At other times the catheter becomes essentially a "heparin-lock," and the patient is allowed to be mobile. While the infant is receiving intermittent infusion, the catheter should be flushed with 2 ml of normal saline, then 2 ml of heparinized saline (100 units/ml) after each use. If there are no infusions put through the line, the catheter should be flushed with heparinized saline twice a day (Table 13-7).

Chronically placed Silastic catheters (Bro-

TABLE 13-7

Heparinization of Broviac/Hickman Catheters

Flushing requirements

1. If the patient is receiving continuous infusions into the catheter, no flushing is required.
2. If the patient is receiving intermittent infusions (i.e., 12-hour TPN, antibiotics) the catheter should be flushed with 2 ml of normal saline, then 2 ml of heparinized saline (100 units/ml) after each use. No additional flushing with heparinized saline is required.
3. If the patient is not receiving any infusions through the catheter, the catheter must be flushed with heparinized saline b.i.d. according to this procedure. It is not necessary to use normal saline for routine flushes.

Supplies

Heparinized saline (100 units/ml)
3 ml syringe
22-gauge 1-inch needle
Sterile 70% isopropyl alcohol pad

Procedure

1. Wash hands thoroughly.
2. Draw up 3 ml of heparinized saline (100 units/ml) using sterile technique.
3. Clamp the catheter.
4. Clean the top of the intermittent injection port with a 70% isopropyl alcohol wipe. Allow to dry.
5. Insert the needle of the syringe containing heparinized saline through the intermittent injection port.
6. Release the occluding clamp.
7. Flush the catheter with 3 ml of heparinized saline (100 units/ml).
8. Clamp the catheter with the occluding clamp while instilling the last 0.5 ml of heparinized saline. This creates positive pressure, which will prevent the backflow of blood into the tip of the catheter.
9. Remove the needle and syringe and discard appropriately.
10. Check that the connections are securely taped.

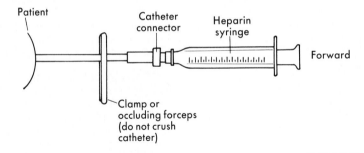

viac) may be used for parenteral medication infusion or blood drawing in addition to TPN administration. The intermittent injection port should be changed at least daily while the patient is in the hospital and any time blood is apparent in its grooves (Table 13-8). If used for blood drawing, the catheter must be handled in a strict, aseptic manner and be appropriately clamped to minimize the risks of air embolism and infectious complications (Table 13-9).

Proper care of the catheter exit site is important and must be carefully taught to the parents before discharge. Dressing changes are initiated after the surgical site is healed and are usually performed every other day (Table 13-10).

Parents need to be fully informed of the signs and symptoms of sepsis, metabolic complications, and embolic phenomena so that they might seek medical assistance before serious complications arise. In addition, they should be taught to recognize catheter complications, in-

TABLE 13-8

Changing the Intermittent Injection Port

Supplies
70% isopropyl alcohol wipes (3)
Intermittent injection port
Syringe/needle filled with 3 ml of heparinized saline
(100 units/ml)

Procedure
1. Wash hands thoroughly.
2. Clamp the catheter.
3. Remove the old intermittent injection port, using an alcohol swab.
4. Using a fresh isopropyl alcohol wipe, clean the threads on the hub of the catheter. Insert a new intermittent injection port.
5. Flush the catheter with 3 ml of heparinized saline (100 units/ml) per heparinization procedure.

cluding breakage or cracking of the catheter (correctable at least for a temporary period) and thrombosis.

SUMMARY

When the fetus is delivered prematurely, controlled nutritional intake via the placenta is abruptly interrupted. Reestablishing adequate nutrition is important for the neonate to be able to respond to environmental stresses and to acute illnesses such as respiratory distress syndrome and sepsis. It is also critical to avoid the long-term sequelae of malnutrition. Since enteral caloric intake may be inadequate for many ill newborns, parenteral nutrition has become an important part of the care of these infants. In most cases

TABLE 13-9

Drawing Blood from the Catheter

Supplies
Sterile syringe/needle containing 3 ml of heparinized saline (100 units/ml)
Sterile syringe/needle containing 5 ml of normal saline
5 ml sterile syringe (1)
Syringes adequate for amount of blood drawn
18-gauge needle
Tubes for blood
70% isopropyl alcohol wipes (3)
Sterile intermittent injection port
Sterile gloves (if patient is receiving parenteral nutrition through double-lumen Broviac)*

Procedure
1. Wash hands thoroughly.
2. Draw up 5 ml of normal saline and 3 ml of heparinized saline (100 units/ml) in separate sterile syringes.
3. Clamp the catheter.
4. Remove the intermittent injection port using an isopropyl alcohol pad and discard. If the patient is receiving a continuous infusion, disconnect the tubing from the catheter and cover the IV tubing with a capped, sterile needle.
5. Attach a 3 ml sterile syringe to the catheter hub. Unclasp the occluding clamp.

6. Aspirate 3 ml of blood.
7. Reclamp the catheter. Remove and discard the first syringe of blood.
8. Attach another syringe to the catheter. Unclasp the catheter and withdraw the appropriate amount of blood for laboratory tests.
9. Clamp the catheter. Remove the syringe of blood to be used for the blood sample.
10. Attach the syringe with 5 ml of normal saline, then release the clamp.
11. Immediately flush the catheter with 3 ml of normal saline. Clamp the catheter with the occluding clamp while instilling the last 0.5 ml of heparinized saline.
12. Fill the appropriate tubes with blood for laboratory tests.
13. Cleanse the end of the catheter with a sterile isopropyl alcohol wipe.
14. If the catheter is being used for continuous infusion, reconnect the IV tubing and set the IV pump if it is being used.
15. If the catheter is not being used for continuous infusion, attach the sterile intermittent injection cap. Flush the catheter with 3 ml of heparinized saline.

*Remember when drawing blood, the clamp must always be on the catheter while the Broviac catheter is open.

TABLE 13-10

Exit Site Care

Supplies

Povidone-iodine scrub/chlorhexidine
10% acetone/70% isopropyl alcohol swabsticks (2)
Povidone-iodine swabsticks (3)
2- by 2-inch gauze pads (4)
Tape

Procedure

1. Wash hands thoroughly.
2. Remove the old dressing. Deposit in a trash basket.
3. Inspect the catheter site and surrounding skin for signs of irritation, leakage, edema, erythema, or altered position of the catheter. Notify the physician if any of the above are present.
4. Secure the catheter to the chest wall, forming a loop so that swabs can easily be used under the catheter.
5. Cleanse the area with acetone/alcohol swabsticks. Always work from the exit site toward the periphery in a circular motion, cleansing a 2- to 3-inch area. Repeat twice using a sterile acetone/alcohol swabstick.
6. Paint the area with a povidone-iodine swabstick, starting at the exit site and working outward in a circular motion until the skin is cleansed 2 to 3 inches around the exit site. Repeat once using a sterile povidone-iodine swabstick. Allow the povidone-iodine to dry or blot dry. Check under the catheter.
7. Using the third sterile povidone-iodine swabstick, cleanse the catheter in a circular motion, starting from the exit site and cleansing 2 to 3 inches of the catheter. Blot dry.
8. Apply a 2- by 2-inch gauze pad.
9. Apply tape.

supplemental nutrition may be delivered via a peripheral vein, but in those with delayed enteral intake it may be necessary to risk mechanical and infectious complications of central catheterization. A neonatal service that uses TPN has the best results if there is an experienced "nutritional" team involving the pediatrician, surgeon, nutritional support nurse, pharmacist, and social worker, with each member playing a vital role to make TPN a safe and effective therapy.

REFERENCES

1. American Academy of Pediatrics Committee on Fetus and Newborn: Vitamin E and the prevention of retinopathy of prematurity, Pediatrics 76:315, 1985.
2. Anderson DW et al: Intravenous lipid emulsion in the treatment of essential fatty acid deficiency: studies in young pigs, Pediatr Res 18:1350, 1984.
3. Auld AM, Bhangananda P, Mehta S: The influence of an early caloric intake with IV glucose on catabolism of premature infants, Pediatrics 37:592, 1966.
3a. Behnke AR, Katch FI, and Katch VL: Routine anthropometry and arm radiography in assessment of nutritional status: its potential, JPEN 2:532, 1978.
4. Cornblath M et al: A controlled study of early fluid administration on survival of low birth weight infants, Pediatrics 38:547, 1966.
5. Dudrick SJ et al: Long term total parenteral nutrition with growth, development and positive nitrogen balance, Surgery 64:134, 1968.
6. Durand M et al: Prospective evaluation of percutaneous central venous Silastic catheters in newborn infants with birth weights of 510 to 3920 grams, Pediatrics 78:245, 1986.
7. Fitzgerald KA and Mackay MW: Calcium and phosphate solubility in neonatal parenteral nutrient solutions containing Trophamine, Am J Hosp Pharm 43:88, 1986.
8. Friedman Z et al: Effect of parenteral fat emulsion on the pulmonary and reticuloendothelial systems in the newborn infant, Pediatrics 61:694, 1978.
9. Georgieff MK and Sasanow SR: Nutritional assessment of the neonate, Clin Perinatol 13:73, 1986.
10. Georgieff MK et al: Effect of neonatal caloric deprivation on head growth and 1-year developmental status in preterm infants, J Pediatr 107:581, 1985.
11. Gilhooly J et al: Central venous silicone Elastomer catheter placement by basilic vein cutdown in neonates, Pediatrics 78:636, 1986.
12. Goldman HI et al: Late effects of early dietary protein intake on low-birth-weight infants, J Pediatr 85:764, 1974.
13. Green HL et al: Evaluation of a pediatric multiple vitamin preparation for total parenteral nutrition. II. Blood levels of vitamins A, D, and E, Pediatrics 77:539, 1986.
14. Hustead VA et al: Relationship of vitamin A (retinal) states to lung disease in the preterm infant, J Pediatr 105:610, 1984.
15. Kushyap S et al: Effects of varying protein and energy intakes on growth and metabolic response in low birth weight infants, J Pediatr 108:955, 1986.
16. Linares J et al: Pathogenesis of catheter sepsis: a prospective study of quantitative and semiquantitative cultures of catheter hub and segments, J Clin Microbiol 21:357, 1985.
17. Phillips B et al: Vitamin E levels in premature infants during and after intravenous multivitamin supplementation, Pediatrics 80:680, 1987.

18. Raihu NCR et al: Milk protein quality in low-birth-weight infants. I. Metabolic responses and effects on growth, Pediatrics 57:659, 1976.

19. Schroeder H et al: Pulmonary fat embolism after intralipid therapy—a post mortem artifact? Light and electron microscopic investigations in low birth weight infants, Acta Paediatr Scand 73:461, 1984.

20. Shenai JP et al: Clinical trial of vitamin A supplementation in infants susceptible to bronchopulmonary dysplasia, J Pediatr 111:269, 1987.

21. Spear ML et al: The effect of fifteen hour fat infusions of varying dosage on bilirubin bonding to albumin, J Parenter Enter Nutr 9:144, 1985.

22. Stahl GE et al: The effect of lipid infusion rate on oxygenation in premature infants, Pediatr Res 18:406A, 1984.

23. Wang EL et al: The management of central intravenous catheter infections, Pediatr Infect Dis 3:110, 1984.

24. Ziegler EE et al: Body composition of the reference fetus, Growth 40:329, 1976.

25. Zlotkin SH and Anderson GH: The development of cystathionase activity during the first year of life, Pediatr Res 16:65, 1982.

SELECTED READINGS

American Academy of Pediatrics, Committee on Nutrition: Nutritional needs of low-birth-weight infants, Pediatrics 75:976, 1985.

Anderson TA and Fomon SJ: Vitamins. In Fomon SJ, editor: Infant nutrition, Philadelphia, 1974, WB Saunders Co.

Coran AG: The long term total intravenous feeding of infants using peripheral veins, J Pediatr Surg 8:801, 1973.

Dorney SFA et al: Improved survival in very short small bowel of infancy with use of long-term parenteral nutrition, J Pediatr 107:521, 1985.

Forlaw L: Parenteral nutrition in the critically ill child, Crit Care Q 3:1, 1981.

Frisancho AR, Klayman JE, and Mitos J: Newborn baby composition and its relationship to linear growth, Am J Clin Nutr 30:704, 1977.

Ghadimi H: Newly devised amino acid solutions for intravenous administration. In Ghadimi H, editor: Total parenteral nutrition: premises and promises, New York, 1974, John Wiley & Sons, Inc.

Hambidge KM: The role of zinc and other trace metals in pediatric nutrition and health, Pediatr Clin North Am 24:95, 1977.

Helms RA et al: Enhanced lipid utilization in infants receiving oral L-carinitine during long-term parenteral nutrition, J Pediatr 109:984, 1986.

Koo WWK et al: Response to aluminum in parenteral nutrition during infancy, J Pediatr 109:877, 1986.

Moran JR and Greene HL: The B vitamins and vitamin C in human nutrition. I. General considerations and "obligatory" B vitamins, Am J Dis Child 133:192, 1979.

Moran JR and Greene HL: The B vitamins and vitamin C in human nutrition. II. "Conditional" B vitamins and vitamin C, Am J Dis Child 133:308, 1979.

Pereira GR, editor: Symposium on perinatal nutrition, Clin Perinatol 13, 1986.

Pettigrew RA et al: Catheter related sepsis in patients on intravenous nutrition: a prospective study of quantitative catheter cultures and guidewire changes for suspected sepsis, Br J Surg 72:52, 1985.

Robin AP and Greig PD: Basic principles of intravenous nutritional support, Clin Chest Med 7:29, 1986.

Snyderman SE: Recommendations of Dr. S. E. Snyderman for parenteral amino acid requirements. In Winters RW and Hasseling EG, editors: Intravenous nutrition in the high risk infant, New York, 1979, John Wiley & Sons, Inc.

Vileisis RA, Inwood RJ, and Hunt CE: Prospective controlled study of parenteral nutrition associated cholestatic jaundice: effect of protein intake, J Pediatr 96:893, 1980.

Wilmore DW and Dudrick SS: Growth and development of an infant receiving all nutrients exclusively by vein, JAMA 203:140, 1968.

Ziegler M et al: Route of pediatric parenteral nutrition: proposed criteria revision, J Pediatr Surg 15:472, 1980.

PART III

Infectious and Hematologic Diseases of the Neonate

CHAPTER 14

Hematologic diseases

ASKOLD D. MOSIJCZUK · CHERYL ELLIS-VAIANI

Understanding fetal and neonatal hematopoiesis is necessary for recognition and proper management of hematologic problems in the newborn. The infant is suddenly transferred from the relative hypoxia of the uterus to an oxygen-rich environment. As a part of the transition to extrauterine existence, the hematopoiesis taking place in the bone marrow at birth virtually ceases and resumes activity when the infant is about 2 months of age. Concurrently, a shift from synthesis of fetal to adult hemoglobin takes place. Additionally, maternal and fetal interactions affect the hematologic system in the newborn. This chapter discusses common hematologic disorders in the neonate: anemia, bleeding diathesis, and polycythemia.

ANEMIA
Physiology

Red blood cells are needed to carry and deliver adequate oxygen to the brain, liver, heart, kidneys, and other organs and tissues in the body. Inadequate delivery of oxygen because of deficiency in the red blood cells causes tissue hypoxia and acidosis. Anemia may be a central cause of hypoxia and acidosis in the newborn or, more commonly, may contribute to these derangements in babies born with pulmonary or cardiac disorders.

Newborns with hyaline membrane disease, pneumonia, and hypoplastic lungs often re-quire transfusions to maintain an optimal hemoglobin concentration to prevent further hypoxia and acidosis.

In more than 90% of term infants, the normal hematocrit range is 48% to 60%, and the normal hemoglobin range is 16 to 20 g/dl (Table 14-1).

In both term and premature infants there can be as much as a 20% difference between the peripheral and the central measurements of hematocrit, with the peripheral measurement being higher as a result of peripheral stasis. Capillary blood, arterial blood, and venous blood reveal respectively lower values, emphasizing the importance of serial measurements from the same source. Arterializing the capillary site by warming the extremity increases the usefulness of capillary samples.

After the first week of extrauterine life, hemoglobin and hematocrit levels decrease as a result of normal bone marrow suppression, reaching a nadir between 2 and 3 months of life. In full-term infants this nadir is approximately 10.7 g of hemoglobin and 31% hematocrit, whereas in premature infants it may reach 9.5 g of hemoglobin for infants weighing 1500 g, and even 8.5 g of hemoglobin for babies weighing less than 1000 g at birth.

NOTE: **The nadir is a normal physiologic process that does not result in hypoxia, acidosis, or other metabolic derangements in an otherwise normal infant; nor will it respond to treatment with iron, folic acid, cyanocobalamin, or vitamin E.**

☐ The opinions and assertions in this chapter are those of the authors and do not necessarily represent those of the Department of the Army or the Department of Defense.

TABLE 14-1 _____

Mean Cord Hemoglobin (Hb) and Hematocrit (Hct) at Birth and Changes in the First Week of Life

	MEAN CORD Hb	MEAN CORD Hct	FIRST WEEK
Full-term and preterm infants (>34 weeks)	16.8 g/dl	53%	No decrease in Hb value
Preterm infants (24-34 weeks)	14-15 g/dl	40%-47%	No decrease in Hb value

Modified from Oski FA: Hematological problems. In Avery, GB, editor: Neonatology: pathophysiology and management of the newborn, Philadelphia, 1975, JB Lippincott Co.

Etiology

Anemia present at birth or in the immediate neonatal period can be caused by blood loss, a hemolytic process, or decreased red blood cell production.

ANEMIA RESULTING FROM BLOOD LOSS

Anemia resulting from blood loss may be a result of occult hemorrhage before birth. The various recognized causes are listed below.

Types of hemorrhage in the newborn*

I. Occult hemorrhage before birth
   A. Fetomaternal
      1. Traumatic amniocentesis
      2. Spontaneous
      3. Following external cephalic version
   B. Twin-to-twin
II. Obstetric accidents and malformation of the placenta and cord
   A. Rupture of a normal umbilical cord
      1. Precipitous delivery
      2. Entanglement
   B. Hematoma of the cord or placenta
   C. Rupture of an abnormal umbilical cord
      1. Varices
      2. Aneurysm
   D. Rupture of anomalous vessels
      1. Aberrant vessel
      2. Velamentous insertion

*From Nathan DG and Oski FA: Hematology of infancy and childhood, vol 1, ed 2, Philadelphia, 1981, WB Saunders Co.

      3. Communicating vessels in multilobed placenta
   E. Incision of placenta during cesarean section
   F. Placenta previa
   G. Abruptio placentae
III. Internal hemorrhage
   A. Intracranial
   B. Giant cephalohematoma, caput succedaneum
   C. Retroperitoneal
   D. Ruptured liver
   E. Ruptured spleen

Frequently, a newborn who has suffered an acute, recent hemorrhage will be pale, in shock, and have a low blood pressure at birth, with a normal hematocrit. However, a repeat hematocrit determination as early as 3 to 6 hours after birth in such an infant will show a significant drop because of hemodilution. Conversely, an infant who has suffered chronic blood loss during gestation, often as a result of prolonged or repeated fetal-to-maternal bleeding, will be pale at birth but usually will show no acute distress. The hematocrit will be low at birth, with microcytic hypochromic indexes on the complete blood count (CBC), reflecting an iron deficiency caused by chronic blood loss. Table 14-2 summarizes the clinical manifestations of a newborn with acute and chronic blood loss.

To document fetal-to-maternal bleeding as a cause of anemia in the newborn, a Betke-

TABLE 14-2

Characteristics of Acute and Chronic Blood Loss in the Newborn

CHARACTERISTICS	ACUTE BLOOD LOSS	CHRONIC BLOOD LOSS
Clinical	Acute distress; pallor; shallow, rapid, and often irregular respiration; tachycardia; weak or absent peripheral pulses; low or absent blood pressure; no hepato-splenomegaly	Marked pallor disproportionate to evidence of distress; on occasion signs of congestive heart failure may be present, including hepatomegaly
Venous pressure	Low	Normal or elevated
Laboratory		
Hemoglobin concentration	May be normal initially, then drops quickly during first 24 hours of life	Low at birth
Red blood cell morphology	Normochromic and macrocytic	Hypochromic and microcytic; anisocytosis and poikilocytosis
Serum iron	Normal at birth	Low at birth
Course	Prompt treatment of anemia and shock is necessary to prevent death	Generally uneventful
Treatment	Intravenous fluids and whole blood; iron therapy later	Iron therapy; packed red blood cells may be necessary occasionally

From Nathan DG and Oski FA: Hematology of infants and childhood, vol 1, ed 2, Philadelphia, 1981, WB Saunders Co.

Kleihauer test should be performed on maternal blood within 24 hours of delivery. This test, also known as the acid elution technique, destroys adult hemoglobin in the maternal cells (ghost cells), while the circulating fetal cells, resistant to the elution, are stained red.

ANEMIA RESULTING FROM A HEMOLYTIC PROCESS

Hemolytic anemias are characterized by shortened red blood cell survival. Normal red blood cell survival in full-term newborns is only 60 to 80 days and may be as low as 30 days in premature infants, as compared with 120 days in adults.[6]

Hemolytic anemias in the neonatal period will usually have a persistently elevated reticulocyte count in the absence of hemorrhage. They are also frequently seen with a declining hemoglobin concentration and jaundice with an elevated indirect bilirubin concentration.

Numerous conditions in the newborn can cause increased red blood cell destruction and shortened red blood cell survival (see outline below).

Causes of a hemolytic process in the neonatal period*

I. Immune
  A. Rh incompatibility
  B. ABO incompatibility
  C. Minor blood group incompatibility
  D. Maternal autoimmune hemolytic anemia
  E. Drug-induced hemolytic anemia

II. Infection
  A. Bacterial sepsis
  B. Congenital infections
    1. Syphilis
    2. Malaria
    3. Cytomegalovirus
    4. Rubella
    5. Toxoplasmosis
    6. Disseminated herpes

III. Disseminated intravascular coagulation

IV. Macro- and microangiopathic hemolytic anemias
  A. Cavernous hemangioma
  B. Large vessel thrombi
  C. Renal artery stenosis
  D. Severe coarctation of aorta

*From Nathan DG and Oski FA: Hematology of infancy and childhood, vol 1, ed 2, Philadelphia, 1981, WB Saunders Co.

Key: ⊕ Rh Positive   ⊖ Rh Negative   ■ Rh Antibody

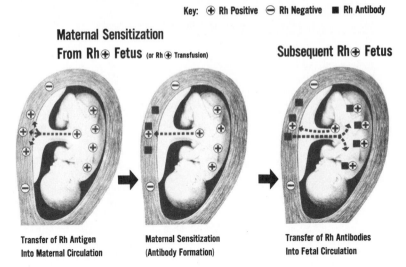

Maternal Sensitization From Rh⊕ Fetus (or Rh⊕ Transfusion)

Subsequent Rh⊕ Fetus

Transfer of Rh Antigen Into Maternal Circulation

Maternal Sensitization (Antibody Formation)

Transfer of Rh Antibodies Into Fetal Circulation

Figure 14-1. Isoimmunization in utero. (Courtesy Ross Laboratories, Columbus, Ohio.)

V. Galactosemia
VI. Prolonged or recurrent acidosis of a metabolic or respiratory nature
VII. Hereditary disorders of the red cell membrane
    A. Hereditary spherocytosis
    B. Hereditary elliptocytosis
    C. Hereditary stomatocytosis
    D. Other rare membrane disorders
VIII. Pyknocytosis
IX. Red cell enzyme deficiencies
    A. Most common
        1. Glucose-6-phosphate dehydrogenase deficiency
        2. Pyruvate kinase deficiency
        3. 5' Nucleotidase deficiency
        4. Glucose phosphate isomerase deficiency
X. Alpha thalassemia syndromes
XI. Alpha-chain structural abnormalities
XII. Gamma thalassemia syndromes
XIII. Gamma-chain structural abnormalities

IMMUNE ANEMIAS

Rh incompatibility. About 85% of the population has the D antigen on their red blood cell membrane, which makes their cells Rh positive, whereas 15% of the population lacks this antigen, making their cells Rh negative. For every 1000 pregnancies, about 90 will have an Rh-positive fetus and an Rh-negative mother. The Rh factor in the fetus may potentially result in the formation of Rh antibodies in the Rh-negative mother directed against the baby's red blood cells. However, only 1 of every 15 pregnancies at risk for Rh disease will actually result in hemolytic disease of the newborn, because Rh immunization of the mother rarely occurs during the first pregnancy. Many of the second infants will have Rh-negative cells, and only a fraction of women at risk will develop antibodies.[6]

In pregnancies affected by Rh hemolytic disease of the newborn, fetal red blood cells containing the D antigen enter the maternal circulation during gestation and evoke the formation of anti-D antibodies. Although both IgM and IgG antibodies are produced by the mother, only the IgG antibodies can cross the placenta and result in hemolysis of fetal red blood cells (Figure 14-1).

The immunoglobin-coated fetal red blood cells are usually destroyed extravascularly in the infant's spleen, where macrophages lining the splenic sinusoids ingest the sensitized red blood cells. This process results in anemia, jaundice

TABLE 14-3 _____

Nonimmune Hydrops Fetalis: Causes and Associations

Fetal
  Hematologic
    Homozygous α-thalassemia
    Chronic fetomaternal transfusion
    Twin-to-twin transfusion (recipient or donor)
    Multiple gestation with "parasitic" fetus
  Cardiovascular
    Severe congenital heart disease (atrial septal
      defect, ventricular septal defect, hypoplastic
      left heart, pulmonary valve insufficiency,
      Ebstein's subaortic stenosis)
    Premature closure of foramen ovale
    Myocarditis
    Large arteriovenous malformation
    Tachyarrhythmias: paroxysmal SVT, atrial flutter
    Bradyarrhythmias: heart block
    Fibroelastosis
  Pulmonary
    Cystic adenomatoid malformation of lung
    Pulmonary lymphangiectasia
    Pulmonary hypoplasia (diaphragmatic hernia)
  Renal
    Congenital nephrosis
    Renal vein thrombosis
  Intrauterine infections
    Syphilis

    Toxoplasmosis
    Cytomegalovirus
    Leptospirosis
    Chagas disease
    Congenital hepatitis
  Congenital anomalies
    Achondroplasia
    E trisomy
    Multiple anomalies
    Turner's syndrome
  Miscellaneous
    Meconium peritonitis
    Fetal neuroblastomatosis
    Dysmaturity
    Tuberous sclerosis
    Storage disease
    Small bowel volvulus
Placental
    Umbilical vein thrombosis
    Chorionic vein thrombosis
    Chorioangioma
Maternal
    Diabetes mellitus
    Toxemia
Idiopathic

From Etches PC and Lemons JA: Pediatrics 64:326, 1979. Reproduced by permission of Pediatrics.

caused by released bilirubin from the destroyed red blood cells, and a compensatory reticulocytosis.

The presence of antibody on the fetal red blood cells can be documented by the direct Coombs' test that is usually positive in Rh hemolytic disease of the newborn.

Clinically, the patient manifests increasing anemia, rapidly rising indirect bilirubin concentration, hepatosplenomegaly, elevated reticulocyte count, and increased nucleated red blood cells. Occasionally, if the hemolytic process is severe, the baby may be stillborn or may have hydrops fetalis at birth.

Rh hemolytic disease is currently rare, since most cases can be prevented by administering anti-D human gamma globulin (RhoGAM) to Rh-negative mothers the first 3 days following delivery or abortion of an Rh-positive infant or fetus. Nonimmune hydrops fetalis has in fact become more frequent than Rh immune hydrops in this country (Table 14-3).

For pregnancies involving an Rh-positive fetus and a previously sensitized mother, amniocentesis should be performed between 21 and 22 weeks gestation to evaluate the severity of fetal hemolysis. This is determined by measuring the bilirubin in the amniotic fluid, which is found by measuring the optical density.

If an amniocentesis indicates severe disease

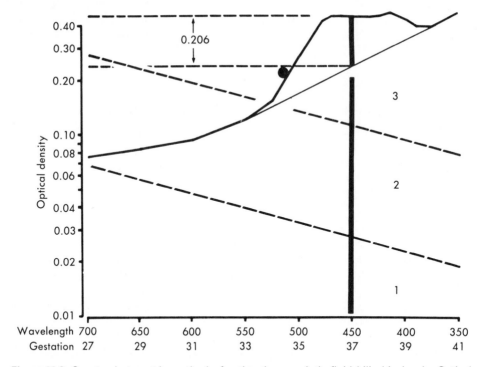

Figure 14-2. Spectrophotometric method of estimating amniotic fluid bilirubin levels. Optical density is measured from wavelength 350 to 700 μm. Optical density rise at 450 mm (because of bilirubin) is measured by rise in optical density at that point above projected baseline. Graph is of amniotic fluid of woman at 34½ weeks gestation. Optical density at 450 mm was 0.206. Value 0.206 is then plotted on graph superimposed in this figure and shown in slanted broken lines that delineate zones 1, 2, and 3. Zone 3 represents severe disease with impending fetal death, zone 2 represents less severe disease, and zone 1 indicates Rh-negative infant or one with mild disease. Calculated optical density must be plotted in this way because density decreases with gestational age. (From Bowman JM and Pollock JM: Pediatrics 35:815, 1965. Reproduced by permission of Pediatrics.)

(zone 3 or 2) or increasing bilirubin concentration at a subsequent testing, an intrauterine transfusion of red blood cells should be given to the fetus, or if the pregnancy is beyond 33 weeks, premature induction of labor is recommended (Figure 14-2).

In Rh-sensitized pregnancies resulting in a live birth and an absence of hydrops fetalis, the major problems are hyperbilirubinemia and the resulting risk of brain damage. The mainstay of treatment is exchange transfusion with Rh-negative type-specific whole blood to re-

move the sensitized Rh-positive erythrocytes, correct the anemia, and wash out bilirubin from the jaundiced infant.

For severely anemic infants with a hemoglobin concentration of less than 12 g/dl, edema, or heptosplenomegaly, an exchange transfusion should be performed immediately. A partial exchange transfusion with 40 ml/kg of packed red cells should be followed by a full exchange transfusion when the infant is stable.[5]

ABO hemolytic disease. Although 15% of pregnancies involve a mother with blood group O and a fetus with blood group A or B, evidence of hemolysis because of ABO incompatibility occurs in only about 3% of these pregnancies. Severe ABO hemolytic disease is rare primarily because of the decreased number of reactive sites on newborn red blood cells as compared with adult A red blood cells. Fewer A or B sites on the newborn red blood cells also explain the weakly reactive direct Coombs' test in ABO hemolytic disease. However, antibodies eluted from neonatal cells react strongly with adult group A or B erythrocytes, in which the A or B sites are close together. This is the basis for the positive indirect Coombs' test result in ABO incompatibility. It is not known why the disease is severe in some infants. Another reason for the relative mildness of ABO hemolytic disease may be a result of maternal anti-A or anti-B antibodies being bound up with the infant A or B substance in the body tissues and therefore not being available to react with newborn red blood cells.

In hemolytic disease resulting from ABO incompatibility, the direct Coombs' test will often be negative, whereas the indirect Coombs' test will be positive. A positive direct Coombs' test result in ABO incompatibility suggests severe hemolysis.

In ABO incompatibility, red blood cell destruction occurs primarily in extravascular sites, as in erythroblastosis fetalis. Contact of sensitized red blood cells with splenic macrophages results in loss of part of the red blood cell membrane, leading to spherocytosis and eventual destruction. It is not known why the spherocytes are not common in Rh disease, where similar mechanisms appear to be operational.

To diagnose clinically significant ABO hemolytic disease, the following conditions should be met:

1. **Indirect hyperbilirubinemia is seen in the first 24 hours of life.**
2. **Mild anemia, reticulocytosis, and nucleated red blood cells are found in the peripheral smear.**
3. **A weakly positive direct Coombs' test**

should be present, or antibody eluted from the infant's red blood cells should react with adult A or B cells.
4. **The mother's serum should contain relatively high levels of anti-A or anti-B antibodies of IgG type.**
5. **Increased numbers of spherocytes and microspherocytes should be present in the peripheral blood of the infant.**

HEMOGLOBINOPATHIES. Hemoglobinopathies can be grouped into defects involving the alpha, beta, or gamma chain. Anemia caused by defects in the gamma chain will be seen at birth, whereas defects involving the beta chain, such as sickle hemoglobin and C hemoglobin, appear later after beta-chain synthesis has replaced gamma-chain synthesis. Alpha-chain mutations rarely cause significant disorders in the newborn.

Occasionally, increased beta-chain synthesis and higher levels of A hemoglobin will be present in the newborn if hemolysis or blood loss occurred in utero. This situation may exist in fetal and maternal blood group incompatibility or with concomitant intrauterine blood loss. If such an infant also has an underlying beta-chain defect such as homozygous sickle cell disease, jaundice, fever, pallor, respiratory distress, and distention may appear at birth. Hemoglobin electrophoresis can be useful in diagnosing these infants.

THALASSEMIAS. All forms of unbalanced hemoglobin synthesis (thalassemia) may be clinically expressed at birth. Alpha thalassemia is best categorized by postulating alpha-chain production to be under the control of four genes:

1. **Absence of one alpha gene, the silent carrier, results in no anemia or other hematologic abnormalities except, possibly, a slightly elevated hemoglobin Bart's.**
2. **Absence of two alpha genes results in alpha thalassemia trait and is seen with microcytosis and hypochromia with no anemia and no jaundice and a slightly elevated hemoglobin Bart's.**
3. **A three-gene defect, hemoglobin H dis-**

ease, causes microcytosis, hypochromia, anemia, and jaundice, and hemoglobin Bart's is apparent.

4. Absence of all four alpha genes results in a fetus with hydrops fetalis and causes only hemoglobin Bart's production that is incompatible with life because of the inability to delivery oxygen to the tissues.

Beta thalassemia (deficient production of beta chains) usually does not cause problems in the immediate newborn period. Since beta chains normally are present in only small amounts at birth, even homozygous beta thalassemia (thalassemia major) can be virtually asymptomatic. With increasing age, the absence of adequate beta-chain production in homozygous beta thalassemia eventuates in the severe hemolytic anemia characteristic of this disease. However, as in hemoglobinopathies involving the beta chain, an additional hemolytic stress or intrauterine hemorrhage can occasionally result in the clinical expression of beta thalassemia in the newborn period.

A hemoglobin electrophoresis may suggest a gene defect in hemoglobin synthesis (thalassemia) in a newborn with anemia, jaundice, elevated reticulocyte count, hypochromia, and microcytosis. A decreased rate of alpha-chain synthesis will cause an elevation of hemoglobin Bart's on hemoglobin electrophoresis. Decreased production of beta chain (beta thalassemia) may cause hemoglobins A_2 or F to increase in infants in whom an additional hemolytic process or blood loss in utero has occurred.

Both trait and homozygous states of beta thalassemia become apparent only after the infant is 2 to 3 months of age as gamma-chain production ceases and converts to the deficient beta-chain production and results in decreased levels of hemoglobin A, relatively increased levels of A_2, and occasionally fetal hemoglobin.

RED BLOOD CELL MEMBRANE DEFECTS. Hereditary spherocytosis, elliptocytosis, and stomatocytosis may manifest clinically as hemolytic anemia in the newborn period.

Most red blood cell membrane defects are difficult to diagnose. The exception is hereditary spherocytosis, since morphologic features (microspherocytes) are present in these infants at birth. An immune process coating the red blood cells such as ABO incompatibility should be eliminated as a cause of spherocytosis before a diagnosis of hereditary spherocytosis is made.

RED BLOOD CELL ENZYME DEFICIENCIES. Glucose-6-phosphate dehydrogenase deficiency is an X-linked abnormality primarily encountered in persons of Mediterranean, Southeast Asian, or African descent. American black men (12%) and women (2%) also may possess an enzyme with decreased activity.

Defects in the glycolytic pathway and pentose-phosphate shunt such as pyruvate kinase and glucose-6-phosphate dehydrogenase deficiency present as a hemolytic anemia with jaundice in the neonatal period. Pyruvate kinase levels, glucose-6-phosphate dehydrogenase levels, and other red blood cell enzyme levels should be measured in newborn blood if these defects are suspected.

Black infants with glucose-6-phosphate dehydrogenase deficiency are usually not affected with severe jaundice unless they are also exposed either prenatally or postnatally to medication with oxidant properties, such as sulfonamides, nitrofurantoin (Furadantin), salicylates, acetanilid, or naphthalene.

IMPAIRED RED CELL PRODUCTION. Several diseases can lead to decreased production of red blood cells and hence anemia in the neonate. *Neonatal leukemia*, a rare disease in this age group, can be seen with leukocytosis, thrombocytopenia, and anemia because of replacement of the bone marrow with leukoblasts. Rubella and other congenital infections can also occasionally result in bone marrow failure and anemia. *Diamond-Blackfan anemia* (pure red cell aplasia) will have isolated anemia caused by isolated failure of erythroid production in the bone marrow. Occasionally other anomalies, such as deformed thumbs, appear in these infants. The mode of inheritance is not known, but autosomal recessive inheritance is suggested. Diamond-Blackfan anemia commonly begins when the infant is between 2 and 3 months of age. *Osteopetrosis* (marble bone disease) is another rare disorder that produces anemia as a result of bone marrow failure. Failure of adequate stem cell production may cause a diminished bone marrow volume and an increased thickness of cortical bone, predisposing the bone to fractures.

Prevention

Some causes of anemia in the neonatal period are preventable. Improved fetal monitoring and obstetric care may prevent anemia caused by blood loss resulting from obstetric accidents, malformations of the placenta and cord, and fetal hemorrhage resulting from dystocia. Administering RhoGAM to Rh-negative women within 72 hours of delivery of an Rh-positive infant (or a fetus if an abortion) prevents most cases of erythroblastosis fetalis. When a previously Rh-sensitized mother is carrying an Rh-positive fetus, amniocentesis performed between 21 and 22 weeks gestation, and if necessary repeated every 2 to 3 weeks, may allow for intrauterine transfusions and possible early delivery of a nonerythroblastotic infant. For sickle cell disease and thalassemias in-utero detection of affected infants currently is possible. Fetal red cells obtained by cordocentesis can be analyzed for abnormal globin-chain synthesis. Fibroblasts obtained by amniocentesis and/or chorionic villous samples can serve as a source of DNA that can be analyzed by restriction endonucleases for the presence or absence of abnormal globin genes.[10,13]

Detecting an affected fetus will ensure adequate planning and preparation by the obstetric and pediatric personnel for the optimal management of the infant in the delivery room and in the nursery.

Data collection
HISTORY

If an infant has anemia, obtaining a family history of anemia is important. This should include questions about relatives with jaundice, anemia, gallstones, stasis ulcers of the legs, splenectomy, or unexplained deaths at an early age.

The racial and ethnic origin of the family should be determined, since hemoglobinopathies and thalassemias are more common in Oriental, black, and Mediterranean people. The perinatal history is extremely important and may considerably narrow the diagnosis.

The mother should be questioned about illnesses during her pregnancy. The obstetric history should be reviewed for possible placental complications or accidents leading to fetal, neonatal, or maternal blood loss. When possible, the placenta should be examined for malformations, tumors, and vascular anastomosis.

SIGNS AND SYMPTOMS

The newborn with suspected anemia should be examined for pallor, hypotension, and tachycardia, which may suggest shock, following acute blood loss. The infant should also be examined for bruising, internal hemorrhage, jaundice, hepatosplenomegaly, signs of intrauterine infection, and congenital anomalies.

Since the newborn with acute anemia may have tachycardia and tachypnea, the presence of arterial hypotension helps distinguish blood loss with impending shock from pulmonary problems. Capsular tears in the liver or spleen are the most frequent sites of internal hemorrhage in the neonate and may follow vigorous cardiac massage during resuscitative efforts. Intracranial hemorrhages (subarachnoid, subdural, and intraventricular) may cause significant anemia, but the identifying symptoms are

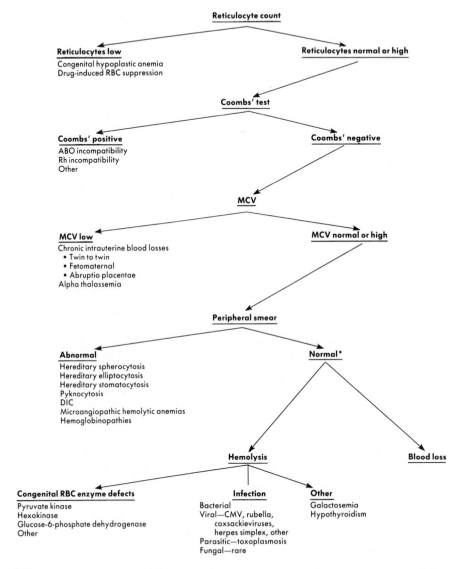

Figure 14-3. Diagnostic approach to anemia in newborn based on reticulocyte count. *Indicates peripheral blood smear with no specifically diagnostic abnormalities. (From Nathan DG and Oski FA: Hematology of infancy and childhood, vol 1, ed 2, Philadelphia, 1981, WB Saunders Co.)

predominantly neurologic. A scalp hemorrhage or an extensive cephalohematoma may cause massive blood loss and a significantly increased hyperbilirubinemia from degradation of the extravasated blood.

The infant with chronic blood loss may demonstrate hepatosplenomegaly, normal or increased central venous pressures, or congestive heart failure.

LABORATORY DATA

All infants should have a central hematocrit determination performed after admittance to the neonatal intensive care unit. Infants with a perinatal history of vaginal spotting, placenta previa or abruptio, emergency cesarean section, cord compression, or asphyxia should have a repeat hematocrit determination performed at 6 to 8 hours of age.

If anemia is confirmed, initial laboratory examinations should include a CBC, red blood cell indexes, a reticulocyte count, direct and indirect Coombs' tests, determination of blood type, and examination of the peripheral blood smear. A reticulocyte count can be used as an essential first step in classifying the infant's anemia (Figure 14-3). Infants with a low reticulocyte count often have decreased red blood cell production because of various forms of bone marrow failure, such as drug-induced red blood cell suppression, Diamond-Blackfan anemia, or congenital infection. Anemic newborns with an elevated reticulocyte count have blood loss or one of the many causes of hemolysis that produces their anemia. If blood loss is absent, further characterization of the hemolytic process can be achieved by examining the results of the Coombs' test, examining the mean corpuscular volume, and examining the peripheral smear for spherocytes, elliptocytes, stomatocytes, schistocytes, and decreased platelets. If the cause of hemolysis is not evident, perform a Heinz body test to look for unstable hemoglobins and obtain red blood cell enzyme measurements to eliminate red blood cell enzyme deficiencies such as pyruvate kinase, glucose-6-phosphate dehydrogenase, and STORCH titers. A more detailed approach to evaluating the anemic newborn is found in Figure 14-3.

Treatment
ANEMIA RESULTING FROM BLOOD LOSS

Usually, the hemoglobin is less than 12 g/dl before signs or symptoms of anemia are present in the newborn. However, an acute blood loss of 20% of the blood volume is sufficient to produce shock in the infant and may not be reflected in the hemoglobin concentration immediately at birth. Repeating the CBC when the infant is between 3 and 6 hours of age shows a decrease in hemoglobin and hematocrit in these cases. If acute blood loss is suspected and the infant is pale and limp at birth, blood pressure should be obtained and monitored, intravenous (IV) fluids at 20 ml/kg started, and oxygen administered. A catheter should be inserted into the umbilical artery to measure blood gases. Blood should be examined for CBC, reticulocyte count, and Coombs' test, and typed and crossmatched. As soon as it is determined that the infant's condition is caused by acute blood loss, give group O, Rh-negative whole blood at 20 ml/kg or group O, Rh-negative packed red blood cells at 10 ml/kg followed by fresh frozen plasma at 10 ml/kg.

Blood or blood products for transfusion

I. Human albumin (5%)
   A. Expensive
   B. May help reduce pulmonary interstitial fluid by raising serum oncotic pressure
   C. No risk of transmitting serum hepatitis
   D. Crossmatching not necessary
   E. Readily available
II. Fresh frozen plasma, platelets
   A. Given in group- and type-specific manner
III. Whole blood
   A. Heparinized whole blood from placenta
      1. Collected under sterile conditions in 20 ml syringe heparinized by rinsing with 0.1 ml $\frac{1}{1000}$ heparin

2. Collected from large surface vessels without milking; administered within 1 hour without refrigeration and through a blood filter
3. Emergency use only
B. Banked blood
1. Warmed and filtered before administering
2. Clotting factors depleted, red blood cell viability decreased, potassium level high, calcium level low with increased storage time; freshest possible blood used
3. Complete crossmatch requiring up to 1 hour and sample of infant's and mother's blood
4. Partial crossmatch requiring up to 30 minutes and sample of infant's and mother's blood
5. Group-specific unmatched unit requiring less than 15 minutes
6. Unmatched low titer O-packed red blood cells requiring less than 15 minutes

Blood volume can be estimated as 85 ml/kg body weight in a term infant and 100 mg/kg body weight in a preterm infant. Packed red blood cells (2 ml/kg body weight) will raise hemoglobin concentration 0.5 g/dl. A 50% decline in arterial pressure approximates at least a 25% reduction in volume.

Calculate the expected elevation in hematocrit:

$$\text{Packed red blood cells required (ml)} = \frac{(\text{Target Hct} - \text{Existing Hct}) \times \text{Blood volume (ml)}}{75 \text{ or known Hct of donor blood}}$$

Further transfusions of blood should be guided by central venous pressures, arterial blood pressures, and clinical course. Attempts to determine the cause of acute blood loss should be made by reviewing the obstetric history, examining the placenta, examining the infant for a possible site of bleeding, and performing a Betke-Kleihauer test on maternal blood.

There are frequent indications for blood transfusions in the intensive care nursery. In addition to acute or chronic anemia, these may include iatrogenic anemia from frequent blood tests and blood lost in surgery. Stringent recording of blood removed for testing assists the practitioner in identifying the need for blood replacement.

BLOOD TRANSFUSION PROCEDURES

In the neonatal intensive care unit a policy of "double-checking" blood is essential to ensure that the proper blood is administered to the proper infant. Blood should be warmed before administration and administered through a blood filter of at least 40 μm. Blood can be given by gravity, pushed through a large vein, or preferably through a volumetric pump, such as the Imed or Holter. Except in extreme emergencies, blood transfusion is not administered through an indwelling umbilical artery catheter but should be administered by an additional peripheral IV. An infant who receives all nutrition from parenteral sources usually will not tolerate discontinuing that IV without significant hypoglycemia, so an additional peripheral IV is required.

Blood should not hang for more than 4 to 6 hours. Fresh blood can be administered through a 25-gauge needle without significant hemolysis. The rate of blood administration is dependent on the infant's weight, fluid status, and reason for transfusion, but transfusions are routinely given over several hours. An infant whose fluid load is carefully monitored may need the maintenance IV decreased for the period of transfusion to prevent fluid overload.

Infants normally should not receive more than 10 ml/kg of whole blood at one time but should receive multiple small transfusions.

Infants who are mildly anemic at birth or anemic as a result of chronic blood loss and who are in no distress do not require transfusion unless their oxygenation capacity is further compromised by cardiac or pulmonary disease. In the absence of acute symptoms, these infants should be treated with ferrous sulfate in a dose of 6 mg of elemental iron/kg body weight/day in three divided doses for 3 months.

Infants with anemia resulting from a hemolytic process require measures to counteract hyperbilirubinemia and correct the anemia.

Rh HEMOLYTIC DISEASE

If an infant is born with known Rh hemolytic disease, the pediatrician in the delivery room should assess the infant's overall status, measure the vital signs, and detect the presence or absence of pallor, organomegaly, ascites, and edema. The cord blood should be sent for CBC, reticulocyte count, nucleated red blood cell count, blood type, direct Coombs' test, and total and indirect bilirubin concentrations.

If the infant is already edematous, pale, or in shock or the cord hemoglobin is less than 12 g/dl, an immediate partial exchange transfusion with 40 ml/kg of packed red blood cells should be performed. Once the infant's condition is stable, a full double-volume exchange transfusion should be promptly performed. If an immediate exchange transfusion is not indicated, serial observations of the total and indirect bilirubin should be obtained. If the rate of bilirubin rise is such that indirect bilirubin will exceed 20 mg/dl in an otherwise healthy term neonate, an exchange transfusion is indicated.

HEMOGLOBINOPATHIES

The most common hemoglobinopathies, sickle cell disease and hemoglobin C disease, generally do not produce anemia or jaundice during the first weeks of life because both defects occur on the beta-globin chain that is present in only small amounts at birth.[9]

HOMOZYGOUS ALPHA THALASSEMIA. Homozygous alpha thalassemia (four-alpha gene defect) may occasionally occur in Oriental infants and results in stillbirth or death shortly after birth, since the absence of alpha chains produces high levels of hemoglobin Bart's. Hemoglobin Bart's is composed of four gamma chains and has a high affinity for oxygen, resulting in impaired

oxygen release to the tissues. No treatment is available for this condition.

HETEROZYGOUS ALPHA THALASSEMIA. Heterozygous alpha thalassemia, resulting from a three-alpha gene defect (hemoglobin H disease), may present with mild anemia, and jaundice may be seen in the neonatal period, with increased but not lethal levels of hemoglobin Bart's.

As previously noted, patients with even the homozygous form of beta thalassemia may be only slightly anemic at birth, because fetal gamma-chain production masks the inability to produce beta chains and hemoglobin A after birth. Phototherapy usually is required to control the resulting hyperbilirubinemia.

RED BLOOD CELL ENZYME DEFECTS

Red blood cell enzyme defects such as pyruvate kinase deficiency are often mild at birth, with only occasional anemia and hyperbilirubinemia. Occasionally, severe anemia and hydrops have been reported with pyruvate kinase deficiency.

Occasionally, glucose-6-phosphate dehydrogenase deficiency produces sufficient hyperbilirubinemia to require an exchange transfusion, especially in Mediterranean and Oriental people. Black infants with a glucose-6-phosphate dehydrogenase deficiency rarely become sufficiently jaundiced to require an exchange transfusion, unless the infant is infected or has received an oxidant compound such as naphthalene in moth balls.

Complications

Recognized complications of severe anemia include stillbirth, hydrops fetalis, shock, congestive heart failure, further compromise of oxygen delivery to tissues in infants with pulmonary and cardiac lesions, poor feeding, and poor weight gain, especially in premature infants. In addition, hemolytic anemias may result in kernicterus.

Amniocentesis and intrauterine transfusion

for the fetus with Rh hemolytic disease may cause laceration of the fetus's abdominal organs and occasionally death.

Potential hazards of exchange transfusion include metabolic derangements such as hypocalcemia, hypoglycemia, hyperkalemia, and acidosis; cardiac problems such as arrhythmias, volume overload, and arrest; vascular problems caused by air emboli, thrombosis, hemorrhage, and perforation; clotting abnormalities including overheparinization and thrombocytopenia; and infectious complications such as bacteremia, hepatitis, especially non-A, non-B hepatitis, cytomegalovirus, and, rarely, acquired immunodeficiency syndrome (AIDS).

Cardiac arrest from hyperkalemia may result from using blood older than 48 hours, which has a higher potassium content. Hypocalcemia and cardiac arrest may result from donor blood with citrate used as an anticoagulant, because the citrate combines with ionized calcium to produce hypocalcemia.

Similarly, simple transfusions may result in volume overload, congestive heart failure, and previously mentioned infections. Complications of blood transfusions include sensitizing the recipient to foreign blood group antigens and transfusion of antigens in the previously sensitized infant. Proper blood bank procedures and attention to administration of crossmatched blood to the proper individual prevent sensitizing the infant to foreign blood group antigens and transfusing antigens in the previously sensitized infant. Infection can partly be prevented by properly screening donors, careful handling during processing and administration of blood, and giving multiple transfusions from a single donor by using multiple transfusion bags. Currently, blood banks screen blood for hepatitis, syphilis, and human immunodeficiency virus (HIV). Since there is no specific serologic test for non-A, non-B hepatitis, transmission of this infection through transfusions is still a problem. Cytomegalovirus

(CMV) transmission can be reduced by using only CMV-negative blood. It is advisable to limit the number of transfusions only to those that are clearly indicated by the infant's medical condition.

Parent teaching

Genetic counseling is essential for the proper prevention and treatment of some neonatal anemias. Parents who have children with hereditary hemolytic anemia or who are known carriers of an autosomal recessive gene such as beta thalassemia, sickle cell, or hemoglobin C gene should be informed about amniocentesis to detect the homozygous state in the fetus.

Parents at risk for an Rh-sensitized pregnancy should be informed about the availability and role of amniocentesis to diagnose Rh hemolytic disease in the unborn child and monitor the intrauterine course. All Rh-negative mothers should be aware of the availability of Rho-GAM, which should be administered within 72 hours after delivery of an Rh-positive child.

In nurseries in which a larger percentage of newborns is from ethnic groups with a high incidence of glucose-6-phosphate dehydrogenase deficiency (Oriental, Mediterranean, black), screening procedures should be performed on newborns to identify those at risk for hemolysis. Parents of these infants should be instructed to avoid giving potential hemolytic agents to their child such as fava beans, exposure to moth balls, and sulfa medications, and the mother should not be exposed to these agents if the child is to be breastfed. As with other aspects of neonatal care, the family is an essential part of the infant's care, and careful, repeated discussions of the problems, recommended treatment, and expected outcome are necessary. Hematologic conditions or abnormal prenatal events must be explained in physiologic terms. Careful explanations of the need for and importance of follow-up for infants with chronic or hemolytic anemia ideally will result in compliance and in few infants lost to follow-up.

• • •

Anemia in the newborn may be caused by many factors, including blood loss in utero as a result of fetal and maternal bleeding, obstetric accidents, and internal hemorrhage resulting from complicated delivery. In other infants with anemia and jaundice, possible factors are hemolysis as a result of Rh disease, ABO incompatibility, abnormalities of red blood cell membrane, defects in hemoglobin structure and synthesis, red blood cell enzyme deficiencies, and impaired red blood cell production. Personnel in the delivery room must recognize the anemic distressed infant who has acutely lost 20% or more of the blood volume so that proper fluid and blood replacement can be administered. The hydropic infant, because of severe Rh sensitization, likewise requires aggressive management with immediate exchange transfusion. Unconjugated bilirubinemia caused by a hemolytic process in the first days of life poses a threat of kernicterus. There are many causes for hemolysis, and fortunately phototherapy and timely exchange transfusion enable most infants to survive, even if an exact diagnosis cannot be made.

BLEEDING DIATHESIS
Physiology

Formation of a blood clot in response to injury requires the combined interaction of the damaged blood vessel, platelets, and soluble clotting proteins (coagulation factors) found in the plasma. Injury to a blood vessel and surrounding tissue triggers several hemostatic events. Exposed collagen in the blood vessel wall stimulates vessel constriction and adhesion of platelets to the site of injury and forms a primary hemostatic plug. Adherent platelets release substances, primarily adenosine diphosphate, that cause more platelets to aggregate at the site of injury. Simultaneously,

exposure of circulating blood to collagen in the damaged blood vessel activates the clotting factors in the plasma (factors XI and XII) to undergo a sequential series of proteolytic reactions that eventually activate factor X. At the same time, damage to the surrounding tissue at the site of blood vessel injury releases tissue thromboplastin, which, together with factor VII, forms a complex that also activates factor X. Activating the clotting system through tissue thromboplastin occurs outside the blood vessel and is therefore referred to as the extrinsic system. Activation of factors VIII, IX, XI, and XII occurs in the blood vessel and is referred to as the intrinsic system. Both the intrinsic and extrinsic systems require calcium that is always present in sufficient amounts for coagulation, even in severe hypocalcemic states. Once factor X has been activated, further clotting occurs through a common pathway. Activated factor X with factor V, platelet phospholipid, and calcium convert factor II (prothrombin) to thrombin. Thrombin cleaves factor I (fibrinogen) into fibrinopeptides and fibrin monomers that are subsequently polymerized and converted into insoluble fibrin by factor XIII. Fibrin is formed at the site of the primary hemostatic plug (made up of platelets), resulting in a solid clot[12] (Figure 14-4). Antithrombin III prevents excessive conversion of fibrinogin to fibrin by inhibiting the action of thrombin. Simultaneous with the formation of a clot, plasminogen in the plasma and in the blood clot is activated to plasmin. Plasmin eventually dissolves fibrin into fibrin-split products and prevents the clotting system from extending beyond forming a localized clot. Plasminogen and other factors responsible for preventing excessive clot formation and its subsequent dissolution are part of the fibrinolytic system.

SCREENING COAGULATION TESTS

BLEEDING TIME. A small standard incision is made in the skin of the forearm, and the time required for the bleeding to stop (usually 3 to 7 minutes) is known as the bleeding time.

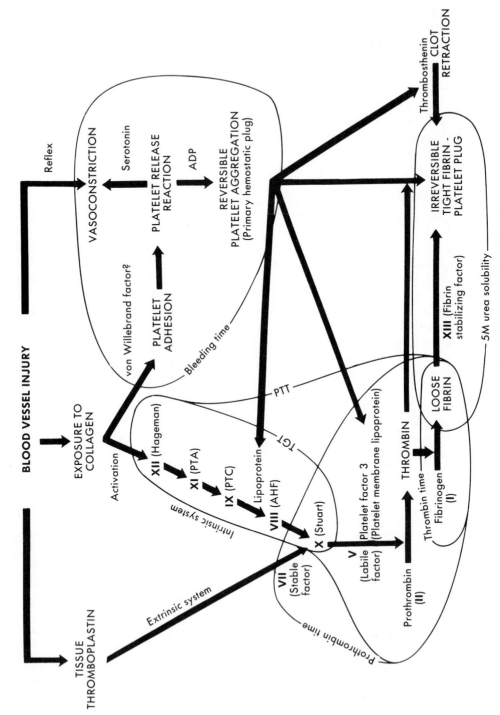

Figure 14-4. Schematic representation of blood coagulation mechanism. (From Strauss HS: Pediatr Clin North Am 19:1011, 1972.)

ACTIVATED PARTIAL THROMBOPLASTIN TIME.
Activated partial thromboplastin time (aPTT) is
performed by placing the patient's anticoagulated
plasma in a test tube, adding kaolin or celite to
activate factor XII, and measuring the time until a
fibrin clot forms.

**Decreased number of platelets, abnormal
platelet function, or abnormalities in the integrity of the blood vessel wall prolong the bleeding time. Defects in the intrinsic system (factors
VIII, IX, XI, and XII) and in the common pathway (factors I, II, V, and X) result in a prolonged
activated PTT.**

PROTHROMBIN TIME. Prothrombin time (PT) is
performed by placing the patient's citrated
plasma in a test tube, adding calcium and tissue
thromboplastin, and measuring the time until the
formation of a fibrin clot. This in effect bypasses
the intrinsic system and measures factor VII (extrinsic system) and the integrity of the common
pathway.

**Defects in factor VII or in the common path-
way prolong the PT.**

THROMBIN TIME. Thrombin time measures the
last step in the coagulation system, the conversion
of fibrinogen to fibrin. A known amount of thrombin is added to citrated patient plasma, and the
time until a fibrin clot is formed is measured.
**Deficient amounts of fibrinogen, defective fi-
brinogen molecules, anticoagulants such as
heparin, or excessive amounts of fibrin-split
products in the patient's plasma prolong the
thrombin time.**

Several coagulation factors are present in decreased amounts in newborn infants, especially in
premature infants. Vitamin K–dependent factors,
II, VII, IX, and X, are usually decreased because
of decreased liver production and decreased vitamin K levels in the neonate. Even after vitamin
K has been administered to the newborn, these
factors may be low for several weeks and even
several months in the case of factor IX. Other
clotting factors that are usually low in newborns
are factors XI, XII, and XIII. However, factors I
(fibrinogen), V, and VIII, as well as platelets, are

in or near the normal range for children and
adults. Despite deficiencies in many of the clotting factors, newborn blood appears to be hyper-
coagulable. This is probably because of low levels
of antithrombin III, a naturally occurring plasma
anticoagulant factor, in newborns.

**Because of the low plasma levels of several
clotting factors, activated PTT and PT are physiologically prolonged in the newborn. Although
exact normal ranges have not been established,
a PT prolonged by more than 50% of adult
control values, or an activated PTT prolonged
by more than 100% of adult control values, is
usually abnormal. Thrombin time is only
slightly (1 to 2 seconds) prolonged above adult
control values because fibrinogen levels in the
newborn are at adult values, but the newborn
fibrinogen molecule may be different from the
adult molecule (fetal fibrinogen). Bleeding
time is the same as in adults, reflecting normal
numbers of platelets.**

Bleeding problems in the newborn are often
the result of local trauma associated with a difficult delivery and not necessarily caused by defects
in the hemostatic mechanism. However, severe
physiologic deficiencies in clotting factors of the
newborn can aggravate the severity of bleeding.

**Intracranial hemorrhage, cephalhematomas,
subdural bleeding, bruising of the presenting
fetal part, localized petechiae, and hepatic,
adrenal, or renal hemorrhages are often the
result of traumatic delivery. Screening coagulation tests—PT, PTT, and platelet count—often
are normal in these infants.**

**Hemorrhages may result from an indwelling
umbilical catheter that is being overzealously
flushed with a heparinized solution. In overheparinization, thrombin time is markedly prolonged, PT and PTT are moderately prolonged,
and fibrinogen and factors V and VIII are unaffected.**

**Pathologic derangements in the coagulation
system often produce other types of bleeding:
(1) generalized petechiae; (2) bleeding from
mucosal surfaces; (3) bleeding from circumci-**

sion; (4) prolonged bleeding from venipuncture, heel stick sites, and an endotracheal tube; or (5) delayed bleeding from the umbilical stump.

Etiology

Most neonatal hemorrhages caused by a defect in the coagulation system can be organized into four broad categories: (1) inherited defects of the coagulation factors, (2) accentuation of the physiologically occurring coagulation factor deficiencies characteristic of the newborn period, (3) transitory disturbances as a result of an associated disease, and (4) quantitative and qualitative platelet abnormalities.

INHERITED DEFECTS OF THE COAGULATION FACTORS

Since none of the clotting factors crosses the placenta, classic hemophilia A (factor VIII deficiency) and severe hemophilia B (factor IX deficiency) can be diagnosed in the newborn. Mild hemophilia B cannot be diagnosed at birth, because factor IX is normally low in the first months of life.

A low factor VIII in the newborn is always abnormal. Besides classic hemophilia A and severe von Willebrand's disease, disseminated intravascular coagulation (DIC) is the other frequent cause of factor VIII deficiency.

Other coagulation factor deficiencies are rare and even when present usually do not cause hemorrhage in the newborn period. Neonates with congenital factor XIII deficiency are an exception, and blood usually oozes from the umbilical stump. Routine coagulation screening tests are normal, since the PT and the PTT monitor the appearance of the fibrin clot, whether or not this clot has been further cross-linked and stabilized by factor XIII. In these cases performing a clot solubility test determines whether the fibrin clot has been cross-linked by the action of factor XIII.

For unknown reasons, babies with even severe forms of hemophilia A or B do not usually manifest bleeding in the first weeks of life. Although spontaneous intracranial hemorrhage has been described, bleeding if present is usually caused by surgical trauma such as circumcision. Severe hemophiliacs usually will not demonstrate recurrent bleeding episodes such as hemarthrosis until mid to late infancy.

Abnormal bleeding after circumcision should be investigated, even if there is no family history of hemophilia, since spontaneous mutations occur rarely and result in hemophilia. Neonates with hemophilia who do not manifest bleeding usually look healthy, and the only abnormality on the coagulation screening tests is a markedly prolonged PTT.

ACCENTUATION OF THE NORMALLY OCCURRING COAGULATION FACTOR DEFICIENCY IN THE NEWBORN PERIOD

Vitamin K deficiency (hemorrhagic disease of the newborn) occurs in approximately 0.5% to 1% of newborns and is a result of accentuation of the normally low level of vitamin K–dependent factors II, VII, IX, and X in the first days of life. The PT and PTT are prolonged. It is thought that hemorrhagic disease is caused by negligible stores of vitamin K, limited oral intake, and absent intestinal bacterial flora to produce vitamin K during the infant's first days of life. Breastfed babies have an even greater risk of vitamin K deficiency, since breast milk has much less vitamin K than cow's milk. Bleeding resulting from a vitamin K deficiency may occur on the first day of life, but usually occurs on the second or third day, and rarely after 4 weeks.

Immature capacity of the liver to synthesize factors II, VII, IX, and X may contribute to bleeding from DIC in which, besides prolonging the PT and PTT, platelets are usually decreased and the infant usually appears ill.

In vitamin K deficiency the infant usually appears healthy but will manifest bleeding from the gastrointestinal tract, umbilical cord, circumcision site, venipuncture sites, and nose, as well as generalized ecchymoses.

In the premature infant, even in the presence of a prophylactic dose of vitamin K, hepatic synthesis of vitamin K–dependent factors may be minimal because of immaturity.

Infants unable to tolerate oral feedings are also at a great risk for vitamin K deficiency. Infants receiving milk-substitute formulas or total parenteral nutrition, or infants with malabsorption disorders (cystic fibrosis, biliary atresia) should receive supplementation with water-soluble vitamin K.

Hemorrhagic disease of the newborn is usually preventable by the prophylactic parenteral administration of 0.5 to 1 mg of vitamin K_1 (phytonadione) to the newborn in the first hour of life. The efficacy of oral vitamin K_1, especially in the exclusively breastfed infant, is unclear at this time.

When hemorrhage occurs as a result of vitamin K deficiency, two additional factors may be present: (1) prophylactic vitamin K may not have been given or (2) the mother may have been on warfarin-sodium (Coumadin) or phenytoin (Dilantin) drug therapy during her pregnancy. Both warfarin sodium and phenytoin cross the placenta and impair vitamin K production in the newborn.

Large doses of vitamin K synthetics such as menadione, hykinone, and menadiol sodium diphosphate (Synkavite) may contribute to hemolytic anemia, hyperbilirubinemia, and kernicterus and are contraindicated in the newborn.

TRANSITORY DEFECTS RESULTING FROM AN ASSOCIATED DISEASE

DIC is an acquired pathologic process manifested by the intravascular consumption of platelets and various plasma clotting factors, especially factors I (fibrinogen), II (prothrombin), V, VIII, and XIII. Several underlying disorders and disease processes can trigger diffuse intravascular clotting. The consumption of platelets and clotting factors usually results in generalized bleeding diathesis. In addition, activation of the clotting mechanism results in fibrin deposited in small vessels, which results in further destruction of platelets, lysis of red blood cells (microangiopathic anemia), occasional thromboses in larger vessels, and activation of the fibrinolytic system leading to the formation of fibrin-split products. These fibrin-split products function as anticoagulants and contribute to further bleeding.

In severely affected infants the laboratory diagnosis of DIC is usually not difficult, because the platelet count is markedly reduced and PT and PTT are markedly prolonged. In milder cases of DIC the wide range of normal values for PT and PTT, especially in premature infants, occasionally requires measuring fibrinogen concentration, fibrin-split products, and thrombin time, besides measuring the platelet count, PT, and PTT. Fibrinogen concentration is usually low, fibrin-split products may be present, and the thrombin time is usually prolonged in DIC. Red blood cell fragmentation (schistocytes) is usually seen on a peripheral smear. Measuring other clotting factors such as V, VIII, IX, X, XI, and XIII is usually not necessary but is useful when attempting to differentiate bleeding caused by DIC from that caused by severe liver disease. With DIC factors V and VIII are usually low, whereas with liver disease factor V may be normal and factor VIII is usually elevated (Table 14-4).

Infants with DIC frequently appear ill and usually have generalized bleeding from puncture sites, the gastrointestinal tract, central nervous system (CNS), and skin. Occasionally, large-vessel thrombosis may occur (probably as a result of low antithrombin III levels in neonates), resulting in gangrene of the affected parts.

PLATELET ABNORMALITIES

A platelet count below $150,000/mm^3$ is always abnormal and should be investigated, even though clinical bleeding may not occur until the count is below $50,000/mm^3$. Thrombocytopenia in an infant that appears well suggests immune-mediated platelet destruction, whereas throm-

TABLE 14-4

Clinical and Laboratory Findings in Neonatal Bleeding Caused by Liver Disease, Vitamin K Deficiency, or DIC

	LIVER DISEASE	VITAMIN K DEFICIENCY	DIC
Clinical appearance	Ill	Often well	Ill
Hepatosplenomegaly	Present	Absent	Present
Platelets	Normal or decreased	Normal	Decreased
PT	Prolonged	Prolonged	Prolonged
PTT	Prolonged	Prolonged	Prolonged
TT	Prolonged	Normal	Prolonged
Fibrinogen	Low or normal	Normal	Low
Factor V	Low or normal	Normal	Low
Factor VIII	Normal	Normal	Low
FDP	Normal or increased	Normal	Increased
Fibrin monomer	Absent	Absent	Present

bocytopenia in an infant that appears ill is usually because of microangiopathic consumption of platelets.

Decreased platelet production as a result of bone marrow failure is unusual in the newborn (see the following outline).

Etiologic classification of neonatal thrombocytopenia*

I. Immune disorders
   A. Passive (acquired from mother)
      1. ITP
      2. Drug-induced thrombocytopenia
      3. Systemic lupus erythematosus
   B. Active
      1. Isoimmune—platelet group incompatibility
      2. Associated with erythroblastosis fetalis—because of the disease or exchange transfusion
II. Infections (? mediated in part by intravascular coagulation)
   A. Bacterial
      1. Generalized sepsis
      2. Congenital syphilis

   B. Viral
      1. Cytomegalic inclusion disease
      2. Disseminated herpes simplex
      3. Rubella syndrome
   C. Protozoal—congenital toxoplasmosis
III. Drugs (administered to mother)—nonimmune mechanisms (e.g., tolbutamide)
IV. Congenital megakaryocytic hypoplasia
   A. Isolated—congenital hypoplastic thrombocytopenia
   B. Associated with absent radii, microcephaly, rubella syndrome, pancytopenia, and congenital anomalies (Fanconi's anemia)
   C. Associated with pancytopenia but no congenital anomalies
   D. Associated with trisomy syndromes—D_1 (13), E (18)
V. Bone marrow disease
   A. Congenital leukemia
VI. Disseminated intravascular coagulation (DIC)
   A. Sepsis
   B. Obstetric complications
      1. Abruptio placentae
      2. Eclampsia
      3. Amniotic fluid embolism
      4. Dead twin fetus
   C. Anoxia
   D. Stasis
      1. Giant hemangioma (including placental chorangioma)

*From Oski FA: Hematological problems. In Avery GB, editor: Neonatology: pathophysiology and management of the newborn, Philadelphia, 1975, JB Lippincott Co.

2. Renal vein thrombosis
3. Polycythemia
VII. Inherited (chronic) thrombocytopenia
   A. Sex-linked
      1. Pure
      2. Aldrich's syndrome
   B. Autosomal
      1. Pure—dominant or recessive
      2. May-Hegglin anomaly—dominant
VIII. Miscellaneous
   A. Thrombotic thrombocytopenic purpura
   B. Inherited metabolic disorders
      1. Glycinemia
      2. Methylmalonic acidemia
      3. Isovaleric acidemia
   C. Congenital thyrotoxicosis

IMMUNE-MEDIATED THROMBOCYTOPENIA. Idiopathic thrombocytopenic purpura in the mother, even with a normal maternal platelet count, may result in the passage of maternal IgG antiplatelet antibodies across the placenta, leading to destruction of the newborn's platelets and neonatal thrombocytopenia.

Occasionally, women with thrombocytopenia because of systemic lupus erythematosus may similarly pass antiplatelet antibodies to the fetus, resulting in neonatal thrombocytopenia. Thrombocytopenia in the newborn may last for several weeks, although serious bleeding manifestations, such as intracranial bleeding, usually do not occur after the first week of life. Only a transitory rise in platelet count occurs from platelet transfusions until the antibody has disappeared.

Infants affected with passively acquired immune idiopathic thrombocytopenic purpura appear healthy except for generalized petechiae and a platelet count that may be less than 10,000/mm³. If the infant shows increasing petechiae or other bleeding, treatment with high-dose IV immune gamma globulin (IVIGG) is recommended (0.4 g/kg/dose, repeated in 24 hours if necessary). Other treatment modalities have included prednisone (2 mg/kg/day in three to four divided doses), platelet transfusions (usually of only transient benefit), and ex- change transfusion to remove sensitized platelets followed by platelet transfusion.

Maternal antibody is usually cleared from the infant's circulation between 1 and 3 months of age so follow-up is necessary at least until that time.

ISOIMMUNE NEONATAL THROMBOCYTOPENIA. As with neonatal thrombocytopenia resulting from maternal idiopathic thrombocytopenic purpura or systemic lupus erythematosus, infants born with isoimmune thrombocytopenia clinically appear well except for bruising and petechiae. Mothers of these infants, unlike mothers of infants with idiopathic thrombocytopenic purpura and systemic lupus erythematosus, have no bleeding history and have a normal platelet count. The antibodies in the newborn responsible for the low platelet count are maternal IgG directed against specific antigens on the infant's platelets inherited from the father but absent from maternal platelets. Usually, the culprit is platelet-specific PLA_1 antigen, which is present on the baby's platelets, the father's platelets, and in 98% of the population. The mother lacks this antigen and therefore mounts an immune response that results in maternal IgG antibodies coating the newborn platelets and leading to their destruction.

Both first-born infants and subsequent newborns can be affected with isoimmune thrombocytopenia. The diagnosis can be made on clinical grounds; however, serologic tests for demonstrating anti-PLA_1 antibodies are available. The affected infant looks healthy except for petechiae, bruises, and an isolated thrombocytopenia. If the platelet count is below 30,000/mm³ or if signs of bleeding in addition to mild cutaneous hemorrhage are present, the baby should be treated with high-dose IVIGG. The risk of CNS bleeding may be as high as 10% to 15%, but usually this occurs only during the first week of life, even though the thrombocytopenia may last for 2 to 3 months.

Other treatment methods are controversial. Splenectomy is contraindicated, and giving random blood bank platelets is usually not

effective, but such transfusions should be given in an emergency situation. Steroids may not cause a rise in the platelet count but may be helpful when given to the mother before delivery.

THROMBOCYTOPENIA RESULTING FROM OTHER CAUSES OF INCREASED PLATELET DESTRUCTION. As discussed previously, DIC often results in decreased numbers of platelets and may sometimes be the most prominent coagulation abnormality. Occasionally, bacterial infection and intrauterine infection caused by rubella or cytomegalovirus may cause thrombocytopenia by decreasing platelet survival. Renal vein thrombosis and necrotizing enterocolitis may cause thrombocytopenia.

In thrombocytopenic newborns who obviously appear ill, sepsis must be ruled out as the underlying cause. Many intensive care nurseries currently obtain periodic platelet determinations in premature infants who appear ill to identify such serious processes as DIC, necrotizing enterocolitis, or renal vein thrombosis.

Hyperviscosity syndrome may cause thrombocytopenia.

Hemangiomas may cause increased destruction of platelets. Giant hemangiomas (Kasabach-Merritt syndrome) can trap and destroy many platelets. The platelet count from blood taken in the hemangioma will be higher than that of blood taken from other sites.

Abrupt swelling and tenseness of the hemangioma generally precede hemorrhage. Suggested treatments include steroids, radiation therapy, or both.

Other causes of thrombocytopenia in the newborn include (1) congenital leukemia; (2) bone marrow malignancy including neuroblastoma and Letterer-Siwe disease; (3) osteopetrosis; (4) selective aplasia of megakaryocytes, such as thrombocytopenia absent radii (TAR) syndrome, and amegakaryocytic thrombocytopenia; (5) inborn errors of metabolism, such as isovaleric acidemia, methylmalonic aciduria, and ketotic hyperglycemia; (6) tolbutamide; (7) massive splenomegaly

with hypersplenism; and (8) exchange transfusion of platelet-poor blood.

Prevention
HEMORRHAGIC DISEASE OF THE NEWBORN

Parenterally administering 0.5 to 1 mg of vitamin K_1 (phytonadione) to all newborns within 1 hour of birth prevents virtually all cases of hemorrhagic disease of the newborn (vitamin K deficiency). Administering vitamin K to the mother prenatally has no advantage over neonatal administration.

HEMOPHILIA A AND B

Hemophilia A and B are sex-linked recessive disorders occurring almost exclusively in males. Determining the sex of the fetus by amniocentesis rules out this disease if the fetus is a female, and a 50% probability of the disease will exist if the fetus is a male.

Fetal blood samples can be obtained in male fetuses at risk that allow diagnosing severe hemophilia A in utero at 20 weeks gestation by measuring factor VIII in fetal blood.

Most causes of neonatal thrombocytopenia are not preventable. However, awareness of a previously affected infant with immune thrombocytopenia allows for optimal preparation for delivery of a possibly affected infant. Other forms of thrombocytopenia and bleeding resulting from DIC are usually not preventable or predictable.

Data collection
HISTORY

If a newborn is bleeding, the following historical data are useful.

If hemorrhagic disease is suspected in the newborn, was vitamin K given to the infant in the delivery room or nursery? A history of other than a normal delivery situation (e.g., outside of hospital, cesarean section, or unexpected resuscitation) may contribute to the failure of vitamin K administration. In addition, prolonged antibiotic administration may contribute to vitamin K deficiency by eliminating the normal intestinal flora. Infants whose mothers are receiving anticonvulsant medication for epilepsy are especially prone to severe vitamin K deficiency.

If hemophilia is suspected, is there a family history of bleeding, especially into the joints in male relatives? A family history of bleeding in both males and females increases the possibility of von Willebrand's disease, which is autosomal dominant and therefore affects both sexes.

If DIC is suspected, were there any obstetric complications in the delivery? Was this a complicated delivery with possible asphyxia in the newborn? Was the mother ill during the last trimester of pregnancy, especially at the time of delivery?

If thrombocytopenia or platelet function disorder is suspected, is there a previous history of bleeding in the mother because of idiopathic thrombocytopenia or systemic lupus erythematosus? Was the mother taking medication during her pregnancy, such as tolbutamide, aspirin, or salicylate-containing over-the-counter preparations (e.g., Alka Seltzer)? (Prolonged bleeding resulting from platelet dysfunction may occur with aspirin, and aspirin can cross the placenta and similarly affect newborn platelets.) Was the mother ill during her pregnancy, especially during the first trimester (rubella, syphilis, toxoplasmosis, or cytomegalovirus)? What is the mother's platelet count? If normal, suspect isoimmune thrombocytopenia. Is there a family history of thrombocytopenia? If so, is it associated with any other disorders?

SIGNS AND SYMPTOMS OF BLEEDING

The health care provider must determine whether the bleeding is localized, such as with trauma because of a difficult delivery, or if the bleeding is generalized, which would suggest a bleeding diathesis.

Scattered "stress" petechiae on the head and shoulders of an otherwise normal infant are often seen in a traumatic or premature delivery and must be differentiated from the widespread, profuse, and often raised petechiae of an infant with thrombocytopenia. A platelet count is very helpful in these situations. Stress petechiae result from a temporary increase in superior vena caval pressure during vertex deliveries.[8] The obstetric team should establish whether the bleeding is confined primarily to the skin in the form of generalized petechiae and purpuric lesions (platelet defect) or if the bleeding is in the form of large bruises and other organ bleeding (coagulation factor depletion).

APPEARANCE. Does the infant appear well or ill? An infant who looks well suggests a platelet function defect, hemophilia or other hereditary factor deficiencies, and vitamin K deficiency as a cause of bleeding. An infant who appears ill suggests sepsis, congenital viral infection, acute infection (gram-negative bacteria), or DIC as a cause of bleeding.

Hepatomegaly with jaundice suggests sepsis, DIC, and possible neonatal leukemia as a cause of bleeding.

UNUSUAL PHYSICAL FINDINGS. Unusual physical findings associated with bleeding disorders are (1) absent radii in the TAR syndrome; (2) microcephaly, congenital heart disease, and chorioretinitis in congenital infection; and (3) giant hemangioma.

LABORATORY DATA

The PT, PTT, platelet count, and fibrinogen should be obtained in all infants suspected of a bleeding diathesis. Obtaining a bleeding time is useful if a platelet function defect is suspected. Specific factor assays or other tests such as fibrin-split products and fibrin monomer should be obtained if DIC is suspected but cannot be differentiated easily from liver disease.

The following abnormalities in screening

tests are most often found in bleeding new-borns:

- If the PT is normal, the PTT is abnormally prolonged, and the platelet count is normal, suspect hemophilia A or B or deficiency in factor XI.
- If the PT and PTT are prolonged and the platelet count is normal, suspect vitamin K deficiency as the most likely cause if the infant is well or liver disease if the infant is ill.
- If the PT and PTT are prolonged and the platelet count is low, suspect DIC.
- If the PT and PTT are normal and the platelet count is low, suspect immune thrombocytopenia if the infant appears well, and renal vein thrombosis, necrotizing enterocolitis, or DIC if the infant is ill.

Treatment
HEMORRHAGIC DISEASE OF THE NEWBORN

Treating a bleeding newborn with suspected vitamin K deficiency consists of IV administration of 1 mg of vitamin K_1 (phytonadione). If a vitamin K deficiency was the cause of the bleeding, bleeding will stop within several hours and the PT and PTT will be markedly improved but not fully corrected. An empiric trial of administering 1 mg of vitamin K should be considered in any newborn with unexplained bleeding, especially if the appropriate laboratory support is not available. If bleeding is severe or if the infant does not respond to vitamin K_1, administer 10 ml/kg of fresh frozen plasma IV.

HEREDITARY COAGULATION FACTOR DEFICIENCY

HEMOPHILIA A (FACTOR VIII DEFICIENCY). If the infant has hemophilia A, give factor VIII concentrate, preferably a monoclonal antibody–derived product (Hyland M, Monoclate) or a wet heat–treated product (Humate, Koate HS) to minimize the risk of non-A, non-B hepatitis, at 20 to 50 units/kg body weight IV in an emer-

gency or 1 pack of cryoprecipitate/3 kg body weight or fresh frozen plasma at 10 ml/kg body weight IV. One cryoprecipitate pack equals 100 units of factor VIII, and 1 ml of frozen plasma equals 1 unit of factor VIII.

VON WILLEBRAND'S DISEASE. In an infant with bleeding due to severe von Willebrand's disease, give 1 pack of cryoprecipitate/3 kg body weight or fresh frozen plasma at 10 ml/kg body weight IV.

HEMOPHILIA B (FACTOR IX DEFICIENCY). If a neonate has hemophilia B, give Profil IX (if available, to diminish the risk of non-A, non-B hepatitis) or factor IX concentrate (Konyne) at 30 to 90 units/kg body weight or fresh frozen plasma at 10 ml/kg body weight IV.

AFIBRINOGENEMIA. If the infant has afibrinogenemia, give 1 pack of cryoprecipitate/3 kg body weight or fresh frozen plasma at 10 ml/kg body weight IV.

OTHER OR UNKNOWN DEFICIENCIES. In the event that the infant has other or unknown deficiencies, give fresh frozen plasma at 10 ml/kg body weight IV.

DISSEMINATED INTRAVASCULAR COAGULOPATHY

Treatment for DIC requires correcting the underlying event or process that originally triggers the clotting cascade. Reversal of shock, hypoxia, acidosis, or sepsis may make further treatment unnecessary. The infant, and not the clotting abnormalities, must be treated.

If the triggering event is relieved and the baby has severe DIC, give platelet transfusions and fresh frozen plasma. The bleeding infant with DIC should receive platelet transfusions (1 unit/5 kg body weight) for the associated thrombocytopenia and clotting factor replacement (fresh frozen plasma at 10 ml/kg infant body weight) or cryoprecipitate, which contains large quantities of fibrinogen and factor VIII for clotting factor replacement. CAUTION: Prothrombin complex concentrates, such as Konyne and Proplex, which contain factors II, VII,

TRIGGER EVENTS

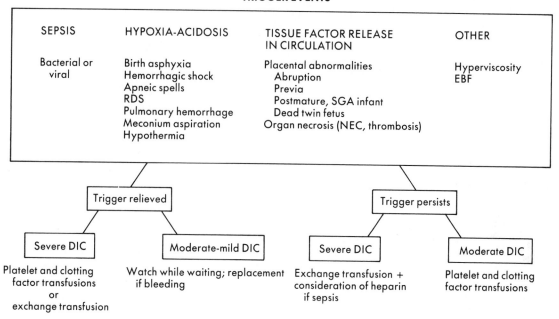

Figure 14-5. Schematic outline for management of infant with disseminated intravascular coagulopathy (DIC). Severe DIC—clinical bleeding, platelets less than 50,000, and fibrinogen less than 100 mg/dl. (From Hathaway WE and Bonnar J: Perinatal coagulation, New York, 1978, Grune & Stratton, Inc. By permission.)

IX, and X, should not be used because of their clot-promoting effect, which may result in serious thromboses. If the infant does not improve, consider exchange transfusion (double volume) using citrate phosphate dextrose whole blood.

Exchange transfusion with fresh whole blood is a reasonable method of attempting to manage DIC in neonates not responding to replacement of platelets, and clotting factors. A two-volume exchange with fresh blood drawn in heparin or citrate or packed red blood cells mixed with fresh frozen plasma and platelet concentrate removes circulating fibrin-split products and activated clotting factors, and

provides the normal number of platelets and labile clotting factors. Although this approach is promising, it must be critically evaluated in control trials before it can be fully recommended. Further guidelines for therapy of DIC are found in Figure 14-5.

If the infant has mild DIC, observe the patient closely and transfuse with fresh frozen plasma and platelets if bleeding occurs. If the triggering event persists and the baby has severe DIC, perform exchange transfusion (as described previously) and consider heparinization if the infant is septic. Administering heparin to infants with DIC, either before or following initial replacement with platelets and clotting factors, attempts to arrest further clotting and consumption. This approach has met with success in some centers.[4]

Heparinization is accomplished by giving the infant 100 units of heparin/kg loading dose IV followed by continuous infusion of heparin at 15 to 25 units/kg/hr. However, because of possible increased bleeding resulting from heparinization, many medical personnel have advised against the routine use of heparin in infants with DIC, except in those with purpura fulminans or with prominent thrombotic manifestations, or with severe hemorrhage uncontrolled by replacement of platelets and clotting factors or exchange transfusion.

If the triggering event persists and the infant has moderate DIC, give platelets and factor transfusions (as described previously).

If large-vessel thrombosis, gangrene, or purpura fulminans occurs, administer 100 units of heparin/kg loading dose IV followed by continuous heparin IV infusion at 15 to 25 units/kg/hr and monitor the effect on DIC by measuring fibrinogen levels and platelet counts.

Adequate heparinization for large-vessel thrombosis results in a prolonged PTT to twice that of normal adult controls. Since both heparin and DIC prolong the PT, PTT, and thrombin time, measuring the fibrinogen level and platelet count is useful. With continuing DIC, fibrinogen and platelets will remain low, whereas favorable response to heparin is heralded by an increased fibrinogen level and platelet count.

PLATELET ABNORMALITIES

Isoimmune thrombocytopenia has an 80% chance of recurrence in subsequent pregnancies. For this reason, some medical authorities recommend performing a cesarean section for all future deliveries. Alternatively, a sample of fetal blood for platelet count can be used to decide the need for a cesarean section; a count above 30,000/mm[3] may allow for a safe vaginal delivery. Once a thrombocytopenic baby is delivered, further management is guided by the severity of bleeding. Increasing petechiae, bruising, or other bleeding are an indicator for high-dose IVIGG. A time-tested alternative to IV gamma globulin is plateletpheresing the mother for 1 to 2 units of platelets just before delivery if an affected fetus is suspected and transfusing the infant soon after delivery if prominent bleeding manifestations appear. Transfusing the isoimmune, thrombocytopenic infant with 1 unit of washed maternal platelets usually elevates the platelet count to more than 100,000/mm[3]. The subsequent fall in platelet count is usually gradual over 7 days, in keeping with the reported normal platelet survival curve. Although the platelet count usually falls to pretransfusion levels, risk of serious bleeding after the first few days is small; babies may go home and be watched closely as outpatients.

If high-dose gamma globulin or maternal platelets are not available, blood bank platelets may be transfused at 10 ml/kg infant weight. Usually, however, such transfusions will not be helpful. Other medical personnel recommend a short course of steroids given to the mother before and during labor in the hope of decreasing the severity of the immunization of subsequent offspring.

In a bleeding newborn with thrombocytopenia caused by maternal idiopathic thrombocytopenic purpura or lupus erythematosus, treatment with high-dose IVIGG should be tried. If bleeding does not cease, perform an exchange transfusion on the baby in an attempt to remove antibodies, and transfuse with fresh platelets. Administer 2 mg/kg body weight/day of prednisone. A short course of steroids given to the mother before and during labor may decrease the severity of thrombocytopenia in the infant.

An infant with bleeding resulting from a platelet function defect should be given platelet transfusions at 10 ml/kg body weight.

Parent teaching

Bleeding problems in the newborn require meticulous counseling and explaining to parents about the disease process, their infant's progress, and the need for follow-up. Genetic counseling and amniocentesis for subsequent pregnancies when an inherited disease (such as hemophilia) is a possibility should be suggested to the parents. The possibility of immune thrombocytopenia recurring in subsequent infants should be explained to parents to aid their decisions about future childbearing.

POLYCYTHEMIA
Physiology

Polycythemia in the newborn is an increase above 65% in the venous hematocrit. This occurs in approximately 4% of the newborn population of Colorado.[13] Above a 65% hematocrit, blood flow becomes increasingly sluggish and hyperviscous, increasing exponentially with an increased rise in the hematocrit.

Although polycythemia is the principal cause of hyperviscosity in the newborn, decreased red blood cell deformability (common in the newborn and aggravated by acidosis and hypoxia), elevated plasma proteins, and hyperlipidemia may cause or contribute to hyperviscosity of newborn blood. Occasionally, infants with a venous hematocrit between 62% and 64% have hyperviscous blood. These factors account for the slightly higher incidence of hyperviscosity as opposed to the incidence of polycythemia in the newborn population.[13]

Etiology

Neonatal hyperviscosity may be a result of (1) polycythemia, the most important cause; (2) decreased red blood cell deformability; and (3) abnormalities in plasma proteins (Figure 14-6).

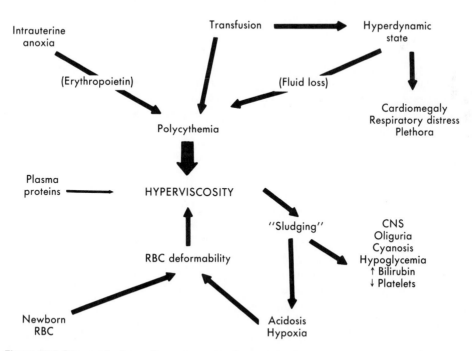

Figure 14-6. Proposed schema for cause and pathogenesis of symptomatic hyperviscosity states in neonate. (From Gross GP, Hathaway WE, and McGaughey HR: J Pediatr 82:1004, 1973.)

Polycythemia may be caused by intrauterine hypoxia and growth retardation that may increase erythropoietin production. The highest incidence of polycythemia is in term and postterm infants who are small-for-gestational-age (SGA). The second highest incidence of polycythemia is in postterm infants who are large-for-gestational-age (LGA), especially infants of diabetic mothers. The greatest number of infants with polycythemia, however, is term infants appropriate-for-gestational-age (AGA). Preterm infants of less than 34 weeks gestation are not affected. Infants with chromosomal abnormalities such as Down's syndrome have a high incidence of polycythemia.

Placental transfusions are an additional cause of polycythemia and occur as a result of (1) obstetric manipulations (i.e., cord clamping that is delayed more than 60 seconds after birth, "milking" or "stripping" the cord, or holding the baby below the level of the placenta); (2) transfusion from twin to twin (In monozygotic twins, a difference in hemoglobin greater than 4 g/dl suggests twin-to-twin transfusion.); or (3) maternal-fetal transfusion.

Decreased red blood cell deformability occurs because of (1) hypoxia, (2) acidosis, (3) hypothermia, (4) hypoglycemia, (5) primary red blood cell abnormalities (i.e., spherocytosis), or (6) low deformable newborn red blood cells, which contribute to hyperviscosity. Abnormalities in plasma proteins, elevated plasma proteins, and elevated fibrinogen levels also cause hyperviscosity.

Prevention

Since polycythemia and hyperviscosity occur with increased frequency in SGA infants, improved prenatal care to reduce the incidence of intrauterine growth retardation helps decrease the incidence of polycythemia. To prevent excessive placental transfusion of blood to the infant, obstetric manipulations that transfuse unknown quantities of blood should be avoided. Optimal management of high-risk deliveries in the delivery room and nursery to prevent hypoxia, hypothermia, acidosis, and hypoglycemia will decrease the impact of these abnormalities on red blood cell deformability and, consequently, hyperviscosity.

Data collection
HISTORY

In an infant with hyperviscosity because of polycythemia, conditions associated with an increased risk of placental insufficiency and chronic fetal hypoxia, resulting in SGA polycythemic infants, should be determined (i.e., a maternal history of preeclampsia, smoking, hypertension, or evidence of maternal-fetal bleeding). In the case of twins, twin-to-twin transfusion must be ruled out as a cause of polycythemia; hematocrit determinations should be obtained from both twins.

A history of obstetric manipulations at birth is often difficult to ascertain from the maternal and newborn delivery room records, yet a history of delayed cord clamping, "milking," or "stripping" helps. Review the records for evidence of stressful delivery, such as the Apgar scores (hypoxia and acidosis), temperature in the delivery room or on admittance to the nursery (hypothermia), and the blood glucose test value (hypoglycemia). In LGA babies evidence of maternal diabetes should be sought. Review the prenatal history for insulin-dependent or gestational diabetes, and review the family history for evidence of chromosomal abnormalities.

SIGNS AND SYMPTOMS

Polycythemia and hyperviscosity cause a variety of signs and symptoms involving the cardiac, respiratory, and neurologic systems.

Common clinical manifestations include[3]:
1. **Plethora with peripheral cyanosis or, occasionally, pallor**
2. **Respiratory distress (tachypnea, retractions, grunting, and flaring nares) that results from diminished pulmonary compliance as a result of an engorged vasculature stiffening the lungs**
3. **Cardiomegaly, congestive heart failure**

4. Neurologic symptoms (lethargy, jitteriness, focal and generalized seizures, abnormal electroencephalogram) that may result from suboptimal brain perfusion because of hyperviscosity
5. Metabolic derangements, such as hypoglycemia and hyperbilirubinemia
6. Thromboembolic conditions such as oliguria resulting from acute tubular necrosis, cerebral infarcts (with subsequent cerebral palsy), or symptoms of necrotizing enterocolitis

Although infants with polycythemia frequently have antecedent or associated abnormalities, such as being SGA or having a difficult delivery that may result in similar symptoms, most medical authorities agree that hyperviscosity may cause the previously mentioned derangements.

LABORATORY DATA

Measuring umbilical venous hematocrit is more reliable than measuring capillary hematocrit or even peripheral venous hematocrit from the antecubital fossa.[12] Some investigators have found that an umbilical vein hematocrit equal to or greater than 63% was frequently associated with hyperviscosity and correlated better with the presence of symptoms than did a peripheral venous hematocrit obtained from the antecubital veins or capillary heel stick hematocrit.[11]

Even though increased umbilical vein hematocrit may be the best indicator of polycythemia and hyperviscosity, most medical personnel recommend evaluating a newborn suspected of hyperviscosity in the following manner:

1. Obtain a capillary hematocrit when the infant is 4 to 6 hours of age. A warmed heel helps decrease falsely high values.
2. If the capillary hematocrit is equal to or greater than 70%, obtain a venous hematocrit (i.e., antecubital fossa). A capillary hematocrit equal to or greater than 70% is often associated with a venous hematocrit equal to or greater than 65%, a value above which hyperviscosity is most likely to exist.
3. If the venous hematocrit is equal to or greater than 65% to 70%, partial exchange transfusion should be considered.

Treatment

Although many centers recommend treating polycythemia (infants with a venous hematocrit equal to or greater than 65%) by partial exchange transfusion, it is controversial. Polycythemia and hyperviscosity may result in permanent neurological sequelae, and symptomatic infants with polycythemia have shown quick and dramatic improvement following partial exchange. However, many infants with venous hematocrits equal to or greater than 65% are completely asymptomatic and show no neurologic abnormalities on follow-up examinations. Furthermore, a peripheral venous hematocrit equal to or greater than 65% is not necessarily predictive of a more central hematocrit equal to or greater than 65%, such as will be obtained by sampling umbilical venous blood. This is especially true if the peripheral venous hematocrit was obtained from antecubital veins that are small or if the blood was obtained with much difficulty and delay. Until more recent data become available, it is probably best to determine both the umbilical venous hematocrit and viscosity before deciding whether to perform a partial exchange transfusion in an asymptomatic infant. In a symptomatic infant, most medical authorities recommend partial exchange transfusion when a venous hematocrit is equal to or greater than 65%.

Once it has been decided to perform a partial exchange transfusion, blood should be removed in 5 to 10 ml increments from the umbilical vein and an equal amount of Plasmanate should be reinfused. Five percent albumin can also be used for replacement.

Treatment with partial exchange transfusion

should be calculated to reduce the central hematocrit to between 50% and 55%[3]:

Volume of exchange (ml) =

$$\text{Weight} \times (80 \text{ ml/kg}) \times \frac{\text{Observed Hct} - \text{Desired Hct}}{\text{Observed Hct}}$$

Complications

Complications of polycythemia and hyperviscosity include respiratory distress, congestive heart failure, hypoglycemia, hyperbilirubinemia, neurologic signs, and sequelae such as significant motor and mental retardation, as well as cerebral infarcts and cerebral palsy at an older age.[1,3] Thromboembolic conditions, cerebral artery thrombosis, necrotizing enterocolitis, and acute tubular necrosis are also complications of polycythemia and hyperviscosity. Other complications of treatment are the same as the risks of umbilical venous catheterization: (1) portal vein thrombosis, (2) phlebitis of the portal vein, and (3) decreased plasma volume if phlebotomy is used alone.

Infants that do not receive an exchange transfusion may show increased irritability; tremulousness; and decreased spontaneous movement, alert state, and orientation to sound and light in the first 2 weeks of life.

The prognosis for infants with polycythemia even after treatment is guarded, with motor and/or mental retardation possible. Long-term benefits of polycythemia treatment have not been documented.

Parent teaching

Prospective parents should be advised to seek prenatal care and avoid smoking and other risk factors associated with placental insufficiency resulting in SGA infants.

Since parents are participating more in the conduct of normal labor, it is important to teach them about the risks to the neonate of placental transfusion from obstetric manipulations such as delayed cord clamping, "milking" the cord,

and holding the baby below the placenta. The principle of "a little is good, so more is better" has no place in the hemodynamics of the neonate.

• • •

Polycythemia of the newborn is always associated with hyperviscosity and is the principal cause of hyperviscosity syndrome in the newborn period. Treatment of this disorder may include partial exchange transfusion with 5% albumin or Plasmanate. Currently, it is not clear whether all babies with polycythemia and hyperviscosity should receive exchange transfusion or only those who are symptomatic.

ACKNOWLEDGMENT

We would like to thank William E. Hathaway for his review and comments.

REFERENCES

1. Amit M and Camfield PR: Neonatal polycythemia causing multiple cerebral infarcts, Arch Neurol 37: 109, 1980.
2. Bowman JM and Pollock JM: Amniotic fluid spectrophotometry and early delivery in the management of erythroblastosis fetalis, Pediatrics 35:815, 1965.
3. Gross GP, Hathaway WE, and McGaughey HR: Hyperviscosity in the neonate, J Pediatr 82:1004, 1973.
4. Hathaway WE, and Bonnar J: Perinatal coagulation, New York, 1978, Grune & Stratton, Inc.
5. Klaus MH and Fanaroff AA: Care of the high-risk neonate, ed 3, Philadelphia, 1986, WB Saunders Co.
6. Nathan DG and Oski FA: Hematology of infancy and childhood, vol 1, ed 2, Philadelphia, 1981, WB Saunders Co.
7. Oski FA: Hematological problems. In Avery GB, editor: Neonatology: pathophysiology and management of the newborn, Philadelphia, 1975, JB Lippincott Co.
8. Paxson CL: Van-Leewen's newborn medicine, Chicago, 1979, Year Book Medical Publishers, Inc.
9. Pearson HA: Sickle cell syndromes and other hemoglobinopathies. In Miller DR, Baehner RL, and McMillan, CW, editors: Blood diseases of infancy and childhood, ed 5, St Louis, 1984, The CV Mosby Co.
10. Pearson HA and Benz EI: Thalassemia syndromes. In Miller DR, Baehner RL, and McMillan CW, editors: Blood diseases of infancy and childhood, ed 5, St Louis, 1984, The CV Mosby Co.
11. Ramamurthy RS and Brans YW: Neonatal polycythemia: criteria for diagnosis and treatment, Pediatrics 68:168, 1981.

12. Strauss HS: Diagnosis and treatment of inherited bleeding disorders, Pediatr Clin North Am 19:1011, 1972.

13. Wirth FH, Goldberg KE, and Lubchenco, LO: Neonatal hyperviscosity: incidence, Pediatrics 63:833, 1979.

SELECTED READINGS

Alter BP et al: Prenatal diagnosis of hemoglobinopathies, N Engl J Med 295:1437, 1976.

Davies SV et al: Transplacental effect of high dose immunoglobin in idiopathic thrombocytopenia (ITP), Lancet I:1098, 1986.

Firshein SI et al: Prenatal diagnosis of classic hemophilia, N Engl J Med 300:937, 1979.

Sidiropoulos D and Straume B: The treatment of neonatal isoimmune thrombocytopenia with intravenous immunoglobulin (IVIGG), Blut 48:383, 1984.

Stockman JA, Garcia JF, and Oski FA: The anemia of prematurity, N Engl J Med 296:647, 1977.

CHAPTER 15

Jaundice

C. GILBERT FRANK · BARBARA S. TURNER · GERALD B. MERENSTEIN

Jaundice or hyperbilirubinemia is an almost universal occurrence in the neonate although not always of clinical significance. Past experiences have suggested the dangers of excessive levels of unconjugated bilirubin, but precise identification of what constitutes a "safe" level for the individual newborn continues to elude detection and is the subject of much ongoing clinical and laboratory investigation. This chapter will provide the reader with a basic understanding of the multiple causes and contributing factors in the development of hyperbilirubinemia; the diagnosis, clinical significance, and complications of hyperbilirubinemia; and current treatment modalities and their complications.

PHYSIOLOGY

To understand the pathophysiology and clinical significance of hyperbilirubinemia, normal bilirubin metabolism in the newborn must be reviewed (Figure 15-1). Most of the bilirubin (75% to 85%) produced by a newborn infant comes from the breakdown of the heme portion of erythrocyte hemoglobin. The remaining 15% to 25% of bilirubin is derived from nonerythroid heme proteins found principally in the liver and heme precursors in the marrow and extramedullary hemopoietic areas that do not go on to form red blood cells. These other sources of bilirubin are sometimes referred to as "early peak" or "shunt" bilirubin.

Bilirubin metabolism is initiated in the re-

☐ The opinions and assertions in this chapter are those of the authors and do not necessarily represent those of the Department of the Army or the Department of Defense.

ticuloendothelial system in principally the liver and spleen as old or abnormal red blood cells are removed from the circulation. The enzymes, microsomal heme oxygenase and biliverdin reductase, are responsible for the production of bilirubin and carbon monoxide. This bilirubin in its unconjugated or indirect-reacting form is released into the plasma.

At a normal plasma pH, bilirubin is very poorly soluble and binds tightly to circulating albumin that serves as a carrier protein. Albumin contains one high-affinity site for bilirubin and one or more sites of lower affinity. Bilirubin binds to albumin in a molar ratio of between 0.5 and 1 mole of bilirubin per mole of albumin. This ratio may be somewhat lower in the sick, very low birth weight (VLBW) infant. The ability of albumin to bind bilirubin is affected by a number of different factors including plasma pH, free fatty acid levels, and certain drugs.

Bilirubin bound to albumin is transported to the liver. Probably via a plasma membrane carrier mechanism with a greater affinity for bilirubin, it is then transported into the hepatocyte. Once inside the cell, bilirubin again becomes protein bound, but this time it is bound to the Y protein (ligandin) and to a lesser extent to the Z protein. Conjugation occurs within the smooth endoplasmic reticulum of the cell. This reaction catalyzed by the enzyme glucuronyl transferase leads to the formation of bilirubin glucuronides that are water-soluble compounds. In addition to this enzyme, conjugation requires glucuronic acid. Conjugated bilirubin is then actively secreted into bile and passes into the small intestine.

Conjugated bilirubin is not reabsorbed from the intestine, but the bowel lumen of the newborn contains the enzyme beta-glucuronidase, which can convert conjugated bilirubin back into glucuronic acid and unconjugated bilirubin, which may be absorbed. This pathway constitutes the enterohepatic circulation of bilirubin and contributes significantly to the infant's bilirubin load.

The catabolism of 1 g of hemoglobin yields 35 mg of bilirubin. Since the red blood cell of the newborn has a shortened life span of 70 to 90 days (adult: 120 days), a significant bilirubin

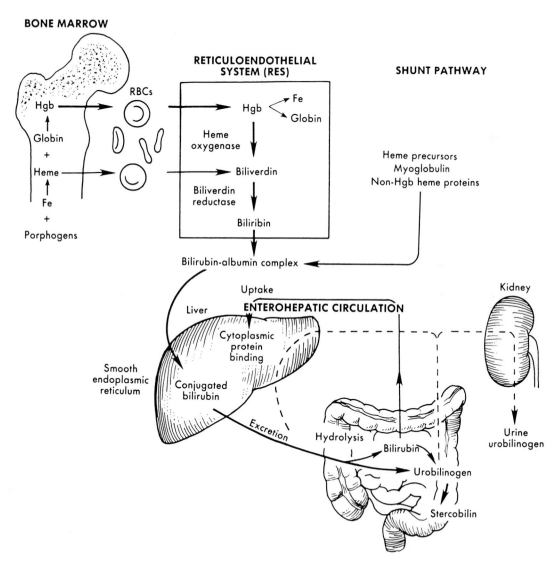

Figure 15-1. Pathways of bilirubin synthesis, transport, and metabolism. (From Gartner LM and Hollander M: Disorders of bilirubin metabolism. In Assali NS, editor: Pathophysiology of gestation, vol 3, Fetal and neonatal disorders, New York, 1972, Academic Press, Inc.)

TABLE 15-1 _____

Factors Affecting Bilirubin-Albumin Binding

FACTOR	MECHANISM
pH (acidosis)	Decreases binding by decreasing affinity at the binding site and increasing tissue affinity
Hematin	Competitively inhibits binding at primary site
Free fatty acids (Intralipid)	Competitively inhibits binding at primary site
Infection	Mechanism not established
Drugs such as sulfa compounds, sodium salicylate, and phenylbutazone	Primarily competitive binding; principally at secondary site; best established for sulfisoxazole
Stabilizers for albumin preparations	Competitively inhibits binding at primary site
X-ray contrast media for cholangiography	Competitively inhibits binding at primary site

load is produced. The breakdown of bilirubin is the only chemical reaction in the body that results in formation of carbon monoxide, a marker sometimes used in studying bilirubin production.

Albumin binding of unconjugated bilirubin may be important in the prevention of toxicity (kernicterus). Once the high-affinity site is saturated, there is a rapid increase in potentially toxic, free (nonbound), unconjugated bilirubin. A bilirubin/albumin molar ratio of 1 corresponds to approximately 8.5 mg bilirubin/g albumin. Although others have been suggested, the only drug demonstrated to carry an increased risk for kernicterus in the human is sulfisoxazole (Table 15-1).

In the hypoglycemic infant glucuronide production may be limited, and thus conjugation is impaired. The presence of beta-glucuronidase in the bowel lumen during fetal life enables

bilirubin to be reabsorbed and transported across the placenta for excretion by the maternal liver.

ETIOLOGY

Chemical hyperbilirubinemia occurs in virtually all newborns. The National Collaborative Perinatal Project[6] found that only about 6% of newborns weighing greater than 2500 g at birth would have serum bilirubin levels greater than 12.9 mg/dl. Pathologic (non-"physiologic") hyperbilirubinemia can be the result of increased production or decreased excretion of bilirubin or occasionally a combination of these two processes (see outline below).

Causes of hyperbilirubinemia

I. Overproduction of bilirubin
   A. Hemolytic disease of the newborn
   B. Hereditary hemolytic anemias
      1. Membrane defects
      2. Hemoglobinopathies
      3. Enzyme defects
   C. Polycythemia
   D. Extravascular blood
      1. Swallowed
      2. Bruising or enclosed hemorrhage (e.g., cephalhematoma)
   E. Increased enterohepatic circulation
   F. Oxytocin-induced labor
II. Undersecretion of bilirubin
   A. Decreased hepatic uptake
      1. Inadequate perfusion of hepatic sinusoids
      2. ? deficiency Y and Z protein
   B. Decreased bilirubin conjugation
      1. Enzyme deficiency
      2. Enzyme inhibition and the Lucey-Driscoll syndrome[8]
   C. Inadequate transport out of hepatocyte
   D. Biliary obstruction
III. Combined overproduction and undersecretion
   A. Bacterial infection
   B. Congenital intrauterine infection
IV. Associated with breastfeeding
   A. Breastfeeding jaundice
   B. Breast milk jaundice
V. Physiologic or developmental jaundice

VI. Miscellaneous
   A. Hypothyroidism
   B. Galactosemia
   C. Infant of diabetic mother

Overproduction of bilirubin
HEMOLYTIC DISEASE OF THE NEWBORN

Hemolytic disease of the newborn may occur when blood group incompatibilities such as Rh, ABO, or in rare instances minor blood groups exist between a mother and her fetus. An Rh-negative mother can become sensitized to the Rh antigen in many ways. For example, sensitization can be caused by an improperly matched blood transfusion or the occurrence of fetal-maternal blood transfusion during pregnancy, delivery, or abortion. Recent data also suggest that sensitization might occur at the time of amniocentesis. The presence of the Rh antigen induces maternal antibody productions, and IgG crosses the placenta into the fetal circulation. There it reacts with the Rh antigen on fetal erythrocytes. These antibody-coated cells are recognized as abnormal and are destroyed by the spleen. This results in increased amounts of hemoglobin requiring metabolic degradation as discussed previously. As the destruction of erythrocytes and production of bilirubin progress, the ability of the fetus to compensate may be surpassed. The wide range of clinical features are discussed elsewhere.

With the widespread use of RhoGAM, the most frequent cause of hemolytic disease of the newborn is ABO blood group incompatibility.

The classic example of hemolytic disease of the newborn has been erythroblastosis fetalis as a result of Rh incompatibility. Of the white population 15% is Rh negative. Fortunately the use of anti-D gamma globulin (RhoGAM), including antenatal administration at 26 to 28 weeks gestation, has markedly decreased the incidence of this serious disease.

The IgG on the surface of the infant's red blood cells is the basis of the positive Coombs' test. Since prior sensitization with the Rh antigen is required for antibody production, the first Rh-positive infant is usually not affected.

ABO incompatibility is limited to mothers of blood group O and affects infants of blood group A or B. All group O individuals have naturally occurring anti-A and anti-B (IgG) antibodies, so previous sensitization is not necessary. Clinical disease is generally milder than that seen with Rh incompatibility.

HEREDITARY HEMOLYTIC ANEMIAS

Erythrocytes with abnormal membranes have abnormal osmotic fragility (generally increased) and an increased rate of splenic destruction. Hemoglobinopathies can be diagnosed by hemoglobin electrophoresis. Individuals with enzyme defects are unable to maintain the integrity of the red blood cells. A precipitating factor for the hemolysis is often not found in infants.

Examples of hemolytic anemias include hereditary spherocytosis and elliptocytosis. The family history may be positive in as many as 80% of cases.

Glucose-6-phosphate dehydrogenase deficiency is the most common enzyme defect. It is more common in certain ethnic groups, including Chinese, Greeks, and blacks. Deficiency of pyruvate kinase may also occur.

POLYCYTHEMIA

Polycythemia (central venous hematocrit >65) is the condition in which an increased red blood cell mass, along with the shortened life span of these cells found in all newborns, results in an increased bilirubin load.

Polycythemia may be idiopathic or may occur as a result of a maternal-fetal transfusion, twin-to-twin transfusion, or delayed clamping of the umbilical cord at the time of delivery.

EXTRAVASCULAR BLOOD

Red blood cells trapped in the enclosed hemorrhages are broken down as resolution occurs.

Clinically, enclosed hemorrhage includes cephalhematoma, subgaleal hemorrhage, cerebral hemorrhage, intraabdominal bleeding, or any occult bleeding. Extensive bruising is associated with higher bilirubin loads as healing occurs. Swallowed maternal blood is another source of increased bilirubin load. Supernatant fluid of stool or gastric juices can be tested by the Apt test. Fetal hemoglobin will resist denaturation by alkali.

INCREASED ENTEROHEPATIC CIRCULATION

The lumen of the newborn's bowel contains the enzyme beta-glucuronidase, which can convert conjugated bilirubin back into its unconjugated form and glucuronic acid.

Meconium contains a substantial amount of bilirubin. It is estimated that there is about 1 mg bilirubin/g meconium, or a total load of 100 to 200 mg. Any delay in the passage of meconium, such as can occur with Hirschsprung's disease (aganglionosis), intestinal atresia, intestinal stenosis (including pyloric), or the meconium plug and meconium ileus syndromes, will increase the bilirubin load that must be metabolized. Pathologic jaundice from these causes is rarely evident in the first 24 to 48 hours of life.

OXYTOCIN-INDUCED LABOR

Cumulative data from multiple studies suggest that the induction of labor with oxytocin results in an increased incidence of hyperbilirubinemia and mean serum bilirubin levels. The mechanism remains unknown but is believed to be increased hemolysis. Observed differences are small, and changes in obstetric practices do not appear to be indicated.

Undersecretion of bilirubin

Infants with normal bilirubin production rates may be unable to remove this load for a variety of possible reasons.

DECREASED HEPATIC UPTAKE OF BILIRUBIN

Diminished hepatic uptake of bilirubin may be a result of inadequate perfusion of hepatic sinusoids or deficient carrier proteins (Y and Z). Certain drugs and compounds such as steroid hormones, free fatty acids, and chloramphenicol may competitively bind to these proteins, creating a functional deficiency.

Inadequate perfusion of hepatic sinusoids occurs when there is a shunt through a persistent ductus venosus or extrahepatic portal vein thrombosis, or an occurrence of hyperviscosity and hypovolemia. This may occur in infants with severe congestive heart failure.

Although Y and Z protein are decreased in other primates, no actual deficiency has yet been demonstrated in the human newborn.

DECREASED BILIRUBIN CONJUGATION

Decreased bilirubin conjugation may be a result of glucuronyl transferase deficiency, as in Crigler-Najjar syndromes I and II or Gilbert's syndrome. It may also be a result of enzyme inhibition, the Lucey-Driscoll syndrome.[8] The serums of some women and their infants contain an increased amount of an as yet unidentified factor that inhibits hepatic conjugation.

Crigler-Najjar syndrome exists in two forms with either complete or partial absence of enzymatic activity. Type I or complete absence is an autosomal recessive disorder. Type II or partial enzyme deficiency is inherited as an autosomal dominant disorder and responds to enzyme induction with phenobarbital. Gilbert's syndrome is another autosomal dominant disorder with partial enzyme activity affecting individuals out of the newborn period with mild bilirubin elevation.

Infants with Lucey-Driscoll syndrome may require exchange transfusion. Dubin-Johnson and Rotor's syndromes are genetically inherited conditions (autosomal recessive and dominant, respectively) in which individuals are able to conjugate bilirubin normally but are unable to excrete it, resulting in direct hyperbilirubinemia.

INADEQUATE TRANSPORT OUT OF THE HEPATOCYTE

Dubin-Johnson and Rotor's syndromes and generalized hepatocellular damage require specialized evaluation, including liver biopsy.

BILIARY OBSTRUCTION

Biliary obstruction often is seen as a diagnostic dilemma between generalized hepatocellular damage and mechanical obstruction.

A variety of disorders can cause cellular damage, including infections such as hepatitis and metabolic disorders such as galactosemia. In a neonatal intensive care unit the most common cause of cellular damage is the use of intravenous alimentation. The mechanism is not well established, but the damage takes at least 2 weeks to develop and is especially prominent in VLBW infants. Biliary atresia or, much less frequently, a choledochal cyst can cause mechanical obstruction to bile flow, resulting in a direct-reacting hyperbilirubinemia.

Combined overproduction and undersecretion

Bacterial infections (sepsis neonatorum) or the occurrence of intrauterine viral infections can result in increased bilirubin production and decreased hepatic clearance. Infants with necrotizing enterocolitis caused by a toxin-producing organism such as certain *Escherichia coli* may develop this form of hepatocellular damage.

Intrauterine infections, including congenital syphilis, toxoplasmosis, rubella, infection caused by cytomegalovirus, herpes simplex, coxsackie B virus, and hepatitis virus, cause clinical jaundice. Infants with these infections will often have additional clinical stigmata of their infection.

Jaundice associated with breastfeeding
BREASTFEEDING JAUNDICE

In general, breastfed infants tend to have slightly higher bilirubin levels than bottle-fed infants, especially on the fifth day of life. It has been postulated that this early jaundice is related to decreased caloric and fluid intake from colostrum[2] and increased enterohepatic circulation due to low stool output and breast milk beta-glucuronidase,[5] although data supporting this are sparse in the literature. In some studies there has been no relationship between the degree of hyperbilirubinemia and the amount of weight lost by the infant.[3]

BREAST MILK JAUNDICE

A small percentage of breastfed infants become jaundiced because of an inhibitor or inhibitory substances found in their mother's breast milk. Initially the inhibitory substance was considered a result of a progestational steroid, 3-alpha-20-beta pregnanediol,[4] but it has not been isolated consistently. Current theory points toward abnormally large amounts of unsaturated fatty acids inhibiting conjugation through an ill-defined mechanism, possibly because of unusually high lipoprotein lipase activity.[1,7,11]

Despite lack of supporting data that breastfed infants are underfed, it is common practice in some institutions to supplement with glucose water or electrolyte solutions after nursing. This does not appear to be necessary and may detract from the mother's establishing successful breastfeeding.

Clinically, infants with breast milk jaundice have an unconjugated hyperbilirubinemia (greater than 12 mg/dl) that becomes exaggerated and persistent by about the fifth day of life. Levels may persist for 4 to 14 days, followed by very gradual declines. Interruption of breastfeeding for 24 to 48 hours results in a prompt fall in bilirubin levels, and resumption of nursing is not accompanied by "rebound" hyperbilirubinemia. This clinical pattern established

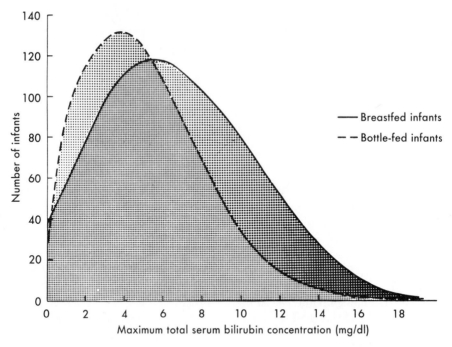

Figure 15-2. Distribution of maximum serum bilirubin concentration in white infants weighing more than 2500 g. Curves were computer generated using exponential I knot spline regression. (From Maisells MJ and Gifford K: Pediatrics 78:837, 1986. Reproduced by permission of Pediatrics.)

the diagnosis of breast milk jaundice. It is essentially a diagnosis of exclusion. There have been no documented cases of kernicterus as a result of breast milk jaundice; but as serum levels in the 15 to 18 mg/dl range are approached, breastfeeding should be interrupted for 48 hours. It is important to support the mother during this period so as not to foster feelings of guilt or inadequacy (Figure 15-2).

Physiologic or developmental jaundice

Physiologic or developmental jaundice is a diagnosis of exclusion. The newborn has a rate of bilirubin production of 8 to 10 mg/kg/24 hours, which is two to two and a half times the production rate in adults. Perfusion of the hepatic sinusoids may be somewhat compromised by incomplete closure of the ductus venous or the presence of extramedullary hemopoietic tissue in the liver. Newborn monkeys have been shown to be deficient in the Y and Z proteins for the first few days of life, and this may also occur in the human newborn. Enterohepatic circulation contributes significantly to the bilirubin load.

The hormonal (estrogen) environment of the infant may inhibit liver function and bilirubin secretion. While a level of 12.9 may define "pathologic" jaundice in the bottlefed infant, levels of up to 14.5 may be physiologic in the breastfed infant.

Physiologic jaundice is partially attributable to a relative deficiency of the enzyme glucuronyl transferase. Enzyme activity increases rapidly after birth independent of the infant's gestational age. A major factor in physiologic

---

CRITERIA THAT RULE OUT THE DIAGNOSIS OF PHYSIOLOGIC JAUNDICE*

1. Clinical jaundice in the first 24 hours of life
2. Total serum bilirubin concentrations increasing by more than 5 mg/dl (85 μmol/L/day)
3. Total serum bilirubin concentration exceeding 12.9 mg/dl (221 μmol/L) in a full-term infant or 15 mg/dl (257 μmol/L) in a premature infant
4. Direct serum bilirubin concentration exceeding 1.5 to 2 mg/dl (26 to 34 μmol/L)
5. Clinical jaundice persisting for more than 1 week in a full-term infant or 2 weeks in a premature infant

From Maisels MJ: Neonatal jaundice. In Avery GB, editor: Neonatology: pathophysiology and management of the newborn, ed 2, Philadelphia, 1981, JB Lippincott Co.
*The absence of these criteria does not imply that the jaundice is physiologic. In the presence of any of these criteria, the jaundice must be investigated further.

---

jaundice remains the increased rate of bilirubin production (see boxed material above).

Miscellaneous
HYPOTHYROIDISM

The mechanism of hyperbilirubinemia in hypothyroidism is not well understood, but in some animal studies thyroxine was needed for the hepatic clearance of bilirubin.

GALACTOSEMIA

The mechanism in galactosemia appears related to a lack of substrate for glucuronidation and the accumulation of abnormal metabolic by-products that are hepatotoxic.

Hypothyroid infants have unconjugated hyperbilirubinemia that may be prolonged. They may fail to show any other signs or symptoms of hypothyroidism until later in their course. Therefore many states now routinely screen for hypothyroidism, galactosemia, and phenylketonuria.

Galactosemia is an autosomal recessive disorder characterized by increased jaundice in infants fed breast milk or lactose-containing formulas. The presence of nonglucose-reducing substances in the urine suggests galactosemia.

INFANT OF A DIABETIC MOTHER

Hyperbilirubinemia in the infant of a diabetic mother is probably related to decreased substrate for glucuronidation. Many of these infants are also delivered slightly prematurely.

PREVENTION

Anti-D gamma globulin (RhoGAM—Ortho Diagnostics) antibody provides passive protection, allowing destruction of the fetal red blood cells and preventing maternal production of anti-Rh antibodies that might affect subsequent Rh-positive pregnancies.

Widespread use of RhoGAM has proved effective in preventing the sensitization of Rh-negative mothers following delivery or abortion of Rh-positive infants. Failures may occur if the amount of RhoGAM administered is insufficient compared with the load of fetal red blood cells received or if a significant fetal-maternal hemorrhage occurred before term. There has been some suggestion that RhoGAM be administered to Rh-negative women undergoing amniocentesis.

Early feeding

The physiologic mechanism is not entirely known but may be caused by a decrease in the enterohepatic circulation.

When compared with infants not fed during the first 24 to 48 hours of life, infants fed earlier have lower peak bilirubin levels.

Phenobarbital

Phenobarbital acts as an inducer of microsomal enzymes, increasing the conjugation of bilirubin.

It also has a direct effect to stimulate bile secretion in infants with nonobstructive cholestasis. Phenobarbital also increases the concentration of ligandin. When used in conjunction with phototherapy, it does not increase the rate of decline.

Phenobarbital is effective when given to the mother before delivery. In infants with significant hemolytic disease of the newborn, it appears to slow the rate of rise of bilirubin and decrease the incidence of exchange transfusion. It is also indicated in infants with Crigler-Najjar syndrome type II. Its use is not indicated on a routine prophylactic basis, since such use would overtreat many infants, and other effects may be detrimental.

DATA COLLECTION

The history, physical examination, and laboratory data play an important role in the evaluation of the jaundiced newborn (see outline on p. 327).

History

The evaluation of the jaundiced infant begins with a good familial, perinatal, and neonatal history. The family history should include the occurrence of disorders associated with jaundice in other family members, especially siblings. The perinatal and obstetric history may provide clues or enable the clinician to anticipate possible hyperbilirubinemia. The infant's course since birth may be important.

Signs and symptoms and clinical approach

A wide spectrum of signs and symptoms may occur in the jaundiced infant, often depending on the causes of the jaundice. In the absence of hemolysis, an infant may be asymptomatic with dermal icterus as the only clinical sign. The infant with hemolytic disease of the newborn may show signs of jaundice and pallor in association with severe anemia and hydrops fetalis or may appear entirely normal at birth. Hepatosplenomegaly resulting from congestion and extramedullary he-

mopoiesis may be present. Infants affected by hemolytic disease of the newborn also have pancreatic islet cell hyperplasia and are at increased risk for hypoglycemia. Along with or in the absence of jaundice, pallor, and hepatosplenomegaly, careful physical examination may reveal the presence of a cephalhematoma or other enclosed hemorrhage. The occurrence of petechiae or purpura raises the possibility of intrauterine infection or sepsis. Congenital anomalies should be noted.

Laboratory data

Knowledge of the mother's and infant's blood types and Rh will establish the potential for hemolytic disease. Coombs' test on cord blood is positive in ABO disease. Later testing of the infant's blood in an ABO incompatibility may show it to be Coombs' negative. A decreasing hematocrit and elevated reticulocyte count suggest a hemolytic process, so the clinician should perform a careful examination of the infant's peripheral blood smear. Signs of the hemolysis may be present, including increased numbers of nucleated red blood cells, the presence of fragmented cells, poikilocytosis, and anisocytosis. Microspherocytosis is characteristic of ABO incompatibility and may at times be confused with hereditary spherocytosis. A knowledge of blood types and clinical course will help in differentiating these two. An abnormal white blood cell count or differential, or thrombocytopenia may suggest infection. In addition to jaundice and anemia in the first few days of life, infants with a hemolytic disease are at risk for development of a "late" anemia following discharge from the nursery. Fractionated (total/direct) bilirubin levels and serial levels help establish causes and enable the clinician to follow the rate of bilirubin rise. Protein and albumin determinations allow a gross assessment of adequacy of bilirubin binding. A great deal of clinical and laboratory research has been performed to determine the degree of and sites available for bilirubin-albumin binding. This information may someday enable the clinician to assess the risk for kernicterus and perform an exchange transfusion at the appropriate time, but these determinations are not presently recommended or available for routine use.

Evaluation of unconjugated hyperbilirubinemia in the neonate

  I. History
     A. Family
     B. Perinatal and obstetric
     C. Neonatal
 II. Physical examination
     A. Pallor
     B. Hepatosplenomegaly
     C. Enclosed hemorrhage
     D. Petechiae
     E. Congenital anomalies
III. Laboratory data
     A. All jaundiced infants
        1. Maternal and infant blood type
        2. Coombs' test on cord blood
        3. Total/direct bilirubin (serial measurements)
        4. Complete blood count, including hematocrit, reticulocyte and platelet counts, white blood cell differential, and peripheral smear for red blood cell morphology
        5. Protein, total and/or albumin
        6. Urinalysis, test for reducing substances
        7. Screen for hypothyroidism
     B. Selected cases
        1. Sepsis evaluation
        2. IgM and STORCH titers
        3. Urine cytology for cytomegalovirus
        4. Viral cultures
     C. New techniques
        1. Transcutaneous bilirubinometry
        2. Bilirubin-binding tests

In addition to inherited forms of hyperbilirubinemia, infants of certain ethnic groups, including Chinese, Japanese, Korean, and American Indian, have significantly elevated bilirubin levels.

Items of interest include possible infection during the pregnancy or the use of oxytocin induction for delivery. Also of concern is the occurrence of an asphyxial episode during labor or delivery. Premature infants have higher mean bilirubin levels and a slightly later peak. A history of asphyxia and medication should be obtained. Also of interest is the infant's feeding and stool patterns. The time of onset or detection of jaundice may be important. Jaundice in the first 24 hours of life must always be considered abnormal.

Jaundice in the newborn can usually be detected clinically at a level of 6 to 7 mg/dl. Visible icterus appears first on the head and face and progresses in a cephalocaudal manner. The extremities are the last skin surface to be affected.

Immediate exchange transfusion with O Rh-negative red blood cells may be necessary in Rh incompatibility with a severely affected infant. Hydrops fetalis is rare in hemolytic disease as a result of ABO incompatibility.

There is an increased incidence of jaundice in trisomic syndromes. Jaundice and umbilical hernia are associated with congenital hypothyroidism.

Minimal laboratory evaluation of the jaundiced newborn should include the mother's and infant's blood types, Rh status, and Coombs' test on cord blood. A complete blood count to include reticulocyte and platelet counts, white blood cell count and differential, peripheral smear for red blood cell morphology, and hematocrit should be performed. Infants suspected of bacterial sepsis should receive antibiotic treatment and a complete sepsis evaluation including cultures of blood, urine, and cerebrospinal fluid. Total and direct bilirubin and total protein must be measured. Albumin levels may be determined or estimated from the total protein level (albumin $\cong$ 5/8 total protein). Urinalysis including evaluation for reducing substances may be helpful. Infants suspected of congenital infection should have additional tests including IgM levels and STORCH syndrome titers. Viral cultures and urine cytology for cytomegalovirus may be performed. Newborn screening should be performed for hypothyroidism, galactosemia, and phenylketonuria.

TREATMENT AND INTERVENTION

Treatment is aimed at preventing the complications of kernicterus. Phototherapy and exchange transfusion are widely used.

Phototherapy

Phototherapy is the most commonly employed means of treatment. The indication for phototherapy is to prevent the infant from requiring an exchange transfusion. It is estimated that 10% of newborns in the United States are treated with phototherapy.

Before the initiation of phototherapy in any infant, appropriate evaluation as to the cause of the jaundice must be performed. Indications for the initiation of phototherapy vary widely from nursery to nursery and are dependent to some extent on the individual infant's clinical status.

Phototherapy generally consists of a single quartz halogen lamp or a bank of four to eight cool white, daybright, or special blue fluorescent bulbs covered by a Plexiglas shield and placed 12 to 30 inches from the patient. The spectrum of light at 420 to 460 nm is the most effective, although present research is evaluating green light with a wavelength of 525 nm. The energy output in this spectrum should be checked periodically to ensure efficiency.

Phototherapy, by photoisomerization and photooxidation, results in the formation of more polar, water-soluble bilirubin products. The most important of these reactions appears to be the formation of lumirubin.[9] Lumirubin does not require conjugation and is rapidly excreted in bile and urine. The production of lumirubin is an irreversible reaction that appears to be dose related (Figure 15-3).

The efficacy of phototherapy depends on energy output in the blue spectrum of the lights and

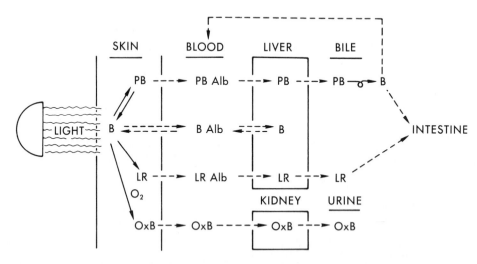

Figure 15-3. General mechanisms of phototherapy for neonatal jaundice. Solid arrows represent chemical reactions; broken arrows represent transport processes. Pigments may be bound to proteins in compartments other than blood. Some excretion of photoisomers, particularly lumirubin, in urine also occurs. *B,* Bilirubin (*Z,Z* isomer); *PB,* photobilirubin (*E,E* and *E,Z* isomers); *LR,* lumirubin (*E* and *Z* isomers; *O* × *B,* bilirubin oxidation products; *Alb,* albumin. (From McDonagh AF and Lightner DA: Pediatrics 75:443, 1985. Reproduced by permission of Pediatrics.)

on the surface area of the infant exposed to those lights.

Animal studies have demonstrated a potential retinal toxicity of light. It is not established that this occurs in the human newborn, but it remains a major concern.

Infants exposed to phototherapy, particularly the low birth weight (LBW) infant and the infant under a radiant warmer, have significant increases in their insensible water loss. These infants also have increased stool water losses and may develop a temporary lactose intolerance.

There are conflicting data in the literature on whether continuous or intermittent administration of phototherapy is most effective.

The concept behind phototherapy arose from the serendipitous observation that infants exposed to sunlight had less jaundice than infants positioned away from the windows.

Phototherapy is not a substitute for exchange transfusion when an exchange is indicated. The decision to treat with phototherapy must be made on an individual basis for each patient.

Special blue lights are the most effective but are not widely used, because they mask the clinical signs of cyanosis and color change in the infant. Many nurseries employ white fluorescent phototherapy bulbs. These are effective and permit better visual monitoring of the patient. The Plexiglas shield absorbs ultraviolet irradiation. Quartz halogen lights are replacing fluorescent lights in many nurseries. A photoreaction occurs in the very outer layers (top 2 mm) of the skin. Once phototherapy has been initiated, serum levels of bilirubin must be monitored frequently (every 4 to 12 hours), because visual assessment of icterus is no longer valid. Hematocrit must also be monitored, especially in infants with hemolytic disease.

To increase exposure, most infants are placed naked under the lights with shielding over the eyes. In the small infant diapers may cover a significant amount of surface area, and some clinicians have found that using a tie-on surgeon's mask as a "bikini bottom" is effective in containing stool and urine. The infant's position should be changed frequently. This permits maximal skin exposure to the lights.

Because of the potential for eye damage, the eyes should be covered while phototherapy is in use. Patches should completely cover the eyes without placing excessive pressure on the eyes and be carefully positioned to avoid occluding the nares. To permit evaluation of the infant's eyes, eye patches should be removed every 4 hours and changed every 8 hours. The patches should be left off during feedings and parental visits.

The infant's temperature should be monitored frequently. Infants in incubators or servocontrolled care centers may become overheated. The servocontrol probe should be shielded by an opaque covering. Infants treated in open cribs may become cold stressed. Fluid balance must be carefully monitored in the infant receiving phototherapy. Weights taken twice a day and close monitoring of intake and output such as urine volume and specific gravity may indicate a need for increased fluids, either orally or intravenously. The presence of reducing substances in the stool can be treated with a nonlactose-containing formula. With continuous phototherapy the infant will receive 18 to 20 hours of light per day with interruptions for feeding, blood drawing, and parental visits. In some studies intermittent schedules such as 15 minutes on and 60 minutes off appear to be as effective as continuous schedules with much less irradiation, but the occurrence of in vitro complications may be greater. Following the cessation of phototherapy bilirubin levels should be followed for at least 24 hours to rule out the occurrence of significant rebound.

Exchange transfusion

An exchange transfusion is indicated for correction of severe anemia, removal of antibody-coated red blood cells in hemolytic disease, or removal of excessive unconjugated bilirubin regardless of its cause. Phototherapy has significantly decreased the need for exchange transfusion. Again, the indications, especially in the VLBW infant, vary from nursery to nursery.

In the infant with severe hemolytic disease, a packed red blood cell exchange transfusion using type O Rh-negative blood may save the infant's life, correct anemia and hypoxemia, and permit successful transition.

Compared with acid-citrate-dextrose blood, citrate-phosphate-dextrose blood has a higher pH, less of an acid load, and longer maintenance of normal 2,3 diphosphoglycerate levels. Despite the acid pH of citrate-phosphate-dextrose blood, most infants do well, because in the liver the citrate is metabolized to bicarbonate.

Administration of 1 g/kg of salt-poor albumin 1 hour before the exchange transfusion has been shown in some studies to increase the efficiency of exchange by about 40%.[10] Aliquot size appears to have no significant effect on the efficiency of the exchange. Smaller aliquots are less stressful to the infant.

Citrate used as part of the anticoagulant solution binds divalent ions such as calcium and magnesium.

Immediately after the exchange, the bilirubin level will be about 45% of the preexchange level. As plasma and tissue levels equilibrate, the bilirubin rises to about 60% of the preexchange level.

It must be stressed that the decision to perform an exchange transfusion must be individualized for each patient.

Central venous pressure must be carefully followed when performing an exchange transfusion with packed red blood cells. If necessary in the delivery room, a slow exchange is performed to reach a hematocrit of 45. Then the infant is transported to the neonatal intensive care unit.

Exchange transfusion trays are commercially available and include a four-way stopcock, necessary tubing and syringes, 10% calcium gluconate, and a plastic bag for discarded blood. Whole blood with a hematocrit of 50% to

55% is used for exchange transfusion. ABO type-specific Rh-negative blood should be used in cases with Rh incompatibility. Type O Rh-specific cells are indicated when ABO incompatibility exists. Citrate-phosphate-dextrose is the anticoagulant most widely used. Fresh blood (<24 hours old) should be insisted on. Albumin priming results in an expansion of plasma volume and should not be used in anemic or edematous infants.

For exchange transfusion the infant should be on a cardiac monitor and restrained in an incubator or on an infant care center with a radiant heater. Generally, 5 to 20 ml aliquots of blood are used, depending on the size and condition of the infant. The initial aliquot should be withdrawn and sent to the laboratory for bilirubin, hematocrit, calcium, and cultures. The rate of exchange is usually 2 to 4 ml/min. Blood used in the exchange should be warmed and mixed in the bag after every 50 to 100 ml. Central venous pressure measurements should be made about every 100 ml and every 50 ml in the hydropic infant.

The infant should be evaluated for hypocalcemia after each 100 ml of the exchange has been completed. Clinical signs and symptoms of hypocalcemia include irritability, tachycardia, or prolongation of the Q-oTc interval. If hypocalcemia is detected, 1 ml of a 10% calcium gluconate solution is slowly infused.

The final aliquot from an exchange should be sent for complete blood count, fractionated bilirubin, calcium ion, electrolytes, culture, and repeat type and crossmatch for potential additional exchange transfusion. In addition to the individuals performing the exchange, one person must keep an accurate record of time, volumes withdrawn and infused, vital signs, and medications administered.

COMPLICATIONS
Hyperbilirubinemia

Hyperbilirubinemia is of clinical concern because of the complication of bilirubin encephalopathy (kernicterus). Kernicterus refers to yellowish staining in nuclear centers of the central nervous system, particularly in the basal ganglia, cerebellum, and hippocampus.

Development of toxicity may be dependent on albumin-bilirubin binding, although interruption of the blood-brain barrier may also play a role. Factors that interfere with albumin-bilirubin binding appear to predispose to the development of kernicterus and have been outlined earlier in this chapter (see Table 15-1). Free unconjugated bilirubin appears to be cytotoxic for central nervous system cells, and uncouples oxidative phosphorylation and reduces protein synthesis in vitro at the mitochondrial level. Once toxicity has occurred, it appears to be irreversible.

Phototherapy

Despite its widespread use since 1958, questions about the safety and side effects of phototherapy remain. The potential for retinal damage, increase in insensible water losses, loose stools, lactose intolerance, temperature elevations, or cold stress have already been discussed. Infants who have an associated cholestatic jaundice and are exposed to phototherapy may develop the "bronze baby syndrome." This is presumably caused by retention of a bilirubin breakdown product produced by phototherapy. Increased platelet turnover and lower mean platelet counts may occur, although the mechanism is unknown. Transient skin rashes and tanning, particularly in black infants, have been reported. Tanning is a result of increased melanin production.

Cell culture studies have demonstrated DNA damage when exposed to phototherapy, especially with intermittent administration. Other potential problems include interference with biologic (circadian) rhythms and with maternal-infant bonding. Although there may be some transient, short-term growth effects, long-term growth effects and development appear unaffected by phototherapy.

A list of complications of phototherapy follows:

1. Potential retinal damage if eyes are exposed
2. Increased insensible water loss
3. Loose bowel movements
4. Temporary lactose intolerance
5. Temperature maintenance (hyperthermia or hypothermia)
6. Bronze baby syndrome
7. Decreased platelet count
8. Transient skin rashes and tanning
9. Potential cellular damage
10. Potential interference with biologic rhythm
11. Potential interference with maternal-infant bonding

Exchange transfusion

Exchange transfusion is a procedure with many potential complications and carries a mortality risk of about 0.5%. Some complications are[*]:

Vascular	Embolization, thrombosis, and necrotizing enterocolitis
Cardiac	Arrhythmias, volume overload, and arrest
Electrolyte	Hypernatremia, hyperkalemia, hypocalcemia, acidosis and alkalosis after exchange
Clotting	Thrombocytopenia, overheparinization, and bleeding
Infection	Bacteremia and blood-borne, viral hepatitis
Others	Hemolysis from old donor blood or from mechanical or thermal injury, perforations of vessels and viscera, hypoglycemia from induced insulin release, and hypothermia from overexposure

Vascular complications are related to the use of umbilical catheters discussed in Chapter 6. Necrotizing enterocolitis has been reported as a post-exchange complication, probably as a result of bowel ischemia during the procedure.

Electrolyte and glucose disturbances are related to the blood preparation used during the

[*]Modified from Odell GB: Neonatal hyperbilirubinemia, New York, 1980, Grune & Stratton, Inc. By permission.

exchange. Acid-citrate-dextrose and citrate-phosphate-dextrose blood have high levels of sodium and glucose and perhaps potassium. Initial hyperglycemia may be followed by reactive hypoglycemia as a result of an insulin response. Although acidic at the time of infusion, a postexchange alkalosis may occur as citrate is metabolized to bicarbonate.

Many of the electrolyte and acid-base disturbances may be avoided by the use of fresh, heparinized blood. Bleeding may occur in the over-heparinized infant but is reversible with protamine sulfate. Thrombocytopenia may occur, especially in the infant requiring repeated exchange transfusions. Bacterial infection is rare, and routine antibiotic prophylaxis is not indicated. Most complications are avoidable if careful attention to technique is observed.

CLINICAL COMPLICATIONS
Hyperbilirubinemia

Early clinical signs of kernicterus include a poor Moro reflex with incomplete flexion of the extremities. Because of the infant's poor sucking ability, feeding may be difficult. In progressive cases the infant develops a high-pitched cry, is hypotonic, and may vomit. Opisthotonic posturing also may occur. In later life, severely affected survivors may manifest choreoathetosis, spastic cerebral palsy, mental retardation, sensory and perceptual deafness, and visual-motor incoordination. More subtle findings may occur in less severely affected infants and may not be apparent during the newborn period. There is speculation that some learning disabilities may be related to hyperbilirubinemia even at what had been previously considered "safe" levels. Unfortunately, the critical level at which bilirubin toxicity occurs in either preterm or term infants has not been established.

Phototherapy

The infant with bronze baby syndrome develops a dark gray-brown discoloration of the skin, urine, and serum. There are generally no clinical symptoms with this syndrome, but there has been at least one reported death. Following cessation of phototherapy, the bronzing gradually resolves. In addition to shielding the eyes, it has been recommended that the gonads be shielded.

Exchange transfusion

The use of freshly collected blood (<72 hours old) will help maintain acceptable potassium levels. Infants with hemolytic disease of the newborn are already at risk for hypoglycemia because of islet cell hyperplasia. Blood glucose levels must be followed closely in the first few hours after an exchange. Heparinized blood must be used within 24 hours of preparation of the unit. In addition to other forms of viral hepatitis, cytomegalovirus may be transmitted to the infant and should be screened for where possible.

PARENT TEACHING

Jaundice and its treatment can be very disturbing to parents. Parents often feel guilty that perhaps something they did or failed to do resulted in their infant's jaundice. Reassurance and support are vital, especially for the nursing mother, who may question her ability to adequately nourish her infant.

Phototherapy is especially distressing and should be explained to the parents before they see the infant under the lights. Eye patches tend to be very disconcerting to most parents. Side effects of phototherapy such as loose or dark-green stools should be explained to parents. Parents may tend to believe that there may be problems with the infant's eyes despite reassurances to the contrary. The lights should be turned off and eye patches removed during visits so normal parent-infant interaction can occur.

Occasionally it will be necessary to follow an infant's bilirubin and/or hematocrit levels on an outpatient basis. The importance of keeping

these outpatient appointments should be stressed.

As with many disorders in newborn infants, a little time spent in careful explanation with the parents can alleviate much fear, guilt, and occasionally anger and help establish a normal family relationship. Causes of jaundice should be explained to the parents, emphasizing that it is usually a transient problem and one to which all infants must adapt following birth. Giving the parents a pamphlet containing information on jaundice and its therapy may help reinforce the instructive efforts.

SUMMARY

Hyperbilirubinemia is a universal problem in newborn infants and must be addressed on a daily basis by everyone providing neonatal care at any level. Causes are many and varied but are best thought of in terms of increased production or decreased secretion of bilirubin. Etiologic factors should be investigated before the onset of therapy. Elevated unconjugated bilirubin is of consequence because of the potential for irreversible central nervous system damage when the bilirubin-albumin binding capacity is exceeded. Unfortunately, testing of this binding capacity and factors affecting it are not yet refined to the point where they are readily available and useful in clinical practice. The relative importance of bilirubin-albumin binding and interruption of the blood-brain barrier remain areas of research interest. Treatment modalities consist mainly of phototherapy and exchange transfusion, procedures that are not entirely without risk.

REFERENCES

1. Cole AP and Hargreaves T: Conjugation inhibitors in early neonatal hyperbilirubinemia, Arch Dis Child 47:415, 1972.
2. Cornwall R and Cornelius CE: Effect of fasting on bilirubin metabolism, N Engl J Med 283:204, 1970.
3. Dahms BB et al: Breast feeding and serum bilirubin values during the first 4 days of life, J Pediatr 83:1049, 1973.
4. Gartner LM and Arias IM: Studies of prolonged neonatal jaundice in the breast-fed infant, J Pediatr 68:54, 1966.
5. Gourley G and Arend R: B-blucuronide and hyperbilirubinemia in breast fed and formula fed babies, Lancet 1:644, 1986.
6. Hardy JB et al: The first year of life: the collaborative perinatal project of the National Institute of Neurological and Communicative Disorders and Stroke, Baltimore, 1979, The Johns Hopkins University Press.
7. Hargreaves T: Effect of fatty acids on bilirubin conjugation, Arch Dis Child 48:446, 1973.
8. Lucey JF, Arias I, and McKay R: Transient familial hyperbilirubinemia, Am J Dis Child 100:787, 1960.
9. McDonagh A and Lightner D: "Like a shrivelled blood orange"—bilirubin, jaundice, and phototherapy, Pediatrics 75:443, 1985.
10. Odell GB, Cohen SN, and Gordes EH: Administration of albumin in the management of hyperbilirubinemia by exchange transfusions, Pediatrics 30:613, 1962.
11. Poland RL, Schultz GE, and Garg G: High milk lipase activity associated with breast milk jaundice, Pediatr Res 14:1328, 1980.

SELECTED READINGS

Allen FM and Diamond LK: Erythroblastosis fetalis including exchange transfusion technique, Boston, 1958, Little, Brown & Co, Inc.

Averbach K and Gartner L: Breast feeding and human milk: their association with jaundice in the neonate, Clin Perinatol 14:89, 1987.

Broderson R: Free bilirubin in blood plasma of the newborn: effects of albumin, fatty acids, pH, displacing drugs and phototherapy. In Stern L, Oh W, and Fris-Hansen B, editors: Intensive care of the newborn, ed 2, New York, 1978, Masson Publishing USA, Inc.

Cashore WJ and Stein L: Neonatal hyperbilirubinemia, Pediatr Clin North Am 29:1191, 1982.

Conley A and Wood B: Albumin administration in exchange transfusion for hyperbilirubinemia, Arch Dis Child 43:151, 1968.

Gartner LM and Hollander M: Disorders of bilirubin metabolism. In Assali NS, editor: Pathophysiology of gestation, vol 3, Fetal and neonatal disorders, New York, 1972, Academic Press, Inc.

Gross SJ: Vitamin E and neonatal bilirubinemia, Pediatrics 64:321, 1979.

Kopelman AE et al: The "bronze" baby syndrome: a complication of phototherapy, J Pediatr 8:466, 1972.

Levine R and Marsels M, editors: Hyperbilirubinemia in the newborn, Report of the Eighty-fifth Ross Conference on Pediatric Research, 1983, Columbus, Ohio.

Levine RL et al: Entry of bilirubin into the brain due to opening of the blood-brain barrier, Pediatrics 69:255, 1982.

Lucey JF: Neonatal jaundice and phototherapy, Pediatr Clin North Am 19:287, 1972.

Maisels MJ: Neonatal jaundice. In Avery GB, editor: Neonatology: pathophysiology and management of the newborn, ed 3, Philadelphia, 1987, JB Lippincott Co.

Maisels MJ and Gifford K: Jaundice in full-term infants, Am J Dis Child 137:561, 1983.

Maisels MJ and Gifford K: Normal serum bilirubin levels in the newborn and the effect of breastfeeding, Pediatrics 78:837, 1986.

Odell GB: Neonatal hyperbilirubinemia, New York, 1980, Grune & Stratton, Inc.

Poland RL and Odell G: Physiologic jaundice: the entero-hepatic circulation of bilirubin, N Engl J Med 284:1, 1971.

Poland RL and Ostrea EM Jr: Neonatal hyperbilirubinemia. In Klaus MH and Fanaroff AA, editors: Care of the high risk neonate, ed 3, Philadelphia, 1986, WB Saunders Co.

Robinson SH: The origins of bilirubin, N Engl J Med 279:143, 1968.

Valaes T: Bilirubin metabolism: review and discussion of inborn errors, Clin Perinatol 3:177, 1976.

Young CY et al: Phenobarbitone prophylaxis for neonatal hyperbilirubinemia, Pediatrics 48:372, 1971.

CHAPTER 16

Infection in the neonate

FREDERIC W. BRUHN · BETTY JONES · JAYNE P. O'DONNELL · GERALD B. MERENSTEIN

The newborn infant is uniquely susceptible to infectious diseases acquired by several routes, including crossing the placenta (prenatal infection), ascending in the perinatal period (natal infection), and shortly after birth while still in the neonatal period (postnatal infection). Causes with particular emphasis on presenting signs and symptoms, laboratory data, treatment, complications, and methods of prevention applicable to the care of the neonate are presented in this chapter. Abbreviations for this chapter are listed on this page.

PATHOPHYSIOLOGY AND PATHOGENESIS

Infections occur when a susceptible host comes in contact with a potentially pathogenic organism. When the encountered organism proliferates and overcomes the host defenses, infection results. Sources of infection in the newborn can be arbitrarily divided into three categories: (1) transplacental acquisition, (2) perinatal acquisition during labor and delivery, and (3) hospital acquisition in the neonatal period from the mother, hospital environment, or personnel.

A diverse group of infectious agents may invade the fetus or newborn. Although certain infections have characteristic associations between the causative agent and the source (e.g., rubella virus plus transplacental acquisition equals a congenital rubella infant), other causative agents may be ac-

quired from several sources and produce variable clinical outcomes (e.g., cytomegalovirus (CMV) plus transplacental acquisition equals a congenital CMV infant, or CMV plus hospital-acquired infection from blood transfusion equals a neonate with CMV pneumonitis).

In general, most infecting organisms listed in Table 16-1 can under the proper circumstances

ABBREVIATIONS

AIDS	Acquired immunodeficiency syndrome
CF	Complement fixation test
CIE	Counter immunoelectrophoresis
CSF	Cerebrospinal fluid
ELISA	Enzyme-linked immunosorbent assay
FA	Fluorescent antibody test
FAMA	Fluorescent antibody to membrane antigen
FTA-ABS	Fluorescent treponemal antibody absorption test
HbsAg	Hepatitis B surface antigen
HIV	Human immunodeficiency virus
IAHA	Immune adherence hemagglutination
IFA	Indirect fluorescent antibody test
IHA	Hemagglutination inhibition test
MHA-TP	Microhemagglutination test for *Treponema pallidum*
RPR	Rapid plasma reagin test
VDRL	Venereal Disease Research Laboratory test

□ The opinions and assertions in this chapter are those of the authors and do not necessarily represent those of the Department of the Army or the Department of Defense.

TABLE 16-1

Common Disease-Producing Agents in the Fetus and Newborn

ORGANISM	TRANSPLACENTAL INFECTION			CONGENITAL DISEASE	NEONATAL DISEASE
	ABORTION	PREMATURE BIRTH	INTRAUTERINE GROWTH RETARDATION		
Bacterial					
Anaerobic bacteria (*Bacteroides, Clostridia, Peptostreptococcus, Veillonella*)	?	?	–	R	R
Escherichia coli	?	?	–	+	+
Group A streptococcus	+	+	–	+	+
Group B streptococcus	+	+	–	+	+
Group D streptococcus	–	–	–	R	+
Haemophilus influenzae	–	–	–	R	+
Klebsiella species	–	–	–	R	R
Listeria monocytogenes	+	+	–	+	+
Neisseria gonorrhoeae	?	+	–	R	+
Neisseria meningitidis	–	–	–	–	+
Proteus species	–	–	–	R	R
Pseudomonas aeruginosa	–	–	–	R	R
Salmonella species	?	+	–	R	+
Shigella species	–	–	–	R	+
Staphylococcus aureus	–	–	–	R	+
Staphylococcus epidermidis	–	–	–	R	R
Viral					
Cytomegalovirus	?	+	+	+	+
Enterovirus (ECHO virus, poliomyelitis, coxsackievirus A and B)	+	?,R	–	R	+
Hepatitis A	–	+	–	–	–
Hepatitis B	–	+	–	R	+
Herpes simplex (type 1 or 2)	+	+	R	R	+
Human immunodeficiency virus	?	?	?	+	+
Measles	+	+	–	R	R
Respiratory syncytial virus	–	–	–	–	+
Rubella	+	+	+	+	R
Varicella	–	–	R	R	+
Fungal					
Candida albicans	–	–	–	+	+
Coccidioides immitis	–	–	–	?	R
Cryptococcus neoformans	–	–	–	R	R
Chlamydial					
Chlamydia trachomatis	–	–	–	–	+

+, Strong evidence for; –, no evidence for; R, rare association; ?, questionable association.

TABLE 16-1—cont'd

Common Disease-Producing Agents in the Fetus and Newborn

| | TRANSPLACENTAL INFECTION | | | | |
ORGANISM	ABORTION	PREMATURE BIRTH	INTRAUTERINE GROWTH RETARDATION	CONGENITAL DISEASE	NEONATAL DISEASE
Spirochetal					
Treponema pallidum	?	+	−	+	+
Borrelia	?	−	−	R	R
Leptospira	?	−	−	R	R
Mycoplasmal					
Mycoplasma hominis	?	−	−	−	R
Mycoplasma pneumoniae	−	−	−	−	R
Ureaplasma urealyticum	?	?	?	?	R
Mycobacterial					
Mycobacterium tuberculosis	?	+	−	R	R
Protozoal					
Plasmodium species	+	+	?	R	R
Pneumocystis carinii	−	−	−	−	R
Toxoplasma gondii	?,R	?,R	?,R	+	+
Trichomonas vaginalis	−	−	−	−	+

cross the placenta or ascend from the birth canal and cause abortion, stillbirth, and disease present at birth or in the neonatal period.

ETIOLOGY

See Table 16-1.

PREVENTION

The main goal is to prevent infections in the fetus and newborn. Unfortunately, few proven measures exist for the prevention of transplacental or perinatal infections acquired during delivery. These measures are important, since most non-bacterial infections (except syphilis and possibly toxoplasmosis and herpes simplex) do not respond to current therapy.

DATA COLLECTION

Thorough data collection for diagnosis of infectious diseases includes a review of the perinatal history, signs and symptoms, and laboratory data.

SPECIFIC INFECTIOUS DISEASES

The following specific infectious diseases are divided by their source of infection.

Transplacental acquisition
ACQUIRED IMMUNODEFICIENCY SYNDROME

PREVENTION. The primary risk to infants for infection with the human immunodeficiency virus (HIV), the causative agent of acquired immunodeficiency syndrome (AIDS), is intrauterine (and possibly intrapartum) exposure to a mother with HIV infection. HIV has been isolated from blood and many bodily fluids. Epidemiologic evidence has implicated only blood, semen, vaginal secretions, and breast milk in transmission. In countries such as the United States where safe alternatives exist, mothers with HIV infection should be discouraged from breastfeeding.

Since the medical history and examination

cannot reliably identify all patients infected with HIV (or other blood-borne pathogens) and since during delivery and initial care of the infant perinatal care providers are exposed to large amounts of maternal blood, precautions (e.g., gloves) should be consistently used for *all* patients when handling the placenta or infant until all maternal blood has been washed away.

DATA COLLECTION

History. Infection in the mother is primarily acquired sexually (bisexual partner, hemophiliac partner, prostitution, promiscuity) or via intravenous (IV) drug abuse. Infection may be asymptomatic. Once the mother is infected with HIV, the transmission of infection to her infant is 50% to 60% of births.

Signs and symptoms. Infants infected with HIV in the perinatal period usually develop signs and symptoms within the first 24 months of life. A few infants have remained asymptomatic for as long as 8 years. Manifestations of infection include lymphoid interstitial pneumonia, weight loss, hepatosplenomegaly, generalized lymphadenopathy, thrombocytopenia, and chronic diarrhea.

Opportunistic infections (disseminated candidiasis, *Pneumocystis carinii* pneumonia, disseminated CMV, chronic herpes simplex virus infection, cryptococcosis, toxoplasmosis, and chronic enteritis with *Cryptosporidium*) may also occur.

Serious and recurrent infections with encapsulated organisms (*Haemophilus influenzae, Streptococcus pneumoniae*) have also been described.

Laboratory data. Epidemiologic data frequently provide the basis for considering the diagnosis (e.g., mother in high-risk category). Primary or secondary immunodeficiency disorders must be excluded.

The primary serologic laboratory test is the enzyme-linked immunosorbent assay (ELISA). The Western blot test is frequently used for confirmation of positive ELISA test results. Separation of the child with passively acquired antibody from the infant with active infection is critical but difficult. Acquired antibody is undetectable in 75% of infants by 12 months of age and in most infants by 15 months of age. Infants have also been described with negative serology but active infection. HIV infection, rather than passive transfer of antibody, is presumed if there is rising titers of anti-HIV antibody or there are new HIV-specific antibody bands on tests such as the Western blot. Viral cultures, detection of HIV antigen, or viral nucleic acids may be more definitive tests whose sensitivity and/or specificity remain to be determined.

TREATMENT. Specific successful antiviral treatment is not currently available. Infants with or suspected of having HIV infection should not receive live vaccines. High-dose IV immunoglobulin may be beneficial. Early diagnosis and aggressive treatment of infections is essential.

CYTOMEGALOVIRUS

PREVENTION. There are no practical methods for preventing CMV. Exposure avoidance is virtually impossible because of the ubiquitous and asymptomatic nature of the infections. Avoiding unnecessary blood transfusions or using CMV serum–negative blood donors has proved to be important in minimizing the occurrence of postnatally acquired CMV, particularly in premature infants.

The question frequently arises regarding assignment of staff to infants with the possible diagnosis of cytomegalovirus. Staff members who may be pregnant have heightened concern regarding this issue. Staff members should be aware that many infants with CMV are often asymptomatic and therefore not identified while in the hospital. To avoid any problems, staff members should employ good handwashing technique with all infants. Wearing gloves when handling urine and other secretions is a strategy that can also be employed by staff members who are working in the neonatal intensive care unit (NICU) and are pregnant or attempting to become pregnant. The actual risk of an infected infant transmitting disease to a susceptible health care worker is unknown but probably small.

DATA COLLECTION

History. Congenital infections are represented by a wide spectrum of disease from asymptomatic disease to profoundly symptomatic disease. Infection in the mother is usually asymptomatic.

Signs and symptoms. An infant with CMV is usually asymptomatic. Congenital manifestations include intrauterine growth retardation, neonatal jaundice (>direct fraction), purpura, hepatosplenomegaly, microcephaly, brain damage, intracerebral calcification, chorioretinitis, and progressive sensorineural hearing loss.

Laboratory data. CMV may be cultured from urine, pharyngeal secretions, and peripheral leukocytes. (Isolation of the virus within 2 weeks of birth indicates transplacental acquisition.) A paired sera demonstration of a fourfold titer rise or histopathologic demonstration of characteristic nuclear inclusions in certain tissues may help. Examining the urine for intranuclear inclusions is not helpful.

PARENT TEACHING. The need for good handwashing technique by parents and caretakers of infants with suspected CMV should be included in discharge instructions.

MEASLES

PREVENTION. Since measles outbreaks are currently an unusual occurrence, prevention is rarely a problem.

DATA COLLECTION

History. Medical personnel should evaluate a susceptible mother (i.e., no previous case of measles or measles immunization) in a community where measles cases are present. Characteristic prodromes are a high fever and respiratory problems.

Signs and symptoms. Symptoms of measles include coughing, coryza, conjunctivitis, and Koplik's spots with cephalad to caudad progression of a morbilliform rash in the mother. The infant is often aborted or delivered prematurely.

Laboratory data. Isolation of measles virus is technically difficult and usually not performed. A paired sera (acute and convalescent) demonstration of a fourfold titer rise is diagnostic.

Treatment. See Table 16-2 for passive immunization.

RUBELLA

PREVENTION. Medical personnel should ensure that all mothers have a protective hemagglutination titer before conception. If the woman is susceptible, vaccinate her with rubella vaccine before conception.

All perinatal health care workers should have rubella titers drawn to identify immunity status. Women of childbearing age who do not have immune titers should be encouraged to have rubella immunization.

DATA COLLECTION

History. Rubella in the first 4 to 5 months of pregnancy has a high incidence of sequelae in the infant. A mother with rubella may be relatively asymptomatic or mildly ill with respiratory symptoms with or without a rash.

Signs and symptoms. Congenital manifestations of rubella include intrauterine growth retardation, sensorineural deafness, cataracts, neonatal jaundice (>direct fraction), purpura, hepatosplenomegaly, microcephaly, chronic encephalitis, chorioretinitis, and cardiac defects (especially patent ductus arteriosus and peripheral pulmonic stenosis). Less frequent manifestations include bone lesions and pneumonitis.

Laboratory data. The virus may be isolated from the throat, blood, urine, and cerebrospinal fluid (CSF). A paired sera demonstration of a fourfold titer rise such as a hemagglutination test (IHA) or a fluorescent antibody test (FA) is diagnostic.

PARENT TEACHING. Infants with congenital

TABLE 16-2

Acceptable Methods of Passive Immunization in Newborns

DISEASE	INDICATIONS FOR USE IN NEWBORNS	WHEN TO USE	PRODUCT*	DOSE
Hepatitis A	Active infection in mother or close family contacts	As soon as possible	HISG	0.02-0.04 ml/kg body weight given intramuscularly (IM)
Hepatitis B	Mothers with acute type B infection or mothers who are antigen positive	As soon as possible (within 12 hr)	HBIG	0.5 ml/kg body weight given IM
Measles	Active infection in mother or close household contacts	As soon as possible (within 72 hr of exposure)	HISG	0.25 ml/kg body weight given IM
Tetanus	Inadequately immunized mothers with contaminated infant (e.g., dirty cord)	As soon as possible	TIG	250 units given IM (optimal dose not established)
Varicella	Infant born to a mother who develops lesions less than 5 days before delivery or within 2 days after delivery	Within 72 hr of birth	ZIG	2 ml given IM

Modified from Remington JS and Klein JO, editors: Infectious diseases of the fetus and newborn infant, ed 2, Philadelphia, 1983, WB Saunders Co.
*HISG, Human immune serum globulin; HBIG, hepatitis B immune globulin; TIG, tetanus immune globulin (human); ZIG, zoster immune globulin.

rubella may secrete the virus for many years. This requires that discharge instructions include preventive strategies that need to be employed to decrease the chance of contact of susceptible pregnant women with the infant. Parents need to be informed of their responsibility to ensure that potentially seronegative women of childbearing age avoid direct contact with the infant. The challenge arises to impress this on the family and at the same time avoid ostracizing the infant or impacting negatively on the parent-infant attachment process. In discharge planning with these families, a collaborative approach should be employed using community health, medical, nursing, and social work input and support.

SYPHILIS

PREVENTION. Avoid exposing the mother to syphilis. Monitor the serum early and late in pregnancy and treat the mother for the appropriate stage of disease. (NOTE: When erythromycin is used in penicillin-sensitive women during gestation, failure to establish a cure in the newborn has occurred as a result of poor transplacental passage of erythromycin.)

DATA COLLECTION

History. A congenital infection may be manifested by a multisystem disease. A primary syphilitic chancre on the cervix or rectal mucosa in a mother may be unnoticed.

Signs and symptoms. An infant exposed to syphilis may be asymptomatic at birth. Neonatal manifestations involve virtually all organ systems, including hepatitis, pneumonitis, bone marrow failure, myocarditis, meningitis, nephrotic syndrome, and a rash involving the palms and soles.

Laboratory data. The microscopic darkfield examination identifies spirochetes from non-oral lesions. Nonspecific, nontreponemal reaginic tests, such as Venereal Disease Research Laboratory (VDRL) tests and rapid plasma reagin (RPR) tests, followed serially with a rise or absence of fall following birth are diagnostic. Specific treponemal antibody serologic tests such as a fluorescent treponemal antibody absorption test (FTA-ABS) and a microhemagglutination test for *Treponema pallidum* (MHA-TP) may also be diagnostic, but an FTA-ABS IgM test is unreliable. A long bone x-ray examination showing metaphysitis or periostitis may help in diagnosing syphilis. VDRL tests on CSF are mandatory in all infants suspected of having congenital syphilis. When the diagnosis of active congenital syphilis is equivocal, it is often best to treat and ascertain the diagnosis by serial serologic determinations.

TOXOPLASMOSIS

PREVENTION. Women susceptible to toxoplasmosis should avoid unnecessary exposure to raw meat and cat feces. Using a pair of gloves when emptying the litter box may provide protection if the pregnant woman (or women attempting to become pregnant) must empty the litter box.

DATA COLLECTION

History. Congenital infections are represented by a wide range of disease from asymptomatic disease to profound symptomatic disease. Mothers may have noted an influenza-like illness, posterior cervical adenitis, or chorioretinitis but usually lack accompanying signs or symptoms. A history of exposure to cat feces or ingestion of raw meat may occasionally be obtained.

Signs and symptoms. Manifestations in the newborn may be prematurity, intrauterine growth retardation, hydrocephalus, chorioretinitis, seizures, cerebral calcifications, hepatosplenomegaly, thrombocytopenia, jaundice, generalized lymphadenopathy, and a rash.

Laboratory data. Isolating *Toxoplasma gondii* from blood or body fluids is difficult and tedious. Cysts may be found in the placenta or tissues of a fetus or newborn. Most congenitally infected infants will have a Sabin-Feldman dye test titer greater than 1:1000 at birth.

Perinatal acquisition during labor and delivery
CHLAMYDIA TRACHOMATIS

PREVENTION. Eye prophylaxis with erythromycin (preferred) or tetracycline ophthalmic ointment minimizes the development of conjunctivitis but has no effect on the subsequent development of pneumonitis.

DATA COLLECTION

History. A mother with *Chlamydia trachomatis* is usually asymptomatic during her pregnancy.

Signs and symptoms. Conjunctivitis may be manifested as congestion and edema of the conjunctiva with minimal discharge developing 1 to 2 weeks after birth and lasting several weeks with recurrences particularly after topical therapy. Infants with pneumonitis usually do not have a fever but have a prolonged staccato cough, tachypnea, mild hypoxemia, and eosinophilia. Otitis media and bronchiolitis may also occur.

Laboratory data. Definitive diagnosis is made by isolating the organism in tissue culture cells. Scraping conjunctival epithelial cells and demonstrating characteristic intracytoplasmic inclusion bodies by a Giemsa stain is diagnostic. Suggestive but nonspecific tests include eosinophilia (>300 to $400/m^3$), and elevated IgM serum levels. Serologic tests are generally difficult to perform and not readily available. Direct immunofluorescence of conjunctival scrapings is also diagnostic and is readily available.

ENTEROVIRUS (COXSACKIEVIRUS A AND B, ECHO VIRUS, AND POLIOMYELITIS)

PREVENTION. To prevent *poliomyelitis*, maintain poliomyelitis immunity with active immunization before conception. Passive protection with pooled human serum globulin may help in selected exposures (0.2 ml/kg body weight, given IM). Routine nursery infection control procedures must be observed.

DATA COLLECTION

History. Infection may occur year-round but is more prevalent from June to December in temperate climates. Most *Enterovirus* infections are asymptomatic. Poliomyelitis is rare because of a high vaccine-induced immunity in the United States.

Signs and symptoms. Mothers with *enteroviral infections* are usually mildly ill with fever or diarrhea. Infants may be asymptomatic or have fever or diarrhea. Fulminating encephalomyocarditis or acute hepatic necrosis may occur within several days of birth, but their occurrence is rare.

Laboratory data. The virus may be isolated from the throat, rectum, or CSF. Isolating coxsackievirus A may require suckling mouse inoculation. Serologic screening is impractical because of the large number of serotypes.

GROUP B STREPTOCOCCUS

PREVENTION. Perinatal (before or during labor) treatment of the mother with penicillin appears to prevent group B streptococcus disease in the neonate and may decrease maternal postpartum endometritis.

DATA COLLECTION. See section on bacterial infections and bacterial sepsis.

HEPATITIS B

PREVENTION. Prenatal screening of women for hepatitis B surface antigen (HBsAg) is indicated and cost-effective. Use of active and passive immunization in infants born of HBsAg-positive mothers is indicated (see Tables 16-2 and 16-3).

DATA COLLECTION

History. Mothers who are HBsAg positive because of the chronic carrier state or acute disease before delivery may pass the infection to their infants at delivery.

Women at high risk include women of Asian, Pacific Island, or Alaskan Eskimo descent; women born in Haiti or sub-Saharan Africa; or women with a history of liver disease, IV drug abuse, or frequent exposure to blood in a medical-dental setting.

Signs and symptoms. The neonate with hepatitis B is usually asymptomatic. Occasionally,

---

TABLE 16-3 _____

Acceptable Methods of Active Immunization in Newborns

DISEASE	INDICATIONS FOR USE IN NEWBORNS	WHEN TO USE	PRODUCT	DOSE
Hepatitis B	Infant born to mother positive for HBsAG* at birth	3 separate doses at birth,† 1 month, and 6 months of age (if infant is still HBsAg negative)	Hepatitis B vaccine	10 µg (0.5 ml) given IM at 1, 2, and 8 months of age
Pertussis	To control rare outbreak in nursery	As soon as possible	Pertussis	0.25-0.5 ml administered subcutaneously
Tuberculosis	Selected infants at risk of contracting tuberculosis	As soon as possible	BCG*	0.1 ml given intradermally and divided into two sites over deltoid muscle

*HBsAg, Hepatitis B surface antigen; BCG, Calmette-Guérin bacillus.
†Within the first 7 days.

infected infants demonstrate elevated liver enzymes or acute fulminating hepatitis. Neonatal infection with subsequent chronic carriage has been implicated in the development of primary hepatocellular carcinoma later in life.

Laboratory data. Virtually all infants at risk of acquiring hepatitis from their mother are HBsAg negative at birth. Many untreated infants become HBsAg positive 4 to 12 weeks postnatally and become lifelong asymptomatic carriers or develop hepatitis B.

HERPES SIMPLEX (TYPES 1 AND 2)

PREVENTION. The key to preventing herpes simplex is avoiding exposure. Mothers at risk (especially those with primary genital herpes within 8 weeks of parturition) should be identified, and a cesarean section should be considered in these mothers within 4 to 6 hours of membrane rupture. Treatment with Acyclovir should begin at the first sign of neonatal disease or when infants have been exposed to an active lesion.

Communication is required between obstetric and neonatal staff to determine the status of a family with a history of herpes. Unnecessary restrictions should not be placed on postpartum mothers who are not actively infected. Health professionals need to employ all family-centered strategies used in their institutions with these families unless these are precluded by the need for the infant's treatment.

DATA COLLECTION

History. Disease caused by type 1 herpes simplex is usually spread via the respiratory route, whereas disease caused by type 2 herpes simplex is usually spread via the genital route.

Many mothers who transmit herpes simplex to their newborn infants are asymptomatic. The risk to the infant from recurrent lesions is minimal.

Signs and symptoms. Infants with herpes simplex have a spectrum of illnesses ranging from localized skin lesions to generalized infections involving the liver, lungs, and central nervous system (CNS). This disseminated disease has a high morbidity and mortality.

Laboratory data. A cytologic examination of the base of skin vesicles with a Giemsa stain (Tzanck test) may reveal characteristic but nonspecific giant cells and eosinophilic intranuclear inclusions. The virus may be readily identified on a tissue culture within 24 to 48 hours from the respiratory and genital tracts, blood, urine, and CSF. Rapid viral diagnosis by fluorescent tests is becoming more widely available. Although serologic tests such as complement fixation test (CF), enzyme-linked immunosorbent assay (ELISA), and neutralization are available, they are of little value in the acute clinical situation.

PARENT TEACHING. Families with herpes simplex require consistent and detailed teaching regarding prevention of transmission of herpes to the infant. Breastfeeding mothers can be reassured that they may continue to breastfeed as long as there are no lesions on their breasts. Emphasis should be placed on the need for breastfeeding mothers to check their breasts for lesions.

Parents with active herpes simplex need to employ good handwashing technique while caring for their infants. Parents with oral herpes should avoid kissing their infants while lesions are open and draining.

LISTERIA MONOCYTOGENES

PREVENTION. Pregnant women should avoid drinking unpasteurized milk to prevent *Listeria monocytogenes* infection.

DATA COLLECTION. See section on bacterial infections and bacterial sepsis.

MYCOBACTERIUM TUBERCULOSIS

PREVENTION. Mothers at risk for *Mycobacterium tuberculosis* infection may be identified with a tuberculin test during pregnancy. If the mother is a tuberculin converter (a positive skin test within the past 2 years), a chest x-ray examination should be obtained. If the mother has active tuberculosis, she should be treated with isoniazid and rifampin during pregnancy.

Separate infants of mothers with active disease from the mother until the mother is not contagious (usually negative sputum). Treat high-risk infants with isoniazid (10 mg/kg/day) or a tuberculosis vaccine (*Calmette-Guérin bacillus*) (see Table 16-3).

DATA COLLECTION

History. A strong history of maternal contact with tuberculosis favors the diagnosis. This is especially true in high-risk populations (southeast Asians, American Indians, and families with a known cavitary disease).

Mothers with HIV infection are at an increased risk for developing active tuberculosis.

Signs and symptoms. Mothers may be relatively asymptomatic or have signs and symptoms that are generalized (fever and weight loss) or localized to the respiratory tract. A congenital infection is extremely rare. Nonspecific signs and symptoms such as failure to thrive and unexplained hypothermia or hyperthermia are the most common manifestations in the neonatal period.

Laboratory data. Acid-fast organisms found on smears of gastric aspirates, sputum, CSF, or infected tissues strongly suggest tuberculosis in the neonate. Isolating *Mycobacterium tuberculosis* by culture is diagnostic and should be aggressively sought. The tuberculin test is usually positive (>10 mm induration) in active tuberculosis. However, a positive skin test requires 3 to 12 weeks to manifest itself and is usually negative in the neonate. A chest x-ray examination also is usually negative in the neonate.

MEASLES

See section on transplacental acquisition.

NEISSERIA GONORRHEAE

PREVENTION. Screening high-risk mothers before delivery may identify asymptomatic gonor-

rhea. Treating positive mothers before delivery or exposed infants at delivery is necessary.

Administering silver nitrate, erythromycin, or tetracycline in the eyes is mandatory in all vaginal deliveries.

DATA COLLECTION

History. Mothers with previous venereal disease are a high-risk group, since 80% of the infected women may be asymptomatic.

Signs and symptoms. The predominant manifestation of gonorrhea is ophthalmia neonatorum, although a systemic, blood-borne infection may rarely occur involving the joints, lungs, endocardium, and CNS. Conjunctivitis usually begins 2 to 5 days after birth. Eye prophylaxis minimizes but does not guarantee freedom from infection. Scalp abscess resulting from fetal monitoring has been reported.

Laboratory data. A Gram's stain of purulent eye discharge revealing gram-negative intracellular diplococci is diagnostic. Culture confirmation using fermentation or fluorescence establishes the diagnosis of gonorrhea. The organism is labile, so cultures should be taken to the laboratory and plated immediately. When gonorrhea is diagnosed, other sexually transmitted diseases may be present concomitantly (especially chlamydia).

PLASMODIUM SPECIES

PREVENTION. Exposure of the pregnant mother to mosquitoes in endemic areas should be minimized with protective netting and mosquito repellants. Prophylaxis through administration of chloroquine to the mother may be necessary in selected situations.

DATA COLLECTION

History. Travel to or presence in an endemic area is necessary except in rare situations (e.g., contaminated blood transfusion). Asymptomatic mothers may give birth to infants with *Plasmodium* infection.

Signs and symptoms. A true congenital infection of *Plasmodium* is rare, but onset in the first day of life has been reported. Fever, anemia, and splenomegaly are present in most infected infants. Nonspecific findings include failure to thrive, poor feeding, and diarrhea.

Laboratory data. The malarial parasites may be diagnosed by a Giemsa stain of a thick smear of peripheral blood. Serologic tests do not help in diagnosing an acute infection but may be useful in retrospectively determining the plasmodia species involved.

SYPHILIS

See section on transplacental acquisition.

VARICELLA

PREVENTION. See Table 16-2.

DATA COLLECTION

History. The history of varicella in the mother before conception virtually excludes the diagnosis. Varicella present in the mother with a fever, respiratory symptoms, and characteristic vesicular rash primarily on the trunk within 5 days of delivery threatens a newborn. Preventive measures should be instituted as soon as possible.

Signs and symptoms. Congenital varicella is rare but has followed maternal varicella in the first trimester of pregnancy. Congenital manifestations include limb atrophy, skin scars, and CNS and eye abnormalities. Acute perinatal varicella frequently is a devastating systemic disease.

Laboratory data. The demonstration of multinucleated giant cells containing intranuclear inclusions in skin scrapings on Giemsa stain is nonspecific but helpful. Isolating the virus from the skin lesions or respiratory tract is difficult. A number of serologic tests such as the fluorescent antibody to membrane antigen test (FAMA), immune adherence hemagglutination test (IAHA), enzyme-linked immunosorbent assay test (ELISA), and neutralization test are available but are not helpful in the acute clinical situation. Complement fixation (CF) serologic tests are relatively insensitive.

Bacterial infections

The most serious of the postnatal infections is sepsis caused by the bacteria listed in the boxed material below.

Neonatal sepsis is characterized by systemic signs of infection associated with bacteremia. Meningitis in the neonate is a relatively frequent sequela of bacteremia. In addition, blood-borne bacteria may localize in other tissues, causing focal disease. Two patterns of bacterial disease, early and late onset, have been associated with systemic infections during the neonatal period. This is particularly true for disease caused by group B streptococcus.

EARLY-ONSET DISEASE

Early-onset disease is present as a fulminant, multisystem illness during the first days of life. Many of these infants are premature and have a history of one or more significant obstetric

---

ORGANISMS CAUSING BACTERIAL SEPSIS

Common organisms
Group B streptococcus
Escherichia coli
Haemophilus influenzae (type b and nontypable)

Unusual organisms
Staphylococcus aureus
Staphylococcus epidermidis
Neisseria meningitidis
Streptococcus pneumoniae
Listeria monocytogenes

Rare organisms
Klebsiella pneumoniae
Pseudomonas aeruginosa
Enterobacter species
Serratia marcescens
Group A streptococcus
Group B streptococcus
Anaerobic species

complications, including premature rupture of maternal membranes, premature onset of labor, chorioamnionitis, or peripartum maternal fever. Bacteria responsible for early-onset disease are acquired from the birth canal before delivery. Early-onset bacterial disease has a high mortality.

LATE-ONSET DISEASE

Late-onset disease may occur as early as 5 days of age but is more common after the first week of life. These infants may have a history of obstetric complications, but they are less common than obstetric complications in early-onset disease. Bacteria responsible for late-onset sepsis and meningitis include those acquired from the maternal genital tract and organisms acquired after birth from human contact or from contaminated equipment or material.

BACTERIAL SEPSIS

PREVENTION. The Centers for Disease Control defines all neonatal infections acquired intrapartum or during hospitalization as nosocomial. Infants requiring the specialized care of NICUs are highly suspectible to infections. Prematurity, stress, immature immune systems, and complicated medical and surgical problems contribute to their increased susceptibility. In addition, most infants in the NICU require a variety of invasive diagnostic, therapeutic, and monitoring procedures; many of these procedures bypass natural physical barriers that may allow colonization to occur and a nosocomial infection to develop.

Infection control principles and practices for the prevention of these nosocomial infections are outlined in Table 16-4. Table 16-5 outlines infection control measures and isolation techniques for specific diseases.

DATA COLLECTION

History. Early-onset disease occurs more often in premature membrane rupture, premature onset of labor, chorioamnionitis, peripartum maternal fever, maternal genitourinary tract infection, prematurity, fetal distress, or aspiration by the neonate. Invasive procedures performed on the neonate, such as intubation, catheterization, and surgery, increase the risk for bacterial infection.

Signs and symptoms. In general, signs, par-

Text continued on p. 353.

TABLE 16-4

Infection Control Principles and Practices to Prevent Nosocomial Infection

PRINCIPLE	PRACTICE
Hand washing Hand washing is the most important procedure for controlling infection in the NICU.	1. Before each shift wash hands, wrist, forearms, and elbows with an antiseptic. Scrub hands with a brush or pad for 2-3 minutes and rinse thoroughly. Chlorhexidine, hexachlorophene, and iodophors are the preferred products. 2. Wash hands for 10-15 seconds between infant contacts. Soap and water are adequate unless the infant is infected or contaminated objects have been handled. 3. Use an antiseptic for hand washing before surgical or similar invasive procedures.
Patient placement Overcrowding in the NICU increases risk of cross-contamination.	Provide 4-6 feet intervals between infants.

TABLE 16-4—cont'd

Infection Control Principles and Practices to Prevent Nosocomial Infection

PRINCIPLE	PRACTICE

Skin and cord care
1. The skin, its secretions, and normal flora are natural defense mechanisms that protect against invading pathogens. Manipulating an infant's skin must be minimized.
 	
2. No single method of cord care has proved to prevent colonization or limit disease.
	1. The American Academy of Pediatrics suggests using a dry technique.
	  a. Delay initial cleansing until temperature is stable.
	  b. Use sterile cotton sponges and sterile water or a mild soap to remove blood from face and head, and meconium from perineal area.
	  c. *Do not* touch other areas unless grossly soiled.
	2. Local application of alcohol, triple dye, and various antimicrobial agents is currently used.

Medical devices
1. Medical devices facilitate infections by
  a. Bypassing normal defense mechanisms, providing direct access to blood and deep tissues
  b. Supporting growth of microorganisms and becoming reservoirs from which bacteria can be transmitted with the device to another patient
  c. Providing a "protected site" when placed in deeper tissue, so phagocytosis or defense mechanisms cannot eradicate the organisms
  d. Using sterile medical devices that are occasionally contaminated from the manufacturer or central supply
	1. IV infusion devices predispose infants to phlebitis and bacteremia. Preventive measures include preparing the site with tincture of iodine (2% iodine in 70% alcohol), an iodophor, or 70% alcohol; anchoring the IV securely; performing site assessment and care every 24 hr (routine site care is not necessary with polyurethane dressings); rotating the IV site every 48-72 hr; changing the IV tubing every 24-48 hr on regular IVs; and discontinuing the IV at the first sign of complication.
	2. Arterial lines predispose infants to bacteremia. Preventive measures include aseptically inserting the catheter using gloves, inspecting the site and performing site care every 24 hr, treating the catheter and stopcocks as sterile fields, and minimizing manipulation by drawing all blood specimens at the same time.
	3. Intravascular pressure—monitoring systems predispose infants to septicemia. Preventive measures include replacing the flush solution every 24 hr, replacing the chamber dome, and administering the tubing and continuous flow device (if used) at 48 hr intervals and between each patient.
	4. Respiratory therapy devices increase the risk of contamination. Preventive measures include using aseptic technique during suctioning; dating opened solution for irrigation, humidification, and nebulization, and discarding after 24 hr; ensuring routine replacement and cleaning of all respiratory equipment, including AMBU bags, cascade nebulizers, endotracheal tube adaptors and tubing; and checking sputum cultures and Gram's stains every several days to assess the degree of colonization or infection in the intubated patient.

Continued.

TABLE 16-4—cont'd

Infection Control Principles and Practices to Prevent Nosocomial Infection

PRINCIPLE	PRACTICE
Specimen collection	
Improperly collected specimens cause infection at the site of collection or erroneous diagnosis leading to the administration of the wrong antibiotic or delayed administration of the appropriate antibiotic.	1. Wash hands before collecting specimen. 2. Observe aseptic technique to reduce risk of infection and to avoid contamination of specimen. 3. Deliver specimens to the laboratory immediately. 4. *Do not use femoral sticks.*
Nursery attire	
Personal clothing and unscrubbed skin areas of personnel should not touch infants.	1. Short-sleeved scrub gowns accommodate washing to elbows. 2. Long-sleeved gowns should be worn and changed between handling of infected or potentially infected infants. 3. Sterile gowns are necessary for sterile procedures.
Employee health	
Transmission of disease among patients and employees can occur bidirectionally. Each NICU must establish reasonable guidelines for restriction of assignments based on the employee's potential to transmit disease and the potential risk of acquiring disease.	1. Conditions that commonly restrict personnel from patient care in the NICU are skin lesions and draining wounds, acute respiratory infections, fever, gastroenteritis, active herpes simplex (oral, genital, or paronychial), and herpes zoster. 2. Conditions that are transmitted from infants to personnel are a. Rubella—Obtain rubella titers from women of childbearing age; if a protective level is not present, vaccination should be carried out. b. Cytomegalovirus—CMV is a potential threat to pregnant women. Adherence to good infection control practices may reduce this threat. c. Hepatitis B is usually not a major problem in the NICU, since host infants are not infectious in the early neonatal period. An effective vaccine is available and may be considered for high-risk individuals. (See Tables 16-2 and 16-3.)
Cohorting	
Cohorting is an important infection control measure used primarily during outbreaks or epidemics in the NICU. The object of cohorting is to limit the number of contacts of one infant with other infants and personnel.	1. Group together infants born within the same time frame (usually 24-48 hr) or who are colonized or infected with the same pathogen. These infants should remain together until discharged. 2. Provide nursing care by personnel who do not care for other infants. 3. After all infants in cohort are discharged, clean room before admittance of a new group of infants.

TABLE 16-5

Infection Control Measures and Isolation Techniques for Specific Diseases

DISEASE/ ORGANISM	RECOMMENDED PRECAUTIONS						INFECTIVE MATERIAL	DURATION OF ISOLATION/ PRECAUTION	COMMENTS
	HAND WASHING	PRIVATE ROOM OR COHORT	MASK	GOWN	GLOVES				
AIDS/HIV	X	D	No	(X)	(X)	Blood and body fluids	Duration of illness	Utmost care needed to avoid needle sticks
Adenovirus	X	X	No	(X)	No	Respiratory secretions and feces	Duration of hospitalization	During outbreaks cohort patients suspected of having adenovirus infection
Conjunctivitis Gonococcal (Ophthalmia neonatorum)	X	X	No	No	(X)	Purulent exudate	Until 24 hours after initiation of effective therapy	
Chlamydia	X	No	No	No	(X)	Purulent exudate	Duration of illness	
Coxsackievirus	X	D	No	(X)	(X)	Feces and respiratory secretions	7 days after onset	
Cytomegalovirus	X	No	No	No	(X)	Urine and respiratory secretions	Duration of illness	Counsel pregnant personnel
Diarrhea	X	D	No	(X)	(X)	Feces	Duration of illness	Identify colonized or infected infants by culture; institute cohorting
ECHO virus	X	D	No	(X)	(X)	Feces and respiratory secretions	For 7 days after onset of illness	
Gastroenteritis	X	X	No	(X)	(X)	Feces	Duration of illness	
Hepatitis Type A	X	D	No	(X)	(X)	Feces	For 7 days after onset of illness	
Type B	X	No	No	(X)	(X)	Blood and body fluids	Duration of positivity	Most contagious before symptoms Avoid needle sticks
Herpes simplex	X	X	No	(X)	(X)	Lesions, secretions, urine, and stool	Duration of illness	

X, Recommended at all times; (X), recommended if soiling is likely, or if touching infective materials; D, desirable but optional.

Continued.

TABLE 16-5—cont'd

Infection Control Measures and Isolation Techniques for Specific Diseases

DISEASE/ ORGANISM	RECOMMENDED PRECAUTIONS					INFECTIVE MATERIAL	DURATION OF ISOLATION/ PRECAUTION	COMMENTS
	HAND WASHING	PRIVATE ROOM OR COHORT	MASK	GOWN	GLOVES			
Influenza A or B	X	X	No	(X)	(X)	Respiratory secretions	Duration of illness	Cohort patient suspected of having influenza during outbreak; staff should receive yearly influenza vaccine
Meningitis								
Aseptic	X	D	No	(X)	(X)	Feces	Duration of illness	
Bacterial	X	No	No	No	No			Cohort colonized or infected infants during a nursery outbreak
Necrotizing enterocolitis	X	No	No	(X)	(X)	(?) Feces	Duration of illness	Cohort ill infants
Respiratory syncytial virus	X	X	X	(X)	(X)	Respiratory secretions	Duration of illness	Cohort suspect infants, especially premature infants, during outbreaks

Disease						Infective material	Duration of precautions	Comments
Rubella	X	X	X	No	No	Respiratory secretions	Duration of hospitalization	Infants may shed virus for as long as 2 years; seronegative women should avoid contact
Staphylococcal disease (S. aureus)	X	D	No	(X)	(X)	Purulent exudate	Duration of illness	
Streptococcal disease Group A	X	D	No	(X)	(X)	Respiratory secretions	24 hours after initiation of effective therapy	
Group B	X	D	No	(X)	(X)	Respiratory and genital secretions		Cohort ill and colonized infants during a nursery outbreak
Syphilis	X	No	No	No	(X)	Lesion secretions and blood	24 hours after start of effective therapy	
Toxoplasmosis	X	No	No	No	No		None	
Varicella	X	X	X	X	X	Respiratory and lesion secretions	Until lesions are crusted	Neonates born to mothers with active chickenpox should be placed on isolation precautions at birth; persons who are not susceptible do not need to mask

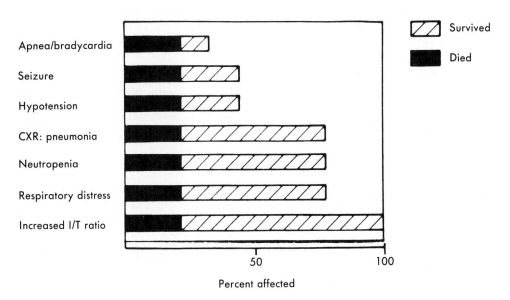

Figure 16-1. Clinical and laboratory findings in nine infants with signs and symptoms of early-onset group B streptococcal disease. (From Nelson SN et al: J Perinatol 6:234, 1986.)

TABLE 16-6

Normal Cerebrospinal Fluid Values in Neonates

	WHITE BLOOD CELLS	POLYMORPHONUCLEAR NEUTROPHILIC (LEUKOCYTES)	PROTEIN (mg/dl)	GLUCOSE (mg/dl)
Premature infants				
Reported means	2-27		75-150	79-83
Reported ranges	0-112		31-292	64-106
Term infants				
Reported means	3-5	2-3	47-67	51-55
Reported ranges	0-90	0-70	17-240	32-78

Modified from Remington JS and Klein JO, editors: Infectious diseases of the fetus and newborn infant, ed 2, Philadelphia, 1983, WB Saunders Co.

ticularly of early-onset disease, are nonspecific and nonlocalizing. Symptoms include temperature instability (hypothermia and/or hyperthermia), respiratory distress (apnea, cyanosis, and tachypnea), lethargy, feeding abnormality (vomiting, increased residuals, and abdominal distention), jaundice (particularly increased direct fraction), seizures, or purpura (Figure 16-1).

Laboratory data. Isolating bacteria from a nonpermissive site (blood, CSF, urine, closed body space) is the most valid method of establishing the diagnosis of bacterial sepsis. Surface cultures (including ear and gastric aspirates) do not establish the presence of active systemic infection but merely indicate colonization. Bacterial antigens or endotoxins may be demonstrated in sera, CSF, urine, or body fluids by a variety of methods (counter immunoelectrophoresis, latex agglutination, and limulus lysate test). Such a demonstration is not totally definitive, nor does it allow determination of the antibiotic sensitivity of the offending organism. The CSF is examined in most infants suspected of sepsis, since meningitis is a frequent manifestation of sepsis in the neonate (Table 16-6).

Several laboratory aids are used in assessing neonatal sepsis, but it must be realized that these tests are nonspecific and occasionally may be misleading. They include the complete blood count (CBC), in which abnormalities in absolute neutrophil count, absolute band count, band/neutrophil ratio, and platelet count may be associated with bacterial sepsis (Figures 16-2 to 16-5). Acute-phase reactants, including C-reactive protein, fibrinogen, haptoglobin, and erythrocyte sedimentation rates, are occasionally useful adjunct tests clinically, and chest x-ray examination and x-ray evaluation of specific indicated areas may also help.

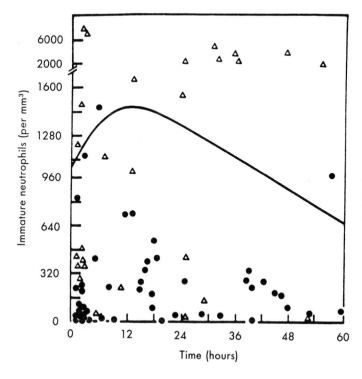

Figure 16-2. Total immature neutrophil counts during first 60 hours of life in infants with sepsis (△) and those delivered of women with pregnancy-induced hypertension (●). (From Engle WD and Rosenfeld CR: J Pediatr 105:982, 1984.)

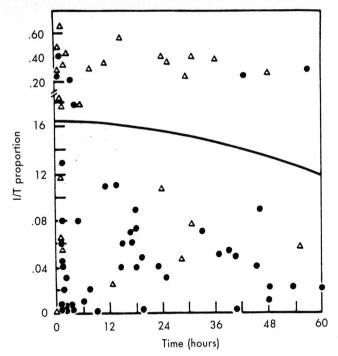

Figure 16-3. Immature to total neutrophil proportion during first 60 hours of life in infants with sepsis (△) and those delivered of women with pregnancy-induced hypertension (●). (From Engle WD and Rosenfeld CR: J Pediatr 105:982, 1984.)

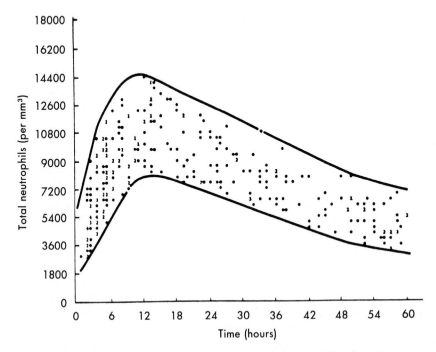

Figure 16-4. Total neutrophil count reference range in first 60 hours of life. Heavy lines represent envelope bounding these data. (From Manroe BL et al: J Pediatr 95:89, 1979.)

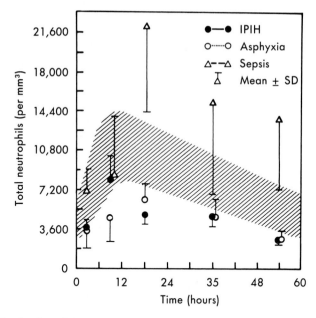

Figure 16-5. Distribution of absolute total neutrophil counts in first 60 hours of life in infants with sepsis (*n* = 13), asphyxia neonatorum (*n* = 12), and those delivered of women with pregnancy-induced hypertension (*IPIH*) (*n* = 20). (From Engle WD and Rosenfeld CR: J Pediatr 105:982, 1984.)

Several other nonspecific laboratory abnormalities may accompany neonatal sepsis, including hypoglycemia, hypocalcemia, thrombocytopenia, and unexplained metabolic acidosis.

TREATMENT

Antibiotics are the cornerstone of the treatment for presumed or confirmed infections in neonates. The indiscriminate or inappropriate use of systemic antibiotics may cause undesirable side effects, may favor the emergence of resistant strains of bacteria, and may alter the normal flora of the newborn.

Adequate and appropriate specimens for culture should be obtained before antibiotic therapy is initiated. Broad-spectrum antibiotic coverage, usually with ampicillin and an aminoglycoside, is commonly initiated pending culture and sensitivity results. Once causative organisms are identified and antibiotic sensitivities established, the most appropriate and least toxic antibiotic or antibiotic combination should be continued for an appropriate period by a suitable route. If adequate cultures are negative after a reasonable period (48 to 72 hours), antibiotic therapy may be discontinued in most situations.

It is important to realize that antibiotics are not the entire solution to treating the infected newborn. Meticulous attention to the treatment of associated conditions such as shock, hypoxemia, thermal abnormalities, electrolyte or acid-base imbalance, adequate nutrition, anemia, drainage of pus, and removal of foreign bodies may be as important as choosing the proper antibiotic. Intravenous immune gamma globulin (IVIGG), 500 mg/kg, especially in the severely neutropenic patient, may be a useful adjunct to antibiotic treatment.

Table 16-7 provides guidelines for choosing

TABLE 16-7

Recommended Therapy for Indicated Conditions

CONDITION	TREATMENT*
Sepsis and/or meningitis	(Value of exchange or granulocyte transfusion for sepsis is controversial)
Initial therapy	IV ampicillin and gentamicin or IV amikacin (If gentamicin-resistant organisms are present in nursery, ampicillin plus cefotaxime is a suitable alternative, particularly if meningitis is present.)
Once specific organisms are identified	
Group B streptococci	IV ampicillin and gentamicin for 14-21 days (Gentamicin may be discontinued if strain is not tolerant.)
Coliform species	IV ampicillin and gentamicin for 21 days (Cefotaxime may replace gentamicin.)
Listeria monocytogenes	IV ampicillin and IV gentamicin for 14-21 days
Enterococci	Same as for *Listeria monocytogenes*
Group A streptococci	IV penicillin G for 14-21 days
Group D streptococci (nonenterococcal)	Same as for group A streptococci
Staphylococcus aureus	IV methicillin for 14-21 days; IV vancomycin for methicillin-resistant strains
Staphylococcus epidermidis	IV vancomycin for 14-21 days
Pseudomonas aeruginosa	IV mezlocillin and IV gentamicin for 14-21 days
Anaerobes	IV chloramphenicol if levels can be monitored (Levels should be in 20-25 μg/ml range.) or IV clindamycin
Pneumonia	
Group B streptococci	Same as for sepsis (Hyaline membrane disease may mimic pneumonitis and vice versa.)
Staphylococcus aureus	Same as for sepsis
Chlamydia trachomatis	PO erythromycin for 14 days
Pneumocystis carinii	PO or IV trimethoprim and sulfamethoxazole or IV pentamidine isethionate
Pertussis	PO erythromycin for 14 days (Clinical course is unchanged but shedding of organism is diminished significantly.)
Other organisms	Same as for sepsis
Skin and soft tissue infections	
Impetigo	IV methicillin or PO dicloxacillin for 7 days (depending on clinical severity)
Group A streptococcal infections	IV penicillin G for 7 days
Breast abscess	IV methicillin and gentamicin for 7 days pending identification of etiologic agent (Change to IV penicillin if *Streptococcus* is etiologic.) (IV ampicillin and/or gentamicin should be used for *Coliform* species pending sensitivities.); value of surgical drainage is individualized
Omphalitis and/or funisitis	IV methicillin for 7 days (Penicillin may be used if infection is caused by group A or B streptococci.)

Modified from Nelson JD: Pocketbook of pediatric antimicrobial therapy, ed 5, Dallas, 1983, Jodone Publishing Co.
*See Table 16-8 for dosages.

TABLE 16-7—cont'd

Recommended Therapy for Indicated Conditions

CONDITION	TREATMENT*
Gastrointestinal infections	
Salmonella species	IV ampicillin for 7-10 days, IV chloramphenicol for 7-10 days, or IV genta-micin for 7-10 days depending on sensitivities (Focal complications of meningitis and arthritis should be monitored closely.)
Shigella species	PO trimethoprim/sulfamethoxazole or PO or IV ampicillin depending on sensitivities
Enteropathogenic *E. coli*	PO colistin, 10-15 mg/kg/day divided q.8h., for 5-7 days
Necrotizing enterocolitis	IV ampicillin and IV gentamicin for 2-3 weeks (If *Pseudomonas* is isolated, IV mezlocillin may be substituted for ampicillin.); supportive measures (gastrointestinal suction) are appropriate
Osteomyelitis or septic arthritis	
Group B streptococci	IV penicillin G for 21 days minimum
Staphylococcus aureus	IV methicillin for 21 days minimum
Coliform species	IV gentamicin for 21 days minimum (IV ampicillin for 21 days minimum if organism is sensitive)
Gonococcus species	IV penicillin G for 10 days
Unknown	IV methicillin and gentamicin for 21 days minimum
Urinary tract infections	Suspect predisposing anatomic defect if urinary tract infection; individualize workup and follow-up
Coliform species	Gentamicin, 3 mg/kg/day divided q.8h., for 10 days
Enterococcus species	Ampicillin, 30 mg/kg/day divided q.8h., for 10 days
Miscellaneous conditions	
"STORCH" infections	
Congenital syphilis	
Without CNS involvement	IM benzathine penicillin for 1-3 doses spaced weekly (Follow-up VDRL tests should revert to negative if treatment is adequate by 1 year.)
With CNS involvement	Parenterally penicillin G, 50,000 units/kg/day, for 10 days
Toxoplasmosis	PO sulfadiazine, 100-120 mg/kg/day divided q.6h., and PO pyrimethamine, 1 mg/kg/day divided q.12h. (Length of treatment is debatable but should be lengthy [i.e., months]. Supplemental folic acid, 1 mg/day, should be added.)
Herpes simplex infections	IV adenine arabinoside, 25 mg/kg/day as 12 hr infusion, for 10 days or IV acyclovir, 30 mg/kg/day as 1 hr infusion divided q.8h., for 10 days
Conjunctivitis	
Chlamydia species	PO erythromycin for 10 days (topical may be ineffective)
Gonococcus species	IV penicillin G for 10 days; cefoxitin for penicillin-resistant strains
Otitis media	
In otherwise normal neonate	PO amoxicillin/clavulinic acid (Augmentin), 40 mg/kg
In neonate with nosocomial infection	PO or IV ampicillin and IV gentamicin (If there is no response to treatment, consider diagnostic tympanocentesis. *S. aureus* and *Coliform* species may be present.)

TABLE 16-8

Antibiotic Dosages for Neonates

ANTIBIOTIC	ROUTE	DAILY DOSAGE AND INTERVALS	
		<7 DAYS OF AGE	>7 DAYS OF AGE
Amikacin sulfate	IV, IM	15 mg/kg/day divided q.12h.	15-22.5 mg/kg/day divided q.8-12h.
Amoxicillin	PO	50 mg/kg/day divided q.12h.	50 mg/kg/day divided q.8h.
Amoxicillin/clavulinic acid	PO	Not recommended	40 mg/kg/day divided q.8h.
Amphotericin B*	IV	0.1 mg/kg over 6 hr infusion initially, increase to 1 mg/kg/day in small increments	Same
Ampicillin			
Meningitis	IV	100 mg/kg/day divided q.12h.	150-200 mg/kg/day divided q.6-8h.
Other indications	IV, IM, PO	50 mg/kg/day divided q.12h.	75 mg/kg/day divided q.8h.
Carbenicillin	IV, IM	200 mg/kg/day divided q.12h.	300-400 mg/kg/day divided q.6-8h.
Cefazolin*	IV, IM	40 mg/kg/day divided q.12h.	40 mg/kg/day divided q.12h.
Cefotaxime	IV, IM	100 mg/kg/day divided q.12h.	150 mg/kg/day divided q.8h.
Cefoxitin	IV	15 mg/kg divided q.8h.	30 mg/kg divided q.6h.
Chloramphenicol succinate (not recommended unless serum concentrations are monitored)	IV, PO	25 mg/kg once daily	25-50 mg/kg/day divided q.12-24h.
Clindamycin*	IV, PO	25 mg/kg divided q.8h.	25-40 mg/kg divided q.6h.
Colistin	PO	4 mg/kg divided q.6h.	Same
Dicloxacillin*	PO	25 mg/kg twice daily	25 mg/kg divided q.8h.
Erythromycin estolate	PO	20 mg/kg/day divided q.12h.	20-30 mg/kg/day divided q.8-12h.
Gentamicin	IV, IM	5 mg/kg/day divided q.12h.	7.5 mg/kg/day divided q.8h.
Kanamycin	IV, IM	15-20 mg/kg/day divided q.12h.	20-30 mg/kg/day divided q.8-12h.
Methicillin	IV, IM	50-75 mg/kg/day divided q.8-12h.	100-150 mg/kg/day divided q.6-8h.
Metronidazole	IV, PO	15 mg/kg loading dose; then 15 mg/kg/day divided q.12h.	Same
Moxalactam	IV, IM	100 mg/kg/day divided q.12h.	150 mg/kg/day divided q.8h.
Nafcillin	IV	40 mg/kg/day divided q.12h.	60-80 mg/kg/day divided q.6-8h.
Neomycin	PO	25 mg/kg divided q.6h.	Same
Nystatin	PO	400,000 units/day divided q.6h.	Same
Mezlocillin	IV, IM	150-225 mg/kg/day divided q.8-12h.	225-300 mg/kg/day divided q.6-8h.
Penicillin G			
Meningitis	IV	100,000-150,000 units/kg/day divided q.8-12h.	150,000-250,000 units/kg/day divided q.6-8h.
Other indications	IV	50,000 units/kg/day divided q.12h.	75,000 units/kg/day divided q.6-8h.
Penicillin G, benzathine	IM	50,000 units/kg (1 dose only)	Same
Penicillin G, procaine	IM	50,000 units/kg/day once daily	Same
Pentamidine isethionate*	IV	4 mg/kg/day for 14 days (Available from CDC, Atlanta, Ga.)	Same
Ticarcillin	IV, IM	150-225 mg/kg/day divided q.8-12h.	225-300 mg/kg/day divided q.6-8h.
Tobramycin	IV, IM	4 mg/kg/day divided q.12h.	6 mg/kg/day divided q.8h.
Trimethoprim/ sulfamethoxazole (TMP/SMX)	IV, PO	10-20 mg/kg/day TMP or 50-100 kg/day SMX	Same
Vancomycin	IV	30 mg/kg/day divided q.12h.	45 mg/kg/day divided q.8h.

*Pharmacokinetics in newborns are not well characterized. These drugs should be used with extra caution in neonates (pediatric infectious disease consultation recommended).

TABLE 16-9

Passage of Antibiotics across the Placenta*

% ANTIBIOTIC IN INDICATED CATEGORY	ANTIBIOTIC
Equal to serum concentration	Amoxicillin
	Ampicillin
	Carbenicillin
	Chloramphenicol
	Methicillin
	Nitrofurantoin
	Penicillin G
	Sulfonamides
	Tetracyclines
	Trimethoprim
50% of serum concentration	Aminoglycosides (exceptions below)
10%-15% of serum concentration	Amikacin
	Cephalosporins
	Clindamycin
	Nafcillin
	Tobramycin
Negligible (less than 10% of serum concentration)	Dicloxacillin
	Erythromycin

*Several factors determine the degree of transfer of antibiotics across the placenta, including lipid solubility, degree of ionization, molecular weight, protein binding, placental maturation, and placental and fetal blood flow.

TABLE 16-10

Passage of Antibiotics into Breast Milk*

% ANTIBIOTIC IN INDICATED CATEGORY	ANTIBIOTIC
Equal to serum concentration	Isoniazid
	Metronidazole
	Sulfonamides
	Trimethoprim
50% of serum concentration	Chloramphenicol
	Erythromycin
	Tetracyclines
Less than 25% of serum concentration	Cefazolin
	Kanamycin
	Nitrofurantoin
	Oxacillin
	Penicillin G
	Penicillin V

*Data on concentrations of antibiotics in human breast milk are sparse. Since most antibiotics are present in breast milk in microgram amounts, they are normally not ingested by the infant in therapeutic amounts.

the proper antibiotic for indicated conditions; Table 16-8 gives the proper dose, route, and frequency of administration of commonly used antibiotics in the newborn nursery. Table 16-9 describes the passage of antibiotics across the placenta, and Table 16-10 describes their passage into breast milk.

COMPLICATIONS

Transplacental infections often result in fetal abnormality or death. Newborns who survive may have long-term sequelae such as developmental, neurologic, motor, sensory, growth, and physical abnormalities.

Before antibiotic use, the mortality from bacterial sepsis was 95% to 100%, but antibiotics and supportive care have reduced the mortality to less than 50%. Debilitated infants (preterm and sick neonates) are at greater risk and have a higher incidence of sepsis than term, healthy neonates. The most common complications of bacterial sepsis are meningitis and septic shock. The outcome is influenced by early recognition and vigorous treatment with appropriate antibiotics and supportive care.

FUNGAL INFECTION

Fungal infections in neonates can cause significant morbidity and mortality. They are usually seen in very low birth weight (VLBW) infants, infants with congenital anomalies requiring surgery, and/or who require multiple or prolonged vascular catheters.

PREVENTION. Since these infants are often colonized at birth, strict adherence to aseptic technique when dealing with central catheters is essential. Antibiotic use should be minimized and limited to treatment of specific illnesses.

DATA COLLECTION

History. VLBW infants, infants requiring surgery, and/or infants requiring invasive procedures such as arterial or venous catheters are at increased risk for fungal infection. The use of lipids increases the risk for infection with lipophilic organisms.

TABLE 16-11

Antifungal Therapy

DRUG	DOSAGE	COMMENTS
Amphotericin B	0.1 to 1 mg/kg/day IV; begin at 0.1 mg/kg and increase daily as tolerated	Nephrotoxic
5-Fluorocytosine (5-FC)	50 to 100 mg/kg/day PO, q.6h.	Hepatotoxic; bone marrow suppression

Signs and symptoms. These may be nonspecific, nonlocalizing, and difficult to differentiate from infants with bacterial sepsis.

Laboratory data. Routine laboratory data, like clinical signs and symptoms, are rarely helpful in differentiating fungal from bacterial infection. Positive cultures from urine or blood indicate systemic infection. Tracheal cultures may be helpful in infants with acquired pneumonia. Urine and buffy coat smear of blood from central catheters should be examined for evidence of budding yeast.

TREATMENT. The treatment of fungal infection will vary from infant to infant. Some infants will respond to simple interventions such as stopping broad-spectrum antibiotics, stopping lipid infusions, or removal of central catheters. Others will require treatment with antifungal agents such as amphotericin B and/ or 5 fluorocytosine (5-FC) (Table 16-11).

PARENT TEACHING

Parents who have infants with viral or bacterial infection require support and information regarding their infant's condition. Questions arise regarding treatment and prognosis, as well as possible long-range effects of the infection. Parents experience significant guilt feelings based on misperceptions regarding what role they had in causing the infection. Health care professionals need to remain sensitive to the crisis that parents are experiencing and address the issues of etiology as well as treatment and prognosis. Valid and factual data as well as information regarding complications and long-term effects should be shared with parents in a timely manner.

Controlling infection in the nursery is of prime importance but does not include excluding the parents from caring for their sick baby. Proper hand washing, gowning, and isolation techniques must be adhered to by everyone. Educating the parents and siblings about the importance of these procedures, along with appropriate reminders, ensures cooperation. With proper precautions, there is no evidence of increased incidence of infection with parent and sibling visits.

All those entering the nursery must be screened for the presence of illness. Anyone with a fever, respiratory symptoms (cough, runny nose, sore throat), gastrointestinal symptoms (nausea, vomiting, diarrhea), or skin lesions should not come in contact with the infant. People with communicable disease (e.g., varicella) or recent exposure to a communicable disease also should not come in contact with the sick neonate.

Daily cord care should be demonstrated, and a return demonstration by the parents should be observed before discharging the infant. Every parent should be taught the signs and symptoms of neonatal illness, because early recognition of signs and symptoms expedites' prompt treatment. Parents must be taught to take axillary temperatures and to read a ther-

mometer. They need to be aware that both hypothermia and hyperthermia may be signs of neonatal illness.

SELECTED READINGS

American Academy of Pediatrics: Report of the Committee on infectious disease, ed 20, Oak Grove Village, Ill, 1986, American Academy of Pediatrics.

American Academy of Pediatrics and American College of Obstetricians and Gynecologists: Guidelines for perinatal care, ed 2, Oak Grove Village, Ill, 1988, American Academy of Pediatrics.

American Academy of Pediatrics Task Force on AIDS: Perinatal HIV infection (AIDS), Pediatrics 82:941, 1988.

Arevelo JA and Washington AE: Cost-effectiveness of prenatal screening and immunization for hepatitis B virus, JAMA 259:365, 1988.

Ascuitto RJ et al: Buffy coat smears of blood drawn through central venous catheters as an aid to rapid diagnosis of systemic fungal infection, J Pediatr 106:445, 1985.

Bailey JE, Kliegman RM, and Fanaroff AA: Disseminated fungal infections in VLBW infants, Pediatrics 73:144, 1984.

Bailey JE et al: Disseminated fungal infections in VLBW infants: therapeutic toxicity, Pediatrics 73:153, 1984.

Bailey JE et al: Fungal colonization in the low birth weight infant, Pediatrics 78:225, 1986.

Boyer KM and Gotoff SP: Prevention of early-onset group B streptococcal disease with selected intrapartum chemoprophylaxis, N Engl J Med 314:1665, 1986.

Brown ZA et al: Effects on infants of a first episode of genital herpes during pregnancy, N Engl J Med 317:1246, 1987.

Burch SM and Chadwick JV: Use of a retroset in the delivery of intravenous medications in the neonate, Neonatal Network 6:51, 1987.

Centers for Disease Control: Guideline for isolation precautions, ed 4, Washington, DC, 1983, US Government Printing Office.

Centers for Disease Control: Classification system for HIV infection in children under 13 years of age, MMWR 36:225, 1987.

Centers for Disease Control: HIV infection in the United States, MMWR 36:801, 1987.

Centers for Disease Control: Update: serologic testing for antibody to HIV, MMWR 36:833, 1988.

Christensen RD et al: Fatal early onset group B streptococcal sepsis with normal leukocyte counts, Pediatr Infect Dis 4:242, 1985.

Engle WD and Rosenfeld CR: Neutropenia in high-risk neonates, J Pediatr 105:982, 1984.

Fischer GW et al: Intravenous immunoglobulin in neonatal group B streptococcal disease, Am J Med 76:117, 1984.

Garner JS and Simmons BP: Guidelines for isolation precautions in hospitals, Infect Control 4(suppl):245, 1983.

Gotoff SP: Immunoprophylaxis and immunotherapy of neonatal group B streptococcal infections, Infection 13(suppl 2):s230, 1985.

Hargrove C: Administration of intravenous medications in the NICU: the development of a procedure, Neonatal Network 6:51, 1987.

Hoff R et al: Seroprevalence of human immunodeficiency virus among childbearing women, N Engl J Med 318:525, 1988.

Kim KS: Efficacy of human immunoglobulin and penicillin G in treatment of experimental group B streptococcal infection, Pediatr Res 21:289, 1987.

Landesman S et al: Serosurvey of HIV infection in parturients, JAMA 258:2701, 1987.

Lepage P et al: Postnatal transmission of HIV from mother to child, Lancet 1:1980, 1987.

Lifson AR: Do alternate modes for transmission of human immunodeficiency virus exist? A review, JAMA 259:1353, 1988.

Long JG and Keyserling HL: Catheter-related infection in infants due to an unusual lipophilic yeast—*Malassezia furfur*, Pediatrics 76:896, 1985.

Manroe BL et al: The neonatal blood count in health and disease. I. Reference values for neutrophilic cells, J Pediatr 95:89, 1979.

Merenstein GB et al: Group B beta hemolytic streptococcus: randomized controlled treatment study at term, Obstet Gynecol 55:315, 1980.

Mok J et al: Infants born to mother seropositive for HIV, Lancet 1:1164, 1987.

Nelson SN, Merenstein GB, and Pierce JR: Early onset group B streptococcal disease, J Perinatol 6:234, 1986.

Pierce JR, Merenstein GB, and Stocker JT: Immediate postpartum cultures in an intensive care nursery, Pediatr Infect Dis 3:510, 1984.

Prober CG et al: Low risk of herpes simplex virus in neonates exposed to the virus at the time of vaginal delivery to mothers with recurrent genital herpes simplex virus infection, N Engl J Med 316:240, 1987.

Wittek AE et al: Asymptomatic shedding of herpes simplex virus from the cervix and lesion site during pregnancy: correlation of antepartum shedding with shedding at delivery, Am J Dis Child 138:439, 1984.

Wong VCW et al: Prevention of the HBsAg carrier state in the newborn infants of mothers who are chronic carriers of HBsAg and HBeAg by administration of hepatitis-B vaccine and hepatitis-B immunoglobulin, Lancet 1:921, 1984.

PART IV

Common Systemic Diseases of the Neonate

CHAPTER 17

Respiratory diseases

MARY I. HAGEDORN · SANDRA L. GARDNER · STEVEN H. ABMAN

Despite the marked improvement in the outcome of premature newborns with respiratory distress over the past decade, significant mortality and high morbidity persist. Much of the improvement in neonatal mortality has been the result of successful treatment and management of respiratory diseases in the neonate. An overview of some of the common respiratory diseases, their treatments, and outcomes are presented in this chapter. General principles and concepts related to respiratory physiology, etiology, and symptomatology are presented, followed by specific disease processes. The chapter also includes current management of these disease processes.

GENERAL PHYSIOLOGY

Any discussion of general respiratory physiology must include some elements of anatomy and embryology and their significance to the clinician (Table 17-1).

Surface-active compounds such as phosphatidylcholine and phosphatidylglycerol stabilize the alveoli. Surface tension forces act on air-fluid interfaces. Surface tension causes a water droplet to "bead up." The surface-active compound (e.g., soap added to a water droplet) reduces the surface tension and allows the droplet to spread out in a thin film. In the lung surface tension forces tend to cause alveoli to collapse. A compound such as surfactant reduces surface tension and allows the alveoli to remain open.

The situation, however, is more complicated than just described. LaPlace detailed the magnitude of the pressure (P) exerted at the surface of an air-liquid interface as equaling twice the surface tension (st) divided by the radius (r) of curvature of the surface $\left(P = \dfrac{2\,st}{r}\right)$. In the absence of surfactant an alveolus with a small radius of curvature has a greater magnitude of pressure at its surface (tending to collapse it) than does an alveolus with a larger radius of curvature. Therefore smaller alveoli would tend to collapse and empty contained gas into larger alveoli.

Surfactant is a substance that modifies surface tension. It decreases surface tension when the radius of curvature is small and increases surface tension when the radius of curvature is greater. An alveolus with a larger radius of curvature has a greater than expected pressure (tending to reduce its volume), and an alveolus with a smaller radius of curvature has less than expected pressure. Therefore the alveoli are stabilized at a uniform radius of curvature (uniform volume).

Surfactant provides a number of useful properties in addition to reducing surface tension, which increases lung compliance, provides alveolar stability, and decreases opening pressure. It also enhances alveolar fluid clearance, decreases precapillary tone, and plays a protective role for the epithelial cell surface. Surfactant is constantly being formed, stored, secreted, and recycled. Conditions that interfere with surfactant metabolism include acidemia, hypoxia, shock, overinflation, underinflation, pulmonary edema, mechanical ventilation, and hypercapnia. Surfactant production is delayed in infants of diabetic mothers in classes of A, B,

TABLE 17-1

Lung Development

STAGE AND MAJOR EVENTS	SIGNIFICANCE
Embryonic (up to 5 weeks) Single ventral outpocketing quickly divides into two lung buds. Mesenchyme surrounds endodermal lung buds, which continue to divide and extend into the mesenchyme. Branching of the airways begins.	Airways begin to differentiate. Branching anomalies (i.e., pulmonary agenesis and sequestered lobe) occur early in fetal life.
Pulmonary arteries invade lung tissue, following the airways, and divide as the airways divide. Pulmonary veins arise independently from the lung parenchyma and return to the left atrium, thus completing the pulmonary circuit.	
Pseudoglandular (5-16 weeks) Progressive airway branching begins. Bronchi and terminal bronchioles form. Muscle fibers, elastic tissue, and early cartilage formation can be seen along the tracheobronchial tree. Mucous glands are found at 12 weeks and increase in number until 25-26 weeks, when cilia begin to develop. Diaphragm develops.	All subdivisions that will form airways are complete by the sixteenth week. Herniation of the diaphragm occurs.
Cannicular (13-25 weeks) Airway changes from glandular to tubular and increases in length and diameter.	Air conducting portion (bronchi and terminal bronchioli) continues luminal development.
20 weeks Fetal airways end in blind pouches lined with cuboid epithelium. A relatively large amount of interstitial mesenchyme is present. Few pulmonary capillaries are present, and they are not closely associated with the respiratory epithelium.	
22-24 weeks Rapid proliferation of the pulmonary capillary bed, an increase of the surface area of the respiratory epithelium, and formation of alveolar ducts and sacculi occur.	Development of the gas exchange portion (the respiratory bronchi and alveolar ducts) begins. Pulmonary vasculature develops most rapidly.
Respiratory epithelium contains cells that become differentiated into type I and type II pneumocytes. Type I pneumocytes produce an extremely thin squamous epithelial layer that lines the alveoli and fuses to the underlying capillary endothelial cells.	By the late fetal period the resulting membrane between the alveoli and capillaries allows sufficient gas exchange to support independent life.
Type II pneumocytes (cuboid cells) are the site of surfactant synthesis and storage.	At 22 weeks surface-active phospholipid (lecithin) can first be detected.

TABLE 17-1—cont'd

Lung Development

STAGE AND MAJOR EVENTS	SIGNIFICANCE
Terminal (24-40 weeks) Lung differentiation: proliferation of the pulmonary vascular bed, creation of new respiratory units (alveolar ducts and alveoli), decrease in amount of interstitial mesenchyme, and fusion of the gas exchange epithelium to the pulmonary capillary epithelium occur.	Before this time the fetal lungs are incapable of supporting adequate gas exchange because of insufficient alveolar surface area and inadequate pulmonary vasculature.
34-36 weeks Phosphatidylglycerol appears, and a dramatic increase in the principal surfactant compound phosphatidylcholine occurs.	Adequate amounts of surface-active material protects against the development of idiopathic respiratory distress syndrome.
Alveolar (postnatal lung development) late fetal life to 8-10 years of age At term the number of airways is complete. There is sufficient respiratory surface for gaseous exchange, and the pulmonary capillary bed is sufficient to carry the gases that have been exchanged.	Although the infant is capable of sustaining respiratory effort and the lung is able to provide oxygenation and ventilation at birth, lung development is still incomplete.
Alveoli continue to increase in number, size, and shape. They enlarge and become deeper to maximize the exposed surface area for gas exchange.	Ongoing lung development implies that infants who have suffered severe lung disease at birth need not become lifelong pulmonary cripples.

and C; infants with erythroblastosis fetalis; and infants who are the smaller of twins. Surfactant production is accelerated in:

1. Infants of diabetic mothers of classes D, F, and R
2. Infants of heroin-addicted mothers
3. Premature rupture of membranes of greater than 48 hours duration
4. Infants of mothers with hypertension
5. Infants subjected to maternal infection
6. Infants suffering from placental insufficiency
7. Infants affected by administration of betamethasone or thyroid hormone to the mother
8. Infants affected by abruptio placentae

The fetal lung is filled with a volume of liquid (20 to 30 ml/kg) equal to the functional residual capacity. This fluid is not amniotic fluid but rather a liquid that has been produced in the lung and discharged through the larynx and mouth into the amniotic fluid. Lung fluid is continuously produced at a rate of approximately 2 to 4 ml/kg/hr.

Because of the movement of lung fluid and its components (notably lecithin) into amniotic fluid, the lecithin/sphingomyelin (L/S) ratio has become a notable clinical tool. Noting a sharp increase in the L/S ratio, Gluck and Kulovich[40] found they could predict infants at risk for idiopathic respiratory distress syndrome (IRDS). In general, L/S ratios of more than 2:1 are not associated with IRDS, whereas ratios of less than 2:1 are associated with it.

During vaginal delivery, approximately one third of the lung fluid may be removed during the thoracic "squeeze" as the infant passes through the birth canal; the remainder of the fluid is removed mainly by the pulmonary lymphatics, although pulmonary capillaries may play a role. During a cesarean section, all of the lung fluid will be removed by the pulmonary lymphatics and capillaries.

The first breath of life, a response to tactile, thermal, chemical, and mechanical stimuli, initiates respiratory effort. The fluid-filled lungs, surface forces, and tissue-sensitive forces are obstacles to the first breath. At birth, gas is substituted for liquid to expand the alveoli. After the alveoli are "opened" during the first few breaths, a film of surface-active material stabilizes the alveoli.

The first breath of life is certainly the most difficult one. During the first breath, a pressure of 60 to 80 cm of water may be required to overcome the effects of the surface tension of the air-liquid interface, particularly the small airways and alveoli. Thus on each subsequent breath less pressure is required to allow for a similar increase in air volume in the lung. The effort of breathing is lessened with subsequent breaths.

GENERAL ETIOLOGY

Respiratory disease may be defined as a progressive impairment of the lungs to exchange gas at the alveolar level. Although the pathologic process causing respiratory disease in the neonate may occur in any portion of the respiratory system (or in other organ systems), the final common pathway in respiratory disease is impairment of gas exchange.

Prematurity is the single most common factor in the occurrence of IRDS. Its incidence is inversely proportioned to gestational age and occurs most frequently in infants of less than 1200 g and 30 weeks gestation. Male infants outnumber female infants 2:1.

The principal factors operating in the development of IRDS in very premature infants are persistence of (or reversion to) the fetal circulatory system and atelectasis. Controversy exists as to which condition exists first. Both conditions tend to perpetuate the other.

Multiple gestations increase the risk of respiratory disease related to lung maturity in the second, third, or more siblings. There is a tendency for the second and subsequent infants to be smaller and suffer perinatal asphyxia. Grand multiparity is associated with increased risk of respiratory disease, particularly when other siblings have had IRDS.

Prenatal maternal complications increase the risk for respiratory disease in the infant. Maternal illnesses such as cardiorespiratory disease, hypoxia, hemorrhage, shock, hypotension, or hypertension result in decreased uterine blood flow with subsequent hypoxia or ischemia at the placental level. Severe maternal anemia causes fetal cardiac depression and respiratory depression. Maternal diabetes may result in preterm delivery because of fetal and maternal indications. There is also a greater incidence of false-positive L/S ratios in diabetic populations. There has been a propensity of infants of diabetic mothers to develop IRDS despite documentation of L/S ratios greater than 2:1. (Despite false-positive readings, the L/S ratio remains the best indication available of fetal lung maturation in all pregnancies.) Abnormal placental conditions (compressed umbilical cord caused by prolapse or breech delivery, placental disease such as infarcts or syphilis, or hemorrhage as a result of placenta previa or abruptio) affect oxygen transfer from mother to fetus and result in an asphyxial insult to the developing fetal lung. Premature rupture of the membranes predisposes the fetus or newborn to the development of infections such as pneumonia, sepsis, or meningitis. Premature or prolonged rupture of the membranes not associated with neonatal infection accelerates fetal lung development and thereby lessens the incidence of IRDS. Prenatal administration of glucocorticoids, maternal toxemia, and maternal heroin addiction also hasten fetal lung maturation.

Factors affecting the fetus during the birthing process may lead to respiratory disease. De-

pression of the respiratory center can be a result of maternal medications that cross the placenta. An infant delivered shortly after administration of maternal analgesia or anesthesia may have only minimal respiratory efforts at birth. Excessive uterine activity, usually as a result of oxytocin induction or augmentation of labor, results in decreased uterine blood flow, late fetal heart rate deceleration, and respiratory depression in the infant at birth. Respiratory disease may be the result of direct trauma to the respiratory center or a cerebral hemorrhage in close proximity to it. Fetal shock caused by difficult labor or dystocia, tight nuchal cord, cerebral hemorrhage, or hemorrhage from the fetal side of the placenta results in central nervous system (CNS) depression and hypoxia. Bleeding results in a generalized hypovolemic condition characterized by decreased oxygen-carrying capacity. Fetal or neonatal asphyxia and blood loss lead to progressive respiratory distress. Delivery by cesarean section prevents one third of the lung fluid from being expelled by the thoracic squeeze of vaginal birth. Thus after cesarean birth all lung fluid must be absorbed through circulatory and lymphatic channels; therefore a greater incidence of transient tachypnea of the newborn may occur as the increased volume of retained fluid is absorbed.

The role of cesarean section in the development of IRDS is still controversial. However, the general consensus is that cesarean section delivery in the absence of fetal distress is not associated with an increased incidence of IRDS. Yet a correlation appears between absence of labor and increased risk of developing IRDS, but the amount of retained lung fluid may be the significant factor.

Obstruction of the airway caused by aspiration of meconium or amniotic fluid occurs either spontaneously at birth or during resuscitative efforts. Although the lungs initially fill with air, subsequent atelectasis occurs as complete airway obstruction prevents further entrance of air. Conversely, a "ball valve" effect or "air-trapping" effect may occur as air is allowed in but is unable to escape because of intermittent obstruction. The presence of amniotic debris, vernix, lanugo, and meconium in the respiratory tract increases the incidence and severity of pulmonary infection. Diaphragmatic paralysis occurs after phrenic nerve injury during birth (usually of a large-for-gestational-age [LGA] infant) and is often associated with Erb's palsy. The paradoxical movement of the paralyzed diaphragm during inspiration and expiration results in inadequate tidal volume and impaired gaseous exchange.

Existing neonatal conditions increase the risk of respiratory disease. Congenital defects that prevent transmission of the stimulus to or from the respiratory center, prevent normal respiratory effort, reduce gas exchange surface area, or hamper the delivery of oxygen to the site of exchange will predispose the infant to respiratory embarrassment. Such defects include heart or great vessel anomalies, diaphragmatic hernia and hypoplastic lung, respiratory tract anomalies (e.g., choanal atresia or tracheoesophageal fistula), chest wall deformities, and CNS defects.

Diseases of the infant can also lead to respiratory disease. Hemolytic disease such as ABO and Rh incompatibility results in anemia and, if severe, in hypovolemic shock. Blood incompatibilities increase respiratory distress by decreasing the oxygen-carrying capacity of the blood. Infections stress the body's systems, increase oxygen requirements, and contribute to an impairment of surfactant production. Chronic lung disease in the form of bronchopulmonary dysplasia (BPD) occurs in 5% to 30% of infants treated with oxygen and mechanical ventilation. Prolonged treatment of IRDS may be necessitated by the severity of the disease but may increase the risk of developing chronic lung disease.

GENERAL PREVENTION
Antepartum

Prevention of respiratory disease begins with prevention of conditions that predispose to respiratory distress. These conditions that constitute "reproductive risks" have been identified and can be categorized as psychosocial, genetic, biophysical, or economic in nature. Once an individual is identified among a high-risk category, comprehensive prenatal care with immediate attention given to maternal complications that arise is crucial (see Chapters 1 and 2).

Intrapartum

Fetal well-being can be assessed by using two tools, electronic monitoring of uterine activity and fetal heart rate and fetal scalp blood sampling. Both enable the practitioner to evaluate how well the fetus withstands the stresses of labor and to make decisions regarding the laboring course.

Electronic fetal heart rate monitoring allows instantaneous fetal heart rate tracings as opposed to the previous method of intermittent evaluation by stethoscope. Fetal heart rate monitoring allows for coincident correlation between uterine contractions and fetal response.

Fetal cardiac response to stress is unlike the older child or adult's response to hypoxia, hypercapnia, and acidosis with tachycardia from sympathetic nervous system discharge. The fetus responds to these same stresses with an initial increase in heart rate. This is quickly followed by bradycardia from parasympathetic stimulation when the hypoxia, hypercapnia, and acidosis persist.

Signs of intrauterine fetal distress include:
1. **Fetal heart rate greater than 160 or less than 100**
2. **Variation from normal fetal heart rhythm (loss of beat-to-beat variability)**
3. **Sudden drop in fetal heart rate between contractions (late deceleration)**
4. **Presence of meconium in vaginal discharge.**

Although there is some controversy regarding normal values of fetal capillary pH, most agree that fetal pH is lower than adult pH and ranges from 7.25 to 7.35.

A pH of 7.20 to 7.24 is considered to show some degree of asphyxia. A fetus with a pH of less than 7.2 is considered to be severely asphyxiated, and immediate treatment or delivery and resuscitation are crucial for fetal viability.

In the absence of severe asphyxia and a requirement for immediate delivery, obstetric maneuvers such as oxygen administration or position changes may be initiated to increase fetal well-being where there is a falling fetal heart rate or capillary pH.

Postpartum

After delivery the infant should be maintained in an environment that minimizes stress and thereby minimizes the oxygen requirement. All infants, but particularly at-risk infants, should be maintained within the narrow parameter of physiologic homeostasis (see Part I).

GENERAL DATA COLLECTION

Since the clinical manifestations of many neonatal illnesses include respiratory symptoms (cardiac, metabolic, neurologic, and hematologic), a systematic and thorough approach to data collection is essential in evaluating an infant in respiratory distress.

History

The perinatal history (antepartum, intrapartum, and postpartum) should be reviewed for risk factors.

Signs and symptoms

Vital signs such as temperature, pulse, respiration, and blood pressure should be checked. Hypothermia and hyperthermia increase oxygen requirements by altering the basal metabolic rate. Hypotension is often associated with respiratory disease.

RESPIRATORY EXAMINATION

Respiratory effort is normally irregular in rate and depth. It is chiefly abdominal, rather than thoracic, with a rate of 30 to 60 breaths/min. Bradypnea is characterized by a rate below 30 breaths/min that is regular (as opposed to periodic or apneic) and may be caused by an insult to the respiratory center of the CNS. Tachypnea, a rate above 60 breaths/min after the first hour of life, is the earliest symptom of respiratory (and often other) diseases. As a compensatory mechanism, tachypnea attempts to maintain alveolar ventilation and gaseous exchange. As a decompensatory mechanism, tachypnea increases oxygen demand, energy output, and the "work" of breathing.

Periodic respirations are cyclic respirations of apnea (5 to 10 seconds) and ventilation (10 to 15 seconds). The average respiratory rate is 30 to 40 breaths/min. Periodic breathing is a common occurrence in small preterm infants as a result of an immature CNS. Apnea is a nonbreathing episode lasting longer than 20 seconds and accompanied by physiologic alterations. The syndrome of apnea is discussed later in this chapter.

Use of accessory muscles of respiration is indicative of a marked increase in the work of breathing. Retractions reflect the inward pull of the thin chest wall on inspiration. Retracting is best observed in relation to the sternum (substernal and suprasternal) and the intercostal, supracostal, and subcostal spaces. The increased negative intrathoracic pressure necessary to ventilate the stiff, noncompliant lung causes the chest wall to retract. This further compromises the lung's expansion. The degree of retraction is directly proportional to the severity of the disease.

Nasal flaring is a compensatory mechanism that attempts to take in more oxygen by increasing the size of the nares and thus decreasing the resistance (by as much as 40%) of the narrow airways. Grunting is forced expiration through a partially closed glottis. The audible grunt may be heard with or without the aid of a stethoscope. As a compensatory mechanism, grunting stabilizes the alveoli by increasing transpulmonary pressure and increases gaseous exchange by delaying expiration.[45]

Color is normally pink after the first breaths of life. Acrocyanosis, peripheral cyanosis of the hands and feet in the first 24 hours of life, is normal. Pallor with poor peripheral circulation may indicate systemic hypotension. Ruddy, plethoric skin color may indicate hyperviscosity or polycythemia, or both, as causes of respiratory symptoms. However, the lack of a deep-red coloring does not rule out polycythemia or hyperviscosity.

Cyanosis, a late and serious sign, is a blue discoloration of the skin, nail beds, and mucous membranes. Differentiation between peripheral cyanosis (of hands and feet) and central cyanosis (of mucous membranes of mouth and generalized body cyanosis) is essential. Since a large decrease in PaO_2 may be tolerated without detectable cyanosis, the lack of cyanosis does not ensure a healthy baby. When hypoxemia reaches a level as to produce frank cyanosis, the insufficiency is usually in advanced stages (see Chapter 8). Therefore cyanosis or its lack is not a reliable sign in the neonate.

Symmetry of the newborn chest is characterized by a relatively round or barrel shape, since the anteroposterior diameter equals the transverse diameter. With prolonged respiratory distress, there is an increase in the anteroposterior diameter, so that the neonate becomes pigeon-chested.

Auscultation of the newborn chest includes comparing and contrasting one side with the other and noting the equality of breath sounds, the presence or absence of rales, rhonchi, or other abnormal sounds. Because of the relatively small size of the newborn's chest, it is hyperresonant, so that breath sounds are widely transmitted. Therefore auscultation cannot always be relied on to detect pathologic conditions (i.e., pneumothorax). Percussion of the chest to determine the presence of air, fluid, or solids may not be useful in the neonate because of small chest size and hyperresonance. Palpation of the neonatal chest wall while the infant is crying may detect gross changes in sound transmission through the chest. Palpation of crepitus in the neck, around the clavicles, or on the chest wall suggests the complication of air leak.

NONRESPIRATORY EXAMINATION

Hypotonia is characterized by a froglike positioning and a lax, open mouth. Progressing from flexion to flaccidity indicates progression of hypoxia and exhaustion from the work of breathing. Cardiac findings such as a murmur, absence of pulses, bounding pulses, palmar pulses, weight gain, hepatosplenomegaly, cyanosis, edema, bradycardia, or tachycardia indicate congestive heart failure or congenital heart defects. A scaphoid abdomen indicates a diaphragmatic hernia.

Laboratory data

Since the clinical presentation of many respiratory and nonrespiratory diseases is the same, a chest x-ray examination may be the only way to differentiate cause and establish the proper diagnosis. X-ray evaluation helps eliminate congenital anomalies (e.g., diaphragmatic hernia with lung hypoplasia, masses, and obstruction) as the cause when acquired respiratory disease (e.g., IRDS, transient tachypnea of the newborn, and pneumonia) is the cause of the distress. X-ray films confirm the presence of pneumothorax or other pulmonary air leaks.

Arterial blood gases are used to demonstrate derangements of oxygenation acid-base balance and to differentiate between respiratory and metabolic components. Initial baseline values are followed by serial observations at least every 15 to 30 minutes after any change in therapy. This may be modified with transcutaneous monitoring. Shunt study may differentiate between lung origin and cardiac origin of respiratory distress. The symptoms of pulmonary disease (cyanosis and low PaO_2) are often alleviated with crying and increased FIO_2 and continuous positive airway pressure. If the same symptoms are cardiac in origin, they remain unchanged or worsen with crying and increased FIO_2 or CPAP. Administration of 100% FIO_2 for 10 minutes or longer may result in an increased PaO_2 (>100 mm Hg), whereas in cardiac disease caused by right-to-left shunting there is no change in PaO_2 after 100% FIO_2 administration. CAUTION: In the presence of severe lung disease with significant right-to-left shunting, cyanosis and PaO_2 may not be changed with 100% FIO_2.

The hematocrit is used to rule out anemia or polycythemia as the cause of the respiratory distress. In anemia, inadequate oxygen content promotes tissue hypoxia. In polycythemia, increased viscosity and sludging of blood flow adversely affect tissue oxygenation.

The white blood cell count and differential aid in diagnosing sepsis as the cause of distress. A blood culture is invaluable in suspected infection and should be obtained before antibiotic therapy. Blood glucose determination to rule out hypoglycemia as a cause is particularly important in infants of diabetic mothers, small-for-gestational-age (SGA) infants, LGA infants, and preterm appropriate-for-gestational-age (AGA) infants. An electrocardiogram, echocardiogram, and cardiac catheterization are used to rule out cardiac abnormalities.

An electroencephalogram and ultrasound examination of the brain help to rule out CNS abnormalities. Serum electrolytes (calcium, sodium, and potassium) aid in eliminating metabolic aberration as the cause of the distress.

GENERAL TREATMENT STRATEGIES

Treatment of any condition should be directed at correction of its underlying cause. Unfortunately, present technology does not allow for therapeutic maneuvers directed at the underlying cause of many neonatal respiratory diseases. In meconium aspiration syndrome, if prevention of the aspiration through thorough suction is to no avail, damage to the neonatal lung results. No therapeutic measure is available at present to augment the healing process. In TTN no therapeutic endeavors are available to aid fluid removal from the neonatal lung field. However, although corrective measures directed at the underlying cause are unavailable, therapy is directed at preventing or alleviating the consequences of the neonatal lung diseases such as hypoxemia and acidemia, allowing healing to take place and reducing iatrogenic complications.

Respiratory support is the hallmark of treatment of neonatal respiratory disease. Respiratory support involves increasing inspired oxygen tensions and providing ventilation if required.

Supplemental oxygen

When the neonate is unable to maintain adequate oxygenation, supplemental oxygen must be provided. Since oxygen is a drug, it must be treated as such and given only for medical indications. Biochemical criteria (PaO_2 <60 mm Hg) and clinical criteria such as respiratory distress, central cyanosis, apnea, asphyxia, and hypotonia are indications to prescribe oxygen.

Regardless of the mode of delivery (hood, ventilator, bag, or mask), safe and effective oxygen administration follows certain principles:

1. No concentration of oxygen has been proved to be "safe." A concentration (e.g., 30%, 40%, 80%, 100%) that is therapeutic for one infant may be toxic for another.

2. To titrate inspired oxygen concentrations to the individual infant's need, arterial PO_2 must be measured and maintained between 50 and 80 mm Hg.

3. Oxygen administration without some form of continuous monitoring of the infant's oxygenation (i.e., arterial blood gases, transcutaneous oxygen monitoring, or pulse oximetry) is dangerous and not recommended.[2]

4. Delivered oxygen should be humidified (30% to 40%), since dry gases are irritating to the airways and humidity decreases insensible water losses.[5] To prevent respiratory therapy equipment from becoming a source of infection, humidifiers and tubing should be replaced at least every 48 hours.

5. Oxygen should be warmed (31° to 34° C [88° to 94° F]) so temperature at the delivery site is the same as the incubator temperature. This prevents cold stress and increased oxygen consumption from blowing cold air in the infant's face.[90]

6. Oxygen concentration must be monitored by continuous or intermittent sampling (at least every hour) and recorded. Oxygen monitors and analyzers should be calibrated every 8 hours.

7. A stable concentration of oxygen is necessary to maintain PaO_2 within normal limits. A sudden increase or decrease in oxygen concentration may result in a disproportionate increase or decrease in PaO_2 caused by vasodilation or vasoconstriction in response to oxygen.[90] Adjustment of supplemental oxygen (particularly lowering FIO_2) must be done slowly to avoid the "flip-flop phenomenon." Hypoxic insult initiates pulmonary vasoconstriction, which causes hypoperfusion and increased pulmonary vascular resistance. The infant should be weaned from supplemental oxygen cautiously[90] (see "rule of seven," p. 166).

8. Observing color, respiratory effort, activity, and circulatory response and monitoring arterial oxygen concentration aid in determining the need for oxygen therapy and for adjustments to it.

9. Clinical observations, FIO_2 concentrations, and time of adjustments must be described, recorded, and reported.

10. Oxygen concentration should be returned to previous levels if clinical ob-

servations of distress and inability to tolerate decreased levels of oxygen occur.

Methods of delivery

For instructions on the bag and mask resuscitation method see Chapter 3.

An oxygen hood is a clear plastic hood that fits over the infant's head to deliver a constant concentration of oxygen. If the infant has sufficient ventilation to maintain a normal arterial carbon dioxide tension, oxygenation by increased inspired oxygen tensions through an oxygen hood may be all the respiratory support that is required. This degree of support is particularly applicable in cases of mild RDS, TTN, meconium aspiration, or neonatal pneumonia.

A blender system is the most reliable way to administer a fixed oxygen concentration via a hood. An appropriately sized hood should be used. If it is too large, the infant may slip out of the hood and FIO_2 may be diluted by leaks; if it is too small, pressure points may develop, especially around the neck. Another source of oxygen must be provided when the infant's head is removed from the hood because of feeding, being held, or suctioning. This secondary source may be set up from the blender source so that the infant's PaO_2 remains constant during suctioning or feedings. The infant may need increased FIO_2 from the secondary source, and this can be easily adjusted according to assessments made with a transcutaneous monitor (TCM) or pulse oximetry; these changes should be recorded.

For both home and hospital use, the nasal cannula provides an acceptable way to administer oxygen to the dependent, older infant who is developing social and motor skills.[95] Oxygen cannulas for neonatal and infant use are now commercially available, or a no. 6, 8, or 10 Fr suction or feeding catheter may be adapted to deliver oxygen.

1. Choose the appropriately sized catheter for the infant.

2. Thread 6 to 8 inches of ligature through two of the small side holes in the distal end of the catheter.

3. Position the catheter across the infant's upper lip with the distal end under the infant's nose. Secure it to the infant's face by taping over the ligature on one cheek and over the proximal end of the catheter to the opposite cheek. Apply Stomahesive directly to the infant's cheeks and tape the ligature and catheter to it to prevent skin irritation.

CAUTION: Neonates are obligatory nasal breathers, so that nasal obstruction (mucus or milk) will decrease the amount of oxygen actually received. Therefore nares should be suctioned as needed. The exact concentrations of oxygen delivered by cannula cannot be measured. Flow rates are titrated by monitoring PaO_2, $TcPO_2$, or pulse oximetry levels and by evaluating the clinical course of pallor, tachypnea, cyanosis, retractions, and body temperature. Oxygen tubing should be long enough to provide opportunities for social and gross motor skill development.

Continuous distending pressure

Application of a continuous distending pressure (CDP) to the lungs increases functional residual capacity. It also increases PaO_2 and improves oxygenation by decreasing intrapulmonary shunting and by improving the match of ventilation and perfusion. The application of CDP improves compliance of the lung and lessens the work of breathing.

In IRDS, where the functional residual capacity is reduced, increased respiratory oxygen tensions via an Oxyhood may not be sufficient to maintain an adequate arterial oxygen tension. More invasive techniques may be required.

Continuous positive airway pressure (CPAP) or continuous negative pressure (CNP) are two methods of delivery of CDP. If the infant cannot maintain a PaO_2 of 60 mm Hg in 0.6 FIO_2, a trial of CPAP, either by the nasal route or through an endotracheal tube, is indicated. Initial levels of CPAP should be in the range of 4 to 5 cm of water. CPAP should be increased to 8 to 10 cm of water by 2 cm increments if required to raise the infant's PaO_2 (as measured by arterial blood gas determinations or transcutaneous monitoring, or both). Arterial blood gas determinations are performed 15 to 30 minutes after initiating CDP and with each adjustment.

If the infant is able to maintain ventilation as indicated by normal arterial carbon dioxide tension, no further respiratory support may be required. Early institution of CDP reduces the need for mechanical ventilation.

Although negative pressure devices, head chambers, and face masks have been used to deliver CDP, using nasal prongs placed in the infant's nares or endotracheal intubation is preferred. A variety of nasal prongs are available. An orogastric tube (feeding tube) should be used for gastric decompression when implementing nasal prongs.

When the infant's PaO_2 is consistently over 70 mm Hg, inspired oxygen concentration and/or CDP may be lowered. Oxygen concentration is usually lowered in 5% to 10% increments to a level of 40% to 60%. CDP is lowered in increments of 1 cm of water to a level of 2 cm of water before discontinuing either prongs or an endotracheal tube. The infant may then be placed into an oxygen hood with the same FIO_2. PaO_2 (or $TcPO_2$) should be checked 15 to 30 minutes after each change.

Pulmonary hygiene

Pulmonary hygiene is normally maintained by ciliary activity, a covering of mucus, and narrowing and dilation of the bronchi with respiration and coughing. Anatomic and physiologic variations in the neonate alter these normal pulmonary mechanisms. The small airway of the neonate has a diameter that is four times smaller than that of the normal adult. Debris that causes only a moderate obstruction for the adult airway causes a disproportionately greater obstruction of the smaller airway of the neonate. Also, the neonate normally has an underdeveloped cough reflex. The sick neonate with insufficient respiratory effort and a weak or nonexistent cry has underventilated lungs. Often the neonate that is attached to multiple life-support systems is cared for in the same position. This localizes secretions in the dependent pulmonary tree and sets the stage for hypostatic pneumonia.

Combined chest physiotherapy and suctioning has become increasingly popular as a treatment modality for infants suffering from IRDS. There is, however, a paucity of literature to substantiate this treatment.

Whenever the normal mechanisms for mobilizing and removing pulmonary secretions are inefficient or inactive, pulmonary hygiene is indicated. Pulmonary hygiene consists of two major components: chest physiotherapy and suctioning. The goals of pulmonary hygiene are:

1. To facilitate removal of pulmonary debris by loosening and mobilizing secretions into the mainstem bronchi for suctioning
2. To maintain a patent airway
3. To promote optimal pulmonary ventilation
4. To prevent pulmonary infection from accumulated secretions

In the neonatal period pulmonary hygiene is indicated for intubated patients with conditions associated with atelectasis, increased secretions, and pulmonary debris (pneumonia, meconium aspiration, IRDS, and bronchopulmonary dysplasia).

CAUTION: The following are guidelines for pulmonary hygiene. These procedures must be individualized.

1. Any manipulation of the sick neonate has the potential for decreasing oxygenation and precipitating hypoxia.[21] Transcutaneous PO_2 readings have demonstrated that pulmonary hygiene and other procedures

(i.e., feeding, peripheral blood drawing, and turning) may effect a transient lowering of oxygen tensions.[62,74] Therefore increased inspired oxygen tensions may need to be provided during these procedures.

2. Pulmonary hygiene with a subsequent rest period should be done before feeding.

3. Percussion over the chest wall should be performed. Percussion over the liver, kidneys, sternum, vertebrae, or stomach should be avoided.

4. Infants receiving chest physiotherapy may appear stressed. Bradycardia, cyanosis, hypotonia, fighting, and struggling are signs of stress that should be observed during pulmonary hygiene. They may indicate either too frequent or too infrequent pulmonary hygiene.

5. Position modifications or deletions may be necessary based on clinical manifestations of stress.

6. The length of time for certain segments and for the procedure as a whole must be kept to a minimum to conserve the neonate's energy and prevent hypoxia. Frequency is determined by individual need and by the amount of secretions and distress.

7. The affected areas are the prime consideration; prophylactic pulmonary hygiene is secondary. The right upper and middle lobes of the lung are the most common sites for the development of secondary pneumonia and atelectasis.[24]

8. Physical assessment and estimates of secretions gauge the effectiveness and frequency of therapy.

9. Communication among care providers maintains continuity in setting priorities, providing adequate pulmonary hygiene, and recognizing what stresses the individual infant.

CHEST PHYSIOTHERAPY

Chest physiotherapy consists of positioning, percussion, and vibration.

POSITIONING. Postural changes use gravity to facilitate the movement of pulmonary debris from smaller to larger bronchi. Specific lung segments must be uppermost and angled so that they drain into their major bronchi (see boxed material on pp. 377 to 380). To facilitate maximal drainage, the infant is positioned 5 to 10 minutes before the onset of percussion and vibration. In the usual course of care, position changes every 1 to 2 hours are a continuum of intermittent postural drainage. Even prone positioning promotes ventilation by increasing lung expansion, increasing PaO_2, and draining the usually dependent posteriorly directed airways.[24,96] If a position is stressful, it should be modified, the amount of time spent in it should be decreased, or it should be deleted according to the infant's tolerance.

PERCUSSION. Percussion of the chest wall with a nontraumatic, cupped device (e.g., padded medicine cup, suction bulb cut in half with padded rim, resuscitation face mask, rubber nursing nipple, or other commercial device) creates a suction action that loosens secretions. The chest wall is gently tapped (for 30 seconds to 1 minute) over the affected area and then prophylactically over other frequently involved segments. Based on the infant's condition and tolerance, 1- to 2-inch segments are percussed. For very small or unstable infants, only one segment may be percussed with each treatment. Notation of the treated area must be exact, so that rotation and treatment of all areas occurs. Frequency varies from 1 to 4 hours depending on the disease process, amount of congestion, and tolerance.

Fractures have been documented in infants with BPD that apparently are the result of vigorous percussion.[25]

VIBRATION. Vibration of the neonatal chest with fingertips, a padded electric toothbrush,

POSTURAL CHANGES TO FACILITATE DRAINAGE

Upper lobes   Position 1: An upright position drains apical segments of the upper lobes.

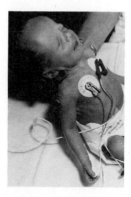

Position 2: A supine position 30° upright angle drains the anterior segments of the upper lobes.

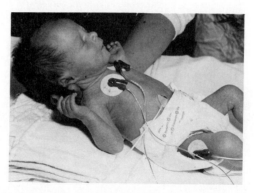

Position 1: A 30° upright angle drains the lateral bronchi of the apical segment of the right lung when infant is on left side and the apical posterior segment of the left lobe when infant is on right side.

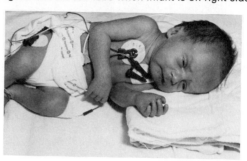

From Dunn D and Lewis AT: Pediatr Clin North Am 20:490, 1973.

Continued.

POSTURAL CHANGES TO FACILITATE DRAINAGE—cont'd

Upper lobes—cont'd   Position 2: A rotation forward 45° drains posterior bronchi of the upper
lobe and apical segments. In addition, rotation to the right also drains
the left posterior segment of the left upper lobe.

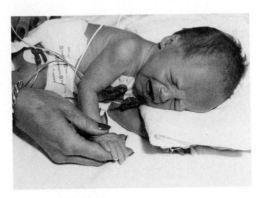

With the right side elevated 45° in the prone position the posterior
segment of the right upper lobe is drained.

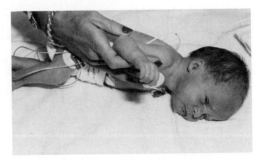

In a supine position the anterior segment of the upper lobes is drained.

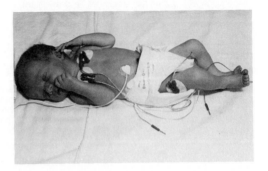

POSTURAL CHANGES TO FACILITATE DRAINAGE—cont'd

Middle lobe and lingula

With the head tilted downward 15° and a 45° rotation to the left the right middle lobe is drained. With the head tilted downward 15° and a 45° rotation to the right the lingula of the left upper lobe is drained.

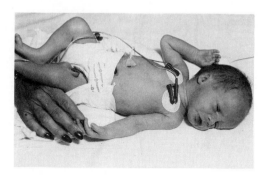

Lower lobes

In a prone position the superior segments of the lower lobes drain.

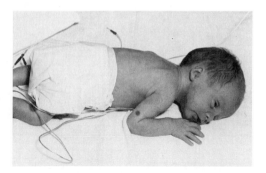

In the supine position with head tilted downward 30° the anterior segments of the lower lobes drain.

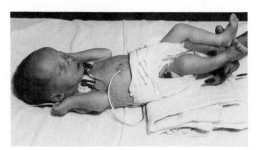

Continued.

POSTURAL CHANGES TO FACILITATE DRAINAGE—cont'd

Lower lobes—cont'd   In side-lying position with the head tilted downward 30° the lateral basal segments are drained. While lying on the right side the medial basal segment of the right side drains.

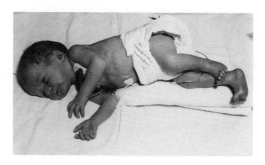

In a prone position with head tilted downward 30° the posterior basal segments of the lower lobes are drained.

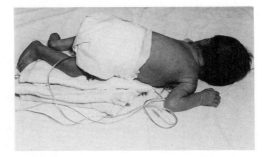

or mechanical vibrator may follow percussion or be performed in lieu of percussion. When done on expiration, vibration of specific lung segments mobilizes secretions. As with percussion, priority is given to involved areas, with prophylactic therapy rotated among the other segments.

The use of positioning, percussion, and vibration increases recovery of the infant's secretions more than the use of gravity alone. Recent studies have shown vibration to be as efficacious for mobilizing secretions as percussion and may be less traumatic and stressful for the infant.[20]

SUCTIONING

Once secretions are loosened and mobilized, they must be removed through the nose and mouth or by tracheal suctioning.

NASO-OROPHARYNGEAL SUCTIONING. When the infant has no artificial airway, suctioning the naso-oropharynx serves two purposes: removing secretions and initiating a cough reflex that mobilizes secretions. With either a suction bulb or catheter, the infant is suctioned immediately after chest physiotherapy. Providing an oxygen source during the procedure is important. Since stimulation of the nares causes reflex inspiration with possible inhalation of oropharyngeal contents, first the mouth and then the nose should be suctioned. The results should be recorded.

CAUTION: Suctioning should be avoided for 30 minutes to 1 hour after feeding unless it is necessary to establish a patent airway. The catheter should be gently inserted upward and back into the nares, never forced. If the catheter is hard to pass or the nares seem blocked, this procedure should be abandoned to prevent swelling and/or trauma.

The catheter may initiate vasovagal stimulation with resultant bradycardia.

ENDOTRACHEAL SUCTIONING (ORAL TUBE OR NASOTRACHEAL TUBE). An artificial airway prevents normal warming, humidifying, and cleansing of the air by the upper airway. The presence of the foreign body, the tube, also increases pulmonary secretions. To maintain a patent airway, sterile endotracheal suction should be performed as assessment indicates (i.e., changes in breath sounds, increased irritability, or labile oxygenation). The pieces of equipment to be prepared are:

1. Sterile suction catheter (of appropriate size; measurement of the length to be passed is essential)
2. Sterile glove
3. Sterile normal saline (without preservative)
4. Stethoscope
5. Suction machine (80 to 100 mm Hg negative pressure)

The sterile catheter and glove package are opened. Sterile normal saline (0.25 to 0.5 ml) is drawn up in a 1 ml syringe. The resuscitation bag is connected to oxygen and the patency is checked so that, if the neonate becomes apneic or bradycardic during the procedure, resuscitation equipment is immediately available. If the infant is on a ventilator equipped with a bag, this may be used for resuscitation if necessary.

Wall suction is adjusted to minimal pressure for effective suctioning. Hands are washed before and after every contact with the neonate. Assessment of the neonate's condition is made before initiating a suction procedure by observing vital signs (pulse and respirations) and color. Auscultation of the chest for adventitious sounds (rales, rhonchi, or wheezing) helps to evaluate the condition and indicate a need for suction. Because suctioning is one of the most stressful procedures performed in infants, suctioning should not be routine, but instead should be based on assessment criteria of breath sounds, oxygenation, etc.

Suction procedure

1. Disconnect and instill 0.25 to 0.5 ml of normal saline into tracheal tube and reconnect baby to ventilator. Saline thins secretions and facilitates their removal from the major bronchi. The amount of saline depends on the size of the infant (<2000 g—0.25 ml; >2000 g—0.5 ml) and the viscosity of secretions.

2. Ventilate with deep inflating breaths. Use six to eight extra breaths at the same oxygen concentration (FIO_2), matching pressure to the ventilator settings. Increase FIO_2 if clinically indicated, using a TCM or oximetry. Hyperoxygenation, increasing the FIO_2 to 100% for ventilation, raises PaO_2 and has been associated with hyperoxia and its attendant consequences (i.e., retinopathy of prematurity). Hyperinflating the lungs helps to minimize hypoxia during suction without the danger of exposure to dangerously elevated PaO_2. Hyperinflation between each suction maneuver and at completion of suctioning restores functional residual capacity and prevents atelectasis. The response to hyperinflation depends on the baby's behavior during the procedure. If the infant is relaxed and at rest, the therapeutic effect of increased PaO_2 occurs; if the infant is fighting and struggling against the bag, the PaO_2 may fall precipitously.[73] Coordinating bag inflation with the infant's normal in-

spiration will tend to minimize struggling and the fall in Pao_2.

3. Put on glove and attach sterile catheter to suction tubing.

4. With ungloved hand, turn infant's head midline. Disconnect from ventilator.

5. Gently pass catheter down endotracheal tube to measured length (this will prevent damage to bronchial mucosa that can occur using method of passing suction catheter until meeting resistance).

6. With ungloved hand occlude suction hole in catheter and withdraw. Use continuous suction so that secretions are not "released" with intermittent suction. Do not use an up-and-down motion while removing the catheter, since this will decrease oxygenation and promote hypoxia. Occlude tracheal tube with catheter for no longer than 5 to 10 seconds because of the danger of prolonged hypoxia. Only one suction attempt should be made before the infant is again ventilated. Assess tolerance of procedure by observing infant's color, heart rate, tone, and activity.

7. Replace on ventilator and hyperinflate with appropriate FIo_2 for six to eight breaths or until adequate oxygenation has been established.

8. Repeat procedure as indicated by results obtained. All suctioning should take place with the head midline, because the catheter is only being passed the length of the endotracheal tube and not to the carina.

9. Suction the nasopharynx and oropharynx.

10. To facilitate pulmonary drainage, improve ventilation, and preserve skin integrity, change infant's position after suctioning. Adequate hydration thins secretions and thus facilitates their removal.

11. Check respirator settings, including alarm system in "on" position. Check tube position to be sure no strain or bend is in the tracheal tube.

12. Reassess infant's condition after procedure by observing vital signs and color and auscultating chest to evaluate effectiveness of therapy. Ensure proper tube placement and adequate bilateral ventilation. Note tolerance of procedure on record, as well as need for increased oxygen or rate during suctioning.

13. Note amount and type of secretions obtained.

NOTE: When two persons are available for suctioning, one remains "sterile" and does the suctioning while the other detaches the tracheal tube from the ventilator, maneuvers the head, and hyperventilates between suctionings.

During pulmonary hygiene, incidences of increased intracranial pressure and hypoxia have been reported.[29] Increased intracranial pressure is inversely related to the hypoxia. As the Pao_2 decreases, the intracranial pressure rises.[28] Transcutaneous monitoring and pulse oximetry are valuable tools in assessing oxygenation status during pulmonary hygiene. If $TcPo_2$ oxygen saturation falls during suction, hyperventilate with a bag until recovery occurs. Muscle relaxation or paralysis with medications may be used to decrease periods of hypoxia or hyperoxia and increased intracranial pressure.

Other aspects of therapy for the neonate with respiratory disease include:

1. Supportive care and monitoring (see Chapters 1 through 8)

2. Nutritional and metabolic care (see Chapters 9 through 13)

3. Infection control and care of hematologic diseases (see Chapters 14 through 16)

4. Care of family—parents and siblings (see Chapters 22 through 25)

Endotracheal intubation

Endotracheal intubation may be accomplished by the orotracheal route or the nasotracheal route. Nasotracheal intubation is more difficult to perform, but it is easier to anchor the tube to prevent accidental extubation. It may be more appropriate for the larger, more vigorous infant. Smaller infants under 1250 g seem to do well with orotracheal tubes.

An endotracheal tube diameter that approximates the diameter of the infant's fifth digit generally fits snugly into the trachea. To measure for an endotracheal tube, the distance from the oral (or nasal) orifice to midway between the glottis and carina may be calculated by multiplying the crown-heel length by 0.2. In an emergency the distance from the lips to midway between the glottis and carina may be approximated by the 7-8-9-10 rule. The distance is 7 cm in a 1 kg infant, 8 cm in a 2 kg infant, 9 cm in a 3 kg infant, and 10 cm in a 4 kg infant.

INTUBATION PROCEDURE

For long-term stability, commercially available endotracheal tube anchors prevent accidental extubation. Some nurseries still prefer fixing tubes with tape or sutures (see Chapter 3).

EXTUBATION PROCEDURE

Assess the infant's condition by observing the heart rate, color, respiratory rate and effort, and auscultating the chest. If the infant's condition is stable, proceed with extubation. Extubate before feeding or empty the stomach to prevent vomiting. Since neonates are obligatory nasal breathers, the nasopharynx must also be suctioned and patent for extubation.

Hyperinflate with deep breaths with the infant's head in the midline and remove the tube on inflation[54] to provide adequate lung expansion and prevent atelectasis, or on expiration[41] so that secretions that have accumulated around the tracheal tube are "blown away" on exhalation and tube removal, or while suctioning to remove secretions that have accumulated around the tube. Place in a warm, humidified oxygen hood at FIO_2 used before extubation.

Reassess the infant's condition, especially for signs of increased work of breathing and distress. Document tube removal and the infant's tolerance. Check arterial blood gases 15 to 20 minutes after extubation to assess oxygenation and ventilation status. Perform a chest x-ray examination to document atelectasis or fully expanded lungs. Continue pulmonary hygiene as long as the infant has secretions. Observe for complications of intubation (see boxed material on p. 384).

Mechanical ventilation

Mechanical ventilation is used in neonates to correct abnormalities in oxygenation ($\downarrow PaO_2$), alveolar ventilation ($\uparrow PaCO_2$), or respiratory effort (apnea or ineffectual respirations). It is not used to treat the primary disease, but frequently it is used to support the infant until the disease is treated or resolved.

Those newborns who meet the following criteria are candidates for assisted ventilation:

I. Blood gases
   A. Severe hypoxemia (PaO_2 <60 mm Hg with FIO_2 of 0.8 on 6 to 8 cm CPAP[51] or PaO_2 <60 mm Hg with FIO_2 >0.4 in infant <1250 g)[28]
   B. Severe hypercapnia ($PaCO_2$ >55 to 65 mm Hg[10,51] with pH <7.10 to 7.20 in infants <1500 g or >1500 g with CPAP)[28]

II. Clinical
   A. Apnea and bradycardia requiring resuscitation in infants with lung disease or unresponsive to CPAP or theophylline therapy in preterm infants with normal lungs
   B. Inefficient respiratory effort such as gasping respirations from asphyxia, narcosis, or primary cardiopulmonary disease
   C. Shock and asphyxia with hypoperfusion and hypotension
   D. IRDS in infants weighing less than 1000 g, frequently making them incapable of maintaining ventilation (In these infants it has been suggested that mechanical ventilation without a trial of CPAP is appropriate.)[28]

VENTILATOR SETTINGS

To individualize assisted ventilation, knowledge of the ventilator capabilities is essential.

INTERMITTENT MANDATORY VENTILATION. Most mechanical ventilators in common use today allow for intermittent mandatory ventilation

(IMV). IMV provides a continuous flow of gas that is available to the infant during spontaneous respirations. Periodic occlusion of the system diverts gas under pressure to the infant. Since IMV provides for spontaneous and mechanical ventilation, only the amount of ventilatory assistance that is needed by the individual infant is provided.

CONTINUOUS DISTENDING PRESSURE. CDP is expressed in centimeters of water. CDP may be given without IMV (CPAP) or with it (positive end expiratory pressure [PEEP]).

The effects of CDP include increased alveolar stability, increased functional residual capacity, decreased risk of atelectasis, increased intrathoracic pressure, and impeded passage of fluid from lung capillaries to alveolar spaces, aiding in

---

COMPLICATIONS OF ENDOTRACHEAL INTUBATION

Immediate

Malposition

Too low	Usually in right mainstem bronchus; no breath sounds in left chest or upper right lobe; atelectasis (Withdraw tube until breath sounds are heard bilaterally and equally.)
Too high	Inadequate ventilation bilaterally, especially at lung bases
Esophagus	Air movement auscultated in stomach with no or inadequate breath sounds

Obstruction

Plug	Partial or complete
Kinking of the tube	
Head position	Flexion or extension with blockage of air flow

Perforation
  Vocal cords
  Trachea
  Pharynx

Infection
Air leak
Increased intracranial pressure
Postextubation

Migratory lobar collapse	Prevent and treat with pulmonary hygiene
Diffuse microatelectasis	In very low birth weight infants may be associated with apnea; treatable by pulmonary hygiene or nasal CPAP, or both

Long term

General	Vocal cord inflammation, stenosis, and eventual dysfunction; tracheoesophageal fistula; subglottic stenosis; tracheal inflammation and stenosis; contributes to bronchopulmonary dysplasia

Specific to the type of tube

Orotracheal	Abnormal dentition; gingival and palatal erosion; palatal grooves
Nasotracheal	Otitis media; erosion of alae nasae and nasal septum; nasal stenosis

the prevention or treatment of pulmonary edema.

PEAK INSPIRATORY PRESSURE. Peak inspiratory pressure (PIP) reflects the maximal amount of positive pressure delivered to the infant on inspiration. It is expressed in centimeters of water pressure.

RATE. The rate reflects how often a volume of gas in the system is delivered to the infant. It is expressed as breaths per minute.

INSPIRATION/EXPIRATION RATIO. The inspiration/expiration ratio (I/E ratio) reflects the relationship between time spent in inspiration and time spent in expiration. When the rate is 60 breaths/min and the total respiratory cycle is 1 second, an I/E ratio of 1:1 means 0.5 seconds is inspiration and 0.5 seconds is expiration. If the I/E ratio is 2:1 with a rate of 60 and the total respiratory cycle is 1 second, inspiration is 0.66 second and expiration is 0.33 second.

Prolonged inspiration may be associated with more efficient ventilation and optimal arterial oxygenation but also has a higher risk of an air leak.[11] Prolonged expiration also improves oxygenation, especially in air-trapping conditions.[11]

MEAN AIRWAY PRESSURE. Mean airway pressure (MAP) is the amount of pressure transmitted to the airway throughout an entire respiratory cycle.[11] Any change in ventilator settings affects the mean airway pressure. MAP is most affected by changes in PEEP, PIP, and I/E ratio.[11,91] MAP is associated with optimal oxygenation ($\uparrow$ PaO_2) and ventilation ($\downarrow$ $PaCO_2$) when pressures range between 6 and 14 cm of water.[11] When MAP exceeds 14 cm of water, there is a progressive deterioration of the blood gases ($\downarrow$ PaO_2, $\uparrow$ $PaCO_2$).[11]

Usual starting pressures for beginning ventilatory support are listed as follows:

FIo₂	**At previous level or 10% higher than previously required concentration**
PEEP	**4 to 6 cm water**
PIP	**16 to 20 cm water**
Rate	**20 to 30 breaths/min**
I/E ratio	**1:1 to 1.5:1**

The inspired oxygen tension is adjusted to provide an adequate arterial oxygen tension. If the infant still has difficulty maintaining an adequate carbon dioxide tension, a faster rate and/or greater inspiratory pressure would be indicated. Table 17-2 lists the usual effects to be expected from changing specific ventilator settings.

To evaluate the efficacy of mechanical ventilation and any adjustments made with the system, continuous monitoring with transcutaneous blood gas monitors or pulse oximeters (see Chapter 6) must be maintained and/or blood gases obtained. Blood gases should be obtained 15 to 30 minutes after beginning ventilatory

---

TABLE 17-2

Usual Effects of Changing Ventilator Settings

INCREASING	Pao₂	Paco₂	pH	CAUSES / COMPLICATIONS
FIo₂	↑	0	0	Oxygen toxicity (bronchopulmonary dysplasia, retrolental fibroplasia); absorption atelectasis
CPAP/PEEP	↑	0 / ↑	0 / ↓	Hypoventilation with respiratory acidosis; decreased cardiac output with metabolic acidosis; air leaks
PIP	↑	↓	↑	Barotrauma with air leaks and bronchopulmonary dysplasia; respiratory alkalosis
Rate	↓	↓	↑	Respiratory alkalosis
I/E ratio (1:1 to 3:1)	↑	0	0	Increased intrapleural pressure; decreased venous return

support or after any change in settings, every 4 to 6 hours if no change is made in ventilator settings, and as needed based on the clinical condition of the infant.

Arterial blood gases should be maintained in the following range (see Chapter 8):

PaO_2	50 to 70 mm Hg
$PaCO_2$	35 to 45 mm Hg
pH	7.35 to 7.45

New therapeutic approaches to neonatal respiratory distress

Based on our current understanding of the central roles of surfactant deficiency and baroinjury in the pathogenesis of acute respiratory distress and the development of chronic lung disease, new therapeutic approaches have been developed in an effort to further attenuate the frequency and severity of lung injury. Clinical trials of such therapeutic modalities as surfactant replacement, high-frequency ventilation (HFV), and extracorporeal membrane oxygenation (ECMO) are currently examining their potential application in the treatment of various neonatal respiratory diseases.

SURFACTANT REPLACEMENT THERAPY

Since surfactant deficiency is the primary abnormality of hyaline membrane disease, the development of an effective clinical strategy for administering exogenous surface-active material to premature infants has been the focus of research efforts for many years. Early clinical trials using nebulized dipalmitoylphosphotidylcholine in human infants with respiratory distress were discouraging.[18,84] However, subsequent studies of the biochemistry and biophysical properties of surfactant demonstrated the important role of other lipids and surfactant-related proteins, leading to renewed interest in its potential clinical use. Subsequent animal studies found that the administration of surfactant into the airway of premature fetal animals prior to ventilation led to marked improvement in gas exchange and survival.[26] Similarly, the delayed administration of

surfactant shortly after the onset of ventilation in preterm animals also resulted in improved ventilation, oxygenation, and survival in comparison with control animals; the best results, however, appeared to be obtained with immediate treatment shortly after birth.[50] Several clinical trials in infants with IRDS have supported these experimental observations. Studies have shown that surfactant harvested from mature bovine lung or human amniotic fluid from normal term pregnancies led to dramatic and rapid improvement in gas exchange, decreased the need for high levels of supplemental oxygen and ventilator therapy, caused less barotrauma, and improved chest x-ray findings in infants treated shortly after birth.[37] Although early problems from blood flow shunting across the patent ductus arteriosus may contribute to some clinical problems, no serious side effects from its clinical use have been reported. Current concerns about possible immunogenicity and negative interactions with endogenous surfactant production require further study. In addition, clinical studies are currently addressing questions related to determining the optimal clinical strategies, such as how much surfactant to administer, how many doses, and what the optimal method of delivery is (i.e., aerosols versus saline suspensions).

HIGH-FREQUENCY VENTILATION

Barotrauma is a major contributing factor to the development of chronic lung disease or death from progressive lung injury in newborns treated with conventional mechanical ventilation. The goal of new ventilatory strategies such as high-frequency ventilation (HFV) is to reduce barotrauma by its application early in the course of IRDS, or to reduce the progression of injury in infants already having advanced pulmonary interstitial emphysema, recurrent pneumothoraxes, or bronchopleural fistula. HFV differs from conventional modes of ventilator support in that it uses smaller tidal volumes at supraphysiologic frequencies, allowing for generation of lower intrathoracic pressure. At high frequencies the calculated tidal volume is less than dead space. Thus the physics of gas flow and exchange are different from the traditional teaching of lung mechanics and are thought to be related to augmented diffusion.[17] Reduction in barotrauma occurs by allowing for ventilation with a very small pressure amplitude around the mean airway pressure in the distal airway. Therefore at high frequencies (commonly 10 to 15 Hertz), the peak inspiratory and expiratory pressures approach mean airway pressure (i.e., lower downstream pressures).

HFV can be achieved by jet ventilators or by oscillators. Jet ventilators deliver short bursts of high-flow gases directly into the proximal airway via a small cannula and have a passive exhalation cycle. Oscillators vibrate columns of air and have active exhalation cycles. Although clinical comparisons of these two methods are still pending, a high incidence of necrotizing tracheitis has been reported with high-frequency jet ventilation.

Animal studies of preterm baboons have demonstrated dramatic effects of homogeneity of ventilation applied shortly after birth in comparison with conventional methods, and the potential application of this method in early IRDS to lessen the incidence of BPD has been suggested. Clinical studies have demonstrated that with HFV it is possible to ventilate infants with severe BPD and pulmonary interstitial emphysema at lower levels than with conventional methods, and improve gas exchange in severely ill neonates. Many questions regarding the clinical use of HFV persist, such as the actual mechanism of gas exchange, its optimal application, the role of intermittent sighs, and its cardiovascular effects.

EXTRACORPOREAL MEMBRANE OXYGENATOR

ECMO is a modification of cardiopulmonary bypass that allows for more prolonged therapy than is traditionally performed in the operating room for cardiac surgery. ECMO establishes a pulmonary bypass circuit, allowing gas exchange to occur outside of the lung by perfusion of blood through a membrane oxygenator. Blood is drawn from a catheter in the right internal jugular vein or right atrium, oxygenated as it crosses the membrane, and then returned to the patient via the right common carotid artery (venoarterial ECMO) or the femoral vein (venovenous). The pump produces a continuous, nonpulsatile flow through the membrane oxygenator as the patient is kept heparinized and continues to be ventilated at low pressures, rates, and oxygen tensions. The goal of this therapy is to "buy time" for the severely injured lung to heal while attenuating ongoing lung injury by decreasing exposure to hyperoxia and barotrauma. Therapy can be continued for several days, until lung recovery appears sufficient to maintain adequate gas tension without ECMO. Early clinical success has been reported in such disorders as severe IRDS, meconium aspiration syndrome, and persistent pulmonary hypertension of the newborn.

Weaning from the ventilator

When the infant's condition improves, ventilatory support is slowly removed. Evidence of improvement includes biochemical parameters and clinical parameters:

1. Arterial blood gases are stable and in the physiologic range.
2. There are spontaneous respiratory efforts against the ventilator when it is connected or against suctioning when the ventilator is disconnected.
3. There is increased activity and muscle tone and progressively decreasing FIO_2 requirement.

With IMV there is a gradual decrease in mechanical ventilation with a corresponding increase in spontaneous respiration. One ventilator setting at a time is changed, and arterial blood gases, transcutaneous, or pulse oximetry values are evaluated to determine the infant's response before another adjustment is made. Since each ventilator parameter has risks and benefits, each parameter must be evaluated before the decision is made as to which one will be lowered. Since high concentrations of oxygen may be toxic to the lungs and hyperoxia may damage the eyes, oxygen is usually lowered first to a level below 80% in 5% to 10% increments. PIP is lowered in 1 to 2 cm increments to a level of 16 cm of water, and rate in 1 to 5 breaths/min increments until the infant is on CPAP alone or has a rate of 5 breaths/min or less. Once adequate oxygenation and ventilation on CPAP alone have been maintained, the infant may be extubated and placed in an oxygen hood. Oxygen should be adjusted with the use of TCM or pulse oximetry.

During the recovery phase of IRDS (approximately 72 hours), changes in lung compliance occur rapidly. Hyperoxia, air leaks, increased intracranial pressure, and decreased cardiac output easily occur if high pressures and high oxygen concentrations are not decreased as rapidly as the lung is recovering.

Infants that are difficult or impossible to wean from the ventilator may have BPD, patent ductus arteriosus, or CNS damage that affects the respiratory control center.

GENERAL COMPLICATIONS
Acute complications

Acute and chronic complications are the result of the disease process or treatment, or both. Beginning with the least invasive therapy and progressing to more complicated ones only as needed accomplishes two goals. It individualizes therapy and minimizes risk of complications. Continuous monitoring of the individual infant's progress is vital in decreasing complications from the disease and from the interventions used to support the infant or to treat the primary condition. Complications of respiratory diseases are:

I. Acute
  A. Sudden deterioration of condition
  B. Air leaks
  C. Central nervous system
    1. Hypoxic-ischemic injury
    2. Increased intracranial pressure
    3. Hemorrhage

  D. Cardiac
    1. Patent ductus arteriosus
    2. Decreased cardiac output
  E. Infection
  F. Bleeding diathesis
  G. Tube
II. Chronic
  A. Oxygen toxicity and barotrauma (BPD)
  B. Hyperoxia (retinopathy of prematurity)
  C. Hypoxia
  D. Tube

Sudden deterioration of the infant's condition is an emergency, and the cause must be found and corrected as soon as possible to minimize further damage. Causes of sudden deterioration are:

I. Tube
  A. Accidental extubation
  B. Accidental disconnection
  C. Plug
II. Machine malfunction
  A. Ventilator or CPAP device
  B. Oxygen blender
  C. Tubing and connections
III. Alarm system "off"
IV. Severe hypoxia
V. Metabolic factors
VI. Air leak
VII. Intraventricular hemorrhage

RESPIRATORY

Management of the infant who has suddenly deteriorated begins with a visual inspection. The oxygen hood, CPAP, or ventilator must be properly connected and free of water. If all connections are intact, the infant must be disconnected from assisted ventilation and connected to a resuscitation bag (that is connected to an oxygen source and kept at the bedside). Manual ventilation matching pressure, rates, and FIO_2 to ventilator settings must be maintained. If the infant improves with these interventions, mechanical failure of the ventilator should be suspected. Assistance to find the mechanical problem or replace the system should

be called for. The baby's respiratory effort must be manually assisted until the problem is solved.

If the infant does not improve with manual ventilation, there is probably a problem with the tube. The infant's condition can be assessed by auscultating the chest for quality of breath sounds. A list of findings and what they suggest follows:

Finding	Possible cause
No air entry bilaterally	Air leak
	Plugged endotracheal tube
	Accidental extubation
Diminished air entry	Air leak
	Endotracheal tube too high
Air entry over stomach	Accidental extubation
Air entry unequal	Air leak
	Endotracheal tube too low
Cardiac point of maximal intensity shifted	Air leak with tension

The endotracheal tube should be suctioned quickly. If there is no improvement in clinical condition or air entry, the tube should be replaced while supporting the infant with bag and mask ventilation. If the tube is too low, it can be repositioned by pulling it back 0.5 to 1 cm. If air entry and clinical condition improve with auscultation, the tube must be secured in the new position and an x-ray examination made for tube placement. If assessment of the chest is suspicious of accidental extubation, the tube must be removed, ventilation with bag and mask administered, and reintubation performed. If the infant does not improve with manual ventilation and the tube is in place, an air leak or intraventricular hemorrhage could be the cause.

Monitors and ventilators are equipped with alarm systems to warn care providers of sudden changes in the infant's condition or in supportive systems. It is imperative that all alarm systems be maintained in the "on" position. Turn-ing the alarms "off" during care for such procedures as suctioning and weighing creates the risk of forgetting to turn them "on" again. In a busy neonatal intensive care unit the compromised infant may not be visually noticed until the hypoxia is so severe that resuscitation is more difficult or impossible. Monitor parameters (both high and low alarm settings) must be individualized for each infant and recorded (see Chapter 6).

The sick neonate may experience a severe hypoxic insult when oxygen is too rapidly altered during caretaking procedures. Feeding, weighing, or turning without an alternative oxygen source may cause a sudden decrease in PaO_2, pulmonary vasoconstriction, hypoperfusion, and an iatrogenic worsening of the condition. Prolonged endotracheal tube suctioning (15 to 20 seconds) causes hypoxia and atelectasis. Care must be organized to conserve energy, minimize hypoxic insults, and maintain the infant in physiologic homeostasis.[65] Alternative oxygen sources must be provided when the usual method of oxygen delivery is disrupted for giving care. Small alterations in FIO_2 prevent rapid increases or decreases in oxygen tension.

METABOLIC FACTORS

Hypoglycemia must never be overlooked as the cause of sudden collapse. Undetected infiltration or disconnection of intravenous (IV) fluids may cause a precipitous drop in blood glucose, with respiratory irregularity, apnea, or seizures. Quickly checking the blood glucose with a reagent strip is always warranted. If low blood glucose is not the cause of the sudden deterioration, it may be a complication of the asphyxial episode. After the infant is stabilized, screening for hypoglycemia and providing adequate fluids and glucose are appropriate (see Chapter 11).

Hypothermia and overwhelming sepsis with their associated metabolic derangements may be the cause of sudden deterioration. Muted response to cold stress is a sequela of asphyxial insult, and cold stress must be avoided after the acute episode. A high level of suspicion for infection should accompany sudden deterioration (see Chapters 5 and 16).

AIR LEAKS

PHYSIOLOGY. When air dissects from an alveolus, it follows the tracheobronchial tree and may accumulate in the mediastinum (pneumomediastinum), in the pleural space (pneumothorax), in the space surrounding the heart (pneumo-

pericardium), or in the peritoneal cavity (pneumoperitoneum). Air leaks are complications of respiratory diseases and treatment strategies.

The free air released from ruptured alveoli may lead to pulmonary interstitial emphysema (PIE) (Figure 17-1). This free air intravasates into interstitial tissue and can compromise pulmonary vascular circulation and decrease ventilation of the lungs. Localized pulmonary interstitial emphysema sometimes resolves spontaneously. Frequently it can continue for weeks or even months. A recent technique of HFV has improved the outcome of these infants.

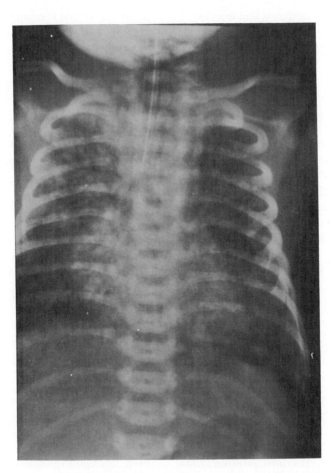

Figure 17-1. Pulmonary interstitial emphysema (PIE).

ETIOLOGIES. Those at increased risk for the development of air leaks fall into three specific categories: healthy term neonates, those with pulmonary diseases, and those receiving positive pressure support (CPAP and IMV).

Healthy term neonates generate pressures of 40 to 80 cm of water for their first breath of life. Therefore a spontaneous air leak is more common in the neonatal period (2% to 10%) than at any other time of life.

Pulmonary diseases such as IRDS as a result of stiff, noncompliant lungs require higher pressures for alveolar ventilation. Aspiration syndromes cause a ball-valve obstruction of debris with distal air trapping (meconium, milk, amniotic fluid, blood, and mucus). Hypoplastic lungs create a risk for air leaks because lung growth and development are abnormal and the lungs are stiff and noncompliant (diaphragmatic hernia and oligohydramnios syndrome). In either congenital lobar or pulmonary interstitial emphysema, alveolar rupture is associated with positive-pressure ventilation.

Positive-pressure ventilation, especially with excessive pressure, results in overdistention with alveolar rupture and air dissection. It occurs in 16% to 36% of infants who are ventilated by CPAP, IMV, or resuscitated with a bag and mask, or with an endotracheal tube and bag.

PREVENTION. Using the least amount of positive pressure to obtain physiologic results decreases the chances of air leaks. Scrupulously clearing the airway before resuscitation and using pressure gauges on resuscitation equipment may prevent aspiration and the possibility of inadvertently using pressure that is too high. Rapid recognition of at-risk infants, clinical manifestations and diagnosis, and emergency treatment improve survival and decrease the long-term sequelae of hypoxia and ischemia.

DATA COLLECTION

History. Pneumothorax or other air leaks should be suspected when any one of the following infants takes a sudden turn for the worse:

1. **A preterm infant with IRDS either with or without positive-pressure support**
2. **A term or postterm infant with meconium-stained amniotic fluid**
3. **An infant with an x-ray picture of interstitial or lobar emphysema**
4. **An infant requiring resuscitation at birth**
5. **An infant receiving CPAP or positive-pressure ventilation**

Signs and symptoms. Asymptomatic air leaks occur in term neonates, frequently require no treatment, and resolve spontaneously in 24 to 48 hours. Gradual onset of symptoms is characterized by increasing difficulty in ventilation, oxygenation, and perfusion. Early clinical manifestations may include restlessness and irritability; lethargy; tachypnea; and use of accessory muscles including grunting, flaring, and retractions. These subtle clinical changes may be unnoticed until the infant progresses to a sudden, profound collapse.

Sudden and severe deterioration in clinical course is characterized by:

1. **Profound generalized cyanosis**
2. **Bradycardia**
3. **Decrease in height of QRS complex on monitor**
4. **Air hunger including gasping and anxious facies**
5. **Diminished or shifted breath sounds**
6. **Chest asymmetry**
7. **Diminished, shifted, or muffled cardiac sounds and point of maximal intensity**
8. **Severe hypotension and poor peripheral perfusion**
9. **Easily palpable liver and spleen**
10. **Subcutaneous emphysema**
11. **Cardiorespiratory arrest**

Laboratory data. Arterial blood gas determinations reveal increasing hypoxemia ($\downarrow$ Pao$_2$), increasing hypercapnia ($\uparrow$ Paco$_2$), and a persistent metabolic acidosis with gradual onset of symptoms. Transillumination of the chest with a fiberoptic probe may reveal hyperlucency of the affected side when compared

with the other side.[58] A chest x-ray examination is the definitive diagnostic technique in air leaks. Since clinical manifestations of many other diseases may be similar to air leaks, the only way to be sure of the diagnosis is to take a chest x-ray examination. Anteroposterior and lateral films must be obtained. Occasionally a decubitus lateral x-ray film may be of value.

TREATMENT. An air leak is a surgical emergency of the chest. Tension within the chest cavity compromises lung excursion and cardiac output; without prompt treatment the infant will not survive. Trained care providers must be immediately available to provide emergency management in any institution that provides positive-pressure ventilatory support.

Evacuation of trapped air to decrease tension and allow proper organ function is the goal of treatment. Pneumomediastinum rarely needs to be treated, but pneumopericardium, a form of pneumomediastinum, may result in cardiac tamponade and need needle aspiration and/or tube drainage. Pneumoperitoneum must be differentiated from a perforated viscus.

A suggested conservative treatment is endotracheal intubation of the affected lung. The tube is advanced 1 to 2 cm beyond the carina in order to occlude the involved lung. This procedure is difficult to perform if the left lung is involved. If the pulmonary interstitial emphysema is localized to one lung or lobe of the lung, differential ventilation or surgical removal of the lobe may be curative. Pneumothorax may be treated with needle aspiration of air. Tube thoracotomy with suction drainage is frequently required.

Immediate supportive care. The head of the bed is elevated 30 to 40 degrees. This decreases the work of breathing by using gravity to localize the air in the upper chest and to push the abdominal organs downward away from the diaphragm.

Oxygen at 100% concentration is administered. The two goals for using 100% oxygen for immediate care are to attempt to improve oxygenation in a severely compromised infant and to use a nitrogen washout technique to increase by as much as sixfold the rate of absorption of the trapped air.[55]

CAUTION: Prolonged administration of 100% oxygen to treat an air leak in term babies has been used. However, exclusive use of 100% oxygen to treat trapped air is not recommended in either the term or preterm baby because of the risk of developing retrolental fibroplasia and the length of time necessary to obtain complete resolution.

The severely compromised infant requires immediate emergency procedures. A diagnostic and therapeutic thoracentesis may be necessary in life-threatening situations where there is not time to wait for x-ray examination.

Needle aspiration. A scalp vein needle (23 to 25 gauge), a three-way stopcock, and a 10 to 20 ml syringe may be used for needle aspiration. The equipment is connected (syringe-stopcock-needle), the chest is prepped for asepsis, and the needle is inserted in the third intercostal space in the anterior axillary line. A slight pop may be felt when the pleura is entered. Air is withdrawn into the syringe and evacuated into the room by turning the stopcock. This procedure is repeated until no more air can be aspirated or until a chest tube can be placed.

Chest tube. Tube thoracotomy is the definitive treatment for pneumothorax. The insertion of a chest tube is an invasive procedure that requires strict surgical technique, with each operator wearing a gown, gloves, mask, and cap. The infant should be appropriately positioned, restrained, and monitored before the chest is prepared for asepsis. Ideally, the anterior chest wall should be prepped a minimum of 3 minutes. If a special tray is not available, a minor suture tray will usually contain the necessary instruments. Necessary equipment is as follows:

Chest tube (no. 8 to 12 Fr Argyle)
Iodine or Betadine scrub solution
Gloves, gown, mask, hat

Sterile drapes

Syringes

Sterile sponges (gauze)

Medicine cups

Lidocaine 1% without epinephrine

Scalpel blades (no. 11 or 15)

Hemostat (mosquito and Kelly)

Scissors

Needle holder

Sterile suture

Sterile connectors (straight)

Tubing

Infant disposable underwater seal drainage system (two- or three-bottle or Pleurevac system)

Suction

Sterile saline

Tape

The insertion site depends on the clinician's preference. In the lateral approach, the site is the fourth to sixth intercostal space on or lateral to the anterior axillary line. In the superior approach, the site is the second or third intercostal space on or just lateral to the midclavicular line[72] (Figure 17-2). Some researchers have documented that the superior approach is more effective for aspiration of pneumothoraxes.[66]

After infiltration of the area with 1% lidocaine, a small incision is made. A purse string suture should be placed around the incision with ends left loose. A curved hemostat is inserted into the incision and opened. The catheter is advanced through the interspace and into the pleural space. The most frequent error on the part of the inexperienced operator is applying too little force to enter the pleural cavity. The purse string is tightened and tied, and then tied to the chest tube. The tube is connected to the underwater drainage system, which may then be connected to a continuous suction (10 to 15 cm of water is most commonly recommended).[67] The tube should be secured with tape and benzoin. An x-ray examination is used to confirm placement of the tube

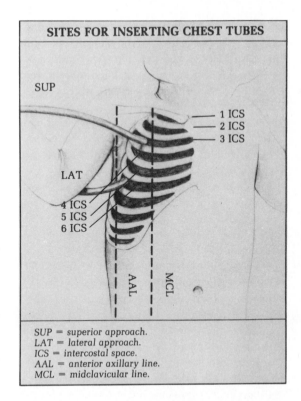

SITES FOR INSERTING CHEST TUBES

SUP · LAT · 1 ICS · 2 ICS · 3 ICS · 4 ICS · 5 ICS · 6 ICS · AAL · MCL

SUP = superior approach.
LAT = lateral approach.
ICS = intercostal space.
AAL = anterior axillary line.
MCL = midclavicular line.

Figure 17-2. Chest tube insertion site. (From Oellrich RG: Pneumothorax, chest tubes and the neonate, MCN 10:31, 1985. Copyright 1985, American Journal of Nursing Co. Reprinted with permission.)

and to evaluate the effectiveness of the therapy.

Complications. In some instances complications have arisen from the placement of chest tubes in neonates. These include hemorrhage, lung perforation, infarction, and phrenic nerve injury with eventration of the diaphragm. Clinical signs of eventration (elevation of the diaphragm into the thoracic cavity) include a shift of the umbilicus upward and toward the affected side.[63,89]

Care of chest tube and drainage system. The chest tube drainage system removes air and fluid material from the pleural space to restore negative pressure and expand the lung. Care providers must be familiar with the operation of the drainage system used in the nursery. The single-bottle water seal system drains air and fluid by gravity and blocks atmospheric air from being drawn into the pleural space. In addition to the water seal, the multiple-bottle systems allow suction to be applied to facilitate drainage and expansion. The Pleurevac system is a single plastic unit divided into three chambers: the collection, water seal, and suction chambers.

Oscillation of fluid in the tube demonstrates effective communication between the pleural space and the drainage bottle. In the small, sick infant intrapleural pressure may only cause fluctuation in the tube at the chest wall. Fluctuation in either the tube or bottle should be observed. Fluctuation may cease as a result of fibrin or blood clots obstructing the tube, kinked or compressed tubing, or the suction apparatus not working properly. Milking and stripping the chest tube every hour expels fluid and clots into the drainage system.

Bubbling in the drainage bottle indicates that air is being removed from the pleural space. Continuous bubbling may indicate an air leak in the system. To locate the source of the leak, the tube is momentarily clamped (beginning close to the chest and working toward the bottle) with a rubber-tipped hemostat. When the clamp is placed between the air leak and the water seal, the bubbling will stop. Patency of the tube, fluctuation, and bubbling should be observed and charted hourly.

Excessive or insufficient fluid in the drainage bottles may interfere with proper function of the drainage system. The bottle may need to be changed, or sterile saline may need to be added.

Frequent turning is important for maximal drainage and lung expansion. Proper stabilizing and positioning of the chest tube is necessary for function, comfort, and prevention of accidental removal. The tubing may be secured by encircling it with an adhesive tab, placing a safety pin through the tape (not the tube), and securing it to the bed. If the tube becomes dislodged, the opening should be covered with sterile gauze and pressure applied until the tube can be replaced.

When the baby is moved for such procedures as x-ray examination and weighing, the tube must be stabilized by holding it close to the chest. If the closed system is disturbed (e.g., broken bottle), the tube should be clamped with a rubber-tipped hemostat that should always be kept at the bedside. The chest tube should be clamped for as short a time as possible. After necessary clamping, vital signs and clinical condition should be closely monitored.

Bottles should be stabilized by being taped to an incubator or warmer so that they are not accidentally broken or picked up. The bottles must always be below the level of the infant's chest to prevent water from being pulled into the pleural space.

Removal of chest tubes. When bubbling has ceased for at least 24 hours and the chest x-ray films show no free air for 12 to 24 hours, the chest tube may be removed. Rapid, sterile removal of the tube is followed by application of a petrolatum gauze pressure dressing.

CNS INSULT

Acute insult to the CNS may result in increased intracranial pressure, hemorrhage, or hypoxic ischemic brain injury (see Chapter 20).

CARDIAC COMPLICATIONS

CDP or IMV may exert sufficient pressure on the pulmonary capillary bed to raise pulmonary artery pressure and interfere with cardiac output.[48] The effect of CDP or IMV on the pulmonary vascular bed and cardiac output may be alleviated by lowering the PIP or PEEP, or both. At times a fluid infusion to increase the intravascular volume may overcome the resistance to the pulmonary blood flow. The effect of MAP on cardiac output is difficult to monitor in most neonatal intensive care units (NICUs), since pulmonary artery or pulmonary wedge pressures are not routinely obtained. Until such time as these measurements are routinely obtained, best CPAP is determined only on clinical grounds.

Patent ductus arteriosus is the most common cardiac complication in neonates with respiratory disease. Most often it is manifested by an increasing oxygen requirement or increased dependency on ventilatory support (see Chapter 18).

INFECTION AND BLEEDING

Procedures such as intubation expose the neonate to the risk of acquired infection. Scrupulous attention to technique when caring for respiratory equipment and performing procedures such as suctioning the endotracheal tube minimizes the risks of infection. Hand washing before and after every contact with the neonate is the best method of preventing hospital-acquired infection in an already compromised, sick neonate. Neonates who are severely ill with respiratory disease may exhibit bleeding diathesis at birth or during the acute phase of their disease. Early recognition and treatment is important (see Part III).

Chronic complications
BRONCHOPULMONARY DYSPLASIA

BPD was first described by Northway and Rosan[71] as serial roentgenographic changes occurring in the lungs of premature infants who survived hyaline membrane disease. BPD also occurs in a variety of conditions, including esophageal atresia, aspiration pneumonia, congenital heart disease, patent ductus arteriosus, and meconium aspiration.[9,47,49,80,83] BPD remains a major clinical problem, with an incidence approaching 20% to 30% in premature infants requiring mechanical ventilation for respiratory distress.[56]

PATHOPHYSIOLOGY. The pathogenesis of BPD is one of constant and recurring lung injury with ongoing repair and healing of the injury. Chronic injury and repair may in itself prolong the need for the very factors that contribute to the development of BPD: oxygen therapy and mechanical ventilation. In IRDS there is injury to the alveolar mucosa, airway mucosa, serum exudation membranes, and fibrin coagulation-forming hyaline membranes. If sufficient hypoxia occurs with resultant damage, the alveolar and airway epithelium and its basement membrane will hemorrhage, and round cell infiltration will begin. Cellular and noncellular debris fill the alveoli and small airways. The obstruction causes microatelectasis, and nonobstructed airways become hyperexpanded and emphysematous.

In the healing and repair process, type II alveolar cells or their precursors multiply and differentiate into type I pneumocytes, which provide alveolar epithelium. Cells of the basal layer of the pseudostratified, ciliated, columnar epithelium lining the airways multiply and migrate to cover the injured airway and rejuvenate the epithelium. During this healing phase the rapidly multiplying and differentiating transitional cells are squamous or cuboidal and therefore appear "metaplastic." Epithelial metaplasia is one of the characteristics of BPD.

As healing occurs, increased inspired oxygen tensions, barotrauma, and infection continue to injure the cells that are taking part in the healing process.

ETIOLOGY. BPD is an iatrogenic disease caused by oxygen toxicity and barotrauma resulting from pressure ventilation. In addition, there is evidence to suggest that fluid overload, infection, ligation of the patent ductus arteriosus, and familial predisposition to asthma also contribute to the development of BPD.[33,69,70]

Oxygen toxicity. BPD has been documented in both long- and short-term exposure to oxygen at both low and high levels (greater than 80%), as well as in infants treated with mechanical ventilation without supplemental oxygen.[70] As a result of these findings, many units have instituted guidelines for oxygen use and monitoring of levels with a TCM or pulse oximetry. In addition, peak pressures should be monitored closely and reduced whenever possible to prevent barotrauma.

Barotrauma. BPD has also been related to barotrauma. BPD has been described in infants who have received peak inspiratory pressures of greater than 35 cm of water[92] and in those with pneumothorax.[68] A decrease in the incidence of BPD has been noted when lower peak inspiratory pressures were used.[82] Although peak inspiratory pressures should be limited whenever possible, some infants with very noncompliant lungs require the use of high pressure for survival. Adequate pressures to inflate the lung should be used to prevent the need for higher oxygen concentrations. Preliminary studies in the use of high-frequency ventilation suggest that this type of ventilation may cause yet another form of barotrauma.

Patent ductus arteriosus. There is a high incidence of BPD among infants with patent ductus arteriosus (PDA)[38] and congestive heart failure.[12,38,49,70] The amount of oxygen and peak inspiratory pressure required to support the neonate through the pulmonary complications of patent ductus arteriosus may result in damage from oxygen toxicity and barotrauma. The increased pulmonary blood flow that occurs may also contribute to pulmonary damage. Because of these findings, medical closure of the ductus with indomethacin or surgical ligation is advocated.

Fluids. BPD has also been detected in infants who have developed symptoms of fluid overload within the first few days of life.[12] Fluid balance in the VLBW infant is complicated by huge insensible water losses and often an intolerance to enteral feedings. Intake, output, and changes in weight must be closely monitored to calculate the fluid needs.

Family history of asthma. Infants who develop BPD may have relatives with asthma that requires hospitalization.[70] The lungs of these infants may be less tolerant of the insults of pulmonary disease, oxygen, pressure, and fluids.

Prematurity. Premature births alone may have a significant effect on pulmonary development, since prematurity results in differences in the development of small airways.[19] As a result, premature infants could be more susceptible to additional damage to the small airways from oxygen,

ventilator pressure, fluids, and circulatory overload. As the survival rate of premature infants of less than 28 weeks gestation increases, the occurrence of BPD may also increase. Despite the fact that management of these risk factors in the development of BPD has improved, BPD is still on the rise, especially in the VLBW and early-gestational-age infant.

PREVENTION. In an attempt to prevent reinjury and allow healing, inspired oxygen tensions should be kept as low as is reasonable to provide adequate arterial oxygen tension. Pressures on the ventilator should be reduced when possible to prevent barotrauma. Infections should be treated with appropriate antibiotic agents.

DATA COLLECTION

History. A history of prematurity, moderate to severe IRDS, intubation with oxygen and positive-pressure ventilation, inability to be weaned from the ventilator, and increasing oxygen requirement at the end of the first week of life are associated with BPD.

Signs and symptoms. Tachypnea, exercise intolerance (feeding and handling), oxygen dependence, and respiratory distress (retractions, nasal flaring, fine rales at the bases or throughout the lung fields) may all be associated with BPD.

Laboratory data. X-ray findings (Figure 17-3) correlate with the stage of disease; however, the pathologic changes are often more severe than the chest x-ray findings indicate.[25,71]

Stage I	Reticulogranular pattern and air bronchogram or IRDS (first 3 days of life)
Stage II	Coarse granular infiltrates that are dense enough to obscure the cardiac markings (first 3 to 10 days of life)
Stage III	Multiple small cyst formation within the opaque lungs and visible cardiac borders (first 10 to 20 days of life)
Stage IV	Irregular larger cyst formation that alternates with areas of increased density (after 28 days of life)

Treatment. The therapeutic goal is to reduce those factors that produce reinjury and to allow the lung to heal so that normal function can be resumed. This process may take weeks or months, even years, in severe lung injuries or in small infants under 1000 g.

Therapy is supportive. Careful attention to fluid balance to prevent fluid overload is important. Early closure of PDA may be beneficial. Usually in BPD the infant's ability to maintain ventilation develops before the ability to maintain adequate oxygenation. Often infants are discharged from the NICU on home oxygen therapy.

Although the pathologic changes in bronchopulmonary dysplasia result in increased airway resistance, there have been few clinical reports on the efficacy of bronchodilators for treating BPD. Bronchodilators may fail to relieve airway obstruction because of relatively poor development of bronchial smooth muscle in preterm infants. Bronchodilators are not often effective in lowering airway resistance in children younger than 12 to 30 months of age.[60,93] In contrast, some improvement in infants with chronic lung disease using bronchodilators has been shown.[15,44,52,85] Bronchodilators such as terbutaline, metaproterenol (Alupent), and albuterol have been used clinically in this population, but little is documented about their effect. Isoproterenol and metaproterenol have been studied and shown to be effective in decreasing airway resistance; metaproterenol also improved compliance and gas exchange.[15,52] Pre-

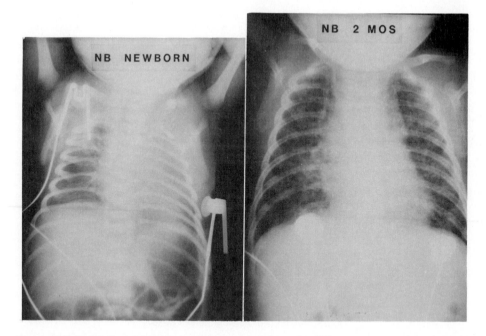

Figure 17-3. Serial chest x-ray films of premature infant with BPD over 2½ year period. Infant's disease process was characterized by multiple hospitalizations for reactive airway disease and pulmonary hypertension. Note progressive lung disease characterized by hyperinflation and eventual clearing of infiltrate by 2½ years of age.   *Continued.*

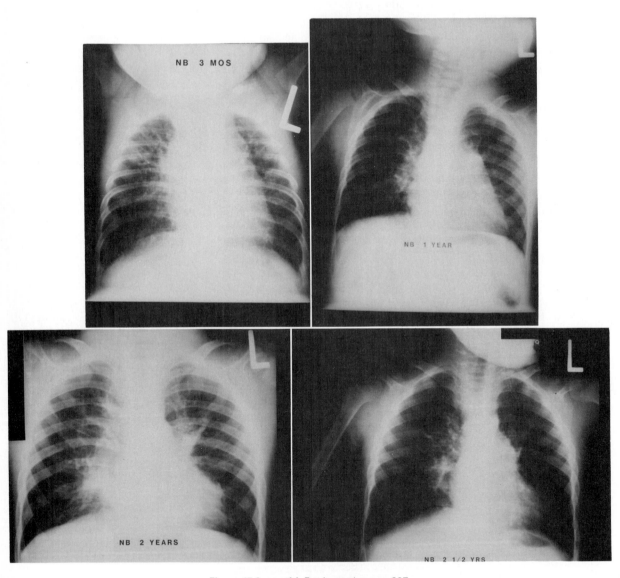

Figure 17-3, cont'd. For legend see p. 397.

term infants with chronic lung disease have been given nebulized bronchodilators in an attempt to reduce airway resistance (Table 17-3).

Theophylline (also studied on a limited basis) is advocated for the ventilator-dependent infant with BPD, because it improves lung compliance and reduces expiratory resistance.[52,85] Methylxanthine therapy promotes weaning of infants with RDS from low rates of ventilatory support.[44] Theophylline has a multisystem effect in the infant[36,97]:

CNS—Stimulation of the CNS at all levels; increased cerebral oxygen consumption; decreased cerebral blood flow

Respiratory—Increased surfactant production, inspiratory drive, respiratory rate, PaO_2 sensitivity

Hematopoietic—Shortened coagulation time

Renal—Increased glomerular filtration rate

Cardiac—Increased heart rate, cardiac contractility, and output

Endocrine—Increased catecholamine and insulin levels

Alimentary—Decreased gastrointestinal motility; increased gastric secretions

Metabolic—Increased glucose levels, ketonuria, and glycosuria

Musculoskeletal—Increased muscle contraction; decreased muscle fatigue

Complications. Complications of BPD include:

1. Progressive interstitial emphysema and cyst formation
2. Air leaks
3. Pulmonary hypertension
4. Cor pulmonale; right-sided heart failure
5. Respiratory infections
6. Bronchiolitis common during first 1 to 2 years of life
7. Fractures from vigorous chest physiotherapy, rickets
8. Requirement for home oxygen therapy

RETINOPATHY OF PREMATURITY (RETROLENTAL FIBROPLASIA)

The association between oxygen administration, prematurity, and subsequent retinal changes often resulting in blindness has been recognized since the 1950s.[53,75] Severe restriction in the use of oxygen with the premature infant resulted in less

TABLE 17-3

Rapid-Acting Bronchodilators Used in Treatment of BPD

BRONCHODILATOR	DOSE	SIDE EFFECTS
Metaproterenol (Alupent)	0.1-0.2 ml in 2 ml of normal saline q.3-4h. (maximum: 0.3 ml)	Tachycardia, tremors, nausea, and vomiting; can cause paradoxical bronchoconstriction
Albuterol (Proventil, Ventolin)	0.1 mg/kg up to 5 mg in 2 ml of normal saline	Same as above
Terbutaline (Brethine)	0.03-0.1 mg/kg/day	Same as above
Medications affecting histamine release		
Cromolyn	10 mg t.i.d.	Urticaria, throat irritation
Theophylline	4 to 6 mg/kg of active theophylline, which should produce a serum level of 8 to 10 μg/ml; maintenance calculated by rate of plasma clearance, usually 3 to 7 mg/kg/day administered every 12 hours	Tachycardia, diuresis arrhythmias, glucosuria, seizures, ketonuria, vomiting, hyperglycemia, jitteriness, hemorrhagic gastritis

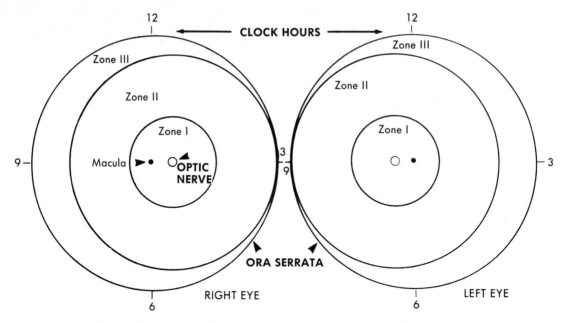

Figure 17-4. International classification of ROP. (From An international classification of retinopathy of prematurity, Arch Ophthamol 102:1131, 1984. Copyright 1984, American Medical Association and courtesy Ross Laboratories, Columbus, Ohio.)

retinopathy of prematurity (ROP), but also in an increased morbidity and mortality.[6,65] With increased survival of the very preterm infant, liberalization of the use of oxygen, and improved technology for support and assisted ventilation, there is a resurgence of ROP.

PHYSIOLOGY. The pathophysiologic process in the development of ROP is not completely understood. Many factors play a role in the pathogenesis. When hyperoxia is involved, it is the pressure in arterial blood (PaO_2) rather than the concentration administered (FIO_2) that is important.

In response to hyperoxia, the retinal vessels constrict. They may permanently constrict and become necrotic (vaso-obliteration). The vessels that have not been obliterated may proliferate in an attempt to reestablish retinal circulation. Proliferatng vessels may extend into the vitreous, causing fluid leakage and/or hemorrhage, with

retinal scar formation, traction on the retina, detachment, and blindness.

The degree of retinal vascularization at birth determines the susceptibility to the insult of hyperoxia. The majority of retinal vascularization is complete by 32 weeks gestation. However, even at 40 weeks the temporal periphery of the retina may still not be completely vascularized.

Early changes may first be evident at the temporal periphery, since this area is the last to be completely vascularized. Proliferation of new vessels may remain localized and spontaneously resolve or may progress to cause total retinal detachment.

ROP is classified by location of disease in the retina (zone), by degree (stage) of vascular abnormality, and by extent of developing vasculature (clock hour)[1,4] (Figure 17-4 and Table 17-4). Changes are first readily seen between 6

TABLE 17-4

Stages of Retinopathy of Prematurity

Stage 1: Demarcation line

A thin white line separates the avascular retina anteriorly from the vascularized retina posteriorly. Abnormal branching vessels lead to the demarcation line, which is flat and lies in the plane of the retina.

Stage 2: Ridge

The ridge has a definite height and width, occupies a volume, and extends up out of the plane of the retina. Its color may change from white to pink. Small, isolated tufts of new vessels may appear posterior to the structure.

Stage 3: Ridge with extraretinal fibrovascular proliferations

To the ridge of stage 2 is added the presence of extraretinal fibrovascular proliferative tissue. Characteristic locations:

1. Continuous with the posterior aspect of the ridge (ragged ridge)
2. Immediately posterior to the ridge but not always appearing to be connected to it
3. Into the vitreous perpendicular to the retinal plane

Stage 4: Retinal detachment

To stage 3 is added unequivocal detachment of the retina caused by exudative effusion of fluid, traction, or both.

"PLUS" disease

Progressive vascular incompetence is noted primarily by increasing dilation and tortuosity of peripheral retinal vessels. Only when posterior veins are enlarged and arterioles are tortuous is the designation "+" added to the ROP stage number (e.g., stage 3 + ROP).

From An international classification of retinopathy of prematurity: Arch Ophthalm. 2:1130, 1984. Copyright 1984, American Medical Association and courtesy Ross Laboratories, Columbus, Ohio.

and 8 weeks of life. Seventy-five percent of mild forms of ROP spontaneously resolve.

ETIOLOGY. ROP is considered primarily a disease of prematurity. The incidence is inversely proportional to birth weight and gestational age. Damage may occur in any preterm infant and has its highest incidence in the infant younger than 28 weeks gestation. Infants weighing less than 1500 g (appropriate weight for gestational age) have the highest incidence of disease (16% to 34%)[42,51] and the highest incidence of blindness (5% to 11%).[42,78]

PREVENTION. Adherence to the principles of oxygen therapy is essential as the first line of defense against developing ROP. Since a baby who is very hyperoxic (PaO_2 >200 mm Hg) will clinically look no different than a baby whose PaO_2 is normal (approximately 80 torr), monitoring of arterial blood gases or transcutaneous oxygen is manda-

tory whenever oxygen is administered. Oxygen tension should be measured 15 to 30 minutes after initiating, altering, or discontinuing therapy.

The usefulness and safety of vitamin E is still unclear. Its use is considered experimental, and its routine administration for the prevention of ROP is not recommended.[3]

DATA COLLECTION. Visualization of the retina is difficult and not predictive of occurring vasoconstriction and retinal changes as a result of hyperoxia. Indirect funduscopic examination by a neonatal ophthalmologist at 6 to 8 weeks may document retinal changes. Contributing factors to the development of ROP are as follows:

1. **Prematurity—very low birth weight (<1500 g)**
2. **Hyperoxia**
3. **Blood transfusions**

4. **Pregnancy complications (hypertension, preeclampsia, diabetes, bleeding, smoking)**
5. **Apnea**
6. **Asphyxia**
7. **Sepsis**
8. **Hypercapnia or hypocapnia**
9. **Ventilatory support (prolonged and with episodes of hypercapnia, hypoxia, or both)**
10. **Multiple gestation**
11. **Nutritional deficiency**

TREATMENT. The best treatment is prevention. NOTE: Even strict adherence to all principles of good care may still not prevent ROP in VLBW infants.

Noninvasive continuous monitoring (TCM and pulse oximetry) enables trending of an infant's fluctuations (hypoxia or hyperoxia) with ventilatory changes, handling, and activity (see Chapter 6). Cryotherapy performed by a qualified, experienced pediatric ophthalmologist appears to be the best treatment.

COMPLICATIONS. When the eyes are not used, microphthalmia (small sunken eyes) results. Glaucoma, strabismus, and late retinal detachment (in teens or early twenties) may develop. Severe myopia may develop as early as 6 months of age. Early detection and correction with lenses is essential to save the child's remaining sight.

PARENT TEACHING. Blindness is defined by most of our society as one of the worst handicaps. Parents will experience grief over this devastating loss and will need help to cope before they will be able to bond to their blind child.

Blind infants are unable to communicate with care providers through the signs and signals of facial expression.[35] Because of the absence of eye language, no cues to infant needs and no feedback of preference, recognition, and delight can be given. Absence of a smile from the blind baby connotes a negative response to the care provider. When care providers understand these behavioral differences, they can assist parents to understand the lack of facial expression. Instead of facial ex-

TABLE 17-5

Incidence of Neurologic Sequelae in Ventilated Infants

INFANT'S STATUS	ALL INFANTS (%)	INFANTS <1500 G (%)
Major neurologic defect	21.2[10]	11[61]
	<21 to 13[62]	23.8[10]
No neurologic defect	80[10,31,61]	44[31]

pression, parents are taught to read the special hand language of their infant as an expression of emotions, intentions, preference, and recognition.[35] Appropriate referrals to occupational therapy, physical therapy, and community resources for extrasensory stimulation for the infant may help avoid developmental delays from insufficient or inappropriate stimulation.

CHRONIC CNS SEQUELAE

If hyperoxia is toxic, hypoxia is just as devastating especially to the brain. For babies receiving ventilation therapy, the degree of hypoxia rather than ventilation itself determines neurologic sequelae. The highest incidence of abnormal findings occurs in infants with intracranial hemorrhage and the lowest birth weights (<1500 g).[10] Accompanying improved survival of VLBW infants is an increase in nonhandicapped survivors (Table 17-5).

Neurologic sequelae are divided into major and minor types. Major neurologic defects such as cerebral palsy, hydrocephalus, seizures, and mental retardation are usually diagnosed in the first 2 years of life. Yet minor defects that are not severely handicapping, such as learning disorders, hyperactivity, minor retardation, altered muscle tone, and fine and gross motor incoordination may not be diagnosed so early. Subtle perceptual problems may be diagnosed in the preschool child or even in the school-age child with inadequate school performance.[31] Cerebral palsy remains the most common neurologic defect in survivors (10% to 26%).[10,31,32]

IDIOPATHIC RESPIRATORY DISTRESS SYNDROME
Pathophysiology

IRDS is a disease of immature lung anatomy and physiology. Anatomically the preterm lung is unable to support oxygenation and ventilation, because alveolar saccules are insufficiently developed, causing a deficient surface area for gas exchange. Also, the pulmonary capillary bed is deficient and the interstitial mesenchyme is present to a greater extent, increasing the distance between the alveolar and the endothelial cell membranes.

Physiologically the volume of surfactant is insufficient to prevent collapse of unstable alveoli. Since the alveoli collapse with each breath, normal functional residual capacity is not established. Because of alveolar collapse, oxygenation and ventilation are insufficient, and each breath requires increased energy output.

Compliance is related to the amount of volume achieved during a given application of pressure. Compliance of the lung is equal to the ratio of the change in volume to the change in pressure. The lung in IRDS has low compliance (i.e., little change in volume is achieved with a relatively great application of pressure), thereby contributing to increased work of breathing. However, the chest wall of the neonate is unfortunately very compliant; a slight application of pressure results in a large change in volume. The infant may not be able to create enough inspiratory pressure to open the alveoli as the chest wall retracts and collapses about the relatively stiff lung. Thus in IRDS the diaphragm contracts, creating an inspiratory pressure that moves less volume into the lung than expected and simultaneously causes large sternal and intercostal retractions of the chest wall.

The increased effort of these opposing forces usually results in hypoxemia and acidemia that cause constriction of the pulmonary vascular (arterial) musculature, severely limiting pulmonary capillary blood flow. The integrity of pulmonary capillary blood flow is critical for the integrity of the alveolar epithelial membrane and the production of surfactant. Without adequate pulmonary capillary blood flow, the type II pneumocytes become deficient in precursor material required for production of surfactant. Lack of surfactant production compounds the deficiency and leads to low compliance. These physiologic factors promote increased work of breathing and aggravate the ongoing ventilatory problems.

In the fetus pulmonary vascular resistance is high, and pulmonary artery blood pressure is greater than systemic blood pressure, causing blood flow from the main pulmonary artery to travel through the open ductus arteriosus to the descending aorta. A second right-to-left shunt occurs across the foramen ovale in the fetus. The high pulmonary vascular resistance is "reactive" to the normal fetal "hypoxemia," since the pulmonary vascular resistance and the pulmonary artery blood pressure decrease as the PaO_2 of the neonate increases. At birth the ductus arteriosus actively constricts in response to the increase in PaO_2 ($PaO_2 > 50$ mm Hg), eliminating blood flow across the ductus and completing the transition to neonatal circulation. The fetal circulatory pattern may persist from birth or be initiated by a transient hypoxemic episode. In the instance of neonatal hypoxemia, the pulmonary vasculature "reacts" by vasoconstriction, raising pulmonary vascular resistance, and the ductus arteriosus "reacts" by relaxing, once again allowing blood flow from the pulmonary artery to the descending aorta, as normally occurs in the fetus. Pulmonary vascular resistance is increased with shunting through the ductus arteriosus. Fetal circulatory patterns are perpetuated by hypoxemia and acidemia and produce systemic hypoxemia that aggravates and perpetuates the condition.

Endothelial damage and alveolar necrosis aggravate the already existing surfactant deficiency. A cyclic deterioration is established, and hypoxia and acidosis persist unless treatment is initiated.

Microscopically, the events that occur in the lung include injury to and death of the alveolar epithelial cells and airway epithelial cells. This injury and death are followed by sloughing of the cells from the respiratory basement membrane, leaving the basement membrane denuded. Exudation of serum follows. Fibrin in the serum clots, and hyaline membranes are formed, covering the denuded basement membranes in the airways and alveolar spaces. If there is sufficient hypoxic damage to the cells and basement membranes, frank hemorrhage may fill the alveolar spaces. These factors serve to decrease the total surface area of the gas exchange membrane. The end result is hypoxemia, acidemia, and increasing respiratory distress.

The entire sequence of events in IRDS is related to the inability to maintain lung expansion and alveolar stability as a result of surfactant deficiency. IRDS evolves from two interrelated problems: atelectasis and persistence of or reversion to the fetal levels of pulmonary hypertension[79] (Figures 17-5 and 17-6).

Etiology

IRDS occurs in infants born prematurely and is a consequence of immature lung anatomy and physiology. In the premature infant or stressed infant, atelectasis from the collapse of the terminal alveoli because of lack of surfactant appears after the first few hours of life. In the premature infant surfactant production is limited, and stores are quickly depleted. Surfactant production may be further diminished by other unfavorable conditions such as high oxygen concentration, poor pulmonary drainage, excessive pulmonary hygiene, or effects of respirator management.

Data collection
HISTORY

A history of prematurity, cesarean section, and/or asphyxial episodes may be seen in infants with IRDS.

PHYSICAL EXAMINATION

Infants with IRDS often show signs of tachypnea, grunting, flaring, and retractions within the first few minutes to hours of life. Pallor or cyanosis may also be present. The trachea is midline, and there is a normal apical pulse. Auscultation of the chest reveals decreased breath sounds and often rales. Many of these infants may be hypotensive.

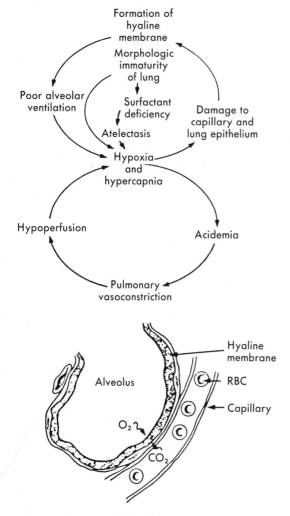

Figure 17-5. Interdependent relationship of factors involved in pathology of RDS. (From Pierog SH and Ferrara A: Medical care of the sick newborn, ed 2, St Louis, 1976, The CV Mosby Co.)

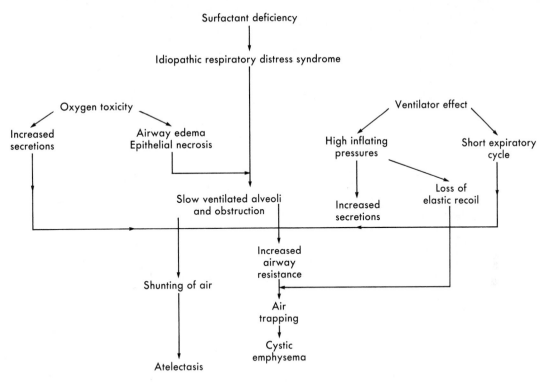

Figure 17-6. Schematic representation of pathogenesis of IRDS.

LABORATORY DATA

A chest x-ray examination reveals a ground-glass appearance that represents areas of collapsed respiratory units adjacent to expanded or even hyperexpanded respiratory units. This can also be described as a bilateral reticulogranular pattern with air bronchograms (Figures 17-7 and 17-8).

Arterial blood gases reveal hypoxemia and often acidemia that may be metabolic, respiratory, or a combination of both (see Chapter 8).

Treatment

Treatment is directed toward:

I. Reducing hypoxemia (see section on general treatment strategies in this chapter and in Chapter 8)

II. Correcting acidemia (see Chapter 8)

III. Increasing the functional residual capacity (see section on general treatment strategies)

IV. Decreasing the work of breathing (see section on general treatment strategies)

V. Continuing physiologic support and maintenance of homeostasis:

A. Maintaining appropriate temperature (see Chapter 5)

B. Monitoring vital signs and arterial blood gases (see Chapters 6 and 8)

C. Providing appropriate fluid, electrolytes, glucose, and calories (see Part II)

D. Observing for complications of disease and treatments (see section on general complications)

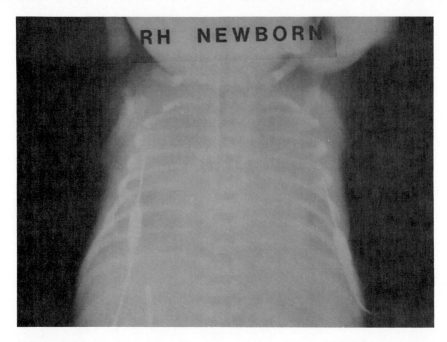

Figure 17-7. Chest x-ray film of 28-week preterm infant with severe IRDS. Note "white out" appearance.

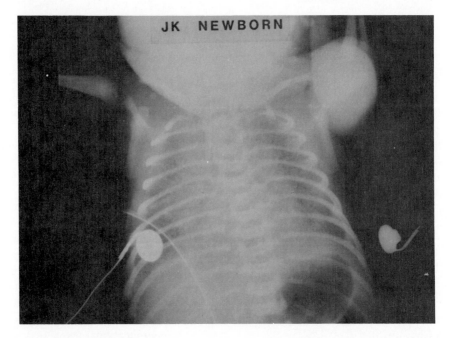

Figure 17-8. Chest x-ray film of 27-week premature infant with IRDS. Note characteristic infiltrate pattern with air bronchograms.

TRANSIENT TACHYPNEA OF THE NEWBORN
Pathophysiology

Transient tachypnea of the newborn (TTN) is the result of delayed reabsorption of normal lung fluid, and thus an alternative name is "wet lung." Lung fluid accumulates in the peribronchiolar lymphatics and the bronchovascular spaces. Thus TTN is an "obstructive" lung disease, whereas IRDS is a "restrictive" lung disease.

Etiology

TTN generally occurs in term or near-term babies with a history of cesarean section or precipitous delivery. In these situations there is a lack of the gradual compression of the chest that perhaps would eliminate some fluid during a normal vaginal delivery. This accumulation of interstitial fluid interferes with the forces that tend to hold the bronchioli open. This interference causes the bronchioli to collapse. The result is air trapping.

Data collection
HISTORY

As previously stated, term or near-term babies with a history of cesarean section or precipitous delivery are predisposed to TTN. Onset is usually 2 to 6 hours after birth.

PHYSICAL EXAMINATION

Respiratory distress including tachypnea, retractions, grunting, and flaring may be seen. Cyanosis in room air may also be present.

LABORATORY DATA

Mild hypoxemia (requiring <40% oxygen) and milk acidemia are usually present. A significant degree of hypoxemia or acidemia will tend to constrict the pulmonary vasculature and aggravate the problem. Chest x-ray examination reveals hyperexpansion with streaky infiltrates radiating from the hilum. These infiltrates are thought to represent interstitial fluid along the bronchovascular spaces. The air trapping causes the appearance of hyperexpansion on the chest x-ray film.

Treatment

In general, support of the patient with TTN requires only the provision of sufficient supplemental oxygen to maintain an arterial oxygen tension of more than 70 to 80 mm Hg and maintenance of usual supportive neonatal care. Although diuretic agents have been advocated, usually little more than general support is necessary while the normal absorption of lung fluid through the lymphatics takes place.

MECONIUM ASPIRATION
Pathophysiology

Before meconium aspiration can occur, meconium must find its way into the amniotic fluid. This condition occurs more often in term or post-term infants when an hypoxic episode is experienced in utero. With fetal asphyxia the anal sphincter relaxes and colonic peristalsis ensues, expelling meconium into the amniotic fluid. Subsequently a second episode of asphyxia occurs during which the infant makes gasping respiratory movements. These movements open the glottis so that meconium flows into the oropharynx and on into the lung.

Etiology

Meconium aspiration produces disease by several mechanisms: meconium may physically obstruct the glottis, trachea, or any number of smaller airways; it promotes development of infection seemingly by increasing the virulence of infecting organisms; the increase in pulmonary vascular resistance caused by asphyxial episode(s) results in increased right-to-left shunting (see Figure 17-9).

Prevention

Before birth, meconium aspiration may be prevented by early recognition of the compromised fetus and appropriate intervention.

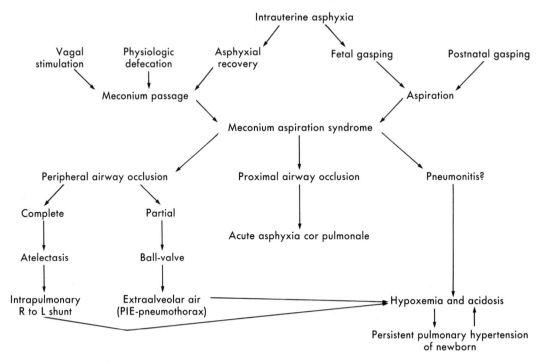

Figure 17-9. Schematic representation of pathogenesis of meconium aspiration syndrome. (Modified from Basick R: Pediatr Clin North Am 24:467, 1977.)

At birth, suction on the perineum may be preventive. On delivery of the head and before delivery of the rest of the body of an infant with meconium-stained fluid, removing meconium, blood, and mucus from the infant's nose, mouth, and pharynx with a DeLee suction trap is essential. This prevents aspiration of the contents into the bronchi with the first gasp of respiration.[16] NOTE: Aspiration of amniotic contents into upper large airways before the first respiratory efforts may occur with the onset of gasping in utero.

After birth, intubation and suction of the trachea may be useful. Pulmonary lavage is not effective and is not recommended.

Data collection
HISTORY

History of asphyxia, intrauterine growth retardation, postterm delivery, and meconium-stained amniotic fluid may be present.

PHYSICAL EXAMINATION

Tachypnea, rales, and cyanosis are seen in mild cases. In moderately severe cases grunting, retractions, and nasal flaring may also be seen. In severe cases the infant is asphyxiated and severely depressed at birth. There is profound cyanosis and pallor, irregular gasping respirations, and an increased anteroposterior diameter of the chest.

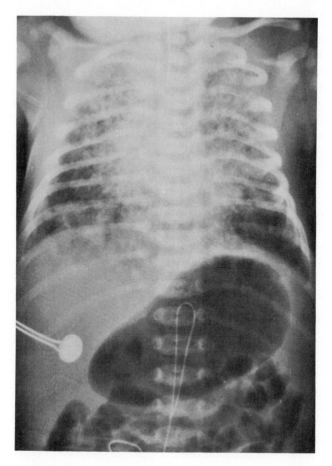

Figure 17-10. Chest x-ray film of infant with meconium aspiration. Note diffuse infiltrates.

LABORATORY DATA

The chest x-ray examination shows marked air trapping and hyperexpansion. There are bilateral, coarse, patchy infiltrates (Figure 17-10). Air leaks are frequently seen.

Severe hypoxemia as a result of ventilation perfusion inequality and right-to-left shunting caused by pulmonary hypertension are usually present. Severe hypercapnia is usually present. Severe acidosis is usually a combined respiratory and metabolic acidosis.

Treatment

Since the major problem in meconium aspiration is hypoxemia, treatment should be directed at improving oxygenation. Mildly affected infants will frequently require only warmed, humidified oxygen by hood. Increasing severity of meconium aspiration will require increased levels of intervention. Some infants will respond to CPAP (4 to 6 cm of water), but others will require full ventilator support. Since these infants are usually term or postterm, they may fight assisted ventilation and require paralyzation to ventilate and oxygenate the lungs adequately. A 0.03 to 0.06 mg/kg/dose of pancuronium bromide (Pavulon) will paralyze the infant. Repeat doses are given as needed. With paralysis, these infants require rapid rates (60 to 80 breaths/min) and high pressure (>30 cm of water). PEEP of 4 to 6 cm of water should also be used.

Mucosal irritation and increased mucosal secretion hamper respiratory and mucociliary clearance efforts. Frequent pulmonary hygiene every 2 to 3 hours will help alleviate this problem.

As with any sick infant, close attention must be given to physiologic support and homeostasis (see also section on general treatment strategies, Chapters 5, 6, and 8, and Part II).

Complications

Persistent fetal circulation is a frequent complication of meconium aspiration, and it compounds the difficulties in oxygenating the infant. An air leak is a complication of both the disease (ball-valve obstruction causing air trapping) and the treatment (CPAP or ventilator support). The underlying asphyxia can be viewed as either a cause or a complication (see Chapter 3).

PERSISTENT PULMONARY HYPERTENSION OF THE NEWBORN (PERSISTENT FETAL CIRCULATION)

Persistent pulmonary hypertension of the newborn (PPHN) is a disease seen primarily in the term and postterm newborn. Infants who present with PPHN have severe pulmonary hypertension with pulmonary artery pressure elevation to levels equal to or higher than systemic pressure and large right-to-left shunts through both the foramen ovale and the ductus arteriosus. This results in respiratory distress, severe hypoxemia, and acidosis, which potentiates pulmonary vasoconstriction. Despite improved identification and aggressive treatment, mortality and morbidity re-

main high. Resultant morbidity in surviving infants includes: chronic lung disease, neurologic sequelae, and pneumothorax.[8,13,27]

Physiology

Once the placental blood source is severed, adequate oxygenation of the newborn depends on inflation of the lungs, closure of the fetal shunts, a decrease in pulmonary vascular resistance, and an increase in pulmonary blood flow. Normally, pulmonary vascular resistance decreases with the first breath of life. When it remains high, successful transition from fetal to neonatal circulation does not occur. In the infant manifesting PPHN, high pulmonary vascular resistance and pulmonary hypertension impede pulmonary blood flow. This leads to hypoxemia, acidemia, and eventually lactic acidosis. The pulmonary arterioles respond to this process with further constriction, promoting an additional decrease in blood flow; thus a cyclic pattern is set up. Pulmonary vascular resistance also maintains higher right-sided pressures in the heart that equal or exceed systemic pressures. This promotes the right-to-left shunting that is characteristic of this disease.[23] PPHN also produces direct and indirect effects on myocardial function. A combination of pressure alterations, hypoxia, and acidemia leads to a cyclic pattern of decreased cardiac output, decreased pulmonary blood flow, and further vasoconstriction (Figures 17-11 through 17-14).

Etiology

PPHN occurs as an idiopathic or unexplained condition. Since full development of the pulmonary arterial musculature occurs late in gestation, persistent PPHN is primarily a condition of the term and postterm infant. In utero development of increased vascular smooth muscle or perinatal factors that cause or contribute to vasospasm are thought to be prime mechanisms of PPHN.

PPHN is also associated with a wide variety of other disorders affecting the cardiac and pulmonary systems: myocardial ischemia,[39] meconium aspiration,[7] transient tachypnea of the newborn,[14]

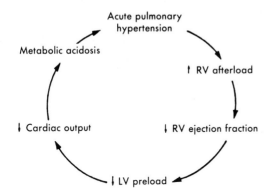

Figure 17-11. Effect of pulmonary hypertension on cardiac output. *RV,* Right ventricle; *LV,* left ventricle. (From Perkin RM and Anas NG: J Pediatr 105:511, 1984.)

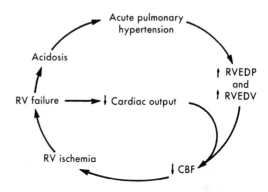

Figure 17-12. Effect of pulmonary hypertension on right ventricular function. *RV,* Right ventricle; *RVEDP,* right ventricular end-diastolic pressure; *RVEDV,* right ventricular end-diastolic volume; *CBF,* coronary blood flow. (From Perkin RM and Anas, NG: J Pediatr 105:511, 1984.)

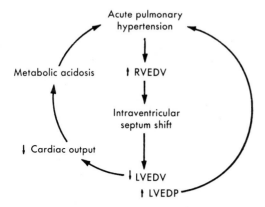

Figure 17-13. Effect of pulmonary hypertension on left ventricular function. *RVEDV,* Right ventricular end-diastolic volume; *LVEDV,* left ventricular end-diastolic volume; *LVEDP,* left ventricular end-diastolic pressure. (From Perkin RM and Anas, NG: J Pediatr 105:511, 1984.)

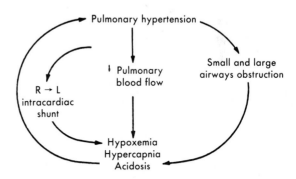

Figure 17-14. Effect of pulmonary hypertension on gas exchange. *R → L,* Right to left. (From Perkin RM and Anas NG: J Pediatr 105:511, 1984.)

pneumonia, alveolar hypoventilation,[86] pulmonary hypoplasia,[81] polycythemia, hypoglycemia, hypocalcemia,[39] sepsis,[87] and maternal ingestion of prostaglandin inhibitors,[77] dilantin,[94] or lithium.[30]

Prevention

Prevention of PPHN includes minimizing intrauterine and perinatal risk factors when possible, maintaining postnatal physiologic homeostasis, and detecting and correcting any underlying abnormality.

Data collection
HISTORY

Risk factors of PPHN are as follows:
I. Intrauterine factors
  A. Fetal hypertension
  B. Chronic in utero hypoxia
  C. Pulmonary hypoplasia (diaphragmatic hernia or oligohydramnios)
  D. In utero ductus arteriosus closure (maternal drugs, i.e., indomethacin or salicylic agents)
  E. Asphyxia
  F. Maternal ingestion of prostaglandin inhibitors, dilantin, or lithium
II. Postnatal factors
  A. Polycythemia
  B. Hypothermia
  C. Hypoglycemia or hypocalcemia
  D. Acidosis
  E. Meconium aspiration syndrome
  F. Parenchymal pulmonary disease
  G. Pneumonia (beta strep)
  H. Transient tachypnea of the newborn
  I. Alveolar hypoventilation
  J. Myocardial dysfunction
  K. Sepsis

There are two major considerations in the history of these infants: (1) the recognition of major disease processes or syndromes that are highly associated with pulmonary hypertension and (2) the timing of the onset of cyanosis and the deterioration of the infant.

PHYSICAL EXAMINATION

The initial clinical presentation is usually a full-term or postterm infant with worsening cyanosis. Tachypnea is a common finding and when accompanied by retractions is indicative of decreased pulmonary compliance. Cyanosis may be either intense at birth or may progressively worsen in association with increased right-to-left shunting. The milder cases of PPHN have minimal tachypnea and cyanosis, frequently associated with stress from crying or feeding. The severe cases are characterized by marked cyanosis, tachypnea, and decreased peripheral perfusion.

Increased pulmonary artery pressure results in the following symptoms[46]:
1. Pulmonic systolic ejection clicks
2. Second heart sound that is single, loud, or narrowly split with a loud pulmonary component
3. Prominent right ventricular impulse that is visible or palpable at the lower left sternal border
4. Soft systolic murmur in the pulmonary area[6]

LABORATORY DATA

The laboratory evaluation of the infant with potential PPHN should include a complete blood count (CBC) with differential, platelet count, chest x-ray examination, and serum glucose, calcium, and arterial blood gas determinations. The CBC is used to detect anemia that could contribute to systemic hypertension, to detect plethora that could lead to increased pulmonary vascular resistance, and to detect an infectious process such as group B sepsis or pneumonia.

Arterial blood gases demonstrate acidosis, hypoxia, and increased $PaCO_2$. If a blood gas is obtained simultaneously in the right radial artery (preductal) and in the descending aorta (postductal), the right-to-left shunt can be documented (preductal PaO_2 > postductal). Simultaneous preductal and postductal transcu-

TABLE 17-6 _____

Diagnostic Tests for PPHN

TEST	USE
Hyperoxia test	If Po_2 does not increase in 100% oxygen, a right-to-left shunt is demonstrated (may be secondary to either PPHN or congenital heart disease).
Comparison of pre- and postductal arterial Po_2	Demonstrates ductal shunting. If negative, it does not rule out PPHN. Most congenital heart disease has no ductal shunting.
Contrast echocardiography "bubble echo"	Demonstrates foramen ovale shunting but should be present in most PPHN.
Hyperoxia-hyperventilation	Most definitive test; if $Po_2 < 50$ mm Hg prehyperventilation and rises to above 100 mm Hg, is almost always PPHN.

From Duara S, Gewitz MH, and Fox WW: Clin Perinatol 11:641, 1984.

taneous oxygen measurements may also be useful in the diagnosis.

The most common radiographic findings associated with PPHN include[46]:

1. Prominent main pulmonary artery segment
2. Mild to moderate cardiomegaly
3. Variable pulmonary vasculature (increased, decreased, or normal)
4. Signs of left ventricular dysfunction that include pulmonary venous congestion and cardiomegaly

The electrocardiogram is usually normal but may demonstrate right ventricular hypertrophy and signs of myocardial ischemia. Echocardiography is helpful in evaluating cardiac structures and ruling out cyanotic lesions. It is often helpful in the evaluation of pulmonary valve pattern for evidence of pulmonary hypertension.

Other diagnostic tests are outlined in Table 17-6.

Treatment

Treatment of PPHN focuses on intervening with or preventing the development of the cyclic pattern previously described.[88] Infants presenting with low systemic blood pressure and cyanosis should have immediate supportive treatment. Intervention is aimed at using various maneuvers to increase pulmonary blood flow.[22,34,76] Pulmonary blood flow should increase if the pulmonary vascular resistance is decreased or if systemic vascular resistance is increased. In both instances right-to-left shunting is impeded. Conventional treatment modalities include direct dilation of pulmonary vasculature through intubation and mechanical ventilation using hyperoxia and hyperventilation, which produce alkalosis. The infant should be ventilated with whatever combination of rate, pressure, and oxygen is needed to lower $Paco_2$ and pH (Tables 17-7 and 17-8). Although the exact mechanism is unknown, alkalosis and/or hypocarbia produce a direct vasodilatory effect on pulmonary vasculature, decreasing pulmonary vascular resistance and thereby improving oxygenation.[34] Large, vigorous infants may require sedation with either phenobarbital (5 to 7 mg/kg), fentanyl (2 to 4 μg/kg),[43,57] or muscle paralysis with pancuronium bromide (0.03 to 0.06 mg/kg/dose) to promote effective ventilation.

In addition to mechanical ventilation, infusion of vasodilators (primarily tolazoline) has been recommended to decrease pulmonary vascular resistance.[59] Tolazoline is a potent vasodilator of the pulmonary and systemic circulation that may be used in the treatment of PPHN. The pulmonary vascular response should be assessed by rapidly (10 to 15 minutes) infusing 1 to 2 mg/kg of tolazoline through a peripheral scalp vein that drains into the superior vena caval system. If the response is favorable (improved PaO_2), a continuous infusion of 0.5 to 1 mg/kg/hr may be instituted. When tolazoline is being used, another IV line is needed to administer fluids and medications to support the systemic blood pressure. The infant must also be observed for gastrointestinal bleeding, pulmonary hemorrhage, and/or systemic hypotension. In the presence of systemic hypotension, volume expansion with albumin, plasma, or blood should be instituted. In the event of hypotension refractory to volume expansion, isoproterenol or dopamine should be considered.

Infusion of vasopressors (dopamine, dobutamine, and isoproterenol) and/or afterload reducers (nitroprusside) have been advocated.[22] Vasopressors decrease the ratio of pulmonary/systemic vascular resistance, thereby decreasing the amount of right-to-left shunting. In addition, they increase cardiac output. Continuous infusions of systemic vasopressors are primarily used to adjunct or counterbalance the hypotension caused by systemic vasodilators. These drugs also increase cardiac output and increase perfusion to vascular beds[22] (Table 17-9).

Some centers are trying new modalities in an attempt to treat PPHN and decrease complications. These treatments for the most part are experimental, with only short-term outcomes

---

TABLE 17-7

pH and PCO_2 Control in PPHN

1. Object is to reduce right-to-left shunt by hyperventilation → increase pH and reduce PCO_2 → reduce pulmonary artery pressure → reduce right-to-left shunt.
2. Each patient seems to have a *critical* level of PCO_2 below which PO_2 begins to rise. The clinician must determine the necessary level of PCO_2 early during treatment.
3. Use PCO_2 levels as low as 16 torr, if necessary, to control PO_2. If PO_2 is not controlled, the prognosis is poor.
4. In the acute, critical stages of the disease, use high ventilator rates and whatever inflating pressure is necessary to decrease PCO_2 to the critical level.
5. Ventilator rates of 100 to 150 breaths/min are recommended during initial therapy to lower the inflating pressure and maintain a low PCO_2.

Modified from Fox WW and Duara S: J Pediatr 103:505, 1983.

TABLE 17-8

Guidelines for Operation of Mechanical Ventilator in PPHN

FACTOR	GOAL	COMMON ERROR
Inspiratory pressure	Level necessary to ↓ PCO_2	Inadequate inspiratory pressure (no movement of chest wall, or decreasing PCO_2); reading on hand manometer may differ from that on ventilator
Ventilator rate	Rapid rates (up to 150 breaths per minute) to ↓ PCO_2, with lowest inspiratory pressure possible	Use of ventilator with maximum rate below level needed to ↓ PCO_2; may require hand ventilation to achieve high rates
Positive end-expiratory pressure	Low values unless pulmonary parenchymal disease exists	Failure to try different levels as patient condition changes
Inspired O_2 concentration	PO_2 > 100 to 120 torr	Weaning too rapidly
Inspiratory-expiratory ratio	Short inspiratory time to prevent air trapping at rapid rates	Inadequate flow rates to achieve short inspiratory time

From Fox WW and Duara S: J Pediatr 103:511, 1983.

available. The alternative to conventional ventilation that is presently being advocated is to produce more normal blood gas values, allowing Pa_{CO_2} to rise to a higher level, rather than the conventional hyperventilation (in an attempt to lower FI_{O_2}, lower pressure, and lessen air leaks, oxygen toxicity, and barotrauma). In addition, altered cerebral hemodynamics due to hypocarbia should be lessened.

Other new treatments include high-frequency ventilation and extracorporeal membrane oxygenator (ECMO). There is also continued research in the area of selective pulmonary vasodilators. As of now, no selective pulmonary vasodilator has been found that is effective in the neonate.[22]

Since maintaining adequate oxygenation is a prime goal of care of infants with PPHN, alterations in "routine" care and handling are essential. Because handling a sick newborn for any reason causes a fall in Pa_{O_2}, the benefits of handling for routine care such as changing linens, weighing, suctioning, and taking vital signs must be balanced against the risk of iatrogenic hypoxia. Pa_{O_2} variations in the newborn are[21]:

TABLE 17-9

Vasopressor Response in the Neonate

DRUG/DOSE	DISADVANTAGES
Dopamine	
<4 μg/kg/min: renal vasodilation, mesenteric and cerebral vasodilation (effects unknown) plus increase in cardiac output	May decrease systemic arterial pressure
5-20 μg/kg/min: increase in cardiac output depending on myocardial norepinephrine	Loss of renal and mesenteric perfusion
>20 μg/kg/min: systemic arterial pressure increases more than pulmonary artery pressure	Cardiac output may decrease
	Myocardial oxygen consumption increases
	Marked increase in left ventricular afterload
	Arrhythmias noted
Dobutamine	
10 μg/kg/min: increases cardiac contractility directly; cardiac output increases depending on myocardial catecholamine stores	No selective renal or mesenteric vasodilation
	Tends to increase skeletal blood flow at the expense of viscera
	Increase in pulmonary artery pressure
Isoproterenol	
0.05-1.0 μg/kg/min: lowers pulmonary vascular resistance in pulmonary hypertensive and vascular disease in child and adult; lowers hypoxemia-induced pulmonary vascular resistance in animal models	Arrhythmias
	No specific vasodilation effects
Nitroprusside	
0.4-5.0 μg/kg/min: cardiac output increases because of decreased left ventricular afterload; systemic vascular resistance (indicated by blood pressure) decreases because of decrease in left ventricular afterload	Systemic vascular resistance remains constant if CO_2 increases

Modified from Drummond W: Clin Perinatol 11:715, 1984.

At rest	± 15 mm Hg variation
While crying	↓ PaO$_2$ by as much as 50 mm Hg
With routine care	↓ PaO$_2$ by as much as 30 mm Hg

Organized, coordinated care and minimizing disturbances are therefore very important. If the baby is not sedated or paralyzed, keeping the infant calm is very important because severe hypoxia will accompany crying. Using pacifiers and decreasing noxious stimuli (i.e., invasive procedures) keeps struggling and crying to a minimum. Continuously monitoring vital signs, blood pressure, and transcutaneous blood gases or pulse oximetry decreases the need for physical manipulation and disturbance.

Complications

Complications are usually associated with treatment and underlying causes, and not primarily with PPHN. Risks of conventional ventilation include air leaks, oxygen toxicity and barotrauma, which can lead to the development of chronic lung disease. Hypocarbia has been known to decrease cerebral blood flow.[13] There has been concern that the prolonged profound hypocarbia produced by hyperventilation could cause severe ischemic damage to the rapidly growing newborn brain. Newer modalities have complications as well. High-frequency ventilation carries a high risk of necrotizing tracheitis and life-threatening hemorrhage.

APNEA
Physiology

The two major control mechanisms that regulate pulmonary ventilation are the neural and chemical systems. The cerebral cortex and brainstem are the governing agents for the neural control system. The peripheral components of this system are found in the upper airway and lung. Respiratory rate and rhythm are regulated by the neural system. The chemical control center is found in the medulla and is sensitive to changes in PaCO$_2$.

The peripheral portion of the chemical system lies in the carotid and aortic vessels and is sensitive to changes in PaCO$_2$.[34] Alveolar ventilation is controlled by the chemical system, and this system is the principal defense against hypoxia. Neonates have a unique response to hypoxemia and carbon dioxide retention. Unlike adults, who have sustained increase in ventilation, infants have a brief period of increased ventilation followed by respiratory depression.

The exact mechanism for regulating ventilation in premature infants has not been well established. It is suggested that this mechanism is immature or inadequate in the premature infant.[34] Apnea of prematurity or primary apnea is not associated with other specific disease entities. The younger the gestational age, the greater the incidence of apnea. Apnea may be associated with hypoxemia, neuronal immaturity, sleep, catecholamine deficiency, and respiratory muscle fatigue.

Etiology

Clinically, various conditions may cause apnea in the premature infant by producing hypoxia and/or altering the sensitivity of peripheral or central chemoreceptors[64] (Table 17-10). Neuronal immaturity seems a plausible cause for apnea. Respiratory efforts are more unstable at a younger gestational age. The decreased response appears to be the result of a general lack of dendritic formation and limited synaptic connections, therefore decreasing the excitatory drive. Another postulation is that apneic episodes are manifestations of synaptic disorders that occur without a motor component. Such phenomena have been confirmed on electroencephalogram. Infants depend on alternating excitation and inhibition to establish rhythmic breathing, and therefore imbalances (e.g., hypoxia, hypoglycemia, or hypocalcemia) may cause respiratory arrest.

Apnea has been noted to appear with greater frequency during sleep and especially during rapid eye movement (REM) or active sleep. Apnea has also been noted in non-REM sleep, but occurs much less frequently. The effects of REM

TABLE 17-10

Causes of Apnea in the Premature Infant

Infection: Pneumonia, sepsis, meningitis

Respiratory distress: RDS, airway obstruction, CPAP application, postextubation, congenital anomalies of the upper airways

Cardiovascular disorders: Patent ductus arteriosus, congestive heart failure

Gastrointestinal disorders: Gastroesophageal reflux, necrotizing enterocolitis

CNS disorders: Depressant drugs, intraventricular hemorrhage, seizure, kernicterus, infection, tumors

Metabolic disorders: Hypoglycemia, hypocalcemia, hyponatremia

Environmental: Rapid increase of environmental temperature, vigorous suctioning, feeding, stooling, stretching

Hematopoietic: Polycythemia, anemia

---

sleep are inhibition of spinal motor neurons, increase in brain activity causing increasing eye movements and muscular twitching, and changes in brain temperature and cerebral blood flow and CNS arousal shown by electroencephalogram changes.

Decreased amounts of peripheral catecholamines in the premature infant have also been postulated as a cause of apnea. This would become critical if hemorrhage or infection was also present in the premature infant and stores were depleted.

The premature infant has a more compliant chest cage and less compliant lungs; this situation results in a greater work load. Respiratory muscle fatigue occurs easily in the absence of fatigue-resistant fibers.

Apnea associated with the sleep state becomes more significant in that premature infants, particularly those less than 32 weeks of gestation, spend 80% of their time asleep. Equally significant is the time spent in REM sleep, the predominant sleep state of premature infants. The percentage of quiet sleep or non-REM sleep will increase from 20% to 60% of the total sleep period by the time an infant is 3 months old.

Secondary apnea may be associated with a particular disease entity or in response to special procedures. Many disorders leading to secondary apnea may exert their influence through hypoxemia and subsequent respiratory center depression.

The majority of secondary apnea arises from four conditions. In IRDS, apnea is related to the degree of parenchymal disease and may result from muscle fatigue. With CNS hemorrhage and seizures, apnea arises from asphyxia with subsequent hypoxemia and respiratory center depression or actual brain injury. Apnea is related to central depression in sepsis. And carbon dioxide retention and hypoxemia associated with the left-to-right shunting of a patent ductus arteriosus may cause apnea. Other associated causes of secondary apnea include metabolic disorders such as hypoglycemia and hypocalcemia, hematologic disorders such as anemia and polycythemia, and drug-related CNS disorders.

Iatrogenic causes of apnea include increased environmental temperature, sudden increases in environmental temperature, vagal response to suctioning of the nasopharynx or to a gavage tube, gastrointestinal reflux, and obstruction of the airway. Reflex apnea occurs when foreign material (milk) is present in the oropharynx. The reflex is protective in that it prevents inhalation of the substance into the airway. Obstruction may occur from improper neck positioning or aspiration.

Prevention

All infants assessed as high risk for apneic spells should be carefully monitored for a period of at least 10 to 12 days. Impedance apnea monitors do not distinguish normal respiratory efforts from gasping movements associated with obstruction. Both heart rate and respiratory rates should be monitored. Alarm systems should be used at all times. A qualified observer is essential.

$TcPO_2$ monitors or pulse oximetry may detect hypoxemic conditions that may lead to apneic spells. In the premature infant younger than 32 weeks gestation this type of apnea is common. Care should be organized to decrease stressful, hypoxic episodes.

Apneic episodes may be prevented or decreased by several means. Gentle tactile stimulation alone has been shown to be effective in decreasing and preventing apneic spells in most premature infants. Noxious stimuli such as vigorous shaking or banging on the incubator should be avoided whenever possible. If tactile stimulus is ineffective and temporary bag and mask ventilation is required, attention should be paid to preventing undue pressure on the lower chin and neck so that the airway remains clear. Too-vigorous bagging may also stimulate pulmonary stretch receptors and induce apnea; therefore it should be avoided. Water bed flotation may decrease the frequency of apnea but generally does not completely eliminate it.

Since increased environmental temperature and sudden changes in temperature have resulted in apneic episodes, prevention includes maintaining the environmental temperature at the lower end of the normal spectrum, particularly if an apneic episode has already occurred. Incubator temperature may require a 0.5° to 1.0° C (1° to 2° F) decrease to counter the problem. Phototherapy may provide sufficient radiant energy to increase the infant's temperature and contribute to the incidence of apnea. Care should be taken to avoid sudden changes in temperature. An infant should not be placed on a cold scale; the infant should be placed in prewarmed incubators or beds. Oxygen should be warmed and humidified before administration.

Careful attention must be paid to prevent airway obstruction. Small neck rolls under the neck and shoulders have been used to decrease neck flexion and prevent airway obstruction when in the supine position. Close monitoring should be done during procedures such as lumbar puncture where accidental airway obstruction may occur.

Data collection

Evaluation of apnea should include studies to rule out treatable causes.

HISTORY

Evaluation of the prenatal and birth history may give a clue to the causes and also provide a basis for further study.

PHYSICAL EXAMINATION

A thorough physical and neurologic examination rules out grossly apparent abnormalities. Observation and documentation of apneic and bradycardic episodes and any relationship to precipitating factors help differentiate primary from secondary apnea.

LABORATORY DATA

A complete blood count helps assess infection and anemia as causes of apnea. Serum glucose, calcium, phosphate, magnesium, sodium, potassium, and chloride levels help assess metabolic causes. Arterial blood gas measurements help assess hypoxemia and metabolic and respiratory contributions to apnea. Blood, urine, and cerebrospinal fluid culture help rule out sepsis as the cause of apnea. The cerebrospinal fluid culture is usually done only when other signs and symptoms of infection are present. Chest x-ray examinations help in assessing cardiac and respiratory causes. The examinations may also rule out aspiration of abdominal contents caused by gastroesophageal reflux. Ultrasound examination of the head and electroencephalogram may be used to rule out intraventricular hemorrhage or other neurologic causes of apnea.

Treatment

Treatment of secondary apnea is aimed at the diagnosis and management of the specific causes. In the treatment of primary apnea (ap-

TABLE 17-11

Methylxanthines Used to Treat Apnea of Prematurity

DRUG	DOSAGE	THERAPEUTIC LEVELS	SIDE EFFECTS
Theophylline	Loading: 5-6 mg/kg Maintenance: 1 mg/kg q.8h. to 3 mg/kg q.12h.	5 to 15, although levels of 3 to 4 μg/ml have been shown to be effective in decreasing apnea	Tachycardia, arrhythmias, diuresis, glucosuria, ketonuria, hyperglycemia, jitteriness, seizures, vomiting, nausea, hemorrhagic gastritis
Caffeine	Loading: 10 mg/kg (20 mg/ kg of caffeine citrate) Maintenance: 2.5 mg/kg/day	Afterload: 8 to 14 μg/ml Maintenance: 7 to 20 μg/ml	See above

nea of prematurity) initial efforts should begin with the least invasive intervention possible. Gentle tactile stimulation is frequently successful, especially with early recognition and intervention. When infants do not immediately respond to external stimuli, bag and mask ventilation must be initiated. Generally, an FIO_2 approximating that used before the spell but not exceeding a 10% increase will alleviate hypoxemia and avoid marked elevations in the arterial PaO_2. The use of the $TcPO_2$ monitor will allow closer following of PaO_2 fluctuation and help prevent complications of oxygen toxicity. Elevation in ambient oxygen concentrations, although decreasing the frequency of apnea, causes prolongation of apnea spells.

Apnea will respond to low pressure (3 to 5 cm of water) nasal CPAP. Mechanical ventilation may be required if the infant fails to respond to lesser measures and continues to have repeated and prolonged apneic episodes. It may also be required in extremely immature, unstable, or debilitated infants.

Methylxanthines (aminophylline, theophylline, and caffeine) are used to treat apnea of prematurity (Table 17-11). They are used only in primary apnea (i.e., when pathologic causes have been eliminated). Treatment should follow a strict protocol, and serum levels must be checked. Methylxanthines are potent cardiac, respiratory, and CNS stimulants and smooth muscle relaxers. Their effect on decreasing the frequency of apnea is related to central stimulation rather than to changes in pulmonary function.

Complications

Side effects of xanthines include gastric irritation, hyperactivity (restlessness, irritability, and wakefulness), myocardial stimulation (tachycardia and hypotension), and increased urinary output.

Prognosis for apnea arising from an underlying cause depends on the outcome of the disease process itself. The prognosis for apnea is generally good in infants who are otherwise well and healthy and for whom the apnea is not prolonged. The prognosis becomes increasingly less favorable with an increased frequency and duration of episodes. Prompt recognition and intervention decrease the possibility of severe complications from hypoxia.

PARENT TEACHING

Parental attachment to the infant with respiratory disease is especially difficult. It is made more difficult if the infant is also premature. Normal interaction is curtailed by the infant's condition and appearance, the environment, and the parent's reaction to these factors. The infant who is in an oxygen hood or being ventilated may give inadequate cues to arouse parental attachment and instead may arouse feelings of grief and loss. A complete discussion of parental attachment is contained in Part V.

The goal of discharge planning is the best possible outcome with the least family disruption. Evaluation of parental readiness to care for their infant is essential to effective teaching and learning. Physical surroundings and preparations for the baby are assessed when possible by a home visit. Parental concerns at bringing home a baby with special care needs must be assessed and discussed. The parents learn to be comfortable in handling and caring for their baby gradually throughout hospitalization. A specially designated or decorated room is used for family visiting and caretaking. Before discharge, the mother and/or father spend the night caring for the infant. Positive reinforcement and praise from the professional staff should be freely given to parents who attend classes and successfully master the tasks of caretaking for their baby.

Special equipment such as oxygen tanks, nasal cannulas, a respirator, and suction equipment for home use must be acquired before discharge. Sources, mode of delivery, and use of equipment must all be taught to parents before discharge. Pulmonary hygiene for infants with prolonged difficulty in handling secretions must also be taught. Written protocols and instructions should be provided to parents whenever possible.[55] Parents must be informed of dosage, route of administration, side effects, and planned duration of use of all medications.

Since fluid and nutritional status is so important to any infant with a chronic condition, nutritional information for parents is required. Infants with tachypnea (BPD) often have difficulty with coordinating suck and swallow. Often smaller, more frequent feedings are necessary when using supplemental oxygen. Alternative feeding methods such as gavage feeding may be necessary to safely provide enough calories with a minimum of work.

Apnea is especially distressing to parents be-

cause of their fears of recurrence once the child goes home. If apnea is related to an underlying disease, treatment of the cause should result in resolution of the apneic episodes. Parents can be reliably assured that recurrence is unlikely unless the disease recurs. With apnea of prematurity, such assurances cannot be offered. However, the assurance can be offered that infants do grow into a regular ventilatory pattern as their respiratory center matures and that all means to protect the infant will be used until that time. Also, the parents can be assured that the infant will not go home until he is ready and the parents are adequately prepared to handle situations that may arise.

Before an infant needing a home monitoring system is discharged from the hospital, the parents must be given adequate support and instruction. Classes on the use of the apnea monitors must include demonstration of the equipment and return demonstrations. Minor equipment checks and repairs should be mastered before discharge. At least two of the caretakers must be proficient in infant cardiopulmonary resuscitation (CPR).

Support by the primary care providers after discharge is essential. Parents must have telephone numbers of the medical facility and personnel they can call 24 hours a day in case of problems or equipment failure.

Anticipatory support includes discussion of potential stress factors related to having an infant on a monitor at home: sibling rivalries, marital stresses, scheduling problems, potential problems with babysitters, and the parent's own fears of the situation. An apnea monitor in the home may provoke anxiety in spite of discussion and instruction.

The parents of every infant who has apneic episodes or serious respiratory disease must be taught CPR. This is a skill that is learned over the course of time by reading written materials and seeing and returning the demonstration. Learning CPR cannot be done on the day of discharge but must be a staged process of indi-

University of Colorado Health Sciences Center
University Hospital
Department of Nursing Service

Standards of Care

Pediatric Respiratory Distress

Pt. = Patient
S.O. = Significant other

Date initiated_____

Date and initial

	Instructed Pt. S.O.	Assess learning			Understands Pt. S.O.

Patient outcome criteria

To include children with upper/lower airway obstruction, pneumonia, bronchiolitis, bronchitis, asthma-reactive airway disease, croup, bronchopulmonary dysplasia, cystic fibrosis.

I. Can name signs of respiratory distress and states what to do if they occur: retractions, nasal flaring, increased respiratory rate (can measure rate and knows normal for child), cyanosis, poor feeding — I

II. Can administer oxygen safely, if prescribed
   A. Verbalizes arrangements for home oxygen, obtaining and refill, payment — A
   B. Can demonstrate use of oxygen equipment: change regulator, adjust liter flow, apply cannula to child's face — B
   C. Can verbalize rules of oxygen safety and discuss written handout with nurse — C
   D. If order is prn, or for portion of day, can verbalize indications or times for use of oxygen — D

III. Demonstrates postural drainage techniques if prescribed; verbalizes purpose and frequency of treatment at home — III

IV. If indicated, can demonstrate CPR on a Resusci-Baby and has discussed written CPR handout with nurse — IV

V. Administers medications safely
   A. Demonstrates safe administration of medication — A
   B. Can identify purpose and side effects of medications — B
   C. Verbalizes understanding of or can read instructions of discharge medications (name, route, dose, length of course of medication)

Continued.

Figure 17-15. Standards of care: pediatric respiratory distress. (Courtesy University of Colorado Health Sciences Center.)

		Date and initial					
		Instructed Pt. S.O.	Assess learning			Understands Pt. S.O.	
Name of medications							
1. _____	1						
2. _____	2						
3. _____	3						
4. _____	4						
VI. Verbalizes an understanding of prescribed diet							
A. Verbalizes food/fluids child is discharged on							
1. Verbalizes how and where to obtain formula/fluids	1						
2. Demonstrates/verbalizes instructions on preparing formula accurately	2						
3. If unable to obtain appropriate formula, parent will _____	3						
B. Verbalizes appropriate intake (_____), symptoms if not tolerating, and resources if diet not tolerated	B						
C. Cystic fibrosis only: verbalizes understanding of interrelationship of diet, stools, and pancreatic enzyme supplement	C						
VII. Verbalizes method for obtaining and location of follow-up care _____	VII						
VIII. Verbalizes understanding of possible/probable effects of hospitalization on infants and children: regression, change in play/eating/sleeping habits, increased dependence, increased sibling rivalry	VIII						

The above information was discussed with:

_____   _____
Name of significant other (S.O.)   Relationship

Nurse	Int	Nurse	Int	Nurse	Int

Figure 17-15, cont'd. For legend see p. 421.

vidual and class instruction. Supplying instructional pamphlets written just for parents aids in initial learning and provides a quick reference. If other family members or babysitters will provide child care during work or evening hours, they too must be able to resuscitate the baby.

Other emergency actions for which parents must be prepared include clearing the infant's airway, calling for help (having emergency phone numbers easily accessible), planning for an alternate communication source (i.e., neighbor's phone), and notifying the community rescue squad of the infant's presence in the home.

Parents must be taught how to recognize signs of illness or significant deterioration in the condition of their infant. In addition to special care needs, parents need information about normal newborn care. Developing realistic expectations and positive parenting skills is as important to these parents as to all new parents.

For the parents of an infant with special respiratory problems, the importance of continuous follow-up care must be emphasized. Follow-up visits should coincide with developmental stages, the natural course of the disease, and expected complications of the disease.

The parents whose child has special respiratory needs must learn a myriad of involved technical information. The primary care provider (frequently the primary nurse) is responsible for organizing, teaching, coordinating, and documenting the information. This nurse is also responsible for assuring that the parents have not only been taught but in fact understand. The special preparation of parents of a baby with respiratory distress may be outlined on a discharge planning tool that is planned and coordinated by the primary nurse (Figure 17-15).

ACKNOWLEDGMENT

We would like to acknowledge and thank William Parry and Mary Baldy for their work as the authors of this chapter in the first edition.

REFERENCES

1. American Academy of Pediatrics: An international classification of retinopathy of prematurity, Pediatrics 74:127, 1984.
2. American Academy of Pediatrics and American College of Obstetricians and Gynecologists: Guidelines for perinatal care, ed 2, Evanston, Ill, 1988, American Academy of Pediatrics.
3. American Academy of Pediatrics, Committee on Fetus and Newborn: Vitamin E and the prevention of retinopathy of premature, Pediatrics 76:315, 1985.
4. American Medical Association: International classification of retinopathy of prematurity, Arch Ophthalmol 102:1130, 1984.
5. Avery GB: Neonatology: pathophysiology and management of newborns, ed 3, Philadelphia, 1986, JB Lippincott Co.
6. Avery ME and Oppenheimer EH: Recent increases in mortality from hyaline membrane disease, J Pediatr 57: 553, 1960.
7. Bacsik R: Meconium aspiration syndrome, Pediatr Clin North Am 24:463, 1977.
8. Ballard R and Leonard C: Developmental follow-up of infants with persistent pulmonary hypertension of the newborn, Clin Perinatol 11:737, 1984.
9. Barnes N et al: Effects of prolonged positive pressure ventilation in infancy, Lancet 2:1096, 1969.
10. Benda G: Five years experience with mechanical ventilation of the preterm infant: complications and outcome, Perinatol Neonatol 4:45, 1980.
11. Boros SJ et al: The effect of independent variations in I:E ratio and end expiratory pressure during mechanical ventilation in hyaline membrane disease: the significance of mean airway pressure, J Pediatr 91:114, 1977.
12. Brown E et al: BPD: possible relationship to pulmonary edema, J Pediatr 92:982, 1978.
13. Bruce D: Effects of hyperventilation on cerebral blood flow and metabolism, Clin Perinatol 11:737, 1984.
14. Bucciarelli R et al: Persistence of fetal cardiopulmonary circulation: one manifestation of transient tachypnea of the newborn, Pediatrics 58:192, 1976.
15. Cabal L et al: Effects of metaproterenol on pulmonary mechanics, oxygenation and ventilation in infants with chronic lung disease, J Pediatr 110:116, 1987.
16. Carson B et al: Combined obstetric and pediatric approach to prevention of meconium aspiration syndrome, Am J Obstet Gynecol 126:712, 1976.
17. Chang H: Mechanisms of gas transport during ventilation with high frequency oscillation, J Appl Physiol 56:533, 1984.
18. Chu J et al: Neonatal pulmonary ischemia, Pediatrics 40:709, 1967.
19. Coates AL et al: Long-term pulmonary sequelae of pre-

mature birth with and without idiopathic respiratory distress syndrome, J Pediatr 90:611, 1977.

20. Curran C and Kachoyeanos M: The effects on neonates of two methods of chest physical therapy, Matern Child Nurs J 4:312, 1979.

21. Dangeman BC et al: The variability of PaO$_2$ in newborn infants in response to routine care, Pediatr Res 10:422, 1976 (abstract).

22. Drummond W: Use of cardiotonic therapy in the management of infants with persistent pulmonary hypertension of the newborn, Clin Perinatol 11:715, 1984.

23. Duara S, Gewitz MH, and Fox WW: Use of mechanical ventilation for clinical management of persistent pulmonary hypertension of the newborn, Clin Perinatol 11:641, 1984.

24. Dunn D and Lewis A: Some important aspects of neonatal nursing related to pulmonary disease and family involvement, Pediatr Clin North Am 20:481, 1973.

25. Edwards DK, Colby TV, and Northway WH: Radiologic pathologic correlations in bronchopulmonary dysplasia, J Pediatr 85:834, 1979.

26. Enhorning G and Robertson B: Lung expansion in the premature rabbit fetus after tracheal deposition of surfactant, Pediatrics 50:58, 1972.

27. Ferrera B et al: Efficacy and neurological outcome of profound hypocapneic alkalosis for the treatment of persistent pulmonary hypertension in infancy, J Pediatr 105:457, 1984.

28. Finer NN and Kelly MA: Optimal ventilation for the neonate. II. Mechanical ventilation, Perinatol Neonatol 7:63, 1983.

29. Finer NN and Tomey PM: Controlled evaluation of muscle relaxation in the ventilated neonate, Pediatrics 67:641, 1981.

30. Fittenberg J: Persistent pulmonary hypertension after lithium intoxication in the newborn, Eur J Pediatr 138:321, 1982.

31. Fitzhardinge PM: Current outcome of NICU population. In Brann AW and Volpe JJ, editors: Report of the seventy-seventh Ross Conference on pediatric research, Columbus, Ohio, 1980, Ross Laboratories.

32. Fitzhardinge PM et al: Mechanical ventilation of infants <1501 grams birthweight: health, growth and neurologic sequelae, J Pediatr 88:531, 1976.

33. Fox W: Bronchopulmonary dysplasia (respirator lung syndrome): clinical course and outpatient therapy, Pediatr Ann 7:40, 1978.

34. Fox WW and Duara S: Persistent pulmonary hypertension in the neonate: diagnosis and treatment, J Pediatr 103:505, 1983.

35. Fraiberg S: Blind infants and their mothers: an examination of the sign system. In Lewis M and Rosenblum L, editors: The effect of the infant on its caregiver, New York, 1974, John Wiley & Sons, Inc.

36. Frank M: Theophylline: a closer look, Neonatal Network 6:7, 1987.

37. Fujiwara T et al: Artificial surfactant therapy in HMD, Lancet 1:55, 1980.

38. Gay J, Daily W, and Meyer B: Ligation of the PDA in premature infants: report of 45 cases, J Pediatr Surg 8:677, 1973.

39. Gersony W: Neonatal pulmonary hypertension: pathophysiology, classification, etiology, Clin Perinatol 11:517, 1984.

40. Gluck L and Kulovich M: Fetal lung development, Pediatr Clin North Am 20:367, 1973.

41. Gregory G: Respiratory care of newborn infants, Pediatr Clin North Am 19:311, 1972.

42. Gunn T: Risk factors in retrolental fibroplasia, Pediatrics 65:1096, 1980.

43. Hansen D and Hickey P: Anesthesia for hypoplastic left heart syndrome: use of high dose fentanyl in 30 neonates, Anesth Analg 65:127, 1986.

44. Harris M et al: Successful extubation of infants with respiratory distress syndrome using aminophylline, J Pediatr 103:303, 1983.

45. Harrison VC, Heese H, and Klein M: The significance of grunting in hyaline membrane disease, Pediatrics 41:549, 1968.

46. Henry G: Noninvasive assessment of cardiac function and pulmonary hypertension in persistent pulmonary hypertension, Clin Perinatol 11:626, 1984.

47. Hodson W et al: BPD: the need for epidemiological studies, J Pediatr 95:848, 1979.

48. Holzman BH and Scarpelli EM: Cardiopulmonary consequences of positive end expiratory pressure, Pediatr Res 13:1112, 1979.

49. Jacob J et al: The contribution of PDA in the neonate with severe RDS, J Pediatr 96:79, 1979.

50. Jobe A et al: Duration and characteristics of treatment of premature lambs with natural surfactant, J Clin Invest 67:370, 1981.

51. Jones MD and Murton LJ: Mechanical ventilation in newborn infants with hyaline membrane disease, Pediatr Ann 1:63, 1977.

52. Kao L: Effect of Isoproterenol inhalation on airway resistance in chronic BPD, Pediatrics 73:509, 1984.

53. Kinsey VE: RLF: cooperative study of retrolental fibroplasia and use of oxygen, Arch Ophthalmol 56:481, 1956.

54. Klaus M and Fanaroff A: Care of the high-risk neonate, ed 3, Philadelphia, 1986, WB Saunders Co.

55. Klaus M and Meyer BP: Oxygen therapy for the newborn, Pediatr Clin North Am 13:725, 1966.

56. Koops B, Abman S, and Accurso F: Outpatient management and followup of BPD, Clin Perinatol 11:101, 1984.

57. Koren G et al: Pediatric fentanyl dosing based on pharmacokinetics during cardiac surgery, Anesth Analg 63:577, 1984.

58. Kuhns LR et al: Diagnosis of pneumothorax and pneumo-

CHAPTER 18

Cardiovascular diseases and surgical interventions

ELAINE DABERKOW · REGINALD L. WASHINGTON

Approximately 1 of every 100 infants born has a congenital heart defect. Some infants have life-threatening defects requiring immediate action within the first few hours and days of life. Others require no intervention until later in life or possibly not at all. It is important for the practitioner to recognize the presence of congenital heart disease, differentiate it from other conditions, and institute appropriate treatment. This chapter is designed to give the reader a clear understanding of neonatal circulation, signs and symptoms of congenital heart disease, and current management practices.

CONGENITAL HEART DISEASE OVERVIEW
Physiology

Profound hemodynamic changes occur with the delivery of the newborn. Rudolph[2] provides an excellent detailed review of this topic. However, because a basic understanding of these physiologic principles is mandatory in understanding congenital heart disease, they are briefly presented here.

FETAL CIRCULATION

Three shunts affect fetal circulation: the ductus venosus, the ductus arteriosus, and the foramen ovale. These three shunts allow mixing of the fetal blood and are important in the development of a normal heart.

The blood with the highest oxygen saturation in the fetus is found in the umbilical veins and is shunted directly to the heart, bypassing the liver through the ductus venosus. Once in the heart, most of this highly saturated blood is shunted directly through the foramen ovale to the left atrium, left ventricle, aorta, and finally the coronary and carotid arteries. Therefore the blood with the highest oxygen saturation is directed to the tissues with the highest oxygen demand—the fetal myocardium and the brain. The desaturated blood returning to the superior vena cava is primarily directed into the right ventricle, main pulmonary artery, ductus arteriosus, and descending aorta where it ultimately enters the placental circulation and is resaturated.

CHANGES THAT OCCUR IN THE FETAL CIRCULATION WITH BIRTH. In utero, the systemic vascular resistance is low primarily because of the low resistance of the placenta. The pulmonary arterioles, which are constricted and hypertrophied, are highly resistant to blood flow. At birth the placenta is removed from the circulation, thereby greatly increasing the systemic vascular resistance. Initiation of respirations produces increased oxygen tension, which decreases pulmonary vascular resistance and increases pulmonary blood flow. In addition, the left atrial pressure increases, closing the foramen ovale and eliminating the right-to-left shunt through the foramen ovale (see Figure 2-1).

The ductus arteriosus is extremely sensitive to the oxygen content of the blood, and the neonatal

PaO$_2$ increases after birth. This increase in oxygen content initiates the constriction of the ductus arteriosus.

Once these changes take place, the newborn's circulation resembles that of an adult. Desaturated blood returns to the heart by the inferior and superior venae cava, enters the right atrium, right ventricle, pulmonary artery, and the pulmonary circulation where oxygen and carbon dioxide are exchanged. This saturated blood then returns to the heart through the pulmonary venous system and enters the left atrium, left ventricle, and ultimately the aorta and systemic arterial system. However, pulmonary vascular resistance and pressures in the right ventricle and pulmonary system remain elevated in the neonate because of the hypertrophy of the pulmonary vessels. This hypertrophy slowly resolves, and the pulmonary vascular resistance and right heart pressures decrease to normal between 1 and 2 months of age.

Etiology

Ninety percent of congenital heart disease is thought to be multifactorially inherited. Multifactorial inheritance involves a genetic predisposition for congenital heart disease interacting with an environmental trigger at a vulnerable time in development. This interaction produces a cardiovascular malformation. The malformation produced varies depending on when the interaction between the environmental trigger and the existing genetic predisposition occurs in embryogenesis. Although multiple environmental triggers exist (including drugs, infectious agents, defects in maternal nutrition or metabolism, and fetal hemodynamics), a specific environmental trigger is

TABLE 18-1

Most Common Environmental Triggers and Specific Defects Associated with Each

POTENTIAL TERATOGENS	FREQUENCY OF CARDIOVASCULAR DISEASE (%)	MOST COMMON MALFORMATIONS
Drugs		
Alcohol	25-30	Ventricular septal defect, patent ductus arteriosus, atrial septal defect
Amphetamines	5-10	Ventricular septal defect, patent ductus arteriosus, atrial septal defect, transposition of great arteries
Anticonvulsants	2-3	Pulmonary stenosis, aortic stenosis, coarctation of aorta, patent ductus arteriosus
Trimethadione	15-30	Transposition of great arteries, Fallot's tetralogy, hypoplastic left heart syndrome
Lithium	10	Ebstein's anomaly, tricuspid atresia, atrial septal defect
Sex hormones	2-4	Ventricular septal defect, transposition of great arteries, Fallot's tetralogy
Infections		
Rubella	35	Peripheral pulmonary artery stenosis, ventricular septal defect, patent ductus arteriosus, atrial septal defect
Maternal conditions		
Diabetes	3-5	Transposition of great arteries, ventricular septal defect, coarctation of aorta
	30-50	Cardiomegaly, myopathy
Lupus erythematosus	?	Heart block

not identified in most cases of congenital heart disease (Table 18-1).

About 8% of congenital heart defects are associated with specific syndromes (e.g., trisomy 21 syndrome and Turner's syndrome) (Table 18-2).

An additional 2% of congenital heart defects predominantly originate because of environmental factors (rubella, maternal anticonvulsant therapy, or maternal alcohol consumption). Approximately 1% of infants in North America have congenital

TABLE 18-2

Chromosomal Aberrations Evident in Neonatal Period that Are Associated with Congenital Heart Disease

POPULATION	INCIDENCE OF CONGENITAL HEART DISEASE (%)	MOST COMMON LESIONS		
		1	2	3
Trisomy 21 syndrome	50	Ventricular septal defect, endocardial cushion defect	Atrial septal defect	Patent ductus arteriosus
Trisomy 18 syndrome	99+	Ventricular septal defect	Patent ductus arteriosus	Pulmonary stenosis
Trisomy 13 syndrome	90	Ventricular septal defect	Patent ductus arteriosus	Dextrocardia
Turner's syndrome	35	Coarctation of aorta	Aortic stenosis	Atrial septal defect

TABLE 18-3

Diagnosis of Infants at Selected Ages*

0-6 DAYS (%)		7-13 DAYS (%)		13-20 DAYS (%)	
Transposition of great arteries	(17)	Coarctation of aorta	(19)	Ventricular septal defect	(20)
Hypoplastic left ventricle	(12)	Ventricular septal defect	(15)	Transposition of great arteries	(17)
Lung disease	(10)	Hypoplastic left ventricle	(11)	Coarctation of aorta	(16)
Tetralogy of Fallot	(9)	Transposition of great arteries	(9)	Tetralogy of Fallot	(8)
Coarctation of aorta	(7)	Tetralogy of Fallot	(6)	Endocardial cushion defect	(6)
Ventricular septal defect	(7)	Heterotaxia	(4)	Heterotaxia	(6)
Pulmonary atresia (with intact ventricular septum)	(7)	Truncus arteriosus	(4)	Patent ductus arteriosus	(4)
Heterotaxia	(6)	Single ventricle	(4)	Total anomalous pulmonary venous return	(3)
Other	(25)	Other	(28)	Other	(20)
TOTAL 896	(100)	TOTAL 210	(100)	TOTAL 116	(100)

From Fyler D et al: Pediatrics 65:391, 1980. Reproduced by permission of Pediatrics.
*NOTE: These numbers are intended as a rough guideline, since there is considerable overlap. Infants with congenital heart disease are often active initially and appear well for several hours or days after birth. In contrast, infants with respiratory distress often have characteristic symptoms within the first several hours after birth.

heart disease. Approximately 50% of these have ventricular septal defect (VSD) alone or in combination with other cardiac abnormalities. Table 18-3 shows the most common congenital heart defects and their time of presentation.

Data collection
HISTORY

A family history of congenital heart disease; a prenatal history of maternal viral infections (rubella and cytomegalovirus) or drug or toxic substance ingestion; asphyxia or dysrhythmias before or at birth; a history of hydrops fetalis; or Rh incompatibility give clues about the most likely diagnosis. The timing of the onset of symptoms may indicate the type of anomaly (see Table 18-3).

CLINICAL PRESENTATION OF INFANTS WITH SEVERE CARDIAC DISEASE

Newborns with severe congenital heart disease usually have one or more of the following signs or symptoms: (1) cyanosis, (2) respiratory distress, (3) congestive heart failure and diminished cardiac output, (4) abnormal cardiac rhythm, and (5) cardiac murmurs. Although cardiac murmurs in the neonatal period do not necessarily indicate severe cardiac disease, they must be carefully evaluated. Absence of a murmur does not exclude cardiac disease. Infants with severe, life-threatening congenital anomalies of the cardiovascular system may not have a murmur.

Each of these previously mentioned categories is considered on an individual basis. The reader is reminded that the differential diagnosis of any individual sign or symptom is important, especially in the neonatal period where there is considerable overlap and several disease entities have identical symptoms. This section individually discusses each sign or symptom and briefly discusses the laboratory evaluation of each.

CYANOSIS. Cyanosis is defined as a bluish discoloration of the skin, nail beds, and mucous membranes resulting from the presence of 3 mg/dl of reduced hemoglobin in the arterial blood or 4 to 5 mg/dl of reduced hemoglobin in the peripheral capillary blood. Cyanosis therefore is dependent on the total hemoglobin concentration and the arterial oxygen saturation, and requires immediate assessment.

When the causes of cyanosis are being considered, the six components of oxygen delivery must be considered individually. These make up the central nervous system (CNS), musculoskeletal system, airways, gas exchange interface in the lungs, hemoglobin, and cardiovascular system. Each of these is only briefly reviewed here. The reader is referred to other sections of this book for a more complete discussion of the individual lesions.

Several disorders of the CNS and neuromuscular system cause poor oxygenation as a result of the abnormal rate or rhythm of respiration. Iatrogenic depression of the cardiovascular system may result from the anesthetic administered to the mother before delivery. Birth trauma can result in either asphyxia or diaphragmatic paralysis and can cause generalized cyanosis. Metabolic abnormalities that cause neuroencephalopathy and resultant cyanosis are hypoglycemia and hypocalcemia.

Several disorders of the lung result in poor oxygenation from alveolar hypoventilation. These disorders include hypoplastic lung, bronchiogenic cysts, pulmonary arteriovenous malformation, atelectasis with resultant lobar emphysema, pneumothorax, aspiration pneumonia, idiopathic respiratory distress syndrome, and shock lung. Differentiating between these disorders and primary cardiac disease is often difficult.

Because the cyanosis depends on the amount of reduced hemoglobin present, any abnormality of the blood that alters either the hemoglobin structure or content may result in cyanosis. Disorders such as polycythemia, hypovolemia, methemoglobinemia, and other hemoglobinopathies may account for cyanosis and must always be considered.

Finally, several disorders of the cardiovascular-pulmonary system may cause cyanosis, even though they do not involve actual structural defects. These disorders include persistent pulmonary hypertension, pulmonary edema, dysrhythmias, and low cardiac output from any cause.

RESPIRATORY DISTRESS. In the newborn period respiratory distress may result from pulmonary venous congestion as a result of a defect in the cardiovascular system, pulmonary disease, or both. This differentiation in the newborn period is often difficult, and infants may have both primary pulmonary disease and cardiac defects.

Most infants with cyanosis from congenital heart disease do not have respiratory distress. If respiratory distress is present, the cyanosis is not proportional to the amount of respiratory distress evaluated from the physical examination and chest x-ray examination. If cyanosis is present and is caused by a fixed right-to-left shunt, increasing inspired oxygen will have little effect on the arterial blood gases. However, if the cyanosis is caused by a diffusion defect in the lungs, the degree of cyanosis decreases with increasing inspired oxygen.

The shunt study is beneficial in differentiating respiratory disease from cyanotic heart disease. Shunt studies are performed by obtaining arterial blood gases (preferably from the right radial artery) when the infant is in room air and then after the infant has been in 100% oxygen for 5 to 10 minutes. If the Pao_2 is greater than 150 torr, the presence of a right-to-left shunt and cyanotic congenital heart disease as the cause of cyanosis is unlikely.

CONGESTIVE HEART FAILURE. Congestive heart failure is a clinical syndrome reflecting the inability of the myocardium to meet the metabolic requirements of the body. Therefore the signs and symptoms of congestive heart failure reflect the decreased cardiac output and decreased tissue perfusion.

Congestive heart failure may be caused by (1) volume overload, (2) pressure overload, (3) cardiomyopathy, or (4) dysrhythmias. However, in the newborn, asphyxia and anemia must also be considered as causes of congestive heart failure.

The common symptoms associated with congestive heart failure can be explained using the physiologic principles previously outlined.

TACHYCARDIA. The heart attempts to compensate for the decrease in cardiac output by increasing either the heart rate or the stroke volume (CO = HR × SV). The newborn has a reduced capacity to increase stroke volume, primarily because the fetal myocardium has relatively few contractile elements and is poorly innervated by the sympathetic nervous system. Therefore the newborn can only increase cardiac output by increasing the heart rate, resulting in tachycardia.

CARDIAC ENLARGEMENT. Dilation and/or hypertrophy of the heart occurs in response to the volume or pressure overload, or the dysfunction associated with cardiomyopathies and dysrhythmias. Dilation of the cardiac chambers is evident on chest x-ray examination, with enlargement of the cardiac silhouette.

TACHYPNEA. Inefficient emptying or overloading of the lungs results in interstitial pulmonary edema. Tachypnea is the first clinical manifestation of pulmonary edema. As pulmonary edema progresses, however, alveolar and bronchiolar edema occur, resulting in intercostal retractions, grunting, nasal flaring, dyspnea, rales, and possibly cyanosis.

GALLOP RHYTHM. The gallop rhythm is an abnormal filling sound due to the dilation of the ventricles. It is heard as a triple rhythm on auscultation.

DECREASED PERIPHERAL PULSES AND MOTTLING OF THE EXTREMITIES. Decreased cardiac output results in a compensatory redistribution of blood flow to vital tissues. Peripheral tissue perfusion is therefore decreased, resulting in mottling of the skin and a grayish or pale skin color, as well as decreased pulses.

DECREASED URINE OUTPUT AND EDEMA. Decreased renal perfusion results in decreased glomerular filtration. This is interpreted by the body as a decrease in intravascular volume, initiating compensatory mechanisms such as vasoconstriction and fluid and sodium retention. In-

fants normally manifest this as weight gain or may have periorbital edema.

DIAPHORESIS. Diaphoresis represents the increased metabolic rate with congestive heart failure and most likely increased activity of the autonomic nervous system. The increased metabolic rate is in response to the increased work load of the heart in failure.

HEPATOMEGALY. The right ventricle in congestive heart failure is less compliant and may not adequately empty, leading to elevated pressures in the right atrium, central venous system, and hepatic system. Hepatomegaly results from hepatic congestion due to the elevated central venous pressure.

DECREASED EXERCISE TOLERANCE. The decreased perfusion to peripheral tissues and the increased energy required by the heart in failure leave little energy reserve for activities such as feeding and crying. The infant may sleep a majority of the time, fall asleep during feedings, and have a weak cry.

FAILURE TO THRIVE AND FEEDING PROBLEMS. Multiple factors contribute to the infant's failure to thrive and feeding difficulties. Tachypnea compromises the infant's ability to feed. The basal metabolic rate increases in infants with congestive heart failure, necessitating a higher caloric intake (150 cal/kg/day or more). The infant must expend more energy to consume the calories but lacks the energy to do so. Additionally, decreased tissue perfusion may curtail the infant's ability to grow.

DIMINISHED CARDIAC OUTPUT. An infant with poor peripheral pulses and skin mottling often has a profound decrease in cardiac output. This is commonly found in infants with coarctation of the aorta or hypoplastic left heart syndrome but may also be noted in asphyxia, metabolic disease, and sepsis.

The "E" class of prostaglandins, such as PGE_1, has been shown to prolong the patency of ductal tissue and is useful in certain "ductal-dependent" lesions (coarctation of the aorta, transposition of the great arteries, and pulmonary atresia) (Table 18-4).

Abnormalities of the cardiac rhythm and murmurs are discussed individually later.

CARDIAC EXAMINATION

See section on specific cardiac lesions.

LABORATORY DATA

ARTERIAL BLOOD GASES. The $PaCO_2$ in cardiac disease is often normal or increased if a primary pulmonary disease is present. Frequent monitoring of blood gases is unnecessary, but the acid-base balance should be monitored closely. The PaO_2 may be normal or greatly decreased, depending on the cardiac lesion and pulmonary status of the infant.

CHEST X-RAY EXAMINATION. The chest x-ray examination may be normal even if life-threatening congenital heart disease is present. However, the degree of pulmonary vascularity helps define the type of congenital heart disease present and is characterized as being increased, normal, or decreased. Likewise, the heart size should be evaluated and is described as being increased, normal, or decreased. The x-ray examination findings or each individual lesion are listed independently.

ELECTROCARDIOGRAM. See the section on specific cardiac lesions.

ECHOCARDIOGRAM. Ultrasonic evaluation of the heart with an echocardiogram is helpful in further defining the type of congenital heart disease present but may not be diagnostic in all cases. The additions of doppler flow interrogation and color flow mapping have greatly increased the accuracy of this tool.

General treatment strategy

Optimal management of infants with heart disease requires specialized expertise. Infants are monitored closely for hypoxia, hypoglycemia, acidosis, and congestive heart failure.

The infant must be kept in an Isolette or warmer in which body temperature is main-

TABLE 18-4

Cardiac Drugs

	ROUTE	DOSE	ONSET OF ACTION	COMMENTS
Atropine	IV	0.01-0.03 mg/kg/dose p.r.n. (maximum 0.4 mg)	Seconds	May cause tachycardia, urinary retention, or hyperthermia
	PO	0.01-0.03 mg/kg/dose q.4-6h. (maximum 0.4 mg)	Minutes	May cause tachycardia
Calcium chloride (10% solution)	IV	0.2-0.3 ml (20-30 mg)/kg/dose q. 10 min p.r.n. (maximum 500 mg)	Minutes	Slow infusion; *must* be IV; potentiates digoxin; bradycardia
Diazoxide (Hyperstat)*	IV	5 mg/kg/dose q. 30 min p.r.n.	1-2 min	May cause hypotension or hyperglycemia
Dobutamine (Dobutrex)†	IV	2-10 μg/kg/min	Minutes	Do not use in IHSS or tetralogy of Fallot; may cause ventricular ectopy, tachycardia, or hypertension Incompatible with alkaline solutions
Dopamine (Intropin)*	IV	5-30 μg/kg/min	Minutes	Often combined with a vasodilator when used at higher doses to counteract alpha vessel constriction; inactivated in alkaline solution
Epinephrine (1:10,000)	IV	0.1 ml/kg/dose (maximum 5 ml/dose) q. 3-5 min p.r.n. (0.01 mg/kg/dose)	Seconds	May cause tachycardia, arrhythmias, or hypertension; not effective if acidosis is present
Furosemide (Lasix)	IV	1-2 mg/kg/dose	5-15 min	May cause metabolic alkalosis + hypokalemia
	PO	1-4 mg/kg/dose	30-60 min	Follow electrolytes: may need KCl supplementation; renal calcification
Hydralazine (Apresoline)	IV	0.1-0.5 mg/kg/dose q.3-6h.	15-30 min	May cause lupuslike syndrome, tachycardia, or hypotension
	PO	0.1-0.5 mg/kg q.6h.; may increase to maximum of 2 mg/kg q.6h.	Often days until titrated effect achieved	Same as above
Hydrochlorothiazide (HydroDiuril)	PO	1-2 mg/kg q.12h.	1-2 hr	May cause electrolyte imbalance; may need KCl supplementation

*Safety and efficacy of these agents in children have not been established.

†Mix: 6 × weight (kg) = milligrams to be added to 100 ml D₅W. Yields: 1 ml/hr = 1 μg/kg/min.
  Example: 6 × 3 kg = 18 mg (dopamine, dobutamine, or Nipride) to be added to 100 ml D₅W.

‡Mix: 0.6 × weight (kg) = milligrams to be added to 100 ml D₅W. Yields: 1 ml/hr = 0.1 μg/kg/min.
  Example: 0.6 × 3 kg = 1.8 mg (Isuprel) to be added to 100 ml D₅W.

†,‡From Pediatric Life Support, Children's Hospital and Medical Center, Seattle, Wash, 1987.

Continued.

TABLE 18-4—cont'd

Cardiac Drugs

	ROUTE	DOSE	ONSET OF ACTION	COMMENTS
Indomethacin	IV	0.1-0.2 μg/kg/dose; may be repeated q.8h. for total of 3 doses		Less effective if administered after 7 days of age; probably will have no effect after 14 days of age
Isoproterenol (Isuprel)‡	IV	0.1-0.4 μg/kg/min	30-60 sec	May cause tachycardia/ventricular tachyarrhythmias; may also cause subendocardial ischemia
Lidocaine (Xylocaine)	IV	IV bolus 1 mg/kg; IV drip 20-50 μg/kg/min		May cause dysrhythmia, CNS agitation, or depression
Nitroprusside (Nipride)†	IV	1-10 μg/kg/min over 10 min to control blood pressure; chronic infusion—2 μg/kg/min (protect from light; change solution q.4h.)	Seconds	May cause hypotension and reflex tachycardia; may cause thiocyanate toxicity, especially if decreased renal function is present
Phentolamine (Regitine)	IV	1-20 μg/kg/min	5-10 min	May cause hypotension; commonly used with an intropic agent
	PO	5 mg/kg/day q.i.d.	N/A	May cause hypotension
Phenytoin (Dilantin)	IV	Load: 3-10 mg/kg over 5 min slow infusion; maintenance: 3-5 mg/kg/day b.i.d.	5-10 min	May cause cardiac depression
	PO	3-5 mg/kg/day b.i.d.	2-4 hr	Therapeutic blood levels (5-20 μg/ml)
Procainamide (Pronestyl)	IV	2 mg/kg/dose over 5 min	1-5 min	May cause hypotension or lupuslike syndrome
	IM	5-8 mg/kg q.6h.	15-30 min	Same as above
Propranolol (Inderal)	IV	Arrhythmias: 0.1-0.15 mg/kg/dose slow IV q.6-8h p.r.n. (maximum single dose, 10 mg); hypercyanotic spell: 0.15-0.25 mg/kg/dose slow IV push q. 15 min (maximum dose 10 mg)	2-5 min	May severely decrease cardiac output
	PO	Arrhythmias: 0.5-1.0 mg/kg/dose t.i.d.-q.i.d. (maximum daily dose 60 mg); hypercyanotic spells: 1-2 mg/kg/dose q.i.d.	30-60 min	See above
Prostaglandin E_1 (Prostin VR)	IV	0.01-0.1 μg/kg/min	Minutes	May cause apnea, fever, or hypotension

TABLE 18-4—cont'd

Cardiac Drugs

	ROUTE	DOSE	ONSET OF ACTION	COMMENTS
Quinidine gluconate (Duraquin)	PO	5-10 mg/kg q.6h.	4-8 hr	May cause gastrointestinal symptoms, hypotension, or blood dyscrasia
Spironolactone (Aldactone)	PO	1-2 mg/kg/day	N/A	Hyperkalemia, gastrointestinal upset, drowsiness
Tolazoline	IV	Test: 1-2 mg/kg slow IV push; maintenance: 1-2 mg/kg/hr	Minutes	May cause hypotension; gastrointestinal or pulmonary hemorrhage
Verapamil (Isoptin)*	IV	0.1-0.2 mg/kg over 1 min q. 30 min p.r.n.	Minutes	Should not be used if heart failure is already present—may cause hypotension; reverse with calcium and a pressor agent
	PO	3-6 mg/kg/day t.i.d.	N/A	Same as above

tained and color changes (pallor and increased cyanosis) may be observed. A cardiorespiratory monitor for continuous cardiac monitoring detects bradycardia, tachycardia, and dysrhythmias. The respiratory effort is assessed for tachypnea, shallow breathing, apnea, retractions, grunting, and nasal flaring. Observe and document activity level such as muscle tone, spontaneous movement, and seizure activity.

MANAGEMENT OF CONGESTIVE HEART FAILURE

The medical management of congestive heart failure attempts to reverse the process outlined previously and helps the heart compensate with increased cardiac output.

Digoxin acts primarily as a positive inotropic (improves contractility) agent but decreases the heart rate and increases urine output (see boxed material on p. 436). This drug should be used with caution if acidosis, myocarditis, or obstructive lesions (e.g., Fallot's tetralogy, subvalvular pulmonary stenosis, and asymmetric septal hypertrophy) are present.

Diuretics such as furosemide (Table 18-4) help decrease total body water (which is increased as a result of congestive heart failure). In general, chronic fluid restriction and low-salt diets are not commonly used in newborns or infants with congestive heart failure.

Infants with congestive heart failure are difficult to feed, and the process is often frustrating. They may have trouble sucking, swallowing, and breathing simultaneously. They may need to rest frequently during a feeding, thus prolonging feeding times, and they may fall asleep exhausted before adequate caloric intake is achieved. Since caloric requirements are higher in infants with congenital heart disease, adequate nutrition must be assured by (1) observing the infant's ability to nipple feed (a soft free-flowing [premature] nipple offers the least resistance to sucking and helps the infant conserve energy), (2) providing adequate calories for growth and if necessary using alternative feeding methods (i.e., gavage) if the infant is sucking poorly, and (3) anticipating the infant's hunger and offering feedings before the

---

DIGOXIN DOSAGES AND COMMON SIDE EFFECTS

Digitalizing schedule

Preterm infant
　IV route: 20-30 μg/kg total dose
　PO route: 30-40 μg/kg total dose
Term infant
　IV route: 30-40 μg/kg total dose
　PO route: 40-50 μg/kg total dose

Total dose is usually divided into three doses giving one half, then one fourth, then one fourth of the total dose q.8h. Check ECG rhythm strip for rate, PR interval, and dysrhythmias before each dose.

Maintenance schedule

Preterm infant
　IV route: 8-10 μg/kg/day
　PO route: 10-12 μg/kg/day
Term infant
　IV route: 10-12 μg/kg/day
　PO route: 12-14 μg/kg/day

Total dose should be divided b.i.d. Allow 12-24 hr between last digitalizing and first maintenance doses. It takes about 6 days to "digitalize" a patient with maintenance doses alone. The sign of digitalis effect is usually prolongation of the PR interval. The first sign of digitalis toxicity is usually vomiting, dysrhythmias, or bradycardia.

---

infant uses energy by crying, (4) positioning the infant in a semierect position for feeding, (5) burping the infant after every half ounce to help minimize vomiting, and (6) weighing the infant daily and checking for appropriate weight gain. Before discharge from the nursery, the infant should be in stable condition (e.g., feeding well and gaining weight appropriately).

An important fact for families to understand is that many infants will not gain weight, or will gain it very slowly because of their cardiac defects, regardless of the method of feeding that is used. The family of an infant in congestive heart failure needs support and teaching. Explanation of the term *congestive heart failure* should be given early on, since it is a frustrating term for parents. The words "heart failure" are often interpreted as "heart attack." It is important that parents understand that saying an infant is in heart failure does not imply that the infant's heart will stop. A simple explanation describing heart failure as a condition in which the heart shows signs of being less able to pump sufficient blood to meet all the needs of the body is helpful in decreasing anxiety for the family.

PATENT DUCTUS ARTERIOSUS
Physiology

The ductus arteriosus is a normal pathway in the fetal circulatory system and allows blood from the right ventricle and pulmonary arterial system to flow into the descending aorta for ultimate delivery to the placenta (Figure 18-1). Functionally, the patent ductus arteriosus (PDA) closes within a few hours to several days after birth, but this closure is often delayed in premature infants. After birth, as a result of a decrease in the pressure of the pulmonary circulation and an increase in the pressure of the aorta, the blood flow through a PDA is predominantly from the aorta to the pulmonary artery (left-to-right shunt). The hemodynamic changes and the resultant clinical manifestations of a PDA depend on the magnitude of the pulmonary vascular resistance and the size of the ductal lumen.

Approximately 15% of infants with PDAs have

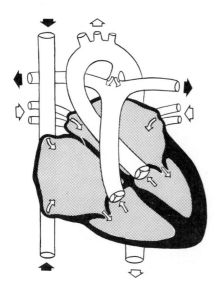

Figure 18-1. Patent ductus arteriosus. (Courtesy Ross Laboratories, Columbus, Ohio.)

additional cardiac defects, including VSDs, coarctations of the aorta, aortic stenosis, or pulmonary stenosis. Rarely, PDA is associated with known syndromes, most commonly rubella.

Data collection
HISTORY

Asphyxial insult or respiratory distress syndrome, inability to wean from a respirator, and an increasing FIO_2 demand usually accompany PDA.

PHYSICAL FINDINGS

Increased flow to the pulmonary circulation and volume overload of the left ventricle are the two major physiologic abnormalities in a PDA.

CYANOSIS. Generally, cyanosis is not present in an isolated PDA, because the predominant shunt is from left to right.

HEART SOUNDS. The majority of infants with PDA have audible murmurs as a result of the left-to-right shunting through the ductus dur-

ing systole. A grade I through III systolic murmur is best heard at the upper left sternal border with radiation to the left axilla and faintly to the back. Although this murmur may occasionally flow into diastole, the classical continuous machinery-like murmur is an unusual occurrence in the newborn period. It is often helpful to briefly disconnect the newborn from the ventilator before auscultating. There are several documented cases of large PDAs in which no murmur was audible.

PULSES. Because of the rapid upstroke and wide pulse pressure, the peripheral pulses are bounding. Pulses are hyperdynamic and easily palpated. Assessment of the pulses should include palpation of palmar, plantar, and calf pulses. The calf pulses are not usually palpable in infants. The presence of an easily palpated pulse in these areas suggests the presence of an aortic run-off lesion, which is most commonly a patent ductus arteriosus.

CONGESTIVE HEART FAILURE. Because of the volume overload of the left ventricle, the infant may show signs of congestive heart failure and pulmonary edema (see section on congestive heart failure).

LABORATORY DATA

ARTERIAL BLOOD GASES. The arterial blood gases are normal.

CHEST X-RAY EXAMINATION. A chest x-ray film appears normal in small shunts. Cardiomegaly is present with increased pulmonary vascularity in large shunts.

ELECTROCARDIOGRAM. The electrocardiogram may be normal, demonstrate left ventricular hypertrophy, or demonstrate combined ventricular hypertrophy. Ischemia is rarely seen.

ECHOCARDIOGRAM. An increased left atrial/aortic ratio suggests a moderate to large left-to-right shunt (i.e., PDA, VSD). An echocardiogram should be performed before medical or surgical closure of the PDA to rule out a ductal-dependent lesion or other associated anomalies. Color flow mapping allows for visualization of the PDA, as well as determination of the direction of blood flow across the PDA (i.e., left to right, right to left, or bidirectional).

CARDIAC CATHETERIZATION. If the echocardiogram has eliminated a ductal-dependent lesion, cardiac catheterization is usually not required before treatment.

Treatment
MEDICAL MANAGEMENT

Asymptomatic infants with PDAs generally do not require medical management or surgical ligation. These infants should be continually monitored for evidence of congestive heart failure, failure to thrive, increasing oxygen requirement, or other complications.

Symptomatic infants weighing less than 1000 g require ductal closure by either ductal ligation or indomethacin therapy. Medical management such as fluid restriction is rarely successful. Indomethacin is administered orally (PO) or intravenously (IV) at a dose of 0.1 to 0.2 mg/kg/dose and may be repeated every 8 hours for a total of three doses. It is much less effective if administered after 7 days of age and probably will have no effect after 14 days of age. Urine output should be continuously monitored, and if there is a dramatic decrease, the drug should be discontinued.

Symptomatic infants weighing more than 1000 g should receive 48 hours of maximal fluid restriction (to the point of decreased weight and urine output). If during that 48-hour period the infant has a decreased oxygen requirement and ventilatory settings, a gradual fluid challenge should be given. If the infant again becomes symptomatic with fluid challenge, or if the infant has made no progress at the end of the 48-hour period, closure of the ductus is recommended.

SURGICAL TREATMENT

Surgical ligation or clipping the ductus arteriosus through a lateral thoracotomy incision is a low-risk procedure when performed by an experienced surgical team.

Complications and residual effects

Complications and residual effects, although rare, include (1) recannulization, (2) recurrent laryngeal or phrenic nerve palsies, or (3) false aneurysms. The surgical mortality in the neonatal period is generally less than 1%.

Prognosis and follow-up

Asymptomatic infants have an excellent prognosis, although close follow-up is necessary because if the ductus remains patent until 9 to 12 months of age, ligation is recommended.

Symptomatic infants with a persistent ductus arteriosus generally experience failure to thrive, continued congestive heart failure, increased oxygen requirements with resultant bronchopulmonary dysplasia, or pulmonary infections.

VENTRICULAR SEPTAL DEFECT
Physiology

VSDs may involve various portions of the ventricular septum and are classified according to the anatomic position that they occupy when viewed from the right ventricle (Figure 18-2).

A VSD may occur as an isolated anomaly or may be part of a more complex cardiac lesion. Only isolated VSDs are discussed in this section. The effect of the VSD on the circulation depends on both the size of the VSD and the relative pulmonary vascular resistance. Pulmonary vascular resistance is nearly systemic immediately after birth but rapidly falls to one-fourth to one-third systemic in the first several days of life.

In a small VSD, the left-to-right shunting at the ventricular level is minimal and the infants are asymptomatic.

Larger VSDs may have a mild to moderate left-to-right shunt, resulting in left ventricular failure and pulmonary edema. Premature infants tend to have lower pulmonary vascular resistance at birth and therefore may be symptomatic. However, infants with severe lung disease (hyaline membrane

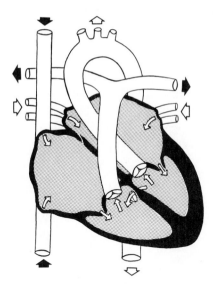

Figure 18-2. Ventricular septal defects. (Courtesy Ross Laboratories, Columbus, Ohio.)

disease, bronchopulmonary dysplasia, or pneumonia) may have elevated pulmonary vascular resistance and therefore minimal left-to-right shunting.

Data collection

See Table 18-1 for infants at increased risk.

PHYSICAL FINDINGS

CYANOSIS. Infants with isolated VSDs are rarely cyanotic in the neonatal period.

HEART SOUNDS. Most infants with VSDs have a heart murmur. The time when this murmur is first audible is dependent on the decrease in the pulmonary vascular resistance and the size of the defect. The murmur is typically a grade II to III/VI systolic murmur heard best at the lower left sternal border. A diastolic flow rumble at the apex indicates a large left-to-right shunt.

CONGESTIVE HEART FAILURE. Congestive heart failure is unusual in the newborn with an isolated VSD. When it occurs, however, it is a result of the volume overload of the left ventricle (see section on congestive heart failure).

LABORATORY DATA

ARTERIAL BLOOD GASES. Arterial blood gases are normal.

CHEST X-RAY EXAMINATION. A chest x-ray film shows a normal to increased heart size with an increased pulmonary vascular flow.

ELECTROCARDIOGRAM. The electrocardiogram in an infant with heart failure is usually normal but may demonstrate ventricular hypertrophy.

ECHOCARDIOGRAM. The M mode is nondiagnostic. A two-dimensional echocardiogram demonstrates a VSD in 90% of the cases. Doppler interrogation of the ventricular septum and/or flow mapping have greatly increased the accuracy of diagnosing a VSD noninvasively. The use of color flow is particularly advantageous in identifying the presence of multiple VSDs and the direction of blood flow across the VSD.

CARDIAC CATHETERIZATION. A cardiac catheterization is diagnostic but not required in the neonatal period unless there is some question regarding the diagnosis or if surgery is being considered.

Treatment
MEDICAL MANAGEMENT

If the patient demonstrates failure to thrive or intractable congestive heart failure with maximal medical management, surgical intervention at any age is necessary (see section on general treatment strategy).

SURGICAL TREATMENT

Surgical treatment of a VSD consists of either suture closure or patching (using pericardium or, more commonly, a synthetic material such as Dacron). In general, a VSD may be approached through a median sternotomy incision through the right atrium and tricuspid valve, therefore avoiding a right ventriculotomy.

Complications and residual effects

Complications and/or residual effects may include (1) a persistent shunt (residual VSD), (2) conduction abnormalities (right bundle-branch block and third-degree heart block), and (3) aortic or tricuspid insufficiency (<1%).

The mortality in infants is approximately 10%, with higher mortality found in the neonatal period. Contraindications to primary VSD closure include the diagnosis of double-outlet right ventricle and multiple muscular VSDs.

Pulmonary artery banding is an alternative to closing the VSD in infants. However, the combined risk of pulmonary banding plus later debanding and VSD closure is about 10%.

Prognosis

Approximately 50% to 75% of small VSDs will spontaneously close.

If a large left-to-right shunt is persistent after 9 to 24 months of age, the infant is susceptible to pulmonary vascular disease.

COARCTATION OF THE AORTA
Physiology

Coarctation of the aorta is a localized constriction of the aorta that usually occurs at the junction of the transverse aortic arch and the descending aorta in the vicinity of the ductus arteriosus (Figure 18-3). However, coarctation can occur anywhere in the aorta from above the aortic valve to the abdominal aorta. The precise location of the coarctation and the presence or absence of associated anomalies affect the clinical presentation. Associated anomalies include PDA, VSD, and bicuspid aortic valve (50%). Coarctation is frequently observed in infants with Turner's syndrome.

Data collection
PHYSICAL FINDINGS

Newborns with critical coarctation of the aorta usually have signs and symptoms of congestive heart failure and low cardiac output. Coarcta-

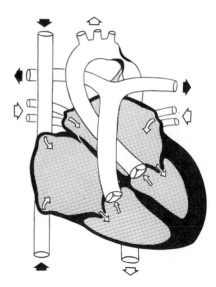

Figure 18-3. Coarctation of aorta. (Courtesy Ross Laboratories, Columbus, Ohio.)

tion of the aorta is a medical and surgical emergency.

CYANOSIS. Generally, cyanosis in the newborn is not present in the isolated coarctation of the aorta.

HEART SOUNDS. Cardiac murmurs are generally not found in an isolated, severe coarctation of the aorta. If other associated cardiac defects are present, however, a murmur may be heard. A soft, grade I to II/VI systolic murmur may be present at the left sternal border, radiating to the left axilla and to the back. A gallop rhythm is usually present. The murmurs of associated anomalies, however, are usually dominant.

PULSES AND BLOOD PRESSURE. The blood pressure proximal to the area of obstruction is higher than the blood pressure distal to the area of obstruction.

The most consistent physical findings in infants with critical coarctation of the aorta is a higher systolic blood pressure (>15 mm Hg) in the upper extremities than in the lower extremities. This blood pressure must be measured with the appropriate-size cuff. In addition, pulses are easily palpable in the upper extremities but are difficult to palpate or are absent in the lower extremities.

CONGESTIVE HEART FAILURE. Congestive heart failure is found in many infants with severe coarctation as a result of a pressure overload on the left ventricle (see section on congestive heart failure).

LABORATORY DATA

ARTERIAL BLOOD GASES. Arterial blood gases are normal.

CHEST X-RAY EXAMINATION. Cardiomegaly may be seen on the x-ray film. Pulmonary vascularity is normal unless associated anomalies are present.

ELECTROCARDIOGRAM. Right ventricular hypertrophy is frequently present. Left ventricular hypertrophy or combined ventricular hypertrophy is rarely seen in the newborn period, and the electrocardiogram may be normal.

ECHOCARDIOGRAM. The area of coarctation can often be visualized using two-dimensional techniques and color flow mapping. Abnormal Doppler blood flow is diagnostic. Cautious interpretation of the findings is suggested.

CARDIAC CATHETERIZATION. Cardiac catheterization is diagnostic and must be performed before any surgical procedure is undertaken to evaluate other associated anomalies.

Treatment
MEDICAL MANAGEMENT

Congestive heart failure should be treated aggressively. Intractable congestive heart failure, acidosis, oliguria, and hypertension are indications for cardiac catheterization and corrective surgery as soon as possible. (See section on general treatment strategy of congenital heart disease.) Balloon dilation of the coarcted site has been performed in the catheterization laboratory at some institutions with variable success.

It is considered an experimental procedure. A significant incidence of aortic wall aneurysm formation has been identified 6 to 12 months later in some genes.

SURGICAL TREATMENT

The surgical procedure of choice for repairing coarctation in infancy is the subclavian flap aortoplasty. A longitudinal incision is made in the aorta across the coarctated site and continued to the end of the distally divided left subclavian artery. The left subclavian artery is used as a patch or flap to increase the diameter of the aorta. This procedure is performed through a lateral thoracotomy incision and has been highly successful in relieving coarctation and providing for future growth of the aorta.

Complications and residual effects

Complications and residual effects include (1) diminished or absent pulses in the left arm, (2) persistent hypertension, (3) Horner's syndrome, (4) paraplegia ($<0.5\%$), and (5) mesenteric vasculitis.

The overall operative mortality is 38% in infancy. However, the high mortality is usually related to the preoperative status and associated lesions. Early detection and referral in addition to the use of prostaglandin E_1 may dramatically reduce this mortality in the future.

Prognosis and follow-up

Infants with mild coarctation require minimal care until later in life. If these patients are medically managed, close follow-up is mandatory, with repeat cardiac catheterization and surgery expected at a later date.

Infants with severe coarctation require prompt medical and surgical treatment. If this therapy is instituted early, the prognosis is generally favorable. Untreated infants with severe coarctation often have a rapidly deteriorating clinical course with left ventricular failure, severe hypertension, or intractable congestive heart failure, and the prognosis is guarded. After surgical repair, frequent follow-up is required to ensure adequate coarctation repair. Repeated cardiac catheterization may be required several months to years after the surgical procedure is completed.

CRITICAL AORTIC STENOSIS
Physiology

Obstruction of the left ventricular outlet may occur below the aortic valve, at the aortic valve, or above the aortic valve (subvalvular, valvular, or supravalvular aortic stenosis) (Figure 18-4). Valvular aortic stenosis is the most common type and is discussed here. A pressure gradient (the pressure difference from the left ventricle to the ascending aorta) of 50 mm Hg or more is indicative of significant aortic stenosis in the newborn.

Data collection
PHYSICAL FINDINGS

Although most infants with aortic stenosis are asymptomatic in the neonatal period, an infant who is symptomatic from critical aortic stenosis needs medical and surgical emergency treatment. The infant with critical aortic stenosis will have pale, gray, cool skin with decreased perfusion and peripheral pulses.

CYANOSIS. Cyanosis is generally not present in isolated valvular aortic stenosis.

HEART SOUNDS. A grade II to IV/VI harsh systolic murmur is typically heard in the upper right sternal border, radiating to the upper left sternal border and faintly to the neck. The intensity of the murmur is unrelated to the severity of the obstruction. An ejection click may be heard at the apex, radiating to the lower left sternal border. A suprasternal notch thrill is palpable.

CONGESTIVE HEART FAILURE. Infants with critical aortic stenosis have congestive heart failure caused by a pressure overload of the left ventricle (see section on congestive heart failure).

LABORATORY DATA

ARTERIAL BLOOD GASES. Arterial blood gases are generally normal.

CHEST X-RAY EXAMINATION. A chest x-ray film shows cardiomegaly with normal pulmonary vascularity.

ELECTROCARDIOGRAM. The electrocardiogram may be normal or demonstrate left ventricular hypertrophy. It is important to remember that there is poor correlation between an electrocardiographic abnormality and the degree of aortic stenosis present.

ECHOCARDIOGRAM. The aortic valve is usually thickened and appears to close abnormally in an echocardiogram. Doppler interrogation can accurately estimate the systolic pressure gradient from the left ventricle to the ascending aorta and identify the level or levels of obstruction.

CARDIAC CATHETERIZATION. Cardiac catheterization is diagnostic and should be performed as soon as possible in all cases of critical aortic stenosis. Some centers are performing balloon dilation of the aortic valve during the cardiac

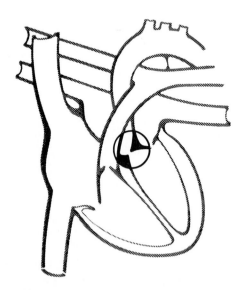

Figure 18-4. Aortic stenosis. (© American Heart Association. Reprinted with permission.)

catheterization; however, this is still considered an experimental procedure.

Treatment
MEDICAL MANAGEMENT

Medical management is usually unsatisfactory, and surgical intervention is necessary for symptomatic critical aortic stenosis in the newborn (see section on general treatment strategies).

SURGICAL TREATMENT

Aortic valvulotomy through a median sternotomy incision is the surgical procedure for correcting critical aortic stenosis in infants. This procedure can usually be accomplished in the newborn with inflow occlusion and circulatory arrest for 1 to 2 minutes. In older infants, cardiopulmonary bypass should be performed. The fused commissures of the valve are incised, permitting the leaflets to open freely during systole.

Complications and residual effects

Complications and residual effects include aortic insufficiency and residual aortic stenosis. The mortality in infancy ranges from 5% to 50%, with the highest risk involving the newborn with critical obstruction. It is hoped that avoidance of a cardiopulmonary bypass operation will reduce the mortality in this group.

Prognosis

Surgery for critical aortic stenosis in the neonatal period is considered a palliative measure for relief of the obstruction. Repeated catheterization and further surgical repair of the valve should be expected in the next several months to years.

CRITICAL PULMONARY STENOSIS WITH INTACT VENTRICULAR SEPTUM
Physiology

In critical pulmonary stenosis with intact ventricular septum, the flow to the pulmonary artery from the right ventricle is obstructed. The obstruction may occur below the valve in the infundibular area, above the valve, or at the valve (subvalvular, supravalvular, or valvular). In valvular stenosis the orifice of the pulmonary valve is markedly narrowed, and the valvular tissue may assume the shape of a cone (Figure 18-5). The pulmonary artery distal to this area of stenosis may be dilated. Because the ventricular septum is intact, the right ventricle is subjected to a marked increase in pressure and becomes hypertrophied. A pressure gradient from the right ventricle to the pulmonary artery of 50 mm Hg or more is indicative of significant pulmonary stenosis in the newborn.

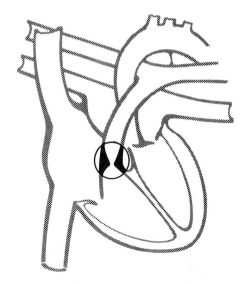

Figure 18-5. Pulmonary stenosis. (© American Heart Association. Reprinted with permission.)

Data collection
PHYSICAL FINDINGS

CYANOSIS. Cyanosis is generally not present in an isolated lesion but may occur in the presence of a right-to-left atrial shunt.

HEART SOUNDS. A harsh, grade II to III/VI systolic murmur is heard in the upper left sternal border, radiating to both axillae and faintly to the back. The diastole is quiet. A murmur of tricuspid insufficiency (Grade I/VI, soft, systolic murmur at the lower left sternal border) may be heard. An ejection click may also be heard at the left sternal border.

CONGESTIVE HEART FAILURE. The infant with critical pulmonary stenosis typically has signs and symptoms of right-sided congestive heart failure resulting from excessive pressure overload (see section on congestive heart failure).

LABORATORY DATA

ARTERIAL BLOOD GASES. Arterial blood gases are generally normal.

CHEST X-RAY EXAMINATION. The chest x-ray film may be normal but usually demonstrates cardiomegaly with normal or decreased pulmonary vascularity.

ELECTROCARDIOGRAM. The electrocardiogram may be normal or demonstrate right ventricular hypertrophy.

ECHOCARDIOGRAM. An abnormal pulmonary valve pattern on a two-dimensional echocardiogram is diagnostic. Doppler interrogation and color flow mapping can accurately estimate the systolic pressure gradient from the right ventricle to the pulmonary artery and identify the level or levels of obstruction.

CARDIAC CATHETERIZATION. Infants suspected of having critical pulmonary stenosis with an intact ventricular septum should undergo cardiac catheterization as soon as possible. Balloon dilation of the pulmonic valve during cardiac catheterization has been successfully performed in many institutions, and in some it is considered the procedure of choice.

Treatment
MEDICAL MANAGEMENT

Surgery is often used in treating severe valvular pulmonary stenosis and is an emergency procedure in any symptomatic newborn. Prostaglandin E_1 has been used successfully to maintain the patency of the ductus arteriosus, thereby allowing adequate pulmonary blood flow until surgery. If balloon dilation has been performed successfully, surgical intervention may be postponed or may not be necessary at all.

SURGICAL TREATMENT

The degree of pulmonary stenosis and the size of the pulmonary arteries determine the surgical approach. If the right ventricle and pulmonary arteries are of adequate size, then pulmonary valvulotomy through a median sternotomy incision is the preferable procedure. This involves incising the pulmonary valve commissures, allowing the leaflets to open freely during systole. Like aortic valvulotomy, this procedure can often be performed under inflow occlusion.

COMPLICATIONS AND RESIDUAL EFFECTS. Complications and residual effects include pulmonary insufficiency and residual pulmonary stenosis. The mortality of pulmonary stenosis is 17% in newborns.

If the right ventricle and pulmonary arteries are too small to allow antegrade flow, then a palliative procedure such as the Blalock-Taussig operation is performed. This procedure consists of bringing down the subclavian artery opposite the aortic arch and anastomosing it to the ipsilateral pulmonary artery.

Complications and residual side effects of Blalock-Taussig shunts include (1) diminished or absent pulses in the affected arm, (2) congestive heart failure from an overlarge shunt, and (3) inadequacy of the shunt. The mortality in this group is higher than in infants with adequately sized right ventricles and pulmonary arteries.

Prognosis

If a palliative shunt has been used, follow-up catheterization and surgical procedures should be anticipated either when the shunt becomes nonfunctional or when total repair is expected. If the lesion has been primarily corrected surgically in the neonatal period, repeated catheterization is routinely performed several months later to evaluate the residual obstruction.

ATRIOVENTRICULAR CANAL ENDOCARDIAL CUSHION DEFECTS
Physiology

The complete type of endocardial cushion defect is characterized by a crescent-shaped atrial septal defect (ASD) involving the most inferior portion of the atrial septum. The anterior leaflet of the mitral valve and the septal leaflet of the tricuspid valve both have clefts and are continuous with each other through the defect. Thus the atrioventricular (AV) valves are represented by a valve common to both sides of the heart. In addition, a VSD is present.

These infants usually have a left-to-right shunt at both the atrial and ventricular levels. In addition, if the cleft in the mitral valve is substantial, mitral insufficiency may also be present. The symptomatology depends on the degree of shunting at the atrial and ventricular levels and the amount of mitral insufficiency present. There is an association between endocardial cushion defects and Down's syndrome.

Data collection
PHYSICAL FINDINGS

CYANOSIS. Generally, cyanosis is not present with an isolated endocardial cushion defect.

HEART SOUNDS. If mitral insufficiency is present, a blowing, systolic, apical murmur with radiation to the left axilla is heard (see section on heart sounds for the ASD and VSD).

CONGESTIVE HEART FAILURE. Congestive heart failure may be present because of volume overload of the ventricles as a result of mitral insufficiency and left-to-right shunting at either the atrial or ventricular level (see section on congestive heart failure).

LABORATORY DATA

ARTERIAL BLOOD GASES. The $PaCO_2$ may be elevated if there is severe mitral insufficiency and pulmonary edema. The pH is usually normal. The PaO_2 is also usually normal.

CHEST X-RAY EXAMINATION. The heart size may be normal or increased. The pulmonary vascularity is generally increased.

ELECTROCARDIOGRAM. An electrocardiogram with a left axis deviation, counterclockwise loop in the frontal plane, and superior axis suggests an endocardial cushion defect.

ECHOCARDIOGRAM. An abnormal mitral valve pattern is seen on an M mode echocardiogram. A two-dimensional echocardiogram with doppler and color flow mapping demonstrates the ASD, VSD, and common AV valves, and the degree of AV valve insufficiency. This technique is diagnostic.

CARDIAC CATHETERIZATION. Cardiac catheterization is diagnostic but generally not performed in the neonatal period in a direct AV canal, unless the infant is refractory to medical management and surgery is anticipated.

Treatment
MEDICAL MANAGEMENT

See general section on medical therapy.

SURGICAL TREATMENT

If the infant does not respond to medical treatment and exhibits congestive heart failure, severe mitral regurgitation, or pulmonary hypertension, surgical repair is necessary. The surgical procedure through a median sternotomy incision involves closing the ASD and VSD, separating the common leaflets of the mitral and tricuspid valves, and reconstructing the mitral valve.

Complications and residual effects

Complications and residual effects include (1) persistent shunt (residual ASD or VSD), (2) conduction abnormalities (dysrhythmias and third-degree heart block), (3) mitral regurgitation, and (4) tricuspid regurgitation. The mortality in infancy is 10% to 25%.

The alternative to total repair is pulmonary

artery banding. This is, however, contraindicated when mitral regurgitation or atrial shunting is severe. The risk of banding plus later debanding and repair approaches the risk of primary total repair.

Prognosis

In the complete endocardial cushion defect, congestive heart failure is a frequent problem and early surgical intervention is generally required. The prognosis of surgical repair in the neonatal period is guarded, with a generally favorable outcome if the surgery can be postponed until the infant is older than 6 months of age. The prognosis is guarded if pulmonary hypertension develops before surgical intervention.

EBSTEIN'S ANOMALY
Physiology

Ebstein's anomaly consists of an abnormally low insertion of the tricuspid valve, incorporating a portion of the right ventricle into the right atrium. The resultant right ventricular cavity is small, and because the elevated pulmonary artery pressure is normally present in the newborn period, the cardiac output from the right ventricle to the pulmonary artery is decreased. This cardiac output generally increases as the pulmonary artery pressure decreases after birth. Tricuspid insufficiency is present in varying degrees in the infant.

Data collection
PHYSICAL FINDINGS

CYANOSIS. The degree of cyanosis is dependent on (1) the amount of right-to-left shunting at the foramen ovale and (2) the amount of blood that enters the pulmonary circulation by the right ventricle. Also, varying degrees of cyanosis are present. In severe cases, the amount of pulmonary blood flow is markedly decreased, and these infants may be deeply cyanotic as well.

HEART SOUNDS. The second heart sound, S_2, is normal in the mildly affected infant, but the pulmonary component of S_2 may be diminished or inaudible in severely affected patients. A nonspecific systolic murmur is usually present and varies from a grade I/VI to a grade V/VI, representing tricuspid insufficiency. Diastolic murmurs, ejection clicks, and triple or quadruple rhythms are frequently heard.

CONGESTIVE HEART FAILURE. Newborns who are symptomatic usually have congestive heart failure resulting from volume overload of the left ventricle (see section on congestive heart failure).

LABORATORY DATA

ARTERIAL BLOOD GASES. The PaO_2 may be normal to very low, depending on the amount of antegrade blood flow through the pulmonary valve. PaO_2 in the low 20s are not uncommon.

CHEST X-RAY EXAMINATION. A chest x-ray film shows cardiomegaly with decreased pulmonary vascularity. Massive cardiomegaly generally indicates severe tricuspid insufficiency.

ELECTROCARDIOGRAM. An electrocardiogram shows abnormal P waves and various degrees of heart block, which are typical. The QRS generally demonstrates a right bundle-branch block. Wolff-Parkinson-White (preexcitation) syndrome is frequently present, and dysrhythmias are common.

ECHOCARDIOGRAM. An echocardiogram with abnormal tricuspid valve patterns on an M mode suggests Ebstein's anomaly. A two-dimensional echocardiogram is diagnostic. Doppler interrogation and color flow mapping are very useful in evaluating the amount of antegrade blood flow through the pulmonary valve and the degree of tricuspid insufficiency present.

CARDIAC CATHETERIZATION. There is an increased risk of dysrhythmias following catheterization. This procedure is not generally performed in the neonatal period unless a question regarding the differential diagnosis exists (to rule out pulmonary atresia).

Treatment
MEDICAL MANAGEMENT

Dysrhythmias, especially supraventricular tachycardia, should be anticipated and appropriately managed (see section on general treatment strategies).

SURGICAL TREATMENT

Surgical treatment for Ebstein's anomaly is rarely indicated in infancy. The procedure through a sternotomy incision involves repositioning the tricuspid valve and an anuloplasty to improve the competency of the valve. In addition, plication of the atrialized ventricle is performed. Replacing the tricuspid valve may be required.

Complications and residual effects

Complications and residual effects include tricuspid insufficiency and dysrhythmias. The mortality in infancy is unknown because of insufficient data.

Prognosis

The prognosis of mild Ebstein's anomaly is generally favorable. Infants with severe Ebstein's anomaly generally improve as the right ventricle output increases. Although surgery has been used successfully in the more severe forms of Ebstein's anomaly, the prognosis is less favorable in patients requiring surgical intervention.

PERSISTENT PULMONARY HYPERTENSION IN THE NEWBORN
Physiology

Infants with abnormally elevated pulmonary vascular resistance have persistent fetal circulation or persistent pulmonary hypertension of the newborn. These infants are generally hypoxic and acidotic but usually do not have severe pulmonary perenchymal disease or underlying cardiac disease. These infants have a right-to-left shunt at the ductal or atrial level.

Data collection
HISTORY

Persistent pulmonary hypertension is usually associated with severe antepartum or peripartum conditions that involve hypoxia reflected by low Apgar scores. These infants are gener-

ally term or near term and are symptomatic within the first hours after birth. Associated findings include hyperviscosity, hypoglycemia, or a congenital diaphragmatic hernia.

PHYSICAL FINDINGS

CYANOSIS. The milder cases of persistent pulmonary hypertension have minimal transient tachypnea and cyanosis associated with stress (crying or feeding). The severe cases have marked cyanosis, tachypnea, acidosis, and decreased peripheral perfusion.

HEART SOUNDS. A loud pulmonary component of S_2 and occasionally a nonspecific systolic ejection murmur are heard.

CONGESTIVE HEART FAILURE. Infants with persistent pulmonary hypertension usually have congestive heart failure because of pressure overload of the right ventricle (see section on congestive heart failure).

LABORATORY DATA

ARTERIAL BLOOD GASES. Arterial blood gases demonstrate acidosis, hypoxia, and increased $PaCO_2$. If a blood gas is obtained simultaneously in the right radial artery (preductal) and in the descending aorta with an umbilical artery catheter (postductal), the right-to-left shunt at the ductal level can be documented. If blood gases are repeated after intubation and pharmacologic intervention (see section on treatment), the amount of hypoxia is often reduced. Simultaneous preductal and postductal transcutaneous oxygen measurement may also be used.

CHEST X-RAY EXAMINATION. A chest x-ray film demonstrates mild to moderate cardiomegaly with normal pulmonary vascular markings. The lung fields may be clear.

ELECTROCARDIOGRAM. The electrocardiogram frequently is normal but may demonstrate right ventricular hypertrophy and signs of myocardial ischemia.

ECHOCARDIOGRAM. An echocardiogram helps to evaluate cardiac structures and rule out cyanotic lesions. Evaluating the pulmonary valve pattern for evidence of pulmonary hypertension is often helpful.

CARDIAC CATHETERIZATION. Cardiac catheterization is usually not performed.

Treatment
MEDICAL MANAGEMENT

Severely affected infants need immediate medical management. Assisted ventilation, IV fluids, bicarbonate to reverse acidosis, and occasionally pulmonary vasodilators (tolazoline) are required. Management is aimed at decreasing pulmonary vascular resistance, increasing systemic vascular resistance, and reducing right-to-left shunting through the foramen ovale and the PDA.

Oxygen is the most potent pulmonary vasodilator. Therefore ventilation with 100% oxygen is useful initially. Large decreases in PaO_2 can lead to increased pulmonary vascular resistance and profound hypoxia. Hyperventilation may be used at rates of 100 to 150 breaths/min to reduce $PaCO_2$, increase pH, and increase PaO_2. Weaning from the ventilator prematurely can cause pulmonary vasoconstriction and an irreversible downward slide in the PaO_2. When normoxia has been maintained for 12 to 24 hours, cautious weaning can be initiated.

Tolazoline may be added when ventilatory management alone is insufficient. Tolazoline is a potent systemic and pulmonary vasodilator. Therefore two IV lines should be used to administer the drug and to administer fluids and medications to support the systemic blood pressure. The pulmonary vascular response to tolazoline should be assessed by rapidly infusing 1 mg/kg through a peripheral IV.

If the response to tolazoline is favorable (easily assessed with a transcutaneous oxygen monitor), a continuous infusion of 0.5 to 1 mg/kg/hr may be instituted. Careful monitoring of the arterial pressure should be maintained, and if the patient becomes hypotensive, the drug should be discontinued. An infusion of albumin or blood should be instituted. In the rare event that hypotension is refractory to conventional therapy, infusion of isoproterenol (Isuprel) or dopamine should be considered (see Chapter 17).

SURGICAL INTERVENTION

Surgery is not performed in infants with persistent pulmonary hypertension.

Prognosis

These infants generally have a favorable prognosis if they respond to the treatments outlined previously and are generally without residual problems following the immediate newborn period.

COMPLETE D-TRANSPOSITION OF THE GREAT ARTERIES
Physiology

Complete d-transposition of the great arteries (Figure 18-6) is one of the most common forms of serious heart disease. The aorta arises from the right ventricle, receives unoxygenated systemic venous blood, and returns this blood to the systemic arterial circulation. The pulmonary artery arises from the left ventricle, receives oxygenated pulmonary venous blood, and returns this blood to the pulmonary circulation. D-transposition can occur by itself or can be associated with other defects (PDA, ASD, VSD, or pulmonary stenosis).

Data collection
HISTORY

Transposition of the great arteries is more prevalent in males and is typically found in infants who are full term.

PHYSICAL FINDINGS

The major physiologic abnormalities in d-transposition of the great arteries are an oxygen deficiency in the tissues and excessive work load of the right and left ventricles. The only mixing of oxygenated and unoxygenated blood occurs in the presence of associated lesions (patent foramen ovale, ASD, VSD, PDA, or collateral circulation). The extent of the mixing depends on

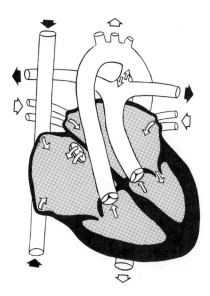

Figure 18-6. Complete transposition of great arteries. (Courtesy Ross Laboratories, Columbus, Ohio.)

the number, size, and position of the anatomic communications, the pressure differential between the two systems, and changes in the systemic and pulmonary vascular resistance.

CYANOSIS. Cyanosis is present in varying degrees, depending on the amount of intercirculatory mixing present. Cyanosis may be mild if the mixing occurs through a significant VSD or PDA. Cyanosis is profound, with intact ventricular septum or a closing PDA. Oxygen therapy will be of limited benefit. Only a certain amount of oxygenated blood is able to reach the systemic circulation, and administration of additional oxygen does not improve this situation. Enlargement of the interatrial communication by balloon septostomy (Rashkind procedure) during cardiac catheterization is critical in establishing adequate intercirculatory mixing for these infants. Alternative or additional management may include surgical removal of the atrial septum (Blalock-Hanlon operation).

Following these palliative procedures, the in-

fant will continue to be cyanotic, especially in times of stress (crying, feeding, or exposure to cold temperatures). If the PaO_2 at rest in room air is not greater than 35 mm torr or if persistent metabolic acidosis is present, inadequate intercardiac mixing should be suspected.

HEART SOUNDS. The aorta arises from the anterior (right) ventricle, and the closure of the aortic valve is easily heard. The S_2 is single with an increased intensity. Murmurs if present are usually those of associated lesions (see section on individual lesions).

CONGESTIVE HEART FAILURE. As a result of the volume and pressure overload experienced by both ventricles, the infant may show signs of congestive heart failure. This is especially true if there is a large VSD or PDA present (see section on congestive heart failure). Digoxin should be used with caution if there is subvalvular pulmonary stenosis present.

LABORATORY DATA

ARTERIAL BLOOD GASES. The pH and $PaCO_2$ are normal. The PaO_2 is typically low (20 to 40 torr), but if a large VSD or PDA is present, the PaO_2 may approach normal levels.

CHEST X-RAY EXAMINATION. A chest x-ray examination may be normal or demonstrate either decreased or increased pulmonary vascularity. The cardiac silhouette may assume the shape of an egg lying on a string. However, this finding is not diagnostic.

ELECTROCARDIOGRAM. The electrocardiogram may be normal or demonstrate right ventricular hypertrophy. Left ventricular hypertrophy and combined ventricular hypertrophy are uncommon.

ECHOCARDIOGRAM. The echocardiogram is extremely useful in establishing the diagnosis and evaluating associated lesions in infants with transposition of the great arteries.

CARDIAC CATHETERIZATION. Cardiac catheterization is diagnostic. A balloon septostomy is mandatory in all cases of transposition of the great arteries to improve interatrial mixing and should be performed regardless of the associated defects present.

Treatment
MEDICAL MANAGEMENT

Following a balloon septostomy, it is not necessary to serially follow arterial blood gases once improvement in the arterial blood gases is demonstrated.

Serial venous and arterial pH measurements should be obtained to rule out the presence of a persistent metabolic acidosis that would suggest inadequate intercardiac mixing. In addition, congestive heart failure should be continually anticipated and treated appropriately if it occurs (see section on general treatment strategies).

SURGICAL TREATMENT

The arterial switch procedure is gaining popularity and in some centers is the treatment of choice for d-transposition of the great arteries. This procedure through a median sternotomy incision involves amputation of the main pulmonary artery and the aorta above the respective valves. The pulmonary artery is anastomosed to the right ventricle, and the aorta is anastomosed to the left ventricle (the aortic valve becomes a functional pulmonary valve, and the pulmonary valve becomes a functional aortic valve). The coronary arteries are resected with a button of surrounding tissue and reanastomosed to the supravalvular area of the ascending aorta.

It is essential in performing this procedure that the left ventricular pressure is systemic. In infants with a VSD, the pressure tends to remain elevated; therefore this procedure may be postponed for several days or even months. However, once the left ventricular pressure decreases below that of the right ventricle, the morbidity and mortality increase dramatically. Therefore infants with an intact ventricular septum require surgery within the first few days of life.

If the arterial switch procedure is not performed and the infant becomes refractory to medical management and exhibits congestive heart failure, failure to thrive, pulmonary hypertension, or severe hypoxia, an alternative surgical procedure is necessary. The most common surgical procedures other than the arterial switch procedure for repair of d-transposition of the great arteries with an intact ventricular septum are the Mustard and the Senning procedures. Both of these procedures performed through a median sternotomy incision involve intraatrial redirection of blood flow. The oxygenated blood returning from the lungs through the pulmonary veins is redirected to the tricuspid valve and right ventricle, while the systemic venous return from inferior and superior venae cava is redirected to the mitral valve and left ventricle.

Complications and residual effects

Complications and residual effects of the arterial switch procedure include (1) dysrhythmias, (2) myocardial ischemia and infarction, and (3) aortic and/or pulmonary supravalvular stenosis.

Complications and residual effects of the Mustard and Senning procedures include (1) dysrhythmias, (2) superior vena cava or inferior vena cava obstruction, (3) tricuspid regurgitation, and (4) pulmonary venous obstruction. This is a severe complication warranting early detection and immediate correction. The mortality in infants is 8% and is even higher in the neonatal period.

Prognosis and follow-up

Without treatment, 30% of these infants die within the first week of life, 50% die within the first month, 70% die within the first 6 months, and 90% die within the first year. With treatment, the mortality is reduced to approximately 20%. The infant should be followed closely to evaluate evidence of increasing cyanosis, failure to thrive, and congestive heart failure. These parameters are used to determine the optimal timing for total surgical correction.

FALLOT'S TETRALOGY
Physiology

Fallot's tetralogy is the most common form of cyanotic congenital heart disease. The four components of Fallot's tetralogy are (1) ventricular septal defect, (2) overriding of the ascending aorta, (3) obstruction to the right ventricular outflow tract, and (4) right ventricular hypertrophy (Figure 18-7).

Data collection
PHYSICAL FINDINGS

Newborns who are symptomatic usually have severe right ventricular outflow tract obstruction.

CYANOSIS. The predominant intercardiac shunt is right to left; therefore most infants with Fallot's tetralogy are cyanotic. However, if the right ventricular outflow obstruction is only mild or moderate, the intercardiac shunt is left to right and the infant initially will be acyanotic.

Infants with Fallot's tetralogy occasionally have a "TET" or hypercyanotic spell. These spells commonly are seen with cyanosis, irritability, pallor, tachypnea, flaccidity, and possible loss of consciousness. TET or hypercyanotic spells may be the result of a transient increase in the obstruction of the right ventricular outflow tract (usually the muscular infundibular area) and usually respond to knee-chest positioning, oxygen, propranolol, or morphine.

HEART SOUNDS. A grade II to III/VI harsh systolic murmur at the mid to upper left sternal border is usually present but is diminished or absent during a TET or hypercyanotic spell. The S_2 is usually loud and single (representing aortic closure).

CONGESTIVE HEART FAILURE. Congestive heart failure is uncommon in Fallot's tetralogy.

LABORATORY DATA

ARTERIAL BLOOD GASES. The $PaCO_2$ and pH are normal. The PaO_2 is normal if the pulmonary stenosis is mild and there is little right-to-left shunting at the ventricular level. If the pulmonary stenosis, however, is more severe, the amount of right-to-left shunting increases and the PaO_2 falls.

CHEST X-RAY EXAMINATION. The classic chest x-ray film of Fallot's tetralogy resembles the shape of a boot with a normal-sized heart. However, the typical chest x-ray examination pattern described is not common in the newborn. Pulmonary vascularity is either normal or decreased.

ELECTROCARDIOGRAM. The electrocardiogram demonstrates right ventricular hypertrophy in infants with Fallot's tetralogy.

ECHOCARDIOGRAM. The echocardiogram is suggestive when the overriding aorta can be demonstrated. Echocardiograms help identify the pulmonary valve to rule out pulmonary atresia. Doppler interrogation helps to define the degree and level of pulmonary stenosis. Color flow mapping identifies the VSD, as well

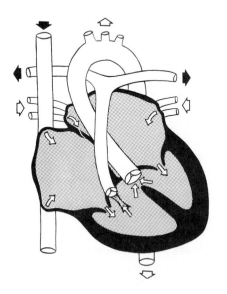

Figure 18-7. Tetralogy of fallot. (Courtesy Ross Laboratories, Columbus, Ohio.)

as the direction of blood flow across the VSD.

CARDIAC CATHETERIZATION. Cardiac catheterization is diagnostic and performed in the newborn when there is a question regarding the differential diagnosis (pulmonary atresia) or in a newborn who is having TET spells.

Treatment
MEDICAL MANAGEMENT

Digoxin is not routinely used in most cases of Fallot's tetralogy, because it may increase the amount of infundibular obstruction present. Propranolol is the preferable drug for treating hypercyanotic infants, although morphine has been used successfully (see section on general treatment strategies).

SURGICAL TREATMENT

Total repair of Fallot's tetralogy involves patch closure of the large VSD and relief of the right ventricular outflow obstruction performed through a median sternotomy incision. Often a pericardial patch across the pulmonary valve annulus is required. The use of homograft conduits for relief of right-sided obstruction has become more common. Contraindications include small size of the child, anomalous left anterior descending coronary artery, and hypoplastic pulmonary arteries.

COMPLICATIONS AND RESIDUAL EFFECTS. Complications and residual side effects include (1) conduction abnormalities (right bundle-branch block and third-degree heart block), (2) residual shunt, (3) residual pulmonary stenosis, and (4) pulmonary insufficiency. The mortality in infants is 5% to 15%.

Total surgical repair of Fallot's tetralogy is not usually recommended in the neonatal period. If surgical intervention is warranted (i.e., the infant is severely hypoxic because of inadequate pulmonary blood flow), a systemic-to-pulmonary shunt is performed. The Blalock-Taussig operation is usually preferred (see previous description of the Blalock-Taussig operation).

Complications and residual effects

Complications and residual effects include (1) diminished or absent pulses in the affected arm, (2) congestive heart failure from an overlarge shunt, and (3) inadequate shunt. The mortality in infancy is 10%.

Prognosis

Early cardiac catheterization with subsequent surgery is recommended if the child is symptomatic or refractory to medical care. Fallot's tetralogy without surgery has a grave prognosis but is improved with surgical correction. However, if surgery is required in early infancy, the results generally are not as favorable.

Parent teaching

Parents should be instructed to place the infant in a knee-chest position during a TET spell and to notify the physician immediately (see general section on parent teaching).

PULMONARY ATRESIA WITH INTACT VENTRICULAR SEPTUM
Physiology

Pulmonary atresia is characterized by complete agenesis of the pulmonary valve. This lesion produces severe signs or symptoms soon after birth and is not compatible with life unless there is an associated interatrial communication and an additional pathway of entry for blood into the pulmonary circulation (PDA). Since the flow to the lungs depends on a PDA, death may occur when this structure closes. The right ventricle is usually hypoplastic but may be normal or dilated, depending on the degree of tricuspid insufficiency present.

Data collection
PHYSICAL FINDINGS

CYANOSIS. Cyanosis is always present in varying degrees, depending on the amount of pulmonary blood flow from the PDA.

HEART SOUNDS. The S_2 is single, and a soft

systolic murmur is heard as a result of either the PDA or tricuspid insufficiency in about one half of the infants with pulmonary atresia.

CONGESTIVE HEART FAILURE. Congestive heart failure is usually present with moderate to severe tricuspid insufficiency (see section on congestive heart failure).

LABORATORY DATA

ARTERIAL BLOOD GASES. The pH and $PaCO_2$ are usually within normal range. The PaO_2, however, is usually very low (20 to 30 torr), unless there is a large shunt at the ductal or bronchial collateral level. In some cases the amount of pulmonary blood flow is insufficient, and the pH may be low, reflecting metabolic acidosis.

CHEST X-RAY EXAMINATION. The heart appears enlarged on x-ray examination if tricuspid insufficiency is present. Pulmonary vascularity is either decreased or normal, depending on the amount of shunting through the PDA.

ELECTROCARDIOGRAM. The electrocardiogram is usually normal but may demonstrate left ventricular hypertrophy. It is important to differentiate this lesion from tricuspid atresia that shows a counterclockwise loop in the frontal planes with a superior axis.

ECHOCARDIOGRAM. The two-dimensional echocardiogram with doppler and color flow mapping can identify absence of blood flow across the pulmonary valve and is diagnostic.

CARDIAC CATHETERIZATION. Cardiac catheterization is diagnostic and should be performed as soon as the diagnosis is suspected. A balloon atrial septostomy is usually performed at the time of catheterization.

Treatment
MEDICAL MANAGEMENT

Prostaglandin E_1 has been used successfully to maintain the ductus arteriosus until surgical intervention (see section on general treatment strategy).

SURGICAL TREATMENT

In most medical centers a systemic-to-pulmonary shunt such as the Blalock-Taussig operation is performed through a lateral thoracotomy incision. However, some institutions are performing a pulmonary valvulotomy or a pulmonary outflow patch procedure in addition to a shunt. This establishes an open pathway through the atretic valve area between the pulmonary artery and the right ventricle. Antegrade blood flow through the right ventricle and pulmonary artery will then promote growth of these areas. The pulmonary valvotomy and pulmonary outflow patch procedures are performed through a median sternotomy incision.

Complications and residual effects

Complications and residual effects of the Blalock-Taussig operation include (1) diminished or absent pulses in the affected arm, (2) congestive heart failure from an overlarge shunt, and (3) inadequate shunt. The mortality in infants is 25%.

Prognosis

Pulmonary atresia is fatal without surgical intervention. If a palliative shunt is used, repeated catheterization and further surgical procedures should be anticipated when the shunt becomes nonfunctional. If primary surgical correction is undertaken in the newborn period, repeated catheterization should be anticipated to evaluate residual obstruction. Despite the development of newer surgical techniques, the prognosis in these infants is guarded.

TOTAL ANOMALOUS PULMONARY VENOUS RETURN
Physiology

Total anomalous pulmonary venous return (TAPVR) is characterized by all the pulmonary veins returning directly or indirectly into the right atrium rather than the left atrium. The presence

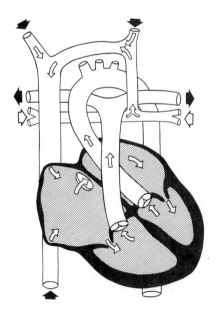

Figure 18-8. Anomalous venous return. (Courtesy Ross Laboratories, Columbus, Ohio.)

of an ASD is necessary to sustain life (Figure 18-8). The four main varieties of TAPVR are (1) supercardiac (most common), in which the drainage to the superior vena cava is through the innominate vein; (2) cardiac, in which the pulmonary veins drain into the coronary sinus or directly into the right atrium; (3) infracardiac, in which the four veins join behind the heart and flow through the diaphragm and connect to the portal venous system; and (4) mixed. Each of the various types of anomalous drainage can occur with or without obstruction along the pulmonary venous pathway. The presence or absence of obstruction profoundly affects the clinical course.

Data collection
PHYSICAL FINDINGS

CYANOSIS. Infants with obstructed or unobstructed TAPVR are typically cyanotic. Because all pulmonary venous return (oxygenated blood) ultimately enters the right atrium (as opposed to the left atrium), a right-to-left shunt at the atrial level is required to sustain life.

HEART SOUNDS. Murmurs are rarely heard in infants with TAPVR and when present are nonspecific.

CONGESTIVE HEART FAILURE. Infants with unobstructed TAPVR usually show signs of congestive heart failure resulting from volume overload of the right ventricle. Infants with obstructed TAPVR generally do not demonstrate evidence of congestive heart failure but typically demonstrate pulmonary venous congestion (see section on congestive heart failure).

LABORATORY DATA

ARTERIAL BLOOD GASES. The pH and $PaCO_2$ are usually normal. The PaO_2 may be within the normal range if there is a large amount of pulmonary blood flow (always associated with severe congestive heart failure). If the pulmonary blood flow is limited, secondary to obstruction of blood flow, the PaO_2 may be low.

CHEST X-RAY EXAMINATION. If the TAPVR is obstructed, the chest x-ray film will demonstrate pulmonary venous congestion without cardiomegaly. If the TAPVR is unobstructed, the chest x-ray film will demonstrate a marked increase in pulmonary vascularity and cardiomegaly.

ELECTROCARDIOGRAM. An electrocardiogram may demonstrate right axis deviation, right ventricular hypertrophy, and right atrial enlargement.

ECHOCARDIOGRAM. An echocardiogram is nondiagnostic. However, the diagnosis of TAPVR is strongly suggested when an extra cavity is seen behind the small left atrium. In addition, a single large pulmonary vein can sometimes be visualized draining into the superior vena cava.

CARDIAC CATHETERIZATION. All infants suspected of having TAPVR should undergo cardiac catheterization as soon as possible. A Rashkind balloon septostomy should be performed at that time to improve intraatrial mixing.

Treatment
MEDICAL MANAGEMENT

Obstructed TAPVR is a surgical emergency. Nonobstructed TAPVR may be medically treated temporarily, although early surgery is generally recommended (see section on general treatment strategy).

SURGICAL TREATMENT

Surgical correction of TAPVR depends on the variety. Supracardiac and infracardiac varieties require surgical reimplantation of the common vein into the left atrium. With color flow mapping, the right-to-left shunting across the atrial septum, as well as the anomalous venous return as it enters through the atrium, superior vena cava, or coronary sinus can be visualized. Infracardiac anomalous veins, however, cannot be visualized with this technique. Intracardiac TAPVR can usually be surgically repaired by realigning the atrial septum during closure of the ASD and directing the anomalous veins to the left atrial side. All repairs are performed through a median sternotomy incision.

Complications and residual effects

Complications and residual effects include pulmonary venous obstruction and dysrhythmias. The mortality varies from 5% to 25% in infancy, depending on the anatomic type.

Prognosis

Infants with nonobstructed TAPVR generally do well if the lesion is recognized early and early corrective surgery is performed. The prognosis for obstructed TAPVR is less favorable despite early surgical intervention.

TRICUSPID ATRESIA
Physiology

In tricuspid atresia there is complete agenesis of the tricuspid valve with no direct communication between the right atrium and right ventricle. Systemic venous blood entering the right atrium is shunted through a patent foramen ovale or ASD

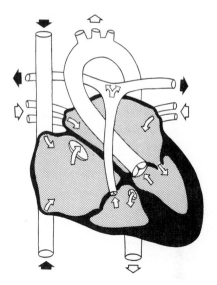

Figure 18-9. Tricuspid atresia. (Courtesy Ross Laboratories, Columbus, Ohio.)

into the left atrium. A VSD is usually present, and the right ventricle and pulmonary arteries may be hypoplastic or normal in size. If the ventricular septum is intact but a large PDA is present, the right ventricular cavity may be hypoplastic and the pulmonary arteries are usually slightly decreased or normal in size (Figure 18-9). Abut 30% of these infants will have transposition of the great arteries.

Data collection
PHYSICAL FINDINGS

CYANOSIS. The degree of cyanosis present varies. Newborns will have marked cyanosis if the pulmonary blood flow is compromised.

HEART SOUNDS. A single S_2 is present in infants with TAPVR. Murmurs of associated shunts (VSD and PDA) are typically present.

CONGESTIVE HEART FAILURE. Congestive heart failure may be present with a large shunt (PDA or VSD) (see section on congestive heart failure).

LABORATORY DATA

ARTERIAL BLOOD GASES. The pH and $PaCO_2$ are usually normal. The PaO_2 may vary from near normal if there is a large VSD or PDA to extremely low if there is limited shunting into the pulmonary system.

CHEST X-RAY EXAMINATION. A chest x-ray film is nondiagnostic and may show a normal heart size or cardiomegaly. Pulmonary vascularity may be normal, decreased, or increased, depending on the degree of pulmonary blood flow.

ELECTROCARDIOGRAM. An electrocardiogram is highly suggestive and usually demonstrates left axis deviation with a counterclockwise loop, a superior axis in the frontal plane, and left ventricular hypertrophy.

ECHOCARDIOGRAM Failure to identify the tricuspid valve echocardiographically is highly suggestive of tricuspid atresia. Color flow mapping can identify the right-to-left shunt at the atrial level and the presence of a VSD and/or PDA.

CARDIAC CATHETERIZATION. Any infant suspected of having tricuspid atresia should undergo immediate cardiac catheterization and a balloon septostomy. A balloon septostomy is performed to improve intraatrial mixing.

Treatment
MEDICAL MANAGEMENT

See section on general treatment strategy.

SURGICAL TREATMENT

When surgery is indicated, the preferred procedure in the neonatal period is a systemic-to-pulmonary shunt such as the Blalock-Taussig operation performed through a lateral thoracotomy incision.

Complications and residual effects include (1) diminished or absent pulses in the affected arm, (2) congestive heart failure from a shunt that is too large, and (3) inadequate shunt.

Definitive repair of tricuspid atresia (Fontan procedure) involves the creation of a communication between the right atrium and pulmonary artery or right ventricular outflow chamber by direct anastomosis or conduit. Closure of the ASD and any VSDs present is also performed. Definitive repair is performed through a median sternotomy incision.

Complications and residual effects

Complications and residual effects include (1) heart failure, (2) pleural effusions, (3) renal or liver failure, (4) persistent shunts, (5) conduit obstruction, and (6) dysrhythmia. The mortality in infancy is unknown, but in older children it approximates 10% to 25%.

Prognosis

The prognosis of tricuspid atresia is guarded. A new surgical technique (Fontan procedure) may improve this prognosis.

TRUNCUS ARTERIOSUS
Physiology

Truncus arteriosus is characterized by one great artery arising from the left and right ventricles,

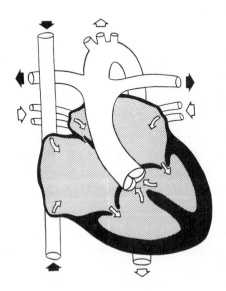

Figure 18-10. Truncus arteriosus. (Courtesy Ross Laboratories, Columbus, Ohio.)

overriding a VSD. This common artery has one valve and gives rise to the pulmonary, coronary, and systemic arteries (Figure 18-10). Truncus arteriosus is classified into three types depending on the origin of the pulmonary arteries:

Type I—A short, main pulmonary artery arises from the common trunk that bifurcates into the right and left pulmonary arteries.

Type II—The right and left pulmonary arteries arise directly from the posterior surface of the common trunk.

Type III—The right and left pulmonary arteries arise directly from the lateral walls of the common trunk.

The ductus arteriosus is absent in approximately 50% of infants with truncus arteriosus. Between 30% and 35% have a right aortic arch.

Data collection
PHYSICAL FINDINGS

In truncus arteriosus the common trunk receives a mixture of unoxygenated blood from the right ventricle and oxygenated blood from the left ventricle. Blood flow to the lungs varies with the type of truncus but is usually increased and at systemic level pressure.

CYANOSIS. Cyanosis is present at birth but varies in intensity according to the amount of pulmonary blood flow. Minimal cyanosis indicates adequate pulmonary blood flow.

HEART SOUNDS. The first heart sound, S_1, will be normal, but the S_2 will be single and loud because of the single valve of the common trunk. A loud systolic ejection click is frequently heard. A loud pansystolic murmur maximal at the lower left sternal border that radiates to the entire precordium is commonly heard. A middiastolic rumble may be present. If the truncal valve is insufficient, a blowing diastolic murmur may be heard. A wide pulse pressure may also be present.

CONGESTIVE HEART FAILURE. Congestive heart failure may be present shortly after birth or appear between 2 and 3 weeks of age. The presence of congestive heart failure depends on the amount of pulmonary blood flow. Persistent high pulmonary arteriolar resistance in the first few weeks of life will decrease pulmonary blood flow, and congestive heart failure will not be present. However, if the truncal valve is severely damaged, congestive heart failure will be present shortly after birth (see section on congestive heart failure).

LABORATORY DATA

ARTERIAL BLOOD GASES. The pH and $Paco_2$ are usually normal. If there is no obstruction to pulmonary blood flow, the Pao_2 may be near normal (usually associated with severe congestive heart failure). If the pulmonary blood flow is restricted, the Pao_2 may be extremely low.

CHEST X-RAY EXAMINATION. Cardiomegaly, displaced pulmonary arteries, and increased vascular markings are typical findings on the chest x-ray film.

ELECTROCARDIOGRAM. Combined ventricular hypertrophy is most often seen in an electrocardiogram. Left atrial enlargement is also commonly found.

ECHOCARDIOGRAM. A two-dimensional echocardiogram is helpful in establishing the diagnosis and in differentiating Fallot's tetralogy from truncus arteriosus. In addition, the echocardiogram is used to identify the number of truncal valve leaflets, the presence of truncal valve insufficiency, and the presence of pulmonary stenosis.

CARDIAC CATHETERIZATION. A cardiac catheterization is diagnostic and should be performed on any infant suspected of having truncus arteriosus.

Treatment
MEDICAL MANAGEMENT

Medical management of these infants consists of stabilizing and treating congestive heart failure when present. Calcium should be closely monitored because of the possibility of DiGeorge syndrome.

SURGICAL TREATMENT

Totally repairing truncus arteriosus is rare in the newborn period. It consists of separating the pulmonary artery from the common trunk, closing the VSD with a patch, and inserting a right ventricular-to-pulmonary artery valved conduit. The use of homograft conduits for repair of truncus arteriosus has become more common. Total repair of truncus arteriosus is performed through a median sternotomy incision.

Complications and residual effects

Complications and side effects include (1) pulmonary vascular disease, (2) residual shunts, (3) truncal valve incompetence, and (4) conduit obstruction. The mortality is 40% to 50% in infancy.

Prognosis

The natural history is dependent on the amount of pulmonary blood flow and the competency of the truncal valve. Without treatment more than half of these infants die before 3 months of age. Survival past 1 year of age ranges from 15% to 30%. Truncus arteriosus is often associated with DiGeorge syndrome, which has a guarded prognosis.

HYPOPLASTIC LEFT HEART SYNDROME
Physiology

Hypoplastic left heart syndrome represents a clinical spectrum that includes severe coarctation of the aorta, severe aortic valve stenosis or atresia, and severe mitral valve stenosis or atresia. The left ventricle and ascending aorta are usually hypoplastic. Coronary blood flow occurs in a retrograde fashion into the small ascending aorta through the PDA. The resultant poor myocardial perfusion leads to rapid decompensation.

Data collection
PHYSICAL FINDINGS

CYANOSIS. These infants are usually not truly cyanotic but rather have severe pallor and a grayish skin color as a result of marked vasoconstriction and congestive heart failure.

HEART SOUNDS. A nonspecific systolic murmur is heard in approximately two thirds of infants with hypoplastic left heart syndrome.

CONGESTIVE HEART FAILURE. Congestive heart failure is present in all cases as a result of right ventricular volume and pressure overload (see section on congestive heart failure).

LABORATORY DATA

ARTERIAL BLOOD GASES. The arterial blood gases are typically normal until the infant begins to deteriorate, at which time the baby will become acidotic.

CHEST X-RAY EXAMINATION. Cardiomegaly with increased pulmonary vascularity and pulmonary edema is seen on the x-ray film.

ELECTROCARDIOGRAM. An electrocardiogram frequently demonstrates right axis deviation and right ventricular hypertrophy. However, the electrocardiogram may be normal.

ECHOCARDIOGRAM. An echocardiogram is usually diagnostic with a small left ventricular cavity and ascending aorta with an abnormal aortic valve pattern.

CARDIAC CATHETERIZATION. Cardiac catheterization is diagnostic. In some cases only an aortic root contrast study using an umbilical artery catheter is required to demonstrate the typical small ascending aorta. If there is a question regarding the differential diagnosis, a heart catheterization is indicated as soon as possible.

Treatment
MEDICAL MANAGEMENT

Hypoplastic left heart syndrome is a lethal lesion, and currently no medical therapy is effective. Surgical intervention offers the only chance of survival (see section on general treatment strategy).

SURGICAL TREATMENT

Recent advances in surgical treatment have made it possible to treat this lesion with a two-staged approach. The mortality is high, but surgery may offer some chance for survival in selected cases. Cardiac transplantation in the newborn is still in the experimental stages.

Prognosis

The prognosis is universally grim. Without surgical intervention, all infants die within several days or weeks of birth. Even with surgical intervention, the mortality is still high.

DYSRHYTHMIAS
Physiology

The development of the cardiac conduction system continues after birth with a steady increase in the sympathetic innervation of the heart. This accounts for the observed heart rate variability and the high frequency of benign dysrhythmias in the newborn. Premature ventricular beats (Figure 18-11), brief episodes of ectopic atrial rhythms, wandering atrial pacemakers (Figure 18-12), and even brief episodes of sinus arrest are all frequently seen in the newborn period. The majority of these dysrhythmias do not require immediate treatment; however, if they persist, the presence of congenital heart disease, sepsis, drug toxicity, persistent hypoxia, adrenal insufficiency, disorders of electrolyte and acid base balance, hypoglycemia, and hypocalcemia should be considered.

All cardiac tissue is capable of generating a spontaneous depolarization. However, the SA node, AV node, and His purkinje system consist of specialized conductive tissue with rapid spontane-

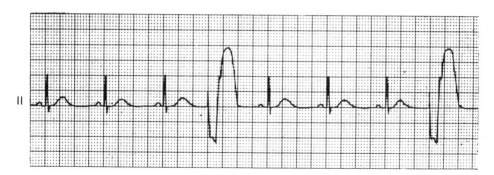

Figure 18-11. Premature ventricular beats.

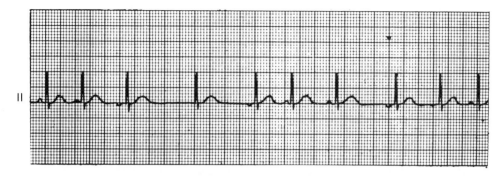

Figure 18-12. Wandering atrial pacemaker with junctional escape (fourth complex).

ous depolarization. The SA node is the normal pacemaker of the heart because it has the fastest rate of spontaneous depolarization. If, however, the spontaneous depolarization of the SA node is delayed or slower than normal, an escape rhythm (Figure 18-12) is generated by either the AV node or His purkinje system (these rhythms are called nodal escape or ventricular escape, respectively). Arrhythmias can also originate from an automatic "ectopic" pacemaker located anywhere in the heart. These ectopic pacemakers become more active in the presence of hypoxia, acidosis, digoxin toxicity, abnormal sympathetic nervous system stimulation, increased wall tension (congestive heart failure), or altered electrolyte balance. Drug therapy for dysrhythmias is based on the ability of certain medications to alter the electrophysiologic properties of cardiac tissue. One class of anti-arrhythmic drugs directly increases the automaticity of certain cardiac fibers. Examples of such drugs include quinidine, procainamide, lidocaine, and phenytoin (see Table 18-4). Other drugs directly or indirectly affect the autonomic nervous system activity. Propranolol is a beta-adrenergic blocker and works in this fashion. Digoxin exerts its chronotropic activity by altering the sympathetic and parasympathetic nervous system response within the heart.

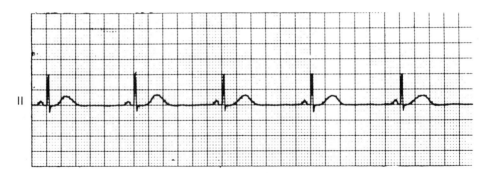

Figure 18-13. Sinus bradycardia.

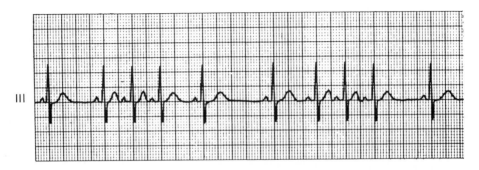

Figure 18-14. Sinus dysrhythmia.

BENIGN ARRHYTHMIAS: SINUS BRADYCARDIA, SINUS TACHYCARDIA, AND SINUS DYSRHYTHMIA

Thirty-five percent to 40% of normal premature infants have brief episodes of sinus bradycardia (Figure 18-13), sinus tachycardia, or sinus dysrhythmia (Figure 18-14) that are benign and require no treatment. Healthy premature and term infants may have heart rates that range from 90 to 200 beats/min. Sustained heart rates (greater than 15 seconds) above or below this range should be evaluated with a 12-lead electrocardiogram and rhythm strip. These are important, because artifact created by the bedside monitors often make accurate interpretations of dysrhythmias impossible.

SUPRAVENTRICULAR TACHYCARDIA

Supraventricular tachycardia (SVT) (Figure 18-15) is the most common tachydysrhythmia in the newborn period. It is the result of either dual AV nodal pathways, rapid conduction through an accessory bundle (Wolff-Parkinson-White syndrome), or the existence of an ectopic atrial pacemaker. SVT is commonly associated with Ebstein's anomaly of the tricuspid valve, L-transposition of the great vessels, cardiomyopathy, or myocarditis. These lesions are present in 10% to 25% of infants with SVT and should be excluded with the appropriate evaluation. Newborns with SVT will have a history of gradually developing congestive heart failure with findings of anxiousness, restlessness, tachypnea, and poor feeding. These symptoms develop after 12 to 24 hours of SVT. SVT often starts and ceases abruptly.

Criteria for SVT include (1) persistent ventricular rate over 200 beats/min, (2) a fixed and regular R-R interval, and (3) little change in heart rate with various activities (crying, feeding, or apnea).

TREATMENT. Various maneuvers may be used to attempt to convert the infant to normal sinus rhythm (NSR). Vagal maneuvers (unilateral carotid pressure, gagging, rectal stimulation) may be attempted but rarely work. Ocular compression should never be used. Stimulation of the diving reflex using an ice bag applied to the infant's face may be attempted. (Caution must be used in this procedure to ensure adequate ventilation for the infant.) Overdrive atrial pacing has been successful in converting SVT to NSR. However, direct-current (DC) cardioversion (1 to 2 watt seconds/kg) is the most effective mode of treatment. The defibrillator must always be in the synchronous mode. If cardioversion is successful, maintenance drug therapy should be initiated.

Traditionally, digoxin has been used to treat

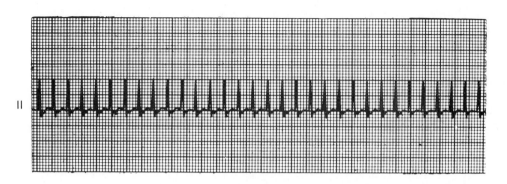

Figure 18-15. Supraventricular tachycardia.

this disorder. Recently, however, it has been suggested that digoxin not be used in Wolff-Parkinson-White syndrome and that this disorder be ruled out before digoxin is used. If not contraindicated, digoxin should be administered IV using standard doses (see box on p. 436).

Propranolol administered IV may be used if the patient is not in congestive heart failure. Beta-blocking agents may inhibit circulating catecholamines, which are needed for the maintenance of adequate cardiac output in the face of congestive heart failure.

Verapamil is a calcium channel blocker and when first introduced was thought to be the drug of choice in SVT. However, recent experience in our institution and others suggests that this drug should not be used as a first-line medication in children under 1 year of age, and should never be used in a patient in congestive heart failure.

If the SVT fails to convert using the methods outlined above, other drugs such as quinidine and procainamide may be required. After conversion to NSR, maintenance drug therapy should be continued for 12 months or longer. Relapses during the first 48 hours are common (70%) and should be anticipated.

Fetal SVT is uncommon, but when present is associated with severe congestive heart failure and hydrops fetalis. Fetal SVT requires aggressive management, including conversion with maternally administered propranolol and digoxin.

ATRIAL FLUTTER AND FIBRILLATION

The presence of atrial flutter (Figure 18-16) usually indicates severe organic heart disease (endocardial fibroelastosis, Ebstein's anomaly of the tricuspid valve, or complex heart defects). Atrial flutter is diagnosed when (1) the atrial rate is greater than 220 beats/min; (2) the P waves are very regular; and (3) there is a characteristic sawtooth pattern, indicating a flutter wave. The ventricular rate will vary depending on the degree of AV block present. Atrial fibrillation is extremely rare and almost always indicates a serious organic heart disease.

TREATMENT. The treatment of atrial flutter or fibrillation is DC cardioversion followed by maintenance therapy with digoxin.

VENTRICULAR TACHYCARDIA

Ventricular tachycardia is frequently associated with severe organic heart disease.

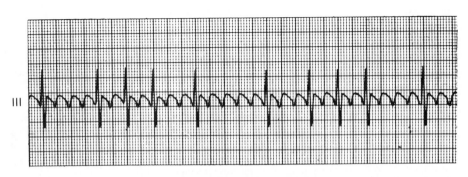

Figure 18-16. Atrial flutter.

TREATMENT. Ventricular tachycardia is best treated with immediate DC cardioversion. Lidocaine may be used as a bolus (1 to 2 mg/kg IV) or as a continuous IV infusion of 20 to 30 μg/min. Following conversion, maintenance therapy should be initiated using phenytoin, Inderal, or tocainide.

COMPLETE ATRIOVENTRICULAR BLOCK

In complete heart block, the ventricular rate is slower than the atrial rate and there is no association between the ventricular and atrial rates. Complete heart block is seen in infants with myocarditis or endocardial fibroelastosis. There is a strong association between congenital heart block and maternal systemic lupus erythematosus (SLE). Often these mothers have no signs or symptoms of lupus, but laboratory confirmation is often possible.

TREATMENT. No treatment is required unless the ventricular rate falls below 50 beats/min or the infant becomes symptomatic, in which case, a pacemaker is required.

PARENT TEACHING

The diagnosis of congenital heart disease in their child is a frightening experience for parents. Depending on the family background, educational level, and emotional state, parents may think their infant will die regardless of the severity of the heart defect. In addition, parents may have an overwhelming sense of guilt at having borne a child with a heart defect. Frequently they ask, "What did I do wrong to cause this?" Therefore comprehensive teaching, reassurance, and support are essential for the well-being of both the infant and the family. Understanding the heart defect aids in decreasing anxiety. Parents should also have a basic understanding of their child's heart defect to provide good care after discharge.

Explain the infant's heart defect to the parents. Draw or show a picture of the heart de-fect, explaining briefly and simply the normal circulation of the heart and how the circulation of their child's heart differs from normal. This explanation should be repeated often for parental understanding and retention. Careful explanation of all tubes, monitors, equipment, and procedures in the nursery also helps decrease parental anxiety.

Heart defects are not visible lesions. Most of these infants will appear quite normal and healthy. It therefore may be difficult for some parents to accept that anything is wrong with their baby. In addition, parents are under great emotional and sometimes physical stress (from labor and delivery), which decreases their ability to hear and retain explanations about the defect. Repetition of explanations is important.

Medical personnel should enhance bonding and decrease the parents' fear of holding or caring for their infant by encouraging interaction with the infant and allowing parents to participate in their infant's care. The parents' confidence in caring for their infant at home is established in the nursery. Parents must feel comfortable caring for their infant and have the opportunity to demonstrate their ability to do so before discharge from the hospital.

Teaching home care of the infant before discharge should be detailed and include medications, signs and symptoms to observe, and guidelines for care. Ideally these should be written instructions. The parents should telephone the physician if the infant demonstrates (1) poor feeding for 1 to 2 days or sweating with feeds, (2) vomiting most of feedings for a 12- to 24-hour period, (3) fast or labored breathing for several hours, (4) decreased activity level, (5) weight loss or failure to gain weight, and (6) frequent respiratory illnesses.

All medications should be explained in detail, including their purpose, action, and administration. Parents should be made aware of the potential adverse effects (side effects) of all of their infant's medications. Parents should be observed giving medications in the nursery before the infant is discharged.

Cyanotic heart disease is particularly disturbing to parents because their infant's skin color is "blue." Parents should be cautioned that their infant will appear blue, especially around the mouth, mucous membranes, hands, and feet, and the blueness will increase with activity such as crying, feeding, and bowel movements. Parents should notify the physician about any of the previously listed symptoms in addition to (1) greatly increased cyanosis, especially if associated with fast or labored breathing, (2) decreased movement in any or all of the extremities, (3) decreased responsiveness or eyes deviating to one side, and (4) seizure activity such as jerking motions or stiffness followed by the infant becoming floppy or limp.

It is important to emphasize to parents that their infant should be treated as normally as possible. There is no activity restriction for infants with heart disease because infants will "self-limit" themselves according to their capacities. It is difficult for parents with a first-born child with heart disease to differentiate "normal baby problems" from cardiac-related problems. For these parents, as well as other parents of children with cardiac defects, it is particularly important to have open communication between the family, the primary care provider, and the cardiologist. Parents should be encouraged to call these medical personnel as needed for support, answers to questions, and reassurance. Support groups of parents whose children have heart defects (such as PATCH) provide information, empathy, and practical tips to parents dealing with medical/surgical interventions for their child's heart defect.

ACKNOWLEDGMENT

We would like to thank David Clark, M.D., F.A.C.S., F.A.C.C., for his contribution to the sections on surgical management.

REFERENCES

1. Fyler D et al: Report of the New England Regional Cardiac Program, Pediatrics 65:377, 1980.
2. Rudolph A: Congenital diseases of the heart; clinical-physiologic considerations of the heart, Chicago, 1974, Year Book Medical Publishers, Inc.

SELECTED READINGS

American Heart Association: If your child has a congenital heart disease: a guide for parents (free on request), Dallas, American Heart Association.

American Heart Association Committee Report: Recommendations for human blood pressure determination by sphygmomanometer, Hypertension 3(4):509A, 1961.

Curley MAQ and Vaughn SM: Assessment and resuscitation of the pediatric patient, Crit Care Nurse 7:26, 1987.

Fink B: Congenital heart disease, Chicago, 1985, Year Book Medical Publishers, Inc.

Friedman WF and George BL: New concepts and drugs for congestive heart failure, Pediatr Clin North Am 31:1197, 1984.

Garson A et al: Parental reactions to children with congenital heart disease, Child Psychiatry Hum Dev 9:86, 1978.

Giovanelli G et al: Hypertension in children and adolescents, New York, 1981, Raven Press.

Gottesfeld IB: The family of the child with congenital heart disease, MCN 4:101, 1979.

Guepes M and Vincent W: Cardiac catheterization and angiography in severe neonatal heart disease, Springfield, Ill, 1974, Charles C Thomas, Publisher.

Guido GW: Septal defects: atrial and ventricular, unit 1, series 3, Cardiovascular disease in the young: nursing intervention, East Norwalk, Conn, 1983, Appleton-Century-Crofts.

Keith J et al: Heart disease in infants and children, New York, 1978, Macmillan Publishing Co., Inc.

Moss S et al: Heart disease in infants, children and adolescents, Baltimore, 1983, Williams & Wilkins.

Ng L: Complete d-transposition of the great arteries, unit 4, series 3, Nursing interventions, East Norwalk, Conn, 1983, Appleton-Century-Crofts.

Park MK and Guntheroth WG: How to read pediatric ECGs, Chicago, 1987, Year Book Medical Publishers, Inc.

Robert RJ: Drug therapy in infants, Philadelphia, 1984, WB Saunders Co.

Rowe MR et al: The neonate with congenital heart disease, Philadelphia, 1981, WB Saunders Co.

Sauer SN: Atrioventricular canal, unit 2, series 3, Cardiovascular disease in the young, nursing intervention, East Norwalk, Conn, 1983, Appleton-Century-Crofts.

Textbook of pediatric advanced life support, Seattle, Children's Hospital Medical Center, 1987.

Tiefenbrunn LJ and Riemenschneider TA: Persistent pulmonary hypertension of the newborn, Am Heart J 3:564, 1986.

Uzark K: Obstructive lesions: pulmonic stenosis, aortic stenosis, coarctation of the aorta, unit 5, series 3, Cardiovascular disease in the young: nursing intervention, East Norwalk, Conn, 1983, Appleton-Century-Crofts.

Viger KH and Collins SA: Tetralogy of Fallot and truncus arteriosus, unit 3, series 3, Cardiovascular disease in the young: nursing intervention, East Norwalk, Conn, 1983, Appleton-Century-Crofts.

Wolterman M and Miller M: Caring for parents in crisis, Nursing Forum 22:34, 1985.

CHAPTER 19

Neonatal nephrology

RONALD PORTMAN · SARA BROWDER · SUSAN M. DISTEFANO

In utero the placenta is the organ responsible for toxin removal and fluid and electrolyte homeostasis. The fetal kidney, however, plays an essential role in the development of the fetus by the generation of amniotic fluid. Postnatally the kidney assumes its role as the regulator of fluid and electrolyte homeostasis through rapid changes in renal function that are clinically difficult to assess. This task is even more difficult in the premature infant whose kidney must perform a role for which it is not ready. Nephrogenesis continues to progress until 36 weeks postconceptional age whether the infant is in utero or ex utero. The genitourinary system has the highest percentage of anomalies, congenital or genetic, of all of the organ systems (10%), and these anomalies frequently present during the neonatal period. The variability in renal function and maturation combined with the high frequency of anomalies makes a prediction of the neonatal kidney's response to an insult very complicated. Our knowledge of these changes is very limited but growing.

In this chapter the anatomic and physiologic development of the kidney and its clinical assessment are presented. Prenatal and postnatal indicators of renal disease are presented, followed by a discussion of the most common and important clinical conditions involving the genitourinary system in the neonatal period.

GENERAL PHYSIOLOGY
Normal development of the kidney[31,46]

The two primitive kidneys, the pronephros and the mesonephros, regress in the human but induce the definitive kidney, the metanephros (Fig-ure 19-1). The pronephros, a solid mass of cells along the nephrogenic cord, is located at the cervical level at approximately 3 weeks gestation. Degeneration of the pronephros begins soon after its formation, and no excretory function occurs. Infection or other insults at this stage in development may result in agenesis or abnormal development of the kidney. The ureter of the pronephros forms the Wolffian, or mesonephric, duct, which induces the formation of the second kidney, the mesonephros. It is speculated that retention of abnormal pronephric tissue may be one cause of mediastinal cysts.

The mesonephros originates at approximately 31 days gestation, evolves from the nephrogenic cord, and forms 40 pairs of thin-walled tubules and glomeruli with excretory function. At the end of the fourth month, these degenerate as the metanephric kidney develops. Portions of the mesonephric duct system retained in males have been shown to form the ducts of the epididymis, the ductus deferens, and the ejaculatory duct. In the female, near-complete degeneration occurs.

The metanephros appears at 31 to 34 days gestation. The ureteric bud or duct grows from the posteromedial wall of the mesonephric duct near its junction with the cloaca. This migrates to the most caudal end of the nephrogenic cord and finally to the lumbar region and rotates medially along the longitudinal axis. Cephalic migration of the kidney to its normal position is due to straightening of the fetus from the curled position. Abnormalities in the ascent or rotation can lead to pelvic kidneys, horseshoe kidneys, or crossed fused ectopia.

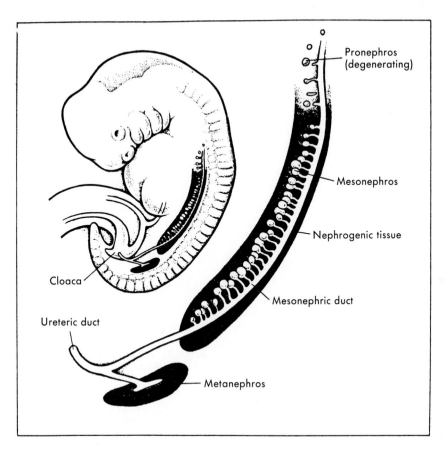

Figure 19-1. Schematic representation of overlapping stages in embryogenesis of human kidney. See text for detailed description. (From Holliday MA: Hosp Pract 13:101, 1978.)

The ureteric bud grows into the metanephric blastema (metanephros), then repeatedly branches dichotomously, determining the number and location of the renal pelvis, calyces, and collecting ducts. The cells of the metanephric blastema clump around the ureteric bud and stimulate the formation of the glomerulus, proximal tubule, loop of Henle, and distal tubule, which then empty into the collecting duct.

Nephrogenesis begins in the renal cortex closest to the medulla (juxtamedullary nephrons). The process continues in a centrifugal pattern with the outermost (superficial cortical) nephrons forming last. The process of forming the lifelong complement of 1 million nephrons in each kidney is complete by 34 to 36 weeks postconceptional age. The kidneys will continue their development at approximately the same rate whether in utero or ex utero. For example, a 28-week gestation premature infant will not complete nephrogenesis for 6 to 8 more weeks (Figure 19-2). How insults such as hypoxia, asphyxia, and various toxins affect this development is not yet clear. The newborn kidney may be relatively protected from these

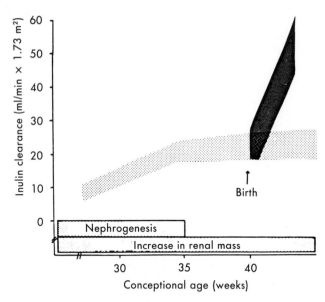

Figure 19-2. Correlation of glomerular filtration rate (GFR) as measured by inulin clearance and postconceptional age. Note marked increase in GFR postnatally. This increase does not occur after 40 weeks unless birth occurs. If birth occurs before nephrogenesis is complete, this increase does not occur until 34 to 36 weeks postconceptional age. (From Guignard JP: Neonatal nephrology. In Holliday MA, Barratt TM, and Vernier RL, editors: Pediatric nephrology, ed 2, © 1987, the Williams & Wilkins Co., Baltimore.)

insults, since the superficial cortical nephrons are not fully developed and the juxtamedullary nephrons are more resistant to hypoxic damage.

GLOMERULAR FILTRATION RATE*

In utero the placenta serves as the major organ for maintenance of body fluid and electrolyte composition and clearance of metabolic wastes. It is not surprising that the percent of cardiac output to the kidneys is low (2.2% to 3.7%) compared with the 25% observed in the adult. Renal blood flow is similarly depressed and distributed mainly to the more mature juxtamedullary nephrons. A high renal vascular resistance is a primary determinant of this reduced flow. The glomerular filtration rate (GFR) is also quite low and increases proportionally with changes in body mass and gestational age. Postnatally there is a dramatic in-

crease in GFR as the kidney assumes its functional role. The GFR doubles in the first 2 weeks of life to 30 to 40 ml/min/1.73 m² (Figures 19-2 and 19-3) and then further increases to the adult normal of 100 to 120 ml/min/1.73 m² by between 1 and 2 years of life. During this period the GFR is increasing at a rate greater than the growth in body mass. Factors responsible for the rise in GFR include an expansion in filtration surface area caused by a greater perfusion of the superficial cortical nephrons and a decrease in renal vascular resistance. Premature infants of less than 34 weeks postconceptional age have a rather stable and low GFR until nephrogenesis is completed. At this point, a threefold to fivefold rise in GFR can be observed (see Figure 19-2). Factors contributing to this phenomenon are not yet determined.

The clinical assessment of GFR is very difficult in a newborn for several reasons. While

*References 5, 6, 19, 29, 53, 54, 56.

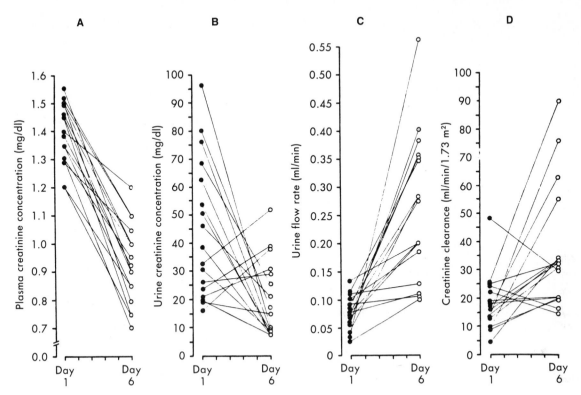

Figure 19-3. **A,** Change in plasma creatinine concentrations on day 1 (*solid circle*) and day 6 (*open circle*) of life. Solid line connects values of individual infant. **B,** Urinary creatinine concentrations. **C,** Urinary flow rate. **D,** GFR as measured by creatinine clearance. Note that increase in GFR is accompanied by decrease in creatinine concentrations as infant excretes maternal creatinine and by increase in urine flow rate. (From Sertel H and Scopes J: Arch Dis Child 48:717, 1973.)

inulin clearances in the infant are accurate, they are not a practical clinical tool. The usual endogenous marker of GFR is the serum creatinine level. At birth, the serum creatinine reflects maternal values as creatinine freely crosses the placenta. As the GFR increases, the creatinine level decreases by 50% to a level of approximately 0.4 mg/dl in the term infant over the first week of life (Figure 19-3). The rate of this decrease can be quite variable depending on the infant's hydration and clinical status. This lack of steady state makes accurate creatinine clearance measurement troublesome. Also, the laboratory measurement of creatinine has a very low sensitivity for any changes in

GFR. For example, in an infant with a normal creatinine of 0.4 mg/dl, the laboratory value may fluctuate from 0.3 to 0.5 mg/dl on the same sample. A true increase in creatinine from 0.4 to 0.5 mg/dl could reflect a decrease in GFR of as much as 25%. However, a rising serum creatinine is never normal.

In an effort to enhance the sensitivity of the serum creatinine, Schwartz et al[53] developed a formula correlating creatinine clearance to body length and plasma creatinine values:

$$\text{GFR (ml/min/1.73 m}^2\text{)} =$$

$$\text{Length (cm)} \times \frac{(0.45)}{\text{Plasma creatinine (mg/dl)}}$$

This method gives the best available estimate of GFR for the term infant until 1 year of age.

The determination of GFR in the preterm infant is much more complicated. The GFR generally does not increase until nephrogenesis is complete. Until this time the infant's creatinine reflects maternal creatinine or creatinine in transfused blood. The only reasonable assessment of renal function in the premature infant is a relative change in creatinine on serial determinations. Values in excess of maternal creatinine or greater than 1.5 mg/dl may be considered abnormal.

If measurement of creatinine clearance is desired, it is best performed by serial timed voids. When the infant voids, Credé's maneuver is performed on the bladder, a timer is set, and a urine bag is applied. At the next void the timer is stopped, Credé's maneuver is performed, and the volume is noted. This can be done two or three times, and an average value used for the clearance result. The clearance formula is:

$$\text{Clearance (ml/min/1.73 m}^2) = \frac{UV}{P} \times \frac{1.73}{BSA}$$

where U is the urine creatinine concentration (milligrams per deciliter), P is the plasma concentration, V is the volume of urine divided by the time of collection in minutes, and BSA is the body surface area in square meters.

URINE FLOW RATE[5,6,19,54,56]

Urine flow in utero is important for its contribution to amniotic fluid and for the development of the urinary tract. Sufficient amniotic fluid volume is critical for fetal development, since compression of the fetus by the uterus can lead to the fetal akinesia syndrome.

The fetal kidney excretes a hypotonic urine (10 ml/kg/hr) with a large sodium content. After birth, the urine flow rate increases in the first week of life (see Figure 19-3). Quite often, infants will void unnoticed in the delivery room. Fifty percent of infants void in the first 12 hours, 92% in the first 24 hours, and 99% in the first 48 hours of life. Causes for failure to void by this time must be carefully evaluated, including abnormalities in volume status or renal function, or anatomic abnormalities such as obstruction. A diuresis occurs in the first 5 days of life as the expanded extracellular fluid volume of the neonate is excreted. A 10% loss of body weight can be normally seen in those first few days of life. Stimuli for this diuresis are unknown but may be related to the rise in renal blood flow and GFR, and possibly to atrial natriuretic factor release.

Oliguria is generally defined as urine output of less than 1 ml/kg/hr. This definition should not be used for the first 48 hours of life, however, since the infant who typically has a poor oral intake may be conserving fluid appropriately. One must not necessarily equate oliguria with an abnormality in renal function. Further assessment of function must be undertaken as previously discussed.

Urine flow is dependent on fluid intake and solute load, as noted in Chapter 10. The neonatal kidney can dilute urine to the same degree as an adult kidney (i.e., 50 mOsm/L); however, the neonate can have difficulty excreting a water load, since it cannot raise the GFR quickly enough to excrete it. This ability to dilute appears to be well developed, since the neonate receives its nutrition in a calorically diluted solution (breast milk) and thus needs to be able to excrete water freely. The term neonatal kidney cannot concentrate well (maximum concentration 700 mOsm/L) because of a low medullary nitrogen content, low peritubular capillary oncotic pressure, inhibition of antidiuretic hormone by prostaglandins, and a short loop of Henle. The kidneys of most infants can fully concentrate by 1 year of age.

SODIUM[5,19,29,55,57]

The fractional excretion of sodium (FENa) is high (15%) in utero and in premature infants but decreases with increasing gestational age

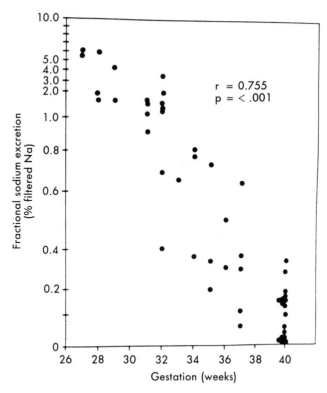

Figure 19-4. Decrease in fractional excretion of sodium occurs with increasing postconceptional age. (From Siegel S and Oh W: Acta Paediatr Scand 65:481, 1976.)

(Figure 19-4). FENa is defined as the clearance of sodium factored by the GFR:

$$\frac{\dfrac{U_{Na}V}{P_{Na}}}{\dfrac{U_{cre}V}{P_{cre}}} \quad \begin{array}{c}\text{On the same}\\ \text{sample,}\\ \longrightarrow\\ \text{volume}\\ \text{cancels}\end{array} \quad \frac{\dfrac{U_{Na}}{P_{Na}}}{\dfrac{U_{cre}}{P_{cre}}} \times 100 = FENa\ (\%)$$

The FENa is 5% to 6% in a 28-week-gestation premature infant, 3% to 5% in a 33-week-gestation infant, and 1% to 3% in a term infant. The extracellular fluid volume is expanded in the newborn, and the aforementioned diuresis is accompanied by a natriuresis. The neonatal kidneys' ability to handle rapid challenges in sodium balance is relatively fixed. The imma-

ture proximal tubule cannot reabsorb adequate amounts of sodium, and thus the distal nephron must compensate with an increase in sodium reabsorption. This is mediated by the increase in the renin, angiotensin, and aldosterone (RAA) levels seen in the newborn.[57] However, this mechanism cannot completely compensate for the increased distal sodium delivery; thus the "salt wasting" of the newborn is observed. Conversely, because of the very high RAA levels, the neonatal kidney cannot increase the FENa rapidly and thus cannot handle a large sodium load. Such a load would lead to edema and volume overload. Prostaglandin levels are also quite high and may also account for the increase in RAA levels. The combination of an increase in prostaglandin production and in the RAA system but with normotension is very similar to the clinical picture seen in patients with Bartter's syndrome. With tubular maturity and increased proximal sodium reabsorption, the RAA and prostaglandin levels gradually fall. Abnormalities in sodium concentration are discussed in Chapter 10. Sodium losses are also increased in the stressed, hypoxic infant as the major oxygen consumption of the kidney is used for sodium reabsorption.

PROXIMAL TUBULAR FUNCTION[6,19,56,61]

The proximal tubule appears to be less well developed anatomically than the glomerulus at birth. Additionally, the neonatal increase in urinary glucose and amino acid excretion have led to the consideration of a possible imbalance of function between the glomeruli and tubules. In fact, there is a balance in each individual nephron for glomerular and tubular function. The tremendous heterogenicity in nephron development can lead to an enhanced delivery of these substrates to certain nephrons. The transport systems are overwhelmed by this filtered load, and thus glucose and amino acids are spilled into the urine. This is termed an increase in "splay." The neonatal expansion of extracellular fluid volume may also lead to a decrease in proximal tubular absorption of these compounds.

Low molecular weight proteins such as beta-2-microglobulin (B_2M) are also absorbed exclusively in the proximal tubule. B_2M is the small subunit of the HLA class I antigen. As cells die, B_2M is released into the circulation and is excreted solely by the kidney. After being freely filtered by the glomerulus, B_2M is 99.9% reabsorbed by the proximal tubule and metabolized to amino acids. Any increase in urinary B_2M levels is suggestive of proximal tubular dysfunction. Whether or not an increased excretion in more premature infants is a marker of tubular immaturity is a matter of some debate. B_2M is, however, a very sensitive marker of damage to the proximal tubule by hypoxia or toxins and has been used clinically for this purpose.[61]

POTASSIUM[5,56]

Potassium levels in the newborn are quite frequently higher than later in childhood (e.g., 5.5 to 6.0 mEq/L). This level is rarely of pathologic significance. The cause of this increase is unknown, but it may be due to a diminished tubular sensitivity to aldosterone.

ACID BASE BALANCE[6,13,19,29,56]

Serum bicarbonate levels are lower in the newborn (19 to 21 mEq/L) as a result of a reduced tubular maximum for bicarbonate reabsorption in the proximal tubule. Another contributing factor is the neonate's expanded extracellular fluid volume that leads to a reduction in sodium and bicarbonate reabsorption in the proximal tubule. Carbonic anhydrase activity is normal in the newborn. The tubular maximum gradually increases to near-adult levels by the first year of life (21 to 24 mEq/L). The ability of the newborn to excrete a hydrogen ion is fairly well preserved, although there may be less net hydrogen excretion in the distal tubule. Urine pH in the newborn is frequently greater than 6, but the appropriateness of urinary pH can only be gauged by comparison with systemic acid base studies. Renal failure, shock, and many inborn errors of metabolism may lead to an increased anion gap metabolic acidosis. Renal tubular acidosis (RTA) may account for a metabolic acidosis with a normal anion gap. RTA can be seen transiently as the neonatal tubule recovers from acute renal failure or renal vein thrombosis.[13] Diarrhea is another common cause of a normal anion gap metabolic acidosis. This can be differentiated from RTA by the use of a urinary anion gap. An increased urinary anion gap signifies RTA; a normal gap signifies gastrointestinal bicarbonate loss.[8]

URIC ACID[29,58]

Serum uric acid levels are elevated in the newborn because of an increase in production. Infants who are stressed have particularly high levels from nucleotide breakdown. There is also a fivefold to sevenfold increase in uric acid

excretion in the newborn over excretion later in life. The fractional excretion of uric acid is 30% at 30 weeks gestation and 18% at 40 weeks gestation as opposed to 5% noted in the adult. Infarcts in the kidney have been noted distal to an obstruction from uric acid. The newborn is relatively protected from this excessive uric acid excretion by the normal alkalinity of the urine improving the solubility of uric acid. Uric acid crystals can appear reddish in the diaper and have been mistaken for blood.

GENERAL ETIOLOGY AND PREVENTION

Although renal anomalies are unpreventable developmental abnormalities, early detection and intervention may prevent further renal damage. Renal involvement is not an uncommon side effect of drugs used in all age groups.[20,27,32,34] When treating the neonate, three categories of drugs deserve attention: diuretics, aminoglycosides, and indomethacin. The neonatal kidney's immature GFR must be considered when one is administering key drugs. Complicating the issue of dosage is the rapid maturation of the neonate's GFR.

Furosemide may have significant side effects when used in the neonate. It is filtered by the glomerulus but primarily secreted in the proximal tubule. An increased dose is required in the newborn because of the low GFR. The loss of potassium through the kidney is well documented and must be treated with potassium supplementation. With furosemide the increased excretion of calcium in urine is associated with renal calcifications, including renal stones and interstitial calcifications, in neonates receiving more than a week of furosemide therapy.[32] This type of calcification is reversed by the addition of a thiazide diuretic that promotes the reabsorption of calcium.

Furosemide is freely used in infants with respiratory distress syndrome and bronchopulmonary dysplasia (BPD). Because of the aforementioned complications and a controlled trial showing benefit in BPD,[34] thiazides should be used as the first drug of choice. If needed, furosemide may then be added to the regimen. Thiazides should always be used with chronic furosemide administration to prevent hypercalciuria. The possibility also exists that the incidence of patent ductus arteriosus (PDA) is increased with the use of furosemide from an increased prostaglandin synthesis.[27]

Aminoglycosides are also excreted by glomerular filtration. Drug levels need to be assessed frequently because of the uncertainty of the rate of renal excretion. The neonatal kidney may be at less risk for nephrotoxicity from aminoglycosides than is the mature kidney, since some protection may be conferred by renal immaturity.

The use of indomethacin in the neonate is not risk-free for the renal system. Renal failure can be induced or exacerbated through the use of indomethacin for the closure of PDA. Studies have shown that prostaglandin synthesis inhibitors may decrease renal blood flow. Also, water excretion may be affected by the removal of the inhibition of prostaglandins on vasopressin effect. Normal renal function often returns a few days after discontinuation of the drug. If renal compromise is already present, surgical management for the PDA should be considered.

GENERAL DATA COLLECTION
History

Fetal swallowing, breathing, and urination are thought to regulate amniotic fluid volume beginning in the second trimester. Abnormalities in these regulatory mechanisms result in alteration of amniotic fluid volume. The quantity of amniotic fluid is the only reliable indication of renal function in the fetus. A clinical change in volume and its subsequent correlation to impaired renal function may be assessed in utero in selected abnormalities.[11,41]

Normally, amniotic fluid volume increases during gestation, peaking at 34 weeks gesta-

TABLE 19-1

Perinatal Indicators of Abnormalities of the Genitourinary Tract

FINDING	SUSPECTED ABNORMALITY
Oligohydramnios	Bilateral renal agenesis, PKD, or dysplasia
	Amnion nodosum
Polyhydramnios	Nephrogenic diabetes insipidus, trisomy 18 or 21, anencephaly, esophageal or duodenal obstruction, Klippel-Feil syndrome
Enlarged placenta (≥25% of infant birth weight)	Congenital nephrotic syndrome
Velamentous insertion of umbilical cord	Increased congenital anomalies
Asphyxia neonatorum	Renal failure
Physical examination	
Hypertension	See text
Skin	
Hemangioma	Hemangioma of kidney or bladder
Edema	Congenital nephrotic syndrome, hydrops fetalis
Eyes	
Phacoma (tubular sclerosis)	Angiomyolipoma of kidney
Retinitis pigmentosa	Medullary cystic disease of kidney
Cataracts	Cystic diseases, Lowe's syndrome, Wilms' tumor
Aniridia	Wilms' tumor
Ears	
Low set or malformed	Increased risk of renal abnormalities, Potter's syndrome
Preauricular pits	Branchio-oto-renal (BOR) syndrome
Skeleton	
Hemihypertrophy	Wilms' tumor
Spina bifida	Neurogenic bladder
Arthrogryposis	Oligohydramnios
Dysplastic nails	Nail-patella syndrome
Abdomen	
Absence of abdominal musculature	Prune belly syndrome
Single umbilical artery	Increased congenital anomalies
Umbilical discharge	Patent urachus
Abdominal mass	See Table 19-6
Pulmonary	
Spontaneous pneumothorax	Increase in renal abnormalities
Pulmonary hypoplasia	Oligohydramnios
Genitourinary—male	
Undescended testes	Prune belly, Noonan's syndrome, Lawrence-Moon-Biedel syndrome
Congenital absence of vas deferens	Renal agenesis or ectopia
Hypospadias	Increase in renal abnormalities
Abnormal urinary stream	Bladder dysfunction or urethral outlet obstruction

Modified from Retek AB: Hosp Pract 11:133, 1976.

TABLE 19-1—cont'd

Perinatal Indicators of Abnormalities of the Genitourinary Tract

FINDING	SUSPECTED ABNORMALITY
Genitourinary—female	
Enlarged clitoris	Adrenogenital syndrome
Cystic mass in urethral region	Ectopic ureterocele, paraurethral cyst
	Sarcoma botryoides
Bulging in vagina	Hydrometrocolpos
Abnormal urinary stream or dribbling	Bladder dysfunction, urethral obstruction
Rectal	
Deficient anal sphincter tone	Neurogenic bladder dysfunction
Dilated prostatic urethra	Posterior urethral valves, prune belly syndrome
Masses	Tumor
Urinalysis	See text

tion. Normal amniotic fluid levels imply adequate renal function and pulmonary development in the fetus. Conversely, pulmonary development is compromised in fetuses with poor renal function because of a compressed diaphragm from urinary tract obstruction and ascites in addition to the uterine "compression" of the fetus seen with oligohydramnios.

Decreased volume, or oligohydramnios, is caused by fetal genitourinary abnormalities such as noted in Table 19-1.[48] The ultrasonographic diagnosis of oligohydramnios involves measuring the largest pocket of fluid in two perpendicular planes. While these criteria are variable in defining oligohydramnios, any assessment of decreased amniotic fluid should be carefully investigated. Fluid pocket measurements of less than 1 cm are associated with perinatal morbidity.[41]

Polyhydramnios, or excessive amniotic fluid, occurs in varying degrees with moderate (2000 ml) to extreme (15,000 ml) increases in fluid volume. A correlation between perinatal outcome and the degree of hydramnios present has been reported. Esophageal abnormalities that inhibit fetal swallowing are implicated as a major etiologic factor in polyhydramnios.

Obviously critical in this prenatal assessment is a family history of renal diseases or syndromes involving the kidneys and a history of prenatal maternal infections, as well as drug, toxin, or medication intake.

Signs and symptoms

Physical findings that are indicators of genitourinary tract abnormalities are outlined in Table 19-1. The table points out the importance of a careful physical examination as a first step in a nephrologic evaluation.[29]

Laboratory data

Ultrasound visualization and amniocentesis are technologies used to assess fetal and amniotic fluid status. Noninvasive in nature, ultrasound creates an image by bouncing sound waves off of a selected target tissue and projecting the image on a screen. This technology plays a vital role in fetal evaluation, allowing an experienced operator to accurately assess fetal age, position, growth, functional and structural abnormalities, and response to the environment. It is also used as a guide for invasive procedures such as amniocentesis.

Amniocentesis, performed during the second

trimester, involves the aspiration of amniotic fluid with a needle transabdominally under ultrasound guidance for safety of the fetus and for increasing the likelihood of a successful tap. Amniocentesis reveals information on fetal lung maturity, presence of fetal chromosomal abnormalities, Rh isoimmunization, as well as prenatal diagnosis of many inherited disorders. The determination of alpha-fetoprotein (AFP), the major serum protein present in early gestation, yields important data from amniocentesis. Produced initially by the yolk sac, levels of AFP peak between 14 and 18 weeks gestation. High concentrations of AFP are associated with open neural tube defects and other conditions such as congenital nephrosis, hydrocele, esophageal atresia, and Meckel's syndrome. Cystinosis can be diagnosed by measuring the cystine content of cells obtained by amniocentesis.

Fetal urinary electrolytes as determined by amniocentesis have recently been studied as biochemical indicators of fetal renal function, but many researchers argue against any relationship between urinary electrolytes and renal function. We would not recommend their use until more convincing data are available.

URINALYSIS[35,56]

A frequently overlooked but very important indicator of renal disease is urinalysis. The perineum should be cleansed with a soapy antibacterial solution and rinsed with water. Sterile gauze or cotton balls are used to dry the perineum after cleansing. A benzoin solution is then applied liberally to the skin to ensure adhesiveness of the sterile urine bag to the perineum. The bag is then applied to the perineum without touching the inner aspect of the urine bag. Urine bags should not be left on the skin for longer than 24 hours, since the adhesive can interrupt the skin integrity, especially in the premature infant. Patients requiring ongoing strict monitoring of urine output should have a fresh urine bag applied to the perineum daily. Allow several minutes for the skin to "breathe"

before placing the new bag. An adhesive-dissolving solution should be applied to the skin before removal of the urine bag to help preserve skin integrity. Conventional pediatric urine bags may be adapted for accurate urine measurement in the extremely premature infant (Figure 19-5).

The specific gravity of the urine in the newborn reflects the ability to concentrate and dilute the urine. As the ability to dilute is fully developed, a specific gravity can be as low as 1.001 to 1.005. Concentration is limited in the term infant, and the maximum specific gravity is usually 1.015 to 1.020. Other components of the urine such as glucose, protein, and dyes can alter the specific gravity. Urine osmolality measurements should be obtained and correlated to serum osmolality if issues of concentration are being considered.

Glucose is found in trace quantities in a term infant's urine but is more frequently noted in the urine of the premature infant. Even minor elevations of plasma glucose concentrations may cause significant glucosuria. This may be quite troublesome during parenteral hyperalimentation, since the large glucose loads may lead to an osmotic diuresis.

Urinary pH is relatively alkalotic at 6. Most neonates can acidify the urine to a pH of 5 if challenged.

Hematuria is not normal in a neonate.[56] The definition of hematuria in older individuals is five or more red blood cells per high-power field. A positive dipstick for heme can be seen with hemoglobinuria noted during hemolytic states and with myoglobinuria noted during severe asphyxia. Inducing a rapid urine flow and alkalinizing the urine to a pH of 7 or higher is important to prevent conversion to ferrihemate, the nephrotoxic breakdown product of these globin molecules. Hematuria may be observed secondary to the trauma of delivery, especially with an enlarged kidney, as in cystic disease or obstruction. Hematuria is most commonly seen in perinatal asphyxia. Other com-

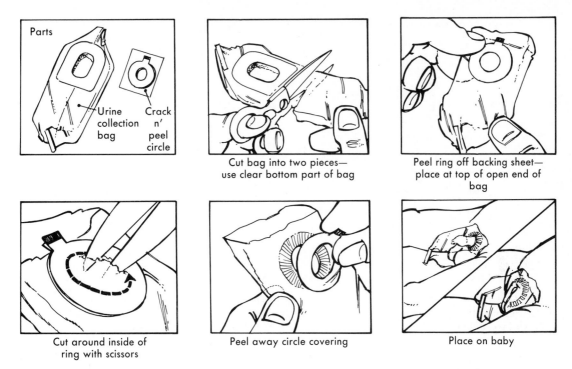

Parts

Urine collection bag   Crack n' peel circle

Cut bag into two pieces— use clear bottom part of bag

Peel ring off backing sheet— place at top of open end of bag

Cut around inside of ring with scissors

Peel away circle covering

Place on baby

Figure 19-5. Urine collection device for premature infant adapted from standard pediatric urine bag and adhesive ring from any transcutaneous oxygen monitoring kit. (Courtesy Ivy Wilson, R.N., B.S.N., of University Children's Hospital at Hermann and Bob Boeye of the University of Texas Health Science Center, Houston.)

mon conditions associated with hematuria include renal vein thrombosis, urinary tract infections, sepsis, embolization to the renal artery (especially from umbilical artery catheters), renal necrosis, hypercalciuria, coagulopathies, and, rarely, congenital glomerulonephritis or nephrosis. Hematuria may also be observed from blood outside of the genitourinary tract that is mixed with urine. This includes blood from a circumcision, perineal irritation, and uterine bleeding due to withdrawal from the effects of maternal hormones. If the hematuria is persistent, it should be evaluated with a urine culture, assessment of proteinuria and urine calcium excretion, measurement of GFR, and an anatomic evaluation of the kidneys such as renal ultrasound.

Pyuria is not infrequently noted in the newborn, especially in females. As many as 25 to 50 white blood cells per high-power field can be observed in the first days of life. Pyuria may be a marker of infection, and a urine culture should be obtained where clinically indicated. However, pyuria may also be seen with stress, fever, sepsis, and other injury to the kidney.

Proteinuria ($\geq$1 plus) is frequently seen in the newborn and is related to gestational age.[35] Protein excretion ranges from 2.3 mg/m^2/hr at 30 weeks gestation to 1.29 mg/m^2/hr at term. Proteinuria is highest in the first day of life but

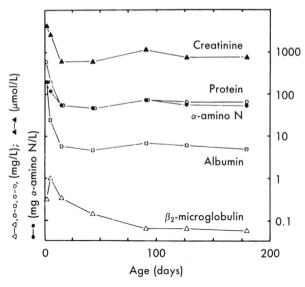

Figure 19-6. Mean urinary concentrations of creatinine (μmol/L), protein (mg/L), alpha-amino nitrogen (mg/L), albumin (mg/L), and B_2M (mg/L) in 41 infants on days 1, 5, 15, 43, 90, 130, and 180 of life. (From Karlsson FA, Hardell LI, and Hellsing K: Acta Paediatr Scand 68:663, 1979.)

then rapidly decreases, as seen in Figure 19-6. Note that B_2M has its peak excretion at 3 to 5 days of life before decreasing. Proteinuria is seen in many renal parenchemal diseases and should be evaluated if it persists. Twenty-four-hour urine collections for protein are difficult to perform in the newborn. Generally, one would see less than 200 mg/m^2 of protein excretion in the neonate but would consider more than 400 mg/m^2/day to be clearly abnormal. Spot urine protein/creatinine ratios should be very effective in assessing proteinuria when normals have been established.

ACUTE RENAL FAILURE*
Pathophysiology

Acute renal failure (ARF) is defined as sudden deterioration of the kidneys' baseline function, resulting in an inability to maintain the body's

*References 12, 21, 26, 29, 42, 59.

fluid and electrolyte homeostasis. This determination is particularly difficult in the newborn.

Etiology

Renal function is adversely affected by multiple insults. Perinatal asphyxia of mild to moderate severity, hypoxemia, hypotension, hypovolemia, acidosis, various medications, and positive-pressure ventilation can cause abnormalities in GFR, urine flow rate, sodium and water excretion, and tubular protein handling (e.g., increased B_2M excretion). These changes may be seen without actual failure of renal function.

Acute renal failure has been reported to occur in up to 8% of neonates admitted to a neonatal intensive care unit (NICU). This is probably an underestimate because of the difficulty in making the diagnosis, especially in nonoliguric cases. A scoring system for diagnosing the severity of perinatal asphyxia suggests that up to 38% of patients with severe asphyxia may have acute renal fail-

TABLE 19-2

Etiology of Acute Renal Failure in the Neonate

	URINARY INDEXES IN OLIGURIC RENAL FAILURE				
	U_{Na} *(mEq/L)*	*FENa (%)*	*RFI*	*U/P cre*	*U/P Osm*
Pretubular	31.4 ± 19.5	0.95 ± 0.55	1.29 ± 0.82	29.2 ± 15.6	> 1.3
Hypotension-sepsis, shock					
Hypovolemia-dehydration, hemorrhage, hypoproteinemia					
Cardiac failure					
Renal artery thrombosis					
Hypoxemia, asphyxia					
Glomerulonephritis					
Mechanical ventilation					
Pressor agents					
Renal parenchymal (tubular)	63.4 ± 34.7	4.25 ± 2.2	11.6 ± 9.6	9.7 ± 3.6	> 1.0
Acute tubular necrosis					
Corticomedullary necrosis					
Asphyxia neonatorum					
Pyelonephritis/interstitial nephritis					
Polycystic kidney disease					
Renal dysplasia/aplasia/hypoplasia					
Intrauterine infection					
Toxins					
Endogenous					
Uric acid					
Hemoglobinuria					
Myeglobinuria					
Exogenous					
Aminoglycosides					
Indomethacin					
Contrast media					
Renal vein thrombosis					
Disseminated intravascular coagulation					
Obstruction					
Urethral obstruction					
Bilateral ureteral obstruction					

Modified from Matthews OP et al: Pediatrics 65:57, 1980. Reproduced by permission of Pediatrics.
U, Urine concentration; *P,* plasma concentration; *FENa,* see text; *cre,* creatinine (mg/dl); *Osm,* osmolarity (mOsm/L); RFI (renal failure index) = $U_{Na} \times$ P/U creatinine.

ure.[12] In fact, asphyxia is the most common cause of acute tubular necrosis in the term neonate (65%); sepsis is the most common cause in the preterm neonate (35%). ARF presents earlier in the term infant and is more likely to be oliguric, whereas the nonoliguric form predominates in the preterm infant and occurs in the second week of life.

Aside from the hypoxia and acidosis, other important contributing factors may be hemoglobinuria, myoglobinuria, and an increase in uric acid excretion. The etiology of ARF is divided into three categories: prerenal, renal parenchymal, and postrenal. Various urinary and blood indexes have been used to separate these entities and are based on the appropriateness of the renal response to a challenge.[42] For example, an infant who is dehydrated with intact tubular function should be avidly conserving sodium and water; thus the FENa would be very low (<1%). If the infant had tubular damage, one would expect the FENa to be greater than 2.5% to 3%. Unfortunately, there are some renal causes such as glomerulonephritis that can give prerenal values for these indexes. When the tubules sense a decrease in filtration, they avidly reabsorb fluid but cannot differentiate between glomerular inflammation and dehydration. Thus, we have categorized these groups into pretubular, tubular, and posttubular causes (Table 19-2). While the use of these indexes is effective in infants and older children, the immaturity of the kidneys in premature infants leads to salt wasting (e.g., FENa of as great as 5% to 7% and abnormalities in water handling that cause difficulty in interpretation). Also, the FENa and renal failure index (RFI) can be affected by salt loading and diuretic therapy.

Inappropriate secretion of antidiuretic hormone may also lead to oliguria; however, these patients have a normal serum creatinine level, hyponatremia, a urine osmolarity that is inappropriately high for the serum osmolarity, and an increase in sodium excretion. Patients with congenital heart disease appear to be especially vulnerable to tubular necrosis after cardiac catheterization and cardiac surgery.

Prevention

Prevention of perinatal asphyxia; management of hypoxemia, hypotension, hypovolemia, and acidosis; and early detection and treatment of infections decrease renal insults.

Data collection

HISTORY

A perinatal history of intrapartal asphyxia and/or hypoxia, hypotension, hypovolemia, acido-sis, infection, or positive-pressure ventilation increases the infant's risk of ARF; cardiac catheterization and/or surgery may have ARF as a sequela.

SIGNS AND SYMPTOMS

Oliguric renal failure would also include a urine flow rate of less than 1 ml/kg/hr after the first 48 hours of life. Nonoliguric forms of ARF have a normal urine flow rate with an increase in creatinine.

LABORATORY DATA

While a good definition does not exist for acute renal failure, the presence of a rising serum creatinine level, when it should be decreasing (see Figure 19-3), is one indicator. Some authors prefer to use an absolute creatinine value of greater than 1.5 mg/dl. The U/P creatinine ratio is helpful and is not affected by diuretics. A fluid challenge of 5 to 10 ml/kg of body weight should be attempted, especially with blood or plasma. Caution must be taken, since these fluids can exacerbate lung disease or heart failure. If heart failure is present, inotropic agents should be considered. A central venous pressure measurement is important and underutilized in measuring the appropriateness of fluid therapy. This is especially important in infants with capillary leak syndrome or with third-space fluids postoperatively. These infants appear fluid overloaded but may be intravascularly depleted. Diuretic administration may be useful therapeutically to remove fluid but does not help diagnostically. An increase in urine output in response to these powerful diuretics does not differentiate between renal involvement and prerenal causes and may in fact dehydrate a patient. Mannitol should be avoided because of its hyperosmolarity and increased risk for intraventricular hemorrhage.

A renal ultrasound evaluation should be performed in all neonates with suspected ARF to assess possible urinary tract obstruction, renal vein thrombosis, and congenital renal abnormalities such as dysplasia, polycystic kidney disease, or aplasia.

Treatment[21,29,59]

Treatment involves removing the cause of the ARF. Prerenal causes require increasing perfusion of the kidney by fluid therapy and restoring cardiac output and blood pressure to normal. Any obstruction or thrombosis needs immediate attention. There is no specific therapy for acute tubular necrosis as yet. Many agents show promise in animal studies, including calcium channel blockers, adenosine triphosphate (ATP), magnesium chloride, or thyroxine, but no controlled trials in humans have as yet been performed. Conservative management must then be undertaken with careful attention to fluid and electrolyte balance, correction of acidosis, avoidance of nephrotoxins, aggressive nutritional therapy, diuretic therapy to maintain urine output, phosphate binders, and cal-cium supplements. Aggressive therapy of any infections is also important, since sepsis can be a fatal event in the patient with renal failure.

Dialysis° should be used only when complications of ARF are no longer medically manageable, including fluid overload, acidosis, hyperkalemia, symptomatic uremia, or prolonged malnutrition, because of the inability to give enough fluid.

In recent years dialysis has become an option for some neonates with chronic or acute renal failure. Both continuous arteriovenous hemofiltration (CAVH) and peritoneal dialysis are feasible for the neonate (Table 19-3). The goal of intervention with CAVH is to provide normal electrolyte balance and fluid removal while the renal system recovers from acute renal failure or profound fluid overload. Because CAVH is

°References 14, 16, 17, 22, 28, 33, 36, 39, 40, 49, 52.

TABLE 19-3 _____

Comparison of the Types of Dialysis for the Neonate

	ADVANTAGES	*COMPLICATIONS/DISADVANTAGES*
Hemodialysis	Most effective form of dialysis	Requires large amount of blood extra-corporeally
		Risk of exsanguination
		Risk of sepsis
		Marked fluid shifts and hypotension
Peritoneal dialysis	No need for vascular access	High risk of peritonitis
	Adaptable for long-term/home care	High risk of leakage at catheter site
	Effective in neonates because of larger peritoneal surface area relative to body weight	Respiratory compromise due to pressure on the diaphragm or hydrothorax
	Effective waste removal without massive fluid shifts	Potential temperature irregularities
		Potential injury to internal organs during catheter insertion
CAVH	Easy vascular access if umbilical vessels are available	Risk of clotted filter membrane
	Rapid removal of fluid in extremely fluid overloaded patients is possible	Risk of electrolyte imbalance
	Requires only small amount of blood extracorporeally	Risk of sepsis
		Risk of blood loss
		Risk of intraventricular hemorrhage/bleeding problems
		Available for acute dialysis only

feasible only in the critical care setting, it is not adaptable to chronic care.

CAVH functions basically through the principle of ultrafiltration via the fibers of a hemofilter.[39,40,49] Commercial CAVH filters are available that take as little as 6 ml of blood to prime. Vascular access can be provided through um-

bilical vessels. The force that drives the system is the neonate's own cardiac output through the umbilical artery. Blood is returned through the umbilical or other large vein (Figure 19-7 and Table 19-4).

Peritoneal dialysis is useful in acute and chronic care; therefore it is the intervention of

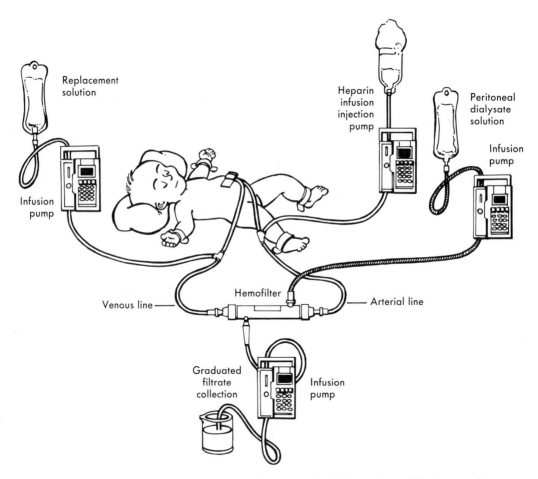

Figure 19-7. Continuous arteriovenous hemofiltration (CAVH) in newborn. Blood access is provided by umbilical artery and venous lines. Infant's own blood pressure forces blood through filter. Blood is heparinized through arterial limb. Replacement solution can be added to arterial or venous limb.[39,40] Amount of fluid removal can be regulated by infusion pump at filter outflow. Continuous arteriovenous hemodiafiltration (CAVHD) can be accomplished by passing peritoneal dialysate through filter via top port (*hatched line*). This allows dialysis as well as ultrafiltration of infant's blood.

choice for the neonate with end-stage renal disease. The goal of chronic peritoneal dialysis treatment in pediatrics is to allow for normal growth and development as well as fluid and electrolyte balance and toxin removal until the time when normal renal function is restored with transplantation.

Peritoneal dialysis functions primarily through the principles of diffusion and ultrafiltration across the peritoneal membrane and begins with the insertion of the dialysis catheter[28] (Figure 19-8 and Table 19-5). Neonatal catheters are commercially available and are best inserted in the operating room. A full cycle of fill, dwell, and drain time usually lasts 1 hour. Dwell volume is gradually increased from 20 to 50 ml/kg per exchange.[36,52]

Before the choice of either type of intervention is made, several ethical concerns must be carefully addressed. Aggressive intervention with dialysis must be viewed as only one option that physicians and parents must consider during this decision-making process. Acute dialysis should be undertaken where reasonable expectations of the infant's recovery are foreseen. Leiberman[39] has reported satisfactory CAVH treatment on almost all the infants in his center. Even though dialysis was effective, a mortality of almost 50% was reported as a result of the underlying disease.

Chronic dialysis is not considered a "standard of care" for the critically ill neonate.[14] Although several centers have begun reporting their results with dialysis in the neonate, the degree of success is not yet clear. These studies must be considered together with results of transplantation in infants. Although peritoneal dialysis with aggressive dietary management[16] can provide some growth for the infant with end-stage renal disease (ESRD), chronic uremia still has well-documented effects on the neurologic development and growth of the infant. Restoration of normal renal function via transplantation has provided catch-up growth

TABLE 19-4 _____

CAVH in the Neonate's Nursing Care Plan

PROBLEMS	NURSING ACTIONS
Potential sepsis	1. Sterile technique to be used at all tubing connections and parts
	2. Occlusive dressings at catheter site
Potential blood loss	1. Assess all tubing connections q.1h. or more frequently p.r.n.
	2. Tape securely all tubing connections
Potential clotted filter	1. Assess filter for blood flow q.1h. and p.r.n.
	2. Titrate heparin infusion to laboratory studies (PT/PTT)
	3. Notify physician of clotted filter, then replace
Rapid fluid shifts	1. Have patient on metabolic bed for continuous weight monitoring
	2. Have drain port connected to infusion pump to control outflow
	3. Have IV fluids available to infuse into inflow line for replacement
	4. Monitor electrolyte values of filtrated blood
Bleeding problems	1. Provide for minimum stimulation if patient has history of IVH
	2. Assess q.1h. or p.r.n. for signs of active bleeding; obtain bleeding studies as ordered
	3. Titrate heparin dose p.r.n. per physician's order
	4. Guiac stools/nasogastric drainage
	5. Dipstick hemofiltrate q.2h.; change filter if positive for blood
Temperature maintenance	1. Provide for infant warmer as needed

and normal development in many infants. Transplantation as an intervention in infants carries its own risks, and there are as yet insufficient data to assess its effectiveness.

The decision to intervene with chronic di-alysis should be made by physicians, parents, and possibly a medical ethics committee. Dialysis should not be started without the goal of ultimate transplantation. All persons involved in the decision making must be aware of the

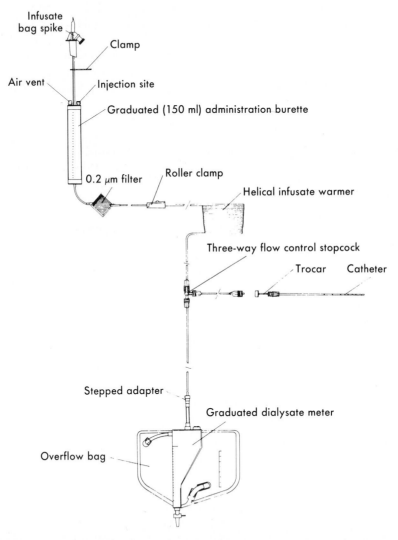

Figure 19-8. Example of commercially available dialysis set for neonatal peritoneal dialysis. Graduated burette in this closed system allows for easily varying amount of dialysate delivered. Helical coils allow dialysate to be warmed in same manner as in exchange transfusion. Graduated meter allows for accurate measurement of outflow. (Copyright Gesco International, San Antonio, Texas, 1987.)

long-term nature of renal failure management, which may extend for months or years into the home and family setting. If dialysis is begun, all should realize that the decision is not irrevocable for either parents or physicians. The prognosis should be openly discussed with the parents, as well as the amount of suffering the infant may have to endure as a result of the many possible life-threatening complications.

The best chance for success lies with an infant with all other organ systems intact and with a good family situation. Finally, the decision-makers, especially the parents, should understand that in light of the experimental nature of intervention, the choice not to intervene in some instances is a valid decision that may be in the infant's best interest. Having said this, we are still optimistic that dialysis and transplanta-

TABLE 19-5

Peritoneal Dialysis in the Neonate's Nursing Care Plan

PROBLEMS	*NURSING ACTIONS*

Potential peritonitis	1. Sterile technique to be used at all tubing connections and bag spikes; all connections are clamped and taped
	2. Assess peritoneal dialysis (PD) fluid with each drain for color, turbidity, and presence of fibrin
	3. Should turbidity exist:
	  a. Obtain cell count, differential, Gram stain, and culture of PD fluid
	  b. Administer antibiotics via dialysate as ordered
	4. Occlusive dressing at catheter site

Potential fluid overload/ dehydration	1. Weigh drain bag after each drain to determine exact outflow record on flowsheet with amount of previous inflow
	2. Weigh neonate at regular intervals during drain to determine real weight of infant
	3. When using 1.5% dialysate, assess for fluid reabsorption:
	  a. Peripheral and dependent edema
	  b. Weight gain
	  c. Failure to drain out all of dwell volume
	4. When using stronger dialysate (up to 4.25%) or very rapid exchanges, assess for:
	  a. Weight loss
	  b. Poor skin turgor and sunken eyes
	  c. Hypotension
	5. Notify physician of weight discrepancies or other symptoms

Potential temperature maintenance problem	1. Warm all PD fluid by blood warmer or heating pad immediately before inflow
Inflow/outflow obstruction	1. Reposition patient, inflow/drain bags 2. Plain radiograph of abdomen to check position of catheter—should be toward pelvis 3. Add heparin to dialysate if fibrin is present
Potential respiratory compromise	1. Carefully clamp all clamps to avoid overfill 2. Position patient with elevated head of bed to reduce pressure on abdomen 3. If distress exists following drain, obtain chest radiograph to rule out pneumonia or hydrothorax

tion will become a very promising treatment modality. Infant transplantation should be performed at a center with experience in this area.

Complications[59]

The mortality of neonates with ARF ranges from 14% to 75%. Patients with the worst prognosis are those with congenital renal anomalies, congenital heart disease, and those requiring dialysis. Patients with nonoliguric forms of ARF have the best prognosis. Recovery of function is unlikely if diffuse cortical necrosis or medullary necrosis has occurred. Reversal of the underlying condition is the most important factor for determining the prognosis. The prognosis also appears to be better if renal perfusion is demonstrated on a ^{99m}Tc glucoheptonate or ^{131}I hippurate nuclear renal scan.[26]

For survivors, chronic renal failure has been seen in as many as 40% of cases. Renal tubular abnormalities (i.e., renal tubular acidosis and concentrating defects) have also been noted. Hypertension can also be seen. Renal growth can be affected, and a kidney can be noted years later to appear hypoplastic or dysplastic.

HYPERTENSION[3,18,23,29]
Physiology

Since nearly universal blood pressure monitoring has occurred, hypertension has been recognized as a significant clinical problem in the neonate cared for in a neonatal intensive care unit (NICU). The incidence of hypertension in healthy term infants appears to be quite low, and the majority of hypertensive infants have a definable etiology. A hypertensive infant may be quite ill, with symptoms similar to those of an infant with sepsis, heart, or lung disease. If the hypertension is properly diagnosed and treated, the outcome may be quite favorable.

Hypertension usually occurs during the first week of life in term infants and during the second week in preterm infants. However, new data suggest that hypertension can occur much later in a sick infant and even after discharge.

The true incidence of hypertension in the newborn has been reported to be between 1.2% and 5% of NICU admissions.

Blood pressures vary by gestational age, body weight, cuff size, and state of alertness. Normal values have been developed by body weight and by postnatal age, but no criteria combining these variables are available. Blood pressure begins low and postnatally increases by 1 to 2 mm Hg/day for the first 3 to 8 days, 1 mm Hg/week for 5 to 7 weeks, and reaches a steady value for the first year of life by 2 months of age.[18,62] Whether the percentile for an infant's blood pressure will track into later childhood or adulthood is still controversial at this point. Normal values for blood pressures in infants are listed in Figure 19-9.

Etiology[3,23]

The causes of hypertension are listed in Table 19-6. Any infant with hypertension must be assumed to have a specific secondary etiology. The most common cause may be a complication of umbilical artery catheterization.

Prevention

Obtaining accurate reliable measurements of blood pressure depends on knowledge of proper equipment usage.[18,62] Under study conditions, the best determinator of blood pressure is the direct arterial measurement, usually through an umbilical artery catheter (UAC). Older techniques such as auscultation, palpation, and flush blood pressure measurements have been replaced by Doppler measurements and, more recently, oscillometry. These latter two measurements have correlated very well with direct arterial measurements for systolic blood pressure but not as well with diastolic blood pressure. Cuff selection is important, since small cuffs give falsely high values. The cuff should completely encircle the extremity and be the largest cuff possible without impinging on the joints of the upper arm or leg. In this way, blood pressures in the arms and legs

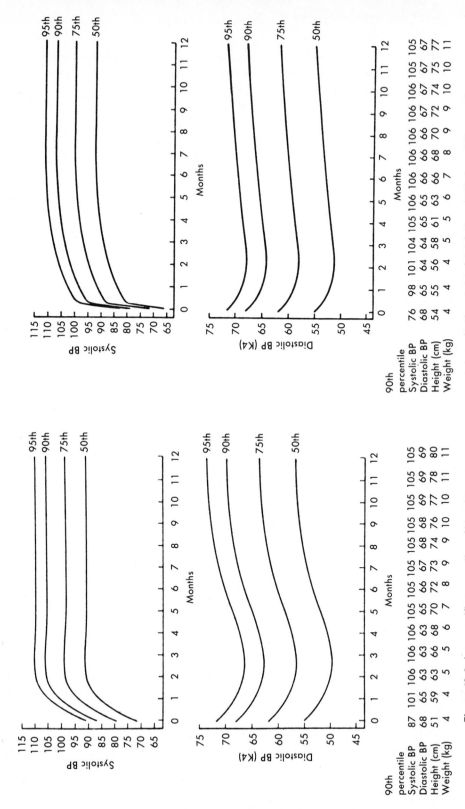

Figure 19-9. Age-specific percentiles of blood pressure measurements in boys (*left*) and girls (*right*). Korotkoff phase IV is used for diastolic blood pressure. Blood pressures exceeding 90th percentile are considered hypertensive unless infant's height and/or weight exceeds 90th percentile. Blood pressures exceeding 95th percentile are always considered hypertensive. (From Report of the Second Task Force on Blood Pressure Control in Children, Pediatrics 79:1, 1987. Reproduced by permission of Pediatrics.)

should be equal. Frequently the same cuff is used for the arm and the leg, with the result that the leg pressures appear to be higher, since the cuff is too small. The size of the cuff and extremity used for measurement should be

---

TABLE 19-6

Etiology of Hypertension in the Neonate

Vascular
Renal artery stenosis
Renal artery thrombosis
Coarctation of the aorta
Hypoplastic abdominal aorta

Renal
Renal dysplasia/hypoplasia
Polycystic kidney disease (autosomal dominant or recessive)
Renal failure
Obstructive uropathy
Reflux nephropathy
Pyelonephritis
Glomerulonephritis
Tumors
   Wilms'
   Neuroblastoma

Endocrine
Adrenogenital syndrome
Cushing's disease
Hyperaldosteronism
Thyrotoxicosis

Other
Closure of abdominal wall defects
Fluid overload
Genitourinary surgery
Hypercalcemia
Increased intracranial pressure
Medications
   Ocular phenylephrine
   Corticosteroids
   Theophylline
   Deoxycorticosterone
Seizures

Modified from Adelman RD: Neonatal hypertension. In Loggie JMH et al, editors: NHLBI workshop on juvenile hypertension, New York, 1983, Biomedical Information Corp.; and Guignard JP: Neonatal nephrology. In Holliday MA, Barratt TM, and Vernier RL, editors: Pediatric nephrology, ed 2, Baltimore, 1987, Williams & Wilkins.

---

documented so that serial measurements will be consistent. The position for measuring blood pressure is always supine. Blood pressures taken on extremities elevated above the level of the heart may give erroneously low values; the converse is true of pressures taken on extremities lower than the level of the heart. Blood pressure can vary greatly with the state of alertness and with crying (Table 19-7). Frequently a sick infant will have the blood pressure measured directly through a UAC as well as by oscillometric techniques. Significant discrepancies between these measurements may be seen, and it is often difficult to discern which one is the "true" blood pressure. Aside from equipment malfunction, discrepancies can be caused by a UAC with a caliber too small for the infant's size, a thrombus at the tip of the catheter, or poor peripheral perfusion.

Judicious use of umbilical catheters (e.g., in infants who need frequent arterial samplings [see Chapter 6]) decreases exposure to catheters in less ill infants who may only need peripheral intravenous (IV) lines for fluid administration.

Data collection
HISTORY

Nearly all hypertensive infants (88%) have had a UAC. The incidence of renal artery thrombosis in patients with indwelling UACs is 3% to 20%; however, only 13% of these infants are clinically diagnosed. Three percent of patients with UACs develop hypertension.[3,23]

SIGNS AND SYMPTOMS

Any infant exceeding the 95th percentile for blood pressure is considered to be hypertensive. Thus 5% of the population would be hypertensive on initial screening. For the term infant, any blood pressure exceeding 95 mm Hg systolic or 75 mm Hg diastolic is considered hypertensive. In premature infants the definition is less well defined but is considered to be 80 mm Hg systolic and 50 mm Hg diastolic.[3]

TABLE 19-7

Effect of State of Alertness on Systemic Blood Pressure in the Newborn

	SYSTOLIC BLOOD PRESSURE (mm Hg)	DIASTOLIC BLOOD PRESSURE (mm Hg)
Quiet sleep	73 ± 10	46 ± 8
Active sleep	77 ± 10	46 ± 8
Awake	79 ± 9	52 ± 8
Awake and sucking	85 ± 10	55 ± 7

From Adelman RD: Neonatal hypertension. In Loggie JMH et al, editors: NHLBI workshop on juvenile hypertension, New York, 1983, Biomedical Information Corp.

Blood pressure measurements should be taken in all extremities to seek evidence for coarctation of the aorta.

The symptoms of hypertension may be severe but very nonspecific. Hypertension presents with respiratory distress in 50% of infants; patent ductus arteriosus in 50%; neurologic symptoms such as seizures, tremor, and abnormalities in tone in 30%; and congestive heart failure in 40%. Intracranial hemorrhage, hemiparesis, hepatosplenomegaly, and cyanosis may also occur.[3,23] However, approximately 50% of infants are asymptomatic.

Effects of hypertension (e.g., hypertensive retinopathy) should also be evaluated, including a fundoscopic examination by an ophthalmologist and cardiac evaluation for evidence of hypertensive damage.

LABORATORY DATA

Evaluation should consist of a study of renal anatomy with ultrasound. If this is unrevealing, a renal scan or angiography should be performed. Serum creatinine levels are usually normal or slightly elevated. Urinalysis may be normal, but hematuria and proteinuria may be noted (either as a sign of the cause of hypertension or as a result of the hypertension). Peripheral renin activities are generally elevated but must be compared with age-matched normal values.[57]

Treatment[3,23]

Hypertension should be treated in the neonate, especially if it exceeds the definition of severe hypertension (>110 mm Hg systolic). However, normalization of blood pressure should not be sought, since an excessive lowering of blood pressure may also be detrimental. A definable cause, such as a urinary tract obstruction, a tumor, or a coarctation should be treated surgically. Rarely, a nephrectomy of the involved kidney has been advocated in medically unmanageable, severe hypertension. Drugs and dosages commonly used in the neonate for blood pressure control are found in Table 19-8. The drugs of choice are propranolol (Inderal), hydralazine (Apresoline), and captopril. Captopril should be used with caution if there is possible unilateral renal artery stenosis, since renal failure has been reported in this situation. For an acute hypertensive crisis, IV hydralazine, IV diazoxide, or oral captopril are the drugs of choice. Sublingual enalapril is currently being evaluated as well.

Complications[3,4,23]

The prognosis is excellent if the blood pressure is well controlled medically or cured surgically. These infants have normal somatic growth and normal development, and most have their antihypertensive medications discontinued after several years of follow-up. Poor renal growth

TABLE 19-8

Antihypertensive Medications for Use in the Neonatal Period*

MEDICATION	DOSE	SCHEDULE	ROUTE	COMMENTS
Propranolol	1-4 mg/kg/dose	b.i.d.-t.i.d.	PO	Contraindicated in heart failure, possibly in BPD, sedation
Hydralazine	0.025-1 mg/kg/dose	b.i.d.	IV	
	0.25-1.5 mg/kg/dose; maximum 4.5 mg/kg/day	b.i.d.-q.i.d.	PO	Tachycardia, sodium retention
	0.1-0.5 mg/kg/dose with beta-blocker 0.4-0.8 mg/kg/dose (sole agent)	q.6h.	IV	
Captopril	0.3-2 mg/kg/dose	t.i.d.	PO	Leukopenia, rash, proteinuria, hyperkalemia, acute renal failure
Diazoxide	1-5 mg/kg/dose	q.4-24h.	IV	Hyperglycemia, fluid retention, hyperuricemia
Sodium nitroprusside	0.5-10 μg/kg/min	Continuous infusion	IV	Keep covered in foil, careful observation for infiltration of IV or varying rate of administration

*No reported experience in the newborn with nifedipine, clonidine (Catapres), labetalol, verapamil, or enalapril. Furosemide (Lasix) and thiazides are not antihypertensive medications, but are used for volume overload.

on the side of the renal artery disease persists, and renal scans tend to be persistently abnormal. Creatinine clearances appear to be normal in most infants.

ABDOMINAL MASS [29,37,38]

Slightly more than half of abdominal masses present during the newborn period are of renal origin. The literature offers no consistent data on the frequency of abdominal masses in infants, but there is general agreement regarding the urgent need to evaluate these patients in an expedient and thorough manner before planning intervention.

The differential diagnosis in the infant with an abdominal mass is shown in Table 19-9.

Data collection
PHYSICAL EXAMINATION

Visualization of the abdomen before manually exploring it allows the examiner to note a mass that may be missed in a tense abdomen. Bi-manual palpation using the flat surface of the fingers while supporting the infant's flank with the other hand allows for exploration of the abdomen during deep palpation. Renal masses are usually smooth to palpation and move with respiration. The size of the mass is not helpful in determining its etiology. Percussion may be used to outline the suspected area, and transillumination is sometimes helpful in identifying hydronephrosis and multicystic kidneys, which are both positive when transilluminated. Some renal masses are quite soft, and excessive pressure during the examination will frequently cause the mass to be missed.

LABORATORY DATA

Ultrasonography is the most desirable diagnostic tool for initial evaluation of an abdominal mass in the newborn. The advantages of this technology include its noninvasive nature, accessibility for bedside studies, recently improved resolution, and relatively low cost.

TABLE 19-9 _____

Neonatal Abdominal Masses

TYPE OF MASS	PERCENT OF TOTAL
Renal masses	55
Hydronephrosis	
Multicystic dysplastic kidney	
Polycystic kidney disease	
Mesoblastic nephroma	
Renal ectopia	
Renal vein thrombosis	
Nephroblastomatosis	
Wilms' tumor	
Genital masses	15
Hydrometrocolpos	
Ovarian cyst	
Gastrointestinal masses	15
Duplication	
Volvulus	
Complicated meconium ileus	
Mesenteric-omental cyst	
"Pseudocyst" proximal to atresia	
Nonrenal retroperitoneal masses	10
Adrenal hemorrhage	
Neuroblastoma	
Teratoma	
Hepatosplenobiliary masses	5
Hemangioendothelioma	
Hepatoblastoma	
Hepatic cyst	
Splenic hematoma	
Choledochal cyst	
Hydrops of gallbladder	

From Kirks DR et al: Radiol Clin North Am 19:527, 1981.

Traditional studies such as IV pyelography are not done in the first weeks of life because of the neonatal kidney's inability to concentrate urine and the decreased GFR. Ultrasound reveals a kidney with communicating cystic masses in hydronephrosis. Renal dysplasia most often is seen as noncommunicating cyst formations on ultrasound. When this diagnostic tool is incapable of differentiating dysplasia and hydronephrosis, renal scintigraphy is indicated. With this modality dysplasia is noted as having no functional activity on a nuclear scan. A hy-

dronephrotic kidney demonstrates "rim" activity with delayed accumulation of the radionuclide in the pelvis and calyces. Selected isotopes (glucoheptonate) used in renal scintigraphy will reveal fine anatomic detail, making this modality a useful tool in assessing renal function in the neonate. Rarely, a percutaneous nephrostogram is performed to determine if cysts are due to obstruction or dysplasia. A voiding cystourethrogram is the method of choice to diagnose vesicoureteral reflux. CT scans can be helpful, especially for differentiating renal masses.

INTRINSIC RENAL PARENCHYMAL ABNORMALITIES [38,46,63]

Renal abnormalities can be classified by the amount of tissue, the differentiation of tissue, and the position of the kidney.

Amount of tissue
PATHOPHYSIOLOGY

Congenital absence or agenesis of renal tissue can occur unilaterally or bilaterally.

BILATERAL AGENESIS. Bilateral agenesis, also known as Potter's disease, is seen rarely, with an incidence of 1 per 4000 births. **The majority of affected infants are male, small-for-gestational-age (SGA), with a history of maternal oligohydramnios.**

Signs and symptoms. The characteristic facial features accompanying Potter's syndrome include wide-set eyes, parrot-beak nose, receding chin, and large, low-set ears with little cartilage. Other associated malformations include pulmonary hypoplasia, hydrocephalus, meningocele, multiple skeletal anomalies, and imperforate anus.

Complications. Death usually occurs within hours to several days as a result of respiratory or renal failure.

UNILATERAL AGENESIS. Unilateral renal agenesis is seen more frequently (1 per 1000 live births) and may present as a solitary kidney on examination with enlargement due to compensatory hypertrophy. Unilateral agenesis has been associated with Turner's syndrome, Poland's syndrome, and VATER syndrome.

Data collection. These patients are often asymptomatic and are diagnosed inadvertently on ultrasound or based on the significant association with malformations of the lower genitourinary tract. There is no need for long-term follow-up in this group.

HYPOPLASIA. Hypoplasia is a deficiency in the amount of renal tissue expressed as an abnormally small kidney. Morphologically the kidney is normal, and renal function is unaffected in the neonatal period. Later in life patients may sometimes outgrow their renal function.

Differentiation of tissue
PATHOPHYSIOLOGY

Abnormalities in renal tissue differentiation are most commonly expressed as dysplastic kidneys. Renal dysplasia is a failure of the metanephrogenic tissue to mature appropriately, frequently because of obstruction of the urinary tract early in gestation. The result is a persistence of immature structures and very little normal-functioning renal tissue.

Renal dysplasia may be seen in one or both kidneys, involving the entire kidney, segments of the kidney, or microscopic areas (foci) of the kidney. Dysplasia is most commonly expressed as cyst formation. Bilateral multicystic dysplastic kidneys are nonfunctional and not compatible with life. Unilateral involvement is both the most common cystic lesion of the neonatal kidney as well as one of the most frequently palpated abdominal masses in the newborn. Unilateral dysplasia shows no predilection for males or females, nor for involvement of the right or left kidney. In the majority of these patients the ureter is absent, atretic, or stenotic. No orifice is found in the bladder. Renal function and structure may be normal in the remaining kidney of infants with unilateral dysplasia; however, frequently ureteropelvic (UPJ) obstruction is present in the contralateral kidney.

DATA COLLECTION

HISTORY. Renal dysplasia is usually sporadic, but some familial cases have been reported.

LABORATORY DATA. A lack of blood flow on a ^{99m}Tc DTPA nuclear renal scan confirms the diagnosis of dysplasia.

TREATMENT

There is generally no need for removal of these kidneys, since they do not cause hypertension, stones, or urinary tract infections, nor do they become malignant. Removal of the kidney is sometimes indicated if its size prevents adequate nutrition.

Position of the kidney
PATHOPHYSIOLOGY

Abnormalities in kidney position are described earlier in the section on normal development. An ectopic kidney frequently located in the pelvis, cross-fused ectopia, and a horseshoe kidney can present as an abdominal mass.

Polycystic kidney disease[9,15,46]
PATHOPHYSIOLOGY

Polycystic kidney disease may present as one of two types in the infant: (1) infantile type, which is autosomal recessive, and (2) adult type, which is autosomal dominant. Traditionally, adult-type disease has not been associated with onset during the first year of life, but recent studies have confirmed both presentations in the infant, and thus an attempt should be made to discontinue use of the terms "infant" and "adult" forms.

Polycystic kidney disease of the recessive type presents with varied severity, but it is always bilateral. The kidneys become enlarged, with a proliferation of renal tubules and dilated collecting tubules. These are no true "cysts," and the kidney has a renoform shape.

Autosomal dominant disease involves cyst formations in any portion of the nephron, Bowman's space, and liver. Rarely, cyst formation in the pancreas and spleen are present. There is a strong association with autosomal dominant polycystic kidney disease (PKD) and cerebral artery aneurysms.

DATA COLLECTION

HISTORY. Recently, criteria for making a definitive diagnosis for both diseases have been developed. Infantile (recessive) disease included patients with the following: (1) congenital hepatic fibrosis on liver biopsy or evidence of portal hypertension, (2) renal histologic studies consistent with collecting tubule ectopia, or (3) a sibling with the disease. Patients diagnosed with adult (dominant) disease had the following: (1) positive parental history or (2) known liver cysts or Berry's aneurysm.[15]

SIGNS AND SYMPTOMS. Both types of polycystic kidney disease can present initially with an abdominal mass. The infant may present with bilateral flank masses, hepatic enlargement, Potter's facies due to oligohydramnios, oliguria, hypoplastic lungs, respiratory distress, and spontaneous pneumothorax. Hypertension is common in both types of the disease.

LABORATORY DATA. Differentiation of autosomal dominant versus recessive type is difficult, since radiographic studies are not consistently accurate in discerning differences.

TREATMENT

Management consists of serial monitoring of blood pressure, renal function, and urine cultures. Neonates with either form of PKD need aggressive treatment of blood pressure with captopril as the drug of choice, treatment of any urinary tract infection, and aggressive nutritional management, including a protein-restricted diet.

HYDRONEPHROSIS [7,44,45,60]
Physiology

The collecting system of the kidney is composed of the ureter, pelvis, and calyces, which function as a system for removing urine from the kidney.

Hydronephrosis, one of the most common abdominal masses in the newborn, involves a dilation of the pelvis and calyces, most often as a result of congenital obstruction. The impaired movement of urine as a result of severe or chronic obstruction may lead to dysplastic and cystic changes that further impair kidney function if the obstruction occurs early in gestation.

Causes of ureteral obstruction include the following:

1. The most common obstruction is at the ureteropelvic junction. The infant presents with a ballooning of the renal pelvis.

2. Obstruction at the ureterovesical junction, also known as congenital megaureter in its primary form, occurs more often in the male infant and more frequently affects the left ureter.

3. Posterior urethral valves (PUVs) in males are the major cause of urethral obstruction. This distal obstruction may result in bladder hypertrophy, hydroureter, and hydronephrosis if severe in nature. Dysplastic changes can be seen if the obstruction occurs early in gestation. The neonate with PUVs is at risk for developing an ascending infection and subsequent renal damage.

4. Prune belly syndrome,[60] also known as Eagle-Barrett syndrome, is a less common cause of obstruction and dilation of the pelves and calyces. There is a strong male predominance. This triad of anomalies includes (a) absence or hypoplasia of the abdominal wall muscles, (b) bilateral cryptorchism, and (c) urinary tract abnormality. The loose, shriveled abdomen is responsible for the "prune belly" appearance, which diminishes with age and does not require surgical correction. Renal dysplasia is usually seen in prune belly syndrome and may range from mild to severe involvement. The enlarged bladder may be seen in conjunction with a patent urachus draining urine. The prostatic urethra is usually hypoplastic.

5. Vesicoureteral reflux is another cause of calyceal dilation not associated with obstruction (see urinary tract infections).

Etiology

The etiology of most types of hydronephrosis is unknown. The etiology of prune belly syndrome remains unclear. Primary prune belly syndrome can be a result of a mesenchymal developmental arrest. A variant of the syndrome can also be seen as a sequelae of an intrauterine distention of the abdomen by an obstructed urinary system. The existence of this secondary cause of prune belly syndrome is controversial.

Prevention

Since the causes of hydronephrosis are unknown, prevention is not possible.

Data collection
HISTORY

A history of oligohydramnios or obstructed urinary system found on ultrasound visualization may be indicative of hydronephrosis.

SIGNS AND SYMPTOMS

Infants may have few if any symptoms, and there are usually no physical findings unless a bladder or kidney is palpated on routine examination. These infants may present with a poor urinary stream and frequently with failure to thrive. Urosepsis may be the most dramatic presentation.

LABORATORY DATA

HYDRONEPHROSIS IN UTERO.[24,25] With the advent of frequent prenatal ultrasound examinations, the finding of a dilated collecting system is not uncommon. Its management is very controversial, and an accurate assessment of fetal renal function is imperative in determining its management. Factors such as (1) amniotic fluid volume, (2) appearance of the kidneys on ultrasound, (3) degree of upper urinary tract dilation, and, most recently, (4) analysis of fetal urine electrolytes may provide information for assessment of fetal renal function.

Ultrasonography is capable of identifying urinary tract dilation between the seventeenth and twenty-fourth weeks of gestation. Dilation does not always imply urinary tract obstruction and must be used in conjunction with the amount of amniotic fluid in determining kidney function. Other conditions such as bilateral vesicoureteral reflux, prune belly syndrome, and primary megaureter may present with dilated collecting systems and are not amenable to in utero surgery. Ultrasound visualization of kidneys supplies other information, such as the appearance and echogenicity of the kidney. Dysplastic kidneys, most of which are caused by early obstruction in utero, often have cortical cysts on ultrasound visualization and an increased echogenicity.

Treatment
HYDRONEPHROSIS IN UTERO

Unilateral obstruction assessed in utero requires no immediate treatment. Close follow-up is indicated, and surgical treatment should be considered postnatally. Bilateral dilated calyces with normal amniotic fluid volume is treated only with observation.

Treatment for bilateral obstruction associated with *decreased* amniotic fluid is dependent on the gestational age of the fetus. In a previable fetus with bilateral obstruction and oligohydramnios, termination of the pregnancy should be considered. When observed, the first intervention should involve karyotype to determine if other anomalies are present. If abnormal, parents are counseled with the option of elective termination or no intervention. Infants who are determined to be viable with oligohydramnios and bilateral obstruction are treated with steroids in utero in an attempt to accelerate lung maturity. The fetus is then delivered at 32 to 34 weeks and surgically corrected ex utero. In infants with dilated collecting systems with initially normal AF volume who on serial ultrasonographic evaluation are shown to have a decreasing AF volume, the infant should be delivered early if viable or, if previable, considered for in utero bladder-AF shunt placement; or termination may be considered. One must remember that the prognosis of any infant requiring end-stage renal disease management is definitely related to the size of the infant when such care is initiated.

TYPES OF HYDRONEPHROSIS

1. Obstruction at the ureteropelvic junction is usually surgically repaired.
2. Obstruction at the ureterovesical junction is also surgically corrected. Surgical correction involves excising the stenotic segment in the obstructed megaureter as well as ureteric reimplantation and is successful in the large majority of infants.
3. Management of PUV is dependent on the age at presentation and the infant's condition. After initial stabilization of the infant, relief of obstruction with a catheter provides quick decompression. Generally, fulguration of the valves is done after 1 year of age. The use of a vesicostomy versus a higher diversion is controversial.
4. Treatment of prune belly syndrome consists of early decompression and end-stage renal disease (ESRD) treatment. Recent success in dialysis and renal transplantation is improving the outlook for these patients and should be strongly considered as management for these infants if other organ systems are normal.

Complications

The mortality of infants with prune belly syndrome is very high; 20% die within 2 weeks, and 50% within the first 2 years of life.

RENAL VEIN THROMBOSIS[47]
Physiology

Renal vein thrombosis (RVT), an acute life-threatening condition, is seen most frequently in neonatal populations. Affecting males more frequently (1.9:1), RVT is associated with conditions that cause circulatory collapse and decreased oxygenation within the kidney.

Thrombosis most often occurs in the smaller renal veins rather than in the main renal vein.

Etiology

Perinatal causes of neonatal RVT include maternal diabetes, toxemia, maternal thiazide therapy, polycythemia, placental insufficiency, birth asphyxia, prematurity, respiratory distress syndrome, and sepsis. Angiography has also been associated with RVT.

Prevention

Good prenatal care and maintenance of perinatal homeostasis decrease the risk of renal vein thrombosis.

Data collection
HISTORY

A history of perinatal causes of renal vein thrombosis raises the care-provider's suspicion of this condition.

SIGNS AND SYMPTOMS

The involved kidney engorges with blood because of obstruction to blood flow and forms a palpable flank mass. Other clinical symptoms may include hematuria (60% of cases), anemia, oliguria, and thrombocytopenia (less than 75,000 platelets).

LABORATORY DATA

Positive blood on dipstick, urine output of less than 1 ml/kg/hr, and a low platelet count are indicative of renal vein thrombosis.

Treatment

Management includes treatment of the underlying illness, treatment of sepsis if suspected, fluid therapy, and possibly dialysis in selected cases. Heparin therapy remains controversial for RVT. Surgical excision of the thrombus is not usually indicated during the acute phase but may be appropriate at a later time. Rarely, nephrectomy is required.

Complications

Renal tubular dysfunction is often observed after recovery from RVT.

MISCELLANEOUS CAUSES OF ABDOMINAL MASS

Wilms' tumor, also known as nephroblastoma, is the most common intraabdominal tumor seen in children and occurs at a rate of 8-9 per 100,000 births in the United States. It presents in two thirds of patients during the first 3 to 6 months of life. The tumor is described as firm, smooth, and confluent with the kidney or attached to the organ. Ten percent of cases involve both kidneys. This condition has an excellent prognosis with treatment. For most patients, surgical removal of the tumor is followed by irradiation and chemotherapy.

Neuroblastoma is the most common malignant tumor in infancy. The primary site of the tumor may originate from any area of neural crest tissue, with the most common site identified in the adrenal gland. Presenting in the neonate as a palpable abdominal mass, this tumor may also cause urinary obstruction. Prognosis is related to the site of the primary tumor, histologic appearance of the tumor, staging of the disease, and patient's age.

URINARY TRACT INFECTIONS[2,29,30]

Urinary tract infections (UTIs) affect approximately 1% of full-term infants and 3% of premature infants. Male infants are affected much more frequently (five times more) than females. *Escherichia coli* is the organism most often implicated in neonatal UTIs, followed by *Klebsiella*.

Vesicoureteral reflux is a common radiographic finding in infants. Primary reflux is seen in abnormalities of the vesicoureteral junction, ureteral duplication, and ureterocele. Secondary reflux is associated with infection, PUV, and neurogenic diseases.

Etiology

Abnormalities of the urinary tract are responsible for a large number of UTIs in the neonate. Whether the infection is ascending from the bladder or hematogenously spread is a matter of debate. The high association of reflux with UTI makes determining the etiology of reflux a priority for planning appropriate treatment. Reflux is graded on a four-point scale, with grade 4 denoting massive hydronephrosis and hydroureter, and can be diagnosed only by a voiding cystourethrogram (VCUG).

Prevention

Although abnormalities of the urinary tract are not preventable, contamination of the urinary tract by catheterization is preventable.

Data collection
HISTORY

Maternal UTIs have also been associated with neonatal UTIs.

SIGNS AND SYMPTOMS

Symptomatic manifestations include abnormal weight loss during the first days of life, decreased feeding, dehydration, irritability, lethargy, cyanosis, jaundice, and septicemia. In some cases the affected kidneys are palpable. Infected infants may also be asymptomatic.

LABORATORY DATA

Evaluation of a neonate with suspected UTI includes an immediate ultrasound examination to rule out upper tract abnormalities. Urine for culture along with blood cultures and a complete blood count should be obtained.

The optimum method of obtaining urine for culture is a suprapubic aspiration of the bladder. Successful results are dependent on a full bladder in the neonate. Catheterization is not recommended in the neonate because of urethral stricture formation in the male and frequent culture contamination in the female. Urine obtained in a urine bag should not be used for cultures. Skin contamination can frequently yield false-positive cultures; conversely, one drop of povidone-iodine (Betadine) in a urine bag can prevent in vitro bacterial growth.

Grades of reflux are diagnosed by VCUG. Sterile urine is necessary before a VCUG is undertaken.

Treatment

Pyuria (10 to 15 white blood cells per high-power field) can be observed in the neonate normally. Treatment for UTI is indicated when an organism is cultured from the urine. Any growth in a urine sample obtained by suprapubic aspiration should be considered an infection if the procedure was cleanly done. Any aspiration of bowel contents must affect the interpretation of culture results. Antibiotic coverage consists of both ampicillin and an aminoglycoside. Sulfonamides are contraindicated in this patient group because of their potential to complicate hyperbilirubinemia.

Antibiotic therapy should continue for 14 days, with a follow-up urine culture done 3 days after therapy has been discontinued.

Complications

Four to 6 weeks later, a VCUG is used to assess any lower urinary tract abnormalities, specifically reflux. A normal study indicates that antibiotic therapy may be discontinued. These patients should be followed with monthly urine cultures. Patients who demonstrate reflux should be maintained on suppressive antibiotic therapy. VCUG should be repeated in 6 months if reflux was initially present.

NEUROGENIC BLADDER[1,51]
Physiology

Neurogenic bladder is an anatomic interruption of the micturition reflex normally triggered by a full bladder. The bladder may be flaccid and unable to empty urine or spastic and hyperreflexive and unable to store urine. Lower motor neuron deficit causes bladder atony, and upper motor neuron deficit can cause spasticity.

Etiology

Infants with lumbosacral spinal malformations commonly have a urinary tract dysfunction known as neurogenic bladder.

Data collection
HISTORY

Elevated AF levels are associated with spinal malformations such as spina bifida or myelomeningocele.

SIGNS AND SYMPTOMS

Often there is a mixed presentation of symptoms. Diagnosis can begin immediately at the bedside when the newborn has no apparent voiding stream or the urine flow rate falls below expectations without other explanations.

LABORATORY DATA

Further clarification of the diagnosis can be made by a VCUG and also later by cystometric studies.

Treatment

Proper bladder management in the neonate is very important. If a VCUG shows no reflux and the urine appears to flow freely from the bladder with only a small amount of residual urine, no intervention is necessary. However, if the sphincter tone is such that urine is stagnant in the bladder, Credé's maneuver can be performed gently at regular intervals. Credé's method should be performed only after a VCUG has documented the absence of reflux. Surgical intervention is indicated in the neonate with neurogenic bladder when there is severe reflux with renal damage present or recurrent UTI. The urologist can create a vesicostomy to allow the free flow of urine into diapers.

Complications

Early diagnosis and intervention for infants with neurogenic bladder can decrease the risks of the complications associated with this problem. Long-term complications of neurogenic bladder include UTIs and vesicoureteral reflux leading to hydronephrosis, electrolyte imbalances, and permanent damage to the kidney.

Discharge planning for these infants should include strong emphasis on scheduled follow-up of voiding dynamics. Intermittent evaluations over several years will be necessary to assure adequate renal function. In later years the vesicostomy is frequently closed, and clean intermittent catheterization initiated.

PARENT TEACHING

Since many renal problems are secondary to abnormalities, parents need the information that nothing they have done or did not do caused the anomaly. Grief work over the loss of the perfect infant is necessary before attachment and caretaking is possible (see Chapters 22 and 23). Genetic counseling enables parents to make informed choices about subsequent pregnancies.

Most infants with renal problems require accurate intake and output measurement. The importance and necessity of measuring intake and not overfeeding must be stressed to parents, as well as the necessity of saving and weighing diapers. Infants who are fluid restricted may be "difficult" for care providers and parents because they are fussy and irritable. Holding, rocking, and using a pacifier for nonnutritive suckling is helpful in calming these infants. Adherence to the prescribed formula and/or breast milk is very important to regulate sodium intake and fluid retention.

Long-term complications that parents may have to recognize and/or manage must be explained and instructions given in writing. Since abnormalities in renal function and anatomy may be sequelae of renal diseases, follow-up by a pediatric nephrologist and/or urologist for urinalysis, cultures, and other diagnostic tests is important. General health maintenance is also important, because growth failure may be a manifestation of ongoing or recurring renal problems.

The importance of administering antihypertensive medications must be stressed to parents. Since hypertension is often a silent condition, the need for continuation of medications must be thoroughly explained. Side effects of hypertensive medications such as sedation, tachycardia, and excessive weight gain, as well as the necessity of medical follow-up, must also be emphasized.

ACKNOWLEDGMENT

Our sincere gratitude is extended to Stewart Knight for her expert preparation of this manuscript.

REFERENCES

1. Action Committee on Myelodysplasia: Current approaches to the evaluation and management of children with myelomeningocele, Pediatrics 63:663, 1979.
2. Adelman RD: Urinary tract infections in children. In Tune BM and Mendoza SA, editors: Pediatric nephrology, New York, 1984, Churchill-Livingstone, Inc.
3. Adelman RD: Neonatal hypertension. In Loggie JMH et al, editors: NHLBI workshop on juvenile hypertension, New York, 1983, Biomedical Information Corp.
4. Adelman RD: Long-term follow-up of neonatal renovascular hypertension, Pediatr Nephrol 1:35, 1987.
5. Arant BS: Renal disorders of the newborn infant. In Tune BM and Mendoza SA, editors: Pediatric nephrology, New York, 1984, Churchill-Livingstone, Inc.
6. Arant BS: Postnatal development of renal function during the first year of life, Pediatr Nephrol 1:308, 1987.
7. Barratt TM and Manzoni GA: The dilated urinary tract. In Holliday MA, Barratt TM, and Vermier RL, editors: Pediatric nephrology, ed 2, Baltimore, 1987, Williams & Wilkins.
8. Battle DC et al: The use of the urinary anion gap in the diagnosis of hyperchloremic metabolic acidosis, N Engl J Med 318:594, 1988.
9. Blyth H and Ockenden BG: Polycystic disease of the kidneys and liver presenting in childhood, J Med Genet 8:257, 1971.
10. Borzyskowski M and Mundy AR: Management of the neuropathic bladder in childhood, Pediatr Nephrol 2:56, 1988.

11. Boylan P and Parisi V: An overview of hydramnios, Semin Perinatol 10:136, 1986.

12. Carter BS et al: Prediction of perinatal asphyxial severity, Pediatr Res 20:376A, 1986.

13. Chan JCM: Renal tubular acidosis, J Pediatr 102:327, 1983.

14. Cohen C: Ethical and legal considerations in the care of the infant with end stage renal disease whose parents elect conservative therapy, Pediatr Nephrol 1:166, 1987.

15. Cole BR, Conley SB, and Stapleton SB: Polycystic kidney disease presenting in the first year of life, J Pediatr 111:693, 1987.

16. Conley SB: Supplemental nasogastric feedings in infants undergoing continuous peritoneal dialysis. In Fine R, editor: Chronic ambulatory peritoneal dialysis and chronic cycling peritoneal dialysis in children, Boston, 1987, Martinus Nijhoff, Publishers.

17. Conley SB et al: The outcome of end stage renal disease (ESRD) in children less than five years old. Presented at the Society for Pediatric Research, Washington, DC, May 1988.

18. deSwiet M, Fayers P, and Shinebourne EA: Systolic blood pressure in a population of infants in the first year of life: the Brompton study, Pediatrics 65:1028, 1980.

19. Edelmann CM Jr: Developmental renal physiology. In Gruskin AB and Norman ME, editors: Pediatric nephrology, Boston, 1980, Martinus Nijhoff, Publishers.

20. Elinder G et al: Development of glomerular filtration rate in excretion of beta 2 microglobulin in the neonate during gentamycin treatment, Acta Paediatr Scand 72:219, 1983.

21. Engle WD: Evaluation of renal function in acute renal failure in the neonate, Pediatr Clin North Am 33:129, 1986.

22. Fine RN and Gruskin AB, editors: End stage renal diseases in children, Philadelphia, 1984, WB Saunders Co.

23. Friedman AL and Hustead VA: Hypertension in babies following discharge from a neonatal intensive care unit, Pediatr Nephrol 1:30, 1987.

24. Glick PL et al: Management of the fetus with congenital hydronephrosis. II. Prognostic criteria and selection for treatment, J Pediatr Surg 20:376, 1985.

25. Golbus MS et al: Fetal urinary tract obstruction: management and selection for treatment, Semin Perinatol 9:91, 1985.

26. Gordon I and Barratt TM: Imaging the kidneys and urinary tract in the neonate with acute renal failure, Pediatr Nephrol 1:321, 1987.

27. Green TP et al: Furosemide promotes patent ductus arteriosus in premature infants with the respiratory distress syndrome, N Engl J Med 308:743, 1983.

28. Gruskin AB: Developmental aspects of peritoneal dialysis kinetics. In Fine R, editor: Chronic ambulatory peritoneal dialysis and chronic cycling peritoneal dialysis in children, Boston, 1987, Martinus Nijhoff, Publishers.

29. Guignard JP: Neonatal nephrology. In Holliday MA, Barratt TM, and Vernier RL, editors: Pediatric nephrology, ed 2, Baltimore, 1987, Williams & Wilkins.

30. Hellstrom M et al: Renal growth after neonatal urinary tract infection, Pediatr Nephrol 1:269, 1987.

31. Holliday MA: Developmental abnormalities of the kidney in children, Hosp Pract 13:101, 1978.

32. Hufnagle KG et al: Renal calcifications: a complication of long-term furosemide therapy in preterm infants, Pediatrics 70:360, 1982.

33. Kalia A et al: Renal transplantation in the infant and young child, Am J Dis Child 143:47, 1988.

34. Kao LC et al: Use of diuretics in bronchopulmonary dysplasia, Pediatrics 74:37, 1984.

35. Karlsson FA, Hardell LI, and Hellsing K: A prospective study of urinary proteins in early infancy, Acta Paediatr Scand 68:663, 1979.

36. Kohaut EC and Alexander S: Ultrafiltration in the young patient on CAPD. In Moncrief J and Popovich R, editors: CAPD update, New York, 1981, Masson Publishing, USA, Inc.

37. Kirks DR et al: Diagnostic imaging of pediatric abdominal masses: an overview, Radiol Clin North Am 19:527, 1981.

38. Kissane JM: Congenital malformations of the kidney. In Hamburger J, Crosnier T, and Gruenfeld JP, editors: Nephrology, New York, 1979, Wiley-Flammarion.

39. Lieberman K: Continuous arteriovenous hemofiltration in children, Pediatr Nephrol 1:330, 1987.

40. Lieberman K et al: Treatment of acute renal failure in an infant using continuous arteriovenous hemofiltration, J Pediatr 106:646, 1985.

41. Manning FA: Ultrasound in perinatal medicine. In Creasy RF and Resnik R, editors: Maternal and fetal medicine: principles and practice, Philadelphia, 1984, WB Saunders Co.

42. Matthew OP et al: Neonatal renal failure: usefulness of diagnostic indices, Pediatrics 65:57, 1980.

43. McGillivray BC and Hall JG: Nonimmune hydrops fetalis, Pediatr Rev 9:197, 1987.

44. McLean RH, Gearhart JP, and Jeffs R: Neonatal obstructive uropathy, Pediatr Nephrol 2:48, 1988.

45. Parkhouse H and Barrett JM: Investigation of the dilated urinary tract, Pediatr Nephrol 2:43, 1988.

46. Potter EL: Normal and abnormal development of the kidney, Chicago, 1972, Yearbook Medical Publishers, Inc.

47. Rasoulpour M and McLean RH: Renal venous thrombosis in neonates, Am J Dis Child 134:276, 1980.

48. Retik AB: Genitourinary problems in children, Hosp Pract 11:133, 1976.

49. Ronco C et al: Treatment of acute renal failure in newborns by continuous arteriovenous hemofiltration, Kidney Int 29:908, 1986.

50. Rotundo A et al: Progressive encephalopathy in children with chronic renal insufficiency in infancy, Kidney Int 21:489, 1982.

51. Roussan MS: Neurogenic bladder dysfunction, Med Times 109:43, 1981.

52. Salusky IB et al: Experience with continuous cycling peritoneal dialysis during the first year of life, Pediatr Nephrol 1:172, 1987.

53. Schwartz GJ, Feld LG, and Langford DJ: A simple estimate of glomerular filtration rate in full-term infants during the first year of life, J Pediatr 104:849, 1984.

54. Sertel H and Scopes J: Rates of creatinine clearance in babies less than one week of age, Arch Dis Child 48:717, 1973.

55. Siegel S and Oh W: Renal function as a marker of human fetal maturation, Acta Paediatr Scand 65:481, 1976.

56. Springate JE, Fildes RD, and Feld LG: Assessment of renal function in newborn infants, Pediatr Rev 9:51, 1987.

57. Stalker HP et al: Plasma renin activity in healthy children, J Pediatr 89:256, 1976.

58. Stapleton FB: Renal uric acid clearance in human neonates, J Pediatr 103:290, 1983.

59. Stapleton FB, Jones DP, and Green RS: Acute renal failure in neonates: incidence, etiology and outcome, Pediatr Nephrol 1:314, 1987.

60. Straub E and Spranger J: Etiology and pathogenesis of the prune belly syndrome, Kidney Int 20:695, 1981.

61. Tack ED, Perlman JM, and Robson AM: Renal injury in sick newborn infants: a prospective evaluation using urinary beta 2 microglobulin concentrations, Pediatrics 81:432, 1988.

62. Task Force on Blood Pressure Control in Children: Report of the Second Task Force on Blood Pressure Control in Children, 1987, Pediatrics 79:1, 1987.

63. Temple JK and Shapira E: Genetic determinants of renal disease in neonates, Clin Perinatol 8:361, 1981.

64. Warsof SL, Nicolaides KH, and Rodeck C: Immune and nonimmune hydrops, Clin Obstet Gynecol 29:533, 1986.

CHAPTER 20

Neurologic disorders

CHESTER J. MINARCIK, JR. ▪ PATRICIA BEACHY

The developing nervous system provides an ongoing challenge for researchers and clinicians alike. Investigation continues in a wide variety of areas, yet basic mechanisms for a pathophysiologic understanding of common events such as neonatal seizures and intraventricular hemorrhages remain unclear.

Improved neonatal care in recent years has not significantly reduced neurologic residua. How much of this is a reflection of sicker and more immature infants being salvaged is difficult to assess. Primary neurologic disease and secondary neurologic complications from such common conditions as cardiopulmonary disease, metabolic derangements, shock, infection, and coagulopathy still represent major problems encountered in every intensive care nursery.

Serious anomalies still appear with regularity, albeit in small numbers. Newly identified causes for malformations include isoretinoin and valproic acid. There appears to be an acquired immunodeficiency syndrome (AIDS) embryopathy.

This chapter deals with selected topics in neonatal neurology, including congenital malformations, trauma, seizures, and intraventricular hemorrhage. At the conclusion there is a section on early intervention and rehabilitation programs, which are widely used yet rarely assessed.

CONGENITAL MALFORMATIONS
Physiology, etiology, and clinical features

Congenital malformations of the nervous system occur when the usual sequence of maturation and development is interrupted (Table 20-1). By definition, the malformation is present at birth. Causes are multiple and largely unknown. Although strictly destructive lesions (such as hydranencephaly resulting from bilateral carotid artery occlusion) are separate from primary failures of morphogenesis, both may be included in the broad category of congenital malformations. The distinction between the two types lies in an understanding of the causes.

Understanding congenital malformations requires an appreciation of the normal embryologic sequence.[7,9,14] The clinical and pathologic identification of normal and abnormal structures allows for timing of the insult or developmental failure. Once timing is established, an appropriate search for the cause can be made.

NEURAL TUBE DEFECTS

At the end of the first embryonic week the *primitive streak* is present on the rostral surface of the embryo. A second streak, the *notochordal process,* develops alongside the primitive streak. The notochord is responsible for the induction of both the *neural plate* and the *neurenteric canal.* Cells proliferate along the lateral margin of the neural plate to form the *neural folds* around the central *neural groove.*

Cells at the apex of the neural folds comprise the *neural crest.* Schwann cells, piarachnoid cells, sensory ganglia, melanocytes, and various secretory cells arise from the neural crest. The neural folds meet and fuse with the rostral (anterior) and caudal (posterior) ends (neuropore), closing approximately by the end of the fourth embryonic week.

TABLE 20-1

Central Nervous System Development and Related Defects

MATURATIONAL PROCESS	TIME	ASSOCIATED DEFECTS
Neural tube defects (dorsal induction, neurulation)	3-4 weeks	Craniorrhachischisis Anencephaly Myeloschisis Encephalocele Myelomeningocele Arnold-Chiari malformation
Segmentation (ventral induction)	5-6 weeks	Cyclopia Holoprosencephaly Arhinencephaly Septo-optic dysplasia (?) Klippel-Feil syndrome (?) Platybasia (?) Sprengel's deformity (?)
Proliferation	2-4 months	Microcephaly Megacephaly Neurocutaneous syndromes (?)
Migration	3-5+ months	Scizencephaly Lissencephaly Pachygyria (macrogyria) Microgyria (polymicrogyria) Neuronal heterotopias
Neuronal organization and functional organization	6 months	Down's syndrome (?) Mental retardation (?) Genetic epilepsy (?)
Myelination	8 months	Congenital hypomyelination Anoxic/ischemic damage

Failure of development at this stage results in the defects of neurulation (or dorsal induction). The most severe of these defects is craniorrhachischisis, in which there is significant malformation of the brain (as in anencephaly), absence of the posterior skull, and an open spine the full length of the spinal cord.

Anencephaly is similar to craniorrhachischisis without the spinal defect. There is essentially no normal brain tissue above the brainstem and thalami, and parts of those structures are malformed.

Myeloschisis involves the failure of the posterior neural tube to close. No skull defect is present.

Encephaloceles are caused by a limited failure of closure at the rostral (head) end of the neural tube. Extensions of meninges or brain tissue through the skull may occur on the ventral or rostral surface.

Myelomeningoceles (or even the more limited meningoceles) are a limited form of myeloschisis with failure of closure at the caudal (tail) end of the neural tube. The Arnold-Chiari deformities are usually included here. These malformations, often seen with myelomeningoceles, involve structures of the brainstem and cerebellum. Generally, the cerebellar tonsils are pulled down through the foramen magnum, and the brainstem is elongated in later life. Hydrocephalus is common. Symptoms of brainstem involvement worsen. Open myelomeningoceles and anencephaly (any defect in which the spinal or cranial contents are "open" to the outside) will cause an elevation of alpha-feto-protein in the amniotic fluid. This is important in prenatal diagnosis.

SEGMENTATION DEFECTS

After closure of the neural tube, suprasegmental structures are formed. The divisions of the brain into hemispheres, formation of the ventricular system, and formation of the major gyral patterns are all part of this period of development. Major areas of the brain, including the cerebellum, basal ganglia, brainstem nuclei, thalamus, and hypothalamus, form at this time. Defects of segmentation and cleavage occur during this phase of neural development. For unknown reasons, defects of segmentation and cleavage are far less common than defects of neurulation. Since these malformations involve abnormalities of ventral induction rather than dorsal induction (such as neurulation), the face, eyes, nose, mouth, and hair are also involved in the malformation. These features should always be investigated carefully for specific anomalies.

Holoprosencephaly is characterized by a single, midline, lateral ventricle; incomplete or absent interhemispheric fissure; absent olfactory system; midfacial clefts; and hypotelorism. The most severe form of holoprosencephaly is cyclopia, a single fused midline eye and supraorbital proboscis. An intermediate form is cebocephaly, which is phenotypically like trisomy D.

Arhinencephaly involves aplasia of the olfactory bulbs and tracts.

When any of these malformations are suspected or when features suggestive of them are seen, careful examination of the hair, eyes, ears, mouth, and nose may reveal other related anomalies.

Septo-optic dysplasia, with blindness and diabetes insipidus, may also be a malformation in this group.

Certain malformations of the base of the skull, cervical spine, and upper cervical cord are also grouped here, although there is less evidence that their embryogenic cause is the same.

Malformations in this group include Klippel-Feil syndrome, platybasia, and Sprengel's deformity. These congenital malformations cause symptoms and signs related to the base of the skull and upper cervical spine. Short necks, restricted neck motion, and mirror movements of the upper extremities are commonly seen symptoms.

MIGRATION AND CORTICAL ORGANIZATIONAL DEFECTS

A critical aspect of brain development has yet to be described. The remaining development of the brain takes over twice as long as the previously described development and includes cellular proliferation, migration, organization, and myelination. The cells that later form the cerebral cortex begin in the germinal matrix (near the caudate nucleus around the lateral ventricles). These cells then migrate in a radial fashion to their final positions near the surface of the brain. Abnormalities of cellular migration result in collections of gray matter in unusual places (heterotopias), abnormal gyri and sulci, abnormal spaces in the brain, and frequent clinical signs of gray matter dysfunction. Frequently these clinical problems are not apparent in the newborn period. The malformations in this grouping show no characteristic cranial or somatic features, because the timing of the malformations is after the formation of large brain structures, divisions, and connections.[10]

Microcephaly can be understood as a malformation if the pathologic findings leading to microencephaly are taken into consideration. Numerous examples of microcephaly are seen in animal studies in which the animals are exposed to various therapeutic agents or are deprived of specific substances in their diets. When certain toxic substances are present or diet is inadequate, there is a failure of brain growth, resulting in microcephaly. Microcephaly may result from an overall decrease in the number of cells or may be the result of smaller cells. Synaptic connections are impaired, and clinical features that suggest an overall failure of brain development predominate.

Schizencephaly is a malformation in which atypical clefts, most often in the region of the sylvian fissure, are present within the brain substance. The clefts, covered only by meninges, may extend to the surface of the brain. Deep structures such as the thalamus and basal ganglia may be displaced.

Porencephaly is most often thought to be the result of destruction of previously normal tissue. Porencephaly is the occurrence of a cavity within the brain. This theory of porencephaly is confirmed by the identification of porencephalic cysts following strokes or meningitis. Porencephalies are more likely to communicate with the ventricles, whereas schizencephalies are more likely to communicate with the subarachnoid space.

The lissencephalic brain has a very smooth cortex with only a few small fissures and sulci. The brain is small, and the ventricles are enlarged. The organization of the cortex is abnormal with frequent heterotopias. Somatic anomalies (cardiac, renal, gastrointestinal, reproductive, and skeletal) may occasionally occur.

Macrogyria (pachygyria) may be a localized hemispheric malformation or a diffuse malformation. The involved gyri show large, abnormal neurons and dense gliosis. Unusually wide gyri with compressed sulci can be seen.

Microgyria or polymicrogyria occurs as a response to an arrest in neuronal maturation before the fifth gestational month. Cytomegalovirus and maternal carbon monoxide poisoning (at 20 to 24 weeks gestation) have been shown in some instances to produce this malformation, but most often the cause is unknown. Anatomically, areas of very small gyri are present in the involved area.

Agenesis of the corpus callosum most likely represents a midline anomaly and is often seen as a part of a more extensive malformation such as Aicardi's syndrome, in which agenesis of the corpus callosum is accompanied by a chorioretinitis and infantile spasms.

Schizencephaly and other malformations often have associated agenesis of the corpus callosum. In this malformation, there is a large subarachnoid space between the two hemispheres, and the lateral ventricles are displaced laterally (a commonly looked-for sign on a computed tomography (CT) scan). The third ventricle is often dilated. An X-linked form has been reported, but most cases are sporadic. Clinically, the X-linked cases generally show multiple neurologic problems, whereas the isolated malformations of the corpus callosum have been found incidentally at autopsy in patients in whom it was not at all suspect.

Migrational anomalies easily lead to problems of gray matter dysfunction. These problems include seizures, mental retardation, motor dysfunction (cerebral palsy), and sensory dysfunction (blindness or deafness). Common manifestations in the newborn period are seizures, microcephaly, small-for-gestational-age (SGA), abnormal cry, and abnormal transillumination. Findings that are present later in life and probably not seen in neonates are mental retardation and spasticity.

Clinical features of schizencephaly include seizures, retardation, spastic quadriparesis, or minimal findings.

Clinical features of porencephaly include seizures, motor problems, increased intracranial pressure if the cyst is enlarging, and abnormal transillumination if the cyst is superficial. On occasion, no symptoms are perceptible.

Clinical features of lissencephaly include seizures, microcephaly, abnormal cry, small-for-gestational age, polyhydramnios, micrognathia, downward-slanted palpebral fissures, anteverted nares, and prominent forehead and occiput. Later severe spasticity, hypsarrhythmia, and severe mental retardation may develop.

Clinical features of macrogyria include spastic hemiplegia or diplegia (depending on the site of involvement). If the area of involvement is very limited, there may be a paucity of findings. Clinical features of microgyria include ab-

sence of findings in the newborn period. Later spasticity and mental retardation are observable.

Signs and symptoms of absence of the corpus callosum are most often a result of associated malformations and anomalies. These include seizures, mental retardation, hydrocephalus, motor abnormalities, and asynchronous electroencephalogram.

ADDITIONAL DEFECTS

Cerebellar malformations are quite varied. Most often, at least a portion of the cerebellum is preserved, but total absence occurs. Hemispheric aplasia or vermal aplasia are seen, and familial forms have been reported. The Dandy-Walker cyst is another complex malformation involving the cerebellum. In it the fourth ventricle is dilated into a cystic structure. The foramina of Magendie and Lushka are atretic, and hydrocephalus results. The cerebellum is small and displaced upward. Associated anomalies include heterotopias, microgyria, agenesis of the corpus callosum, aqueductal stenosis, and syringomyelia. No specific causes are known. The differential diagnosis includes an arachnoid cyst of the posterior fossa. In the case of an arachnoid cyst, the fourth ventricle is not part of the malformation and is normal, although it may be displaced.

Clinical features of cerebellar malformations include absence of symptoms in the newborn period, cerebellar findings in family members (hypotonia, incoordination, and nystagmus), especially in vermal aplasia, or total absence of symptoms throughout life.

Clinical features of the Dandy-Walker cyst include frequent progressive hydrocephalus, associated malformations that cause additional specific symptoms, possible absence of symptoms in the newborn period, enlargement of the occipital shelf and posterior part of the skull, positive transillumination in a triangular shape, nystagmus, lateral gaze, palsy, abnormalities of respiratory control, and, later in life, ataxia.

Craniosynostosis is the abnormal fusion of the bones of the skull. The causes of this malformation are unknown. The premature closure of sutures may involve one or many sutures, with resulting deformity of the skull. Numerous terms are used to describe the shapes the skull assumes when craniosynostosis is present. Among these terms are plagiocephaly, scaphocephaly, dolichocephaly, keel-shaped deformity, and clover-leaf skull. Any of the atlases of human malformations give striking examples of these deformities.

Craniosynostosis should be suspected in the presence of microcephaly or a misshapen head. Appropriate evaluation requires x-ray films of the skull and a CT scan to define which if any of the sutures are stenosed and what problems might exist with brain structure (pressure or malformation).

Hydrocephalus may occur in many different situations from many separate causes. An inherited, X-linked form exists. Intrauterine infections are another cause. Hydrocephalus may be associated with many of the malformations listed above. Hydrocephalus results when the normal flow of ventriculospinal fluid is obstructed. This may be as the result of an atretic portion of the ventricular system, blockage from the outside, inflammation within the ventricular system causing a permanent blockage, or (very rarely) overproduction of ventriculospinal fluid. Therefore if the cause is an inflammatory process that caused degeneration and destruction of part of the ventricular pathway, hydrocephalus may at times be more appropriately categorized with the destructive lesions. These infectious processes may also be responsible for some of the cases of congenital porencephaly. Vascular occlusion is the other cause thought to be responsible for some malformations in the "destructive lesion" category, including cases of porencephaly, schizencephaly, and hydranencephaly.

Data collection

The diagnosis of malformations of the central nervous system (CNS) may be quite obvious (as in anencephaly) or totally unrecognized during life (as in some cases of agenesis of the corpus callosum). Careful examination of all newborns will result in the identification of most malformations. At times the diagnosis will be suspected not on the basis of the examination, but on the basis of an accompanying sign such as seizures.

When a congenital malformation is suspected, whether or not somatic signs are present, careful evaluation of the status of the CNS is in order. CT scanning is important for a better understanding of the intracranial structures, and electrophysiologic studies (electroencephalogram and evoked potentials) will help assess the functional aspects of the malformation. Clearly, there is no need for these studies in a seriously malformed infant who is not expected to survive.

Two very important tests have become available in recent years that allow for prenatal diagnosis of certain congenital malformations of the nervous system. Ultrasound examination (an abdominal ultrasound scan of the mother) provides an opportunity to identify certain malformations by viewing the fetus during development. Hydrocephalus, encephaloceles, myelomeningoceles, and anencephaly may be identified prenatally. Determination of alpha-fetoprotein in the amniotic fluid allows for the identification of anencephaly and open myelomeningoceles. A nonenclosed nervous system will cause a significant rise in alpha-fetoprotein in the amniotic fluid. Amniocentesis provides the amniotic fluid necessary for this determination. Testing of maternal serum for alpha-fetoprotein is less specific and more controversial. At the present time, the combination of ultrasound examination and amniocentesis provides the most helpful information.

Clinical signs and symptoms have been described for each individual nervous system malformation presented earlier in this chapter.

Treatment

Very limited treatment is available for congenital malformations of the nervous system. A variety of strategies are available for making efforts at reducing secondary complications or providing earlier management to handle these complications more efficiently.

The greatest efforts and accomplishments have been made for those with congenital malformations who might be expected to live productive lives. When secondary complications are managed appropriately, children with myelomeningoceles often become well-adjusted, productive adults. This is not possible when the malformation causes severe retardation.

Some of the malformations are lethal in a short period of time (anencephaly and hydranencephaly) making intervention unnecessary and inappropriate. When intervention results only in increased time of survival without any improvement in profound physical and mental handicaps, the desirability of intervention should be questioned.

Treatment of many of the malformations of the brain is limited to the management of the manifestations of the malformation. These would include seizures, hearing impairment, spasticity, and secondary orthopedic problems. Since the primary defect cannot be changed, it is important to recognize that for many of the conditions, substantial improvement cannot be hoped for.

In certain malformations some specific treatment is indicated. If the encephalocele is small and a large amount of the brain is not contained in the sac, the defect should be closed. Associated neurologic problems such as seizures should be treated.

When treatment is thought to be appropriate, closure of the myelomeningocele should be performed as soon as possible. In this way, the risk of meningitis and ventriculitis can be reduced. Untreated infants often die within the first year of life. Soon after closure of the primary defect, many infants develop hydrocephalus or experience a more severe case of antecedent hydrocephalus. Shunting then becomes necessary. (See boxed material on p. 507 for care of the infant with a ventriculoperitoneal shunt.)

The only situation in which microcephaly could be considered treatable is total craniosynostosis. Generally, skull deformity is also present in these infants with craniosynostosis, but it is always wise to consider the possibility of craniosynostosis in any infant with a small head.

If present, total craniosynostosis should be treated surgically.

The management of congenital hydrocephalus consists primarily of early shunting, as soon after birth as possible. Experimental procedures with fetal surgery in the early 1980s,

---

VENTRICULOPERITONEAL SHUNT

Purpose: To drain excess cerebrospinal fluid (CSF) from the ventricles into the peritoneum in order to relieve intracranial pressure, prevent further damage to the brain, and promote optimal outcome.

I. Positioning
   A. Place an unaffected side (may position on shunt side with "donut" over operative site once incision has healed). Keep head of bed flat to 15° to 30° to prevent too-rapid fluid loss.
   B. Support head carefully when moving infant.
   C. Turn q.2h. from unaffected side of head to back.
II. Shunt site
   A. Use strict aseptic technique when changing dressing.
   B. Pump shunt if and only as directed by neurosurgeon.
   C. Observe for fluid leakage around pump.
III. Observe and document all intake and output. Watch for symptoms of excessive drainage of CSF:
   A. Sunken fontanel
   B. Increased urine output
   C. Increased sodium loss
IV. Observe, document, and report any seizure activity or paresis.
V. Observe for signs of ileus:
   A. Abdominal distention (serially measure abdominal girth)
   B. Absence of bowel sounds
   C. Loss of gastric content by emesis or through orogastric tube
VI. Perform range-of-motion exercises to all extremities.

VII. Observe and assess for symptoms of increased intracranial pressure (shunt failure):
   A. Increasing head circumference (measure head daily)
   B. Full and/or tense fontanel
   C. Sutures palpably more separated
   D. High-pitched, shrill cry
   E. Irritability/sleeplessness
   F. Vomiting
   G. Poor feeding
   H. Nystagmus
   I. Sunset sigh of eyes
   J. Shiny scalp with distended vessels
   K. Hypotonia/hypertonia
VIII. Observe and assess for signs of infection:
   A. Redness or drainage at shunt site
   B. Hypothermia/hyperthermia
   C. Lethargy/irritability
   D. Poor feeding/weight gain
   E. Pallor
IX. Parent teaching
   A. Teach parents and give written copy of signs and symptoms of increased intracranial pressure, infection, and dehydration.
   B. Emphasize importance of notifying physician for any signs and symptoms.
   C. Demonstrate and receive return demonstration of proper head positioning (at rest, lifting, and carrying).
   D. Demonstrate and receive return demonstration of drug administration. Teach parents side effects of medications.
   E. Emphasize importance of follow-up medical care for assessment and medication adjustment.

including fetal ventriculostomy and multiple ventricular taps, held promise for earlier treatment of hydrocephalus.

Outcome was variable, and the procedures were not as reliable as hoped. It was not always possible to distinguish true hydrocephalus from ventriculomegaly without increased pressure. Shunting soon after birth often produces a far better outcome than would be assumed, with minimal motor deficit and only a mild to moderate deficit in intellect.

Monitoring of pregnancies with fetal ultrasound allows for the detection of congenital hydrocephalus. Induction of lung maturation with steroids has been suggested to allow a preterm delivery (with a smaller head) without excessive pulmonary complications. In this way, a permanent shunt can be placed sooner than with term delivery.[4]

Complications

Many of the expected complications are dealt with previously in the sections describing the malformations and their associated problems. It is difficult to separate true complications from problems occurring by nature of the malformation. For example, hydrocephalus following closure of a myelomeningocele is not truly a complication of the procedure or the disease but merely a condition brought out by the procedure.

Malformations carry with them disturbed anatomy and physiology that are reflected in abnormal function. General problems commonly encountered are seizures, retardation, sensorimotor abnormalities, disturbances in primary sensory function such as vision and hearing, orthopedic problems, and vegetative functions. Often the problems are multiple.

The problems encountered are ordinarily explainable on the basis of the malformation. Midline defects in the brain (particularly at the base of the brain) will often have clinical problems involving the hypothalamus. Difficulties in temperature regulation and appetite are seen. If the pituitary gland itself is involved, thyroid and adrenal function may be abnormal, and diabetes insipidis may be present. To some extent, the anatomy predicts the kinds of problems encountered. Involvement of the cortex causes seizures, retardation, and sensorimotor problems. White matter damage can cause spasticity. If the brainstem participates in the malformation, apnea, deafness, sleep disturbance, oculomotor disturbances, and problems with suck and swallowing may be seen. Spinal cord lesions cause quadriplegia or paraplegia. Genitourinary problems and to a lesser extent gastrointestinal problems are also seen.

Apnea and other brainstem findings may occur when the malformation involves the brainstem, as in Arnold-Chiari deformities, Dandy-Walker cysts, occipital encephaloceles, and arachnoid cysts.

Pituitary-hypothalamic dysfunction may manifest itself in impaired temperature regulation, thyroid abnormalities, diabetes insipidus, and adrenal insufficiency.

Most of the complications occur after the newborn period, although the causes are already present at birth. These include seizures, retardation, spasticity, genitourinary problems, and orthopedic problems. In many of these circumstances the problem is already present, but the functional expression, such as ambulation, retardation, and deafness, is lacking. In the infant's follow-up examinations careful attention must be given to those problems likely to develop or intensify with age. When a specific malformation is identified, it is necessary to become familiar with the anticipated problems not only to anticipate them as they appear, but also to lessen any secondary damage that might occur if they go unrecognized.

Parent teaching

Infants with congenital malformations present such a complex variety of problems that parent teaching needs to begin as early as possible. Often parents will know from the time of birth or earlier that a major problem exists. In other circumstances the anomaly will only be detected after appropriate studies are performed.

When nonviability is expected, care should be directed to the emotional needs of the family. There will be questions about etiology and genetics, and these should be dealt with according to the family's wishes.

If serious handicaps are expected and the infant is expected to survive, the parents should be encouraged to participate in the care of the infant from the beginning. Not only will the adjustment occur more easily, but the important aspects of care in special circumstances will be learned more effectively. The social service, nursing, psychologic, and parent education resources of the hospital will be needed. Parent teaching must be individualized according to the anomaly. There may be support groups or specialized clinics available to help not only in the aftercare, but also in parent education.

Parent teaching for the mothers and fathers of infants with congenital anomalies should be started early, involve the parents in the care of the infant, use the resources of the hospital for specialized help, and continue after the baby has gone home from the hospital.

BIRTH INJURIES
Physiology and etiology

Birth injuries (birth trauma) are the direct result of difficulties encountered during the delivery process. They may be minor injuries without expected sequelae or may be the direct cause of death in the neonatal period. Classification of birth injuries are usually etiologic (predisposing factors or mechanisms of injury) or anatomic. An anatomic classification is used in this discussion to illustrate the commonly encountered problems (Table 20-2).

The timing of birth injuries can be used to describe causes. Etiologic classification of birth injuries include uterine injury (antenatal), fetal monitoring procedures, abnormal or difficult presentations, methods of delivery, and multifactorial injuries. It should be recognized that the same injury might be caused in several ways. Thus a cephalhematoma could be the result of forceps delivery or vacuum extraction. A variety of specific predisposing factors increase the risk for birth injury:

1. Macrosomia
2. Cephalopelvic disproportion
3. Dystocia
4. Prematurity

TABLE 20-2

Anatomic Classification of Birth Injuries

SITE OF INJURY	TYPE OF INJURY
Scalp	Caput succedaneum
	Subgaleal hemorrhage
	Cephalhematoma
Skull	Linear fracture
	Depressed fracture
	Occipital osteodiastasis
Intracranial	Epidural hematoma
	Subdural hematoma (laceration of falx, tentorium, or superficial veins)
	Subarachnoid hemorrhage
	Cerebral contusion
	Cerebellar contusion
	Intracerebellar hematoma
Spinal cord (cervical)	Vertebral artery injury
	Intraspinal hemorrhage
	Spinal cord transection or injury
Plexus injuries	Erb's palsy
	Klumpke's paralysis
	Total (mixed) brachial plexus injury
	Horner's syndrome
	Diaphragmatic paralysis
	Lumbosacral plexus injury
Cranial and peripheral nerve injuries	Radial nerve palsy
	Medial nerve palsy
	Sciatic nerve palsy
	Laryngeal nerve palsy
	Diaphragmatic paralysis
	Facial nerve palsy

5. Prolonged or precipitous labor
6. Breech presentation
7. Forceps usage
8. Rotation of fetus
9. Version and extraction
10. Handling following delivery

Multiple factors are often present. When multiple predisposing factors are present, they are often caused by a single underlying maternal disease. A common example would be a premature, macrosomic fetus with a diabetic mother in whom labor is not progressing properly.

The common factors that are present in deliveries complicated by birth injuries are:

1. **Unusual progress of labor**
2. **Unusual size or shape to the fetus (large-for-gestational age and hydrocephalus)**
3. **Problems encountered during delivery (dystocia and forceps application)**
4. **Unusual or unexpected presentations (breech or unexpected twin)**

The maternal history must always be studied for the underlying disease process or conditions that might increase the risk for a birth injury.

Prevention

Most birth injuries may be preventable, at least in theory. Careful attention to risk factors and the appropriate planning of delivery should reduce the incidence of birth injuries to a minimum. Transabdominal ultrasonography allows for pre-delivery awareness of macrosomia, hydrocephalus, and unusual presentations. Particular pregnancies may then be delivered by controlled elective cesarean section to avoid significant birth injury. Care must be taken to avoid substituting a procedure of greater risk. Often a small percentage of significant birth injuries cannot be anticipated until the specific circumstances are encountered during delivery. Emergency cesarean section may provide last-minute salvage, but in these circumstances the injury may truly be unavoidable.

Specific birth injuries
INJURIES TO THE SCALP

The three commonly encountered forms of extracranial hemorrhage (caput succedaneum, subgaleal hemorrhage, and cephalhematoma) are distinguished not only in clinical manifestations, but also in pathophysiology. These three extracranial scalp injuries are included with neurologic birth injuries not because they have associated neurologic problems, but because the question of possible neurologic involvement is often raised by the family or health care providers.

PHYSIOLOGY AND ETIOLOGY. The caput succedaneum is caused by trauma to the scalp, usually during a routine, vertex, vaginal delivery. The caput is the result of hemorrhagic edema superficial to the aponeurosis of the scalp. Spread of the edema is therefore not restricted to suture lines and is soft and pitting because of its superficial location.

Subgaleal hemorrhage is caused by forces that compress and then drag the head through the pelvic outlet. Significant acute blood loss can occur with shock as the presenting symptom. Bleeding may continue after birth with enlargement of the accumulated blood and dissection of the blood along tissue planes into the neck. Such a hemorrhage carries the greatest potential for complications, but fortunately it is the least common form of birth injury to the scalp.

Cephalhematoma is a subperiosteal collection of blood. The cause is uncertain, but its occurrence is more common in primiparous women and in forceps delivery. Males are generally more likely to be affected than females. The firm, tense collection of blood may increase in size after birth, but significant blood loss does not occur.

DATA COLLECTION. With caput succedaneum, physical examination reveals soft, pitting edema that is diffuse and crosses suture lines. There is no need for laboratory tests.

Because the subgaleal collection of blood is under the aponeurosis connecting the occipito-frontalis muscle and superficial to the peri-

osteum, subgaleal hemorrhage crosses suture lines. It is firm but fluctuant to palpation. Vital signs should be carefully monitored for symptoms of shock. The hematocrit should be serially followed, and bilirubin levels should be determined during recovery.

Cephalhematoma may occur anywhere but is most commonly found in the parietal area on one side. Because the location of the blood is subperiosteal, it is confined by suture lines. Symptoms are normally absent. A skull fracture underlying the cephalhematoma is present in 10% to 25% of affected infants. X-ray examination of the skull defines the fracture. An occipital cephalhematoma may be mistaken for an occipital encephalocele. Lack of resolution and associated neurologic deficit aids in distinguishing the more severe pathologic process.

TREATMENT. No treatment is required for any of these three lesions. In subgaleal hemorrhage, treatment of blood loss and shock may be necessary. During resolution the breakdown of the blood may cause hyperbilirubinemia requiring treatment.

PARENT TEACHING. Careful preparation of the parents for the acute side effects of subgaleal hemorrhage is important. Parents should be warned of the possibility of swelling and discoloration of the face, head, and neck. Parents can ignore a cephalhematoma unless localized changes occur, suggesting secondary infection (erythema, induration, or drainage). Cephalhematoma may be evident for 6 to 8 weeks.

SKULL FRACTURES

Three forms of skull fracture should be identified and differentiated: linear fractures, depressed fractures, and occipital osteodiastasis.

PHYSIOLOGY AND ETIOLOGY. Linear skull fracture is the most common type of skull fracture. The result of compression of the skull during delivery, a linear skull fracture most often has no associated injuries and causes no symptoms.

Bleeding may be seen extracranially (common) or intracranially (rare). Intracranial bleeding causes symptoms referable to the bleeding rather than to the fracture itself.

The typical depressed skull fracture is of the "ping-pong" type, an indentation without loss of bony continuity. Forceps are usually the direct cause of injury, which most often is without complication or sequelae. When neurologic signs are present, direct cerebral injury, intracranial bleeding, or free bone fragments should be suspected.

Occipital osteodiastasis is a traumatic separation of the squamous and lateral portions of the occipital bone. It is identified only by autopsy, and posterior fossa subdural hematoma, brainstem compression, and cerebral contusion are common associated injuries.

DATA COLLECTION. A linear skull fracture usually has no signs or symptoms unless intracranial bleeding has occurred. Skull x-ray films most frequently demonstrate a parietal fracture. A depressed skull fracture is usually a palpable "ping-pong" fracture in the parietal area. No other signs and symptoms are present unless they are caused by intracranial bleeding or focal irritation of the cortex. Evaluation with a skull x-ray examination or CT scan is necessary to delineate the fracture and to identify complications.

TREATMENT. No treatment has been developed for a linear skull fracture. The controversy over treatment of a depressed skull fracture centers around the mode of treatment and the necessity for treatment. If free bone fragments are identified, neurosurgical intervention is required. More conservative approaches are indicated when no complications are present. Vacuum extractors and breast pumps have been used with variable success.

COMPLICATIONS. With a linear skull fracture the single complication to be aware of is a "growing" skull fracture. A dural tear may allow leptomeninges to extrude into the fracture site, setting up the possibility of a leptomeningeal cyst. As the cyst enlarges, the edges of the fracture may fail to fuse and even spread apart, giving the appearance of a "growing" fracture. Palpation and x-ray examination demonstrate the lesion. Surgical correction may be required to ensure healing and prevent further complications. With a depressed skull fracture intracranial bleeding and direct cerebral injury with seizures or residual neurologic deficit are rare.

PARENT TEACHING. Parents should be instructed to have the fracture site checked for several months to ensure that reunion of the bone has taken place. Patients will have no other aftercare unless neurosurgical intervention was necessary or complications developed.

INTRACRANIAL BIRTH INJURIES

Three major forms of bleeding occur intracranially: epidural hematoma, subdural hemorrhage, and subarachnoid hemorrhage. Added to these are cerebellar hemorrhages, cerebellar contusions, and cerebral contusions. Each has its own particular set of symptoms and signs, and complications and sequelae. Intraventricular hemorrhage is usually not related to trauma and is covered separately in this chapter.

PHYSIOLOGY AND ETIOLOGY. Epidural hematoma is pathophysiologically difficult to form in newborns because of a relatively thick dura. When present, it is almost always accompanied by a linear skull fracture across the middle meningeal artery.

Subdural hemorrhage is more common in term infants than in preterm infants and occurs from trauma tearing veins and venous sinuses. Four major pathologic entities are defined: laceration of the tentorium, laceration of the falx, laceration of the superficial cerebral vein, and occipital osteodiastasis. Tentorial laceration causes a posterior fossa clot with compression of the brainstem. The straight sinus, Galen's vein, lateral sinus, and infratentorial veins may be involved.

Laceration of the falx is caused by rupture of the inferior sagittal sinus. The laceration usually occurs at the junction of the tentorium and the falx, and the clot appears in the longitudinal cerebral fissure over the corpus callosum. Laceration of superficial cerebral veins causes subdural bleeding over the convexity of the brain. Subarachnoid bleeding or contusion of the brain may also be present.

Subarachnoid hemorrhage is the most common type of neonatal intracranial hemorrhage. In term infants trauma is the most common cause, whereas in preterm infants hypoxia is more often the cause. Small hemorrhages are more common than massive ones and usually result from venous bleeding. Underlying contusion may occur.

Cerebral contusion is uncommon as an isolated event. Focal blunt trauma is necessary to produce a contusion. Pathologically, focal areas of hemorrhage and necrosis are seen. Shearing forces may cause slitlike tears in the white matter.

Cerebellar contusion and intracerebellar hemorrhage are uncommon events generally seen in association with occipital osteodiastasis and infratentorial subdural hemorrhage. These are catastrophic events, as described previously, and most often result in the death of the patient.

DATA COLLECTION. For epidural hemorrhage the signs and symptoms may be diffuse (increased intracranial pressure with a bulging fontanel) or focal or lateralizing seizures, eye deviation, and hemisyndromes. Laboratory tests should include x-ray examination to look for fractures and CT scanning to identify bleeding.

Infants with subdural hemorrhage are neurologically abnormal at birth. Tentorial lacerations and laceration of the falx tend to produce signs by pressure on the brainstem. These signs include skew deviation of the eyes, apnea, coma, or unequal pupils. Nuchal rigidity and opisthotonos are signs of progressive herniation. Signs and symptoms of subdural hemorrhage from laceration of the superficial cere-

bral veins are variable. Small clots may produce no identifiable dysfunction. Typical symptoms are those of focal or lateralized cerebral dysfunction, although increased intracranial pressure may occur. CT scans including views of the posterior fossa should be obtained immediately when a subdural hemorrhage is suspected.

With subarachnoid hemorrhage underlying contusions may cause focal neurologic signs. Often no significant increase in intracranial pressure is found acutely. Irritability and a depressed level of consciousness may persist. Seizures are frequent in term infants, whereas apnea is common in preterm infants. Useful laboratory data include lumbar puncture and CT scan results. Focal signs predominate in cerebral contusions.

TREATMENT. Surgical evacuation of epidural and subdural clots may be necessary as emergency procedures. Subdural taps may be useful in the symptomatic infant with subdural bleeding from laceration of superficial cerebral veins. Many infants with intracranial bleeding may require treatment of seizures.

COMPLICATIONS. The complications of epidural hemorrhage range from none to permanent neurologic deficits with or without seizure. Sequelae of subdural hemorrhage occur in 20% to 25% of affected infants. The most common sequelae are focal neurologic signs. Seizures and hydrocephalus are seen less often. Hydrocephalus is the major potential complication of subarachnoid hemorrhage and directly alters outcome. If hydrocephalus is not present, as many as 90% of affected infants are normal at follow-up. Only 35% to 50% of those in whom hydrocephalus develops will be normal.

PARENT TEACHING. Since the long-term outcome is variable and may be abnormal even in infants normal at the time they leave the nursery, parent teaching must be individualized. The need for appropriate follow-up and intervention must be emphasized. Referral to appropriate support groups may also be helpful.

SPINAL CORD INJURIES

PHYSIOLOGY AND ETIOLOGY. Injuries to the spinal cord (usually the cervical portion) are most often seen in complicated breech deliveries. Before cesarean sections were performed routinely for breech delivery, fatal attempts to deliver vaginally were often associated with interspinal hemorrhage. The breech presentation in conjunction with a hyperextended head is the most dangerous situation and is worsened by a depressed fetus. Traction, rotation, and torsion cause mechanical strain on the vertebral column. Cephalic deliveries are not entirely safe; because of the difference in mechanical forces, a different clinical picture is seen with a higher lesion.

DATA COLLECTION. Clinical manifestations depend on the severity and location of the injury. Clinical syndromes include stillbirth or rapid neonatal death, respiratory failure, and spinal shock syndrome. High cervical cord injuries are more likely to cause stillbirths or rapid death of the neonate. Lower lesions cause an acute cord syndrome. Common signs of spinal shock include flaccid extremities (may just involve the lower extremities if the cervical cord is spared), a sensory level, diaphragmatic breathing, paralyzed abdominal movements, atonic anal sphincter, and distended bladder. Useful laboratory tests include myelography, a CT scan of the spine, and somatosensory-evoked potentials to help determine the extent and site of the lesion. The differential diagnosis includes dysraphism, neuromuscular disease, and cord tumors.

COMPLICATIONS. After the acute phase, chronic lesions include cysts, vascular occlusions, adhesions, and necrosis of the spinal cord. Flaccid or spastic quadriplegia is expected. Some infants with spinal cord injuries will be respiratory dependent. Bowel and bladder problems will continue.

PARENT TEACHING. Parents need to understand fully the implications of severe injury to the spinal cord. Recovery is frequently minimal to nonexistent. Continued specialized care may be required, including ventilator therapy. The overwhelming implications for the family cannot be emphasized strongly enough.

PLEXUS INJURIES

PHYSIOLOGY AND ETIOLOGY. Plexus injuries occur much more commonly than cord injuries and result from lateral traction on the shoulder (vertex deliveries) or the head (breech deliveries). Most often a depressed fetus or dystocia from a large baby is a contributing factor. Inappropriate augmentation of labor is another possible additive cause. Estimates of the incidences of brachial plexus injuries range from 0.5 to 1.9 per 1000 live births. Extremely mild cases may have undetectable findings and may remain unidentified.

Pathologic changes range from edema and hemorrhage of the nerve sheath to actual avulsion of the nerve root from the spinal cord. Of the reported cases of plexus injuries, 90% involve the C5-7 nerve roots and are classified as Erb's palsy. In a small minority of cases, the C4 nerve root is also affected, causing diaphragmatic problems. The site of injury in Erb's palsy is Erb's point where C5 and C6 nerve roots join to form the upper trunk. Total brachial plexus palsy occurs in 8% to 9% of the cases and has findings referable to C5 to T1 (and possibly C4). When T1 is involved, the sympathetic fibers become affected with an ipsilateral Horner's syndrome (ptosis, anhydrosis, and miosis) and possible delay in pigmentation of the iris. Less than 2% of the cases have Klumpke's paralysis involving only C8 to T1. In this form the site of pathologic conditions is the point at which C8 to T1 join to form the lower trunk.

DATA COLLECTION. Signs of brachial plexus palsies vary somewhat, most often because of overlap of the pure clinical syndromes. Shoulder and arm findings are characteristic of a true Erb's palsy. Involvement of the hand and fingers is seen in total forms or Klumpke's paralysis. Table 20-3 lists the specific cord levels involved in various functions that might be addressed.

TABLE 20-3

Brachial Plexus Examination: Distinguishing Features

PART EXAMINED	SPINAL LEVEL
Diaphragm movement (downward)	C4 (C3-5)
Deltoid muscle	C5
Spinatus muscle	C5
Biceps muscle	C5-6
Brachioradialis muscle	C5-6
Supinator of arm	C5-6
Biceps tendon reflex	C5-6
Wrist extensors	C6-7
Long extensor of the digits	C6-7
Triceps tendon reflex	C6-7
Wrist flexors	C7-8, T1
Finger flexors	C7-8, T1
Dilator of iris	T1
Eyelid elevator (full elevation)	T1
Moro reflex (shoulder abduction)	C5
Moro reflex (hand motion)	C8-T1
Palmar grasp	C8-T1

Evaluation of diaphragmatic function by x-ray examination is at times necessary. Myelography may be required to identify nerve root avulsion, which generally should be suspected when recovery does not occur. Electromyography often shows abnormalities early in the course of the injury, suggesting that the process may actually have begun in the last weeks of pregnancy rather than at the time of delivery.

Clinical syndromes of plexus injuries include Erb's palsy, total palsy, and Klumpke's paralysis. Erb's palsy accounts for about 90% of plexus injuries. It involves the upper part of the plexus, C5-7 and occasionally C4. The shoulder and upper arm are involved, and the biceps reflex is decreased. When C4 is involved, diaphragmatic dysfunction is present.

Total palsy occurs in 8% to 9% of the cases. Plexus involvement is diffuse (C5 to T1 and occasionally C4). The upper and lower arm and hand are involved. Horner's syndrome (ptosis, anhydrosis, and miosis) exists when T1 is involved. The diaphragm is affected when C4 is

involved. Biceps and triceps reflexes are decreased.

Klumpke's paralysis is seen in less than 2% of cases. The lower part of the plexus, C8 to T1, is involved. The lower arm and hand are involved. T1 involvement is associated with Horner's syndrome. Triceps reflex is decreased.

TREATMENT. Treatment should include immobilization for 7 to 10 days. Finger and wrist splints may be necessary. Passive range-of-motion exercises follow, and then gradual increase of activity to the affected limb is permitted.

COMPLICATIONS. Associated trauma may occur and should be carefully investigated. Common associated injuries include clavicular fracture, shoulder dislocation, cord injury, facial nerve injury, and humeral fracture. Full recovery of plexus function is seen in 85% to 95% of cases in the first year of life.

PARENT TEACHING. Parents should be taught passive range-of-motion exercises to encourage mobility and prevent contractures. Instructions should begin before discharge from the hospital. Most often the instructions are given by a neonatal nurse or an occupational or physical therapist.

Parents may equate the presence of a brachial plexus injury with poor obstetric care. Most often this will not be the case. The awareness of early changes on electromyography should be used to help families understand that the factors causing injury to the plexus may begin long before the onset of labor.

CRANIAL AND PERIPHERAL NERVE INJURIES

Median and sciatic nerve injuries are usually postnatal and result from brachial and radial artery punctures (median nerve) and inferior gluteal artery spasm (umbilical artery line drug instillation). Recovery is variable.

Median nerve palsy is manifested by decreased pincer grasp, decreased thumb strength, and the continuous flexed position of the fourth finger. Sciatic nerve palsy is manifested by decreased hip abduction and decreased distal joint movement. Hip adduction, flexion, and rotation are normal, since they are controlled by the femoral and obturator nerves.

Radial nerve damage is usually seen in conjunction with a humeral fracture. Prolonged labor is normally present. Congenital bands may also be causative. Recovery takes place in weeks to months.

Radial nerve palsy is manifested by wrist drop (decreased finger and wrist extension) and normal grasp.

Laryngeal nerve palsy may be seen in conjunction with facial or diaphragmatic paralysis. If the paralysis is unilateral, a hoarse cry may be heard. Bilateral involvement causes breathing to be difficult and the vocal cords to remain closed in the midline. It is important to rule out intrinsic brainstem disease. Often the presence of other brainstem findings such as oculomotor problems, apnea, or facial palsy will help clarify this. Evoked potentials, both brainstem auditory and somatosensory, may also help rule out brainstem involvement.

Laryngeal nerve palsy is manifested by difficulty in swallowing (superior branch), difficulty in breathing (bilateral), and difficulty in vocalizing (recurrent branch). Also, the head is held high and flexed laterally with slight rotation.

Diaphragmatic paralysis is most often seen in association with plexus injuries (80% to 90% have an associated plexus injury) and has the same cause. Some series have a mortality of 10% to 20%. Other patients recover fully in 6 to 12 months. Treatment has consisted of using rocking beds, electric pacing of the diaphragm, continuous positive airway pressure, respirators, or plication. Since diaphragmatic paralysis may occur in other conditions such as myotonic dystrophy, attention to the differential diagnosis is important, particularly when an associated brachial plexus problem is not present.

Diaphragmatic paralysis is demonstrated by respiratory difficulty in the first few hours of life. X-ray film shows elevation of the hemidiaphragm with paradoxical movement that may disappear on positive end expiratory pressure or continuous positive airway pressure.

Facial palsy may be part of intrinsic brainstem disease (see previous discussion of laryngeal nerve palsy) or other conditions such as Möbius syndrome, myotonic dystrophy, or facial muscle agenesis. When it is traumatic in origin, facial palsy is thought to be caused by the position of the face on the sacral promontory at the exit of the nerve from the stylomastoid foramen. It is debatable whether forceps delivery increases the incidence. Normally, both the upper (temporofacial) and lower (cervicofacial) branches are involved. Known complications (from lack of total resolution) include contractures and synkinesis. Cosmetic surgical procedures are occasionally necessary but are often delayed for years.

Facial palsy is seen on the left side in 75% of cases. Features include a widened palpebral fissure, flat nasolabial fold, and decreased facial expression.

NEONATAL SEIZURES
Physiology

Seizures are signs of malfunctioning neuronal systems. It is most useful to think of a localized or generalized loss of inhibitory control as the source of the seizure activity. This inhibitory loss may be the result of damage to the developing brain or transient effects such as disturbances in blood flow, glucose availability, or hypoxia. These disturbances may cause paroxysmal electrical activity recorded as seizures on the electroencephalogram (EEG). Ordinarily there are clinical signs that mimic what might, under other circumstances, be normal brain activity but, in the context of the seizure, cause stereotyped, repetitive, and inappropriate activity.

Seizures may be the only manifestation of brain dysfunction, but this is extremely uncommon in the neonate. Most often seizures in the newborn period are the result of a very significant brain insult; the clinical signs of the insult are multiple.

Etiology and data collection

Neonatal seizures may be caused by a variety of acute and chronic stresses on the brain. Table 20-4 lists the general groups of causes of neonatal seizures. The search for a cause proceeds in an orderly, methodic way. Most often the known history of perinatal problems will narrow the differential diagnosis to one or two likely causes. Acute metabolic changes that are likely to cause seizures should be rapidly investigated first.

Sepsis should never be overlooked as a potential cause. The infectious agent (meningitis, encephalitis, empyema, abscess, septic thrombosis, and ventriculitis) may directly affect the CNS. Systemic infection may cause seizures through the complication of shock, coagulopathy, impaired oxygenation, and multisystem organ failure. When the cerebrospinal fluid is examined, not only will the changes associated with infection be identified, but evidence of bleeding (red blood cells) or cell destruction (protein) may also be found.

Structural studies are routinely performed as part of the evaluation. Presently, the most useful studies are CT scans and ultrasound examination.

The infant's history should be carefully reviewed to narrow the possible causes to the most likely ones. Physical examination may further narrow the differential diagnosis. Once these are quickly repeated, blood should be drawn for arterial blood gases, electrolytes, glucose, calcium, and magnesium.

Appropriate cultures, aerobic and anaerobic, must be obtained. Usual culture sites or specimens include blood, urine, spinal fluid, tracheal aspirate, and surface. The cerebrospinal fluid should be examined for red blood cells and white blood cells, organisms (Gram's stain), protein, sugar, and resting opening pressure.

Ultrasound examinations are particularly useful for identifying and following intraventricular bleeding and hydrocephalus. The in-

fant is exposed to no radiation, either immediate or long-term; no complications, either immediate or long-term, have been identified.

TABLE 20-4

Common Causes of Neonatal Seizures

Acute metabolic conditions	Hypocalcemia Hypoglycemia; hyperglycemia Hypomagnesemia Pyridoxine dependency or deficiency Hyponatremia; hypernatremia
Inherited metabolic conditions	Maple syrup urine disease Nonketonic hyperglycemia Hyperprolinemia Galactosemia Urea cycle abnormalities Organic acidemias
Infections	Viral encephalitis, herpes, or enterovirus Congenital infections Bacterial meningitis Sepsis Brain abscess Septic venous thrombosis
Intracranial hemorrhage	Subdural hematoma Cerebral contusion Subarachnoid hemorrhage Epidural hemorrhage Intraventricular hemorrhage

Hypoxic ischemia
Congenital malformations
Neonatal drug withdrawal (e.g., opiates)
Kernicterus
Specific nongenetic syndromes
Benign familial neonatal seizures

The test may be repeated as often as needed and is usually performed at the bedside.

Although it provides better resolution for identifying subtle changes in brain structure, a CT scan exposes the developing brain to significant radiation. The larger the number of "cuts" made, the greater the exposure. The exact amount of radiation varies with the type of machine and length of the study. Short-term effects have not been detected, but the potential for long-term or cumulative effects of radiation exposure has not been determined. In addition, the use of contrast media is often essential for a complete study. This may be contraindicated in newborns with impaired renal function or in those with delicate fluid balance.

Although they provide interesting and helpful information in older patients with seizures, newer imaging techniques such as positron emission tomography have not been widely applied to newborns except as research. The potential hazards of isotopic scanning need further study before positron emission tomography can be put to general use in newborns.

Magnetic resonance imaging produces exceptional detail and is sensitive to changes in cellular composition. Presently the studies often require greater than an hour's time, limiting their practicality in the sick newborn.

CLINICAL SEIZURE TYPES

The application of technology used in the assessment of patients with epilepsy has finally been applied to neonates experiencing seizures. Simultaneous EEG and video recording allow for the accurate diagnosis of difficult-to-assess subtle behaviors, apneic and bradycardic spells, and the jerks and twitches commonly seen in preterm newborns. Many have been surprised to find no correlation between events thought to be seizures and changes on the EEG.[2]

It is now widely accepted that much of what had been called neonatal seizure activity represents nonseizure subcortical or brainstem activ-

TABLE 20-5

Classical Categories of Neonatal Seizures

Clonic	Focal clonic
	Multifocal clonic
	Migratory clonic
Tonic	Unilateral
	Decorticate spells
	Decerebrate spells
Myoclonic	Limited (focal)
	Bilateral
Subtle	Nystagmus*
	Tonic eye deviation†
	Sucking
	Mouthing movements
	Bicycling
	Swimming movements
	Eyelid flutter or blinking*
	Apnea
	Autonomic or vasomotor changes

*Actually clonic movements.
†Actually tonic episodes.

ity that reflects poor brain functioning. Tonic episodes and so-called "subtle" seizures are frequently found to be in this category of "non-seizures."

Focal clonic, migratory clonic, and multifocal clonic seizures are the most likely to have true cortical origins. Eye blinking (a clonic manifestation) may be seen, as may nystagmus. Focal clonic seizures have been seen as an important manifestation of stroke in the neonate.[3] Apnea has been seen as an ictal manifestation without any other evidence of seizure activity, although most apnea is not on this basis.

The lack of ongoing monitoring of brain activity in most neonatal units makes accurate identification of seizures extremely difficult. The best correlation can be obtained by obtaining an EEG during periods of presumed seizure activity. If the activity is confirmed as true seizures, then the same activity or closely related activity is also likely to be true seizure activity.

The traditional categorization of neonatal seizures is presented in Table 20-5. The classification does not have the same significance as the International Classification of Seizures in older individuals. Some general observations may pertain, even with the confusion surrounding the accurate diagnosis of neonatal seizures.

Episodes characterized as tonic and subtle are most likely to be seen in premature infants. Tonic episodes are quite commonly associated with intraventricular hemorrhage. Clonic, multifocal clonic, and migratory clonic seizures are more common in term infants. Myoclonic seizures often indicate a metabolic etiology such as nonketotic hyperglycemia or urea cycle disorder.

Prevention

Many neonatal seizures can be successfully prevented by careful attention to possible metabolic changes expected on the basis of the infant's condition. Hypoglycemia, hypocalcemia, hypomagnesemia, and often hypoxia can be anticipated and controlled.

Seizures resulting from intracranial malformations, infections, or prenatal injury most often cannot be prevented. Inherited metabolic disorders may not be identified until after initial symptoms (often including seizures) appear.

Whether neonatal seizures can be prevented by pretreatment of the mother (in high-risk situations thought likely to result in neonatal seizures) has not been adequately investigated. As progress in antenatal treatment of the fetus continues, this may become an area for further investigation.

Treatment

The rational treatment of neonatal seizures involves a vigorous attempt to achieve four specific goals.

ACUTE TREATMENT

The first goal is acute treatment of prolonged or multiple seizures and status epilepticus. Prolonged seizures and frequent, multiple seizures

TABLE 20-6

Acute Management of Neonatal Seizures

Assess clinical situation—are the episodes seizures?

Draw blood for glucose, calcium, magnesium, blood gas analysis, and electrolytes.

Maintain adequate oxygenation and ventilation.

Perform Dextrostix.

　If Dextrostix <25-45, give 200 mg/kg IV minibolus of glucose.

　If Dextrostix >25-45, give phenobarbital, 20 mg/kg IV.

If seizures continue after 10-20 minutes, the following steps should be taken:

　Give additional doses of phenobarbital, 5 mg/kg each, to a total of 40 mg/kg.

　Give pyridoxine, 50-100 mg IV bolus.

If seizures continue or recur after the above steps:

　Draw phenobarbital level.

　Correct calcium or magnesium if low.

　Give phenytoin, 20 mg/kg IV (no more rapidly than 10-20 mg/min).

If seizures persist or continue with the above treatment:

　Consider major intracranial etiology (malformation, bleed, etc.).

　Repeat metabolic studies (including NH_4) and blood levels of phenobarbital and phenytoin.

　Give diazepam, 0.3 mg/kg IV.

　Be prepared to intubate patient if drug-induced apnea occurs or to maintain ventilatory support.

　Consider giving paraldehyde, titrating with a 4% solution.

Once seizures are under control, maintain phenobarbital levels between 20-30 mg/dl.

Cultures (blood and CSF) should be considered as soon as the infant is stable.

may result in metabolic changes and cardiorespiratory difficulties. Whether or not seizures themselves may cause brain damage is an unanswered question. It seems appropriate to make vigorous efforts to control seizures completely, although this may not always be possible. When the administration of a single drug does not result in lasting control, a second or third should be tried. Table 20-6 outlines a plan for acute management.

The most commonly used drugs for the control of acute seizures and status epilepticus in the newborn are phenobarbital and phenytoin (Table 20-7). Both are given in loading doses of 20 mg/kg. In most infants this load achieves a blood level within the therapeutic range. Since both drugs are always given intravenously (IV) for this indication, the blood level is promptly achieved. When these antiepileptic drugs are unsuccessful in bringing the seizure(s) under control, alternate drugs such as paraldehyde or diazepam may be used.[12] Diazepam is given IV in a dose of 0.3 mg/kg.

CORRECTION

The second goal is correction of underlying remediable causes. This goal is often more important than the first goal, since some seizures induced by metabolic abnormalities cannot be controlled with antiepileptic drugs until the metabolic derangement is corrected. It is especially inappropriate to treat a newborn with antiepileptic drugs before correctable causes have been excluded.

After the drawing of blood for glucose, calcium, magnesium, electrolytes, and blood gas determination, therapy may begin. It is always proper to administer glucose. Inspired oxygen concentration may be raised temporarily if hypoxia is suspected. The IV administration of 50 to 100 mg pyridoxine should ideally be done under electroencephalogram monitoring. In this way the true causes of pyridoxine dependency or deficiency can be detected.

PREVENTION

Prevention of further seizures is the third goal. Seizure prophylaxis is an admirable goal for patients of all ages, but it is often not easily achieved in newborns. Often in spite of the appropriate and vigorous administration of several antiepileptic drugs, seizures persist for several days only to remit spontaneously and never return. Despite this rather frequent observation, attempts to provide adequate seizure prophylaxis seem justified.

Phenobarbital remains the most studied and most used drug for seizure control in the newborn. Since the half-life of phenobarbital is long, it is not necessary to give routine maintenance doses on a fixed schedule.

Phenytoin is also used extensively. Although it may be very useful in acute treatment, phenytoin is often quite difficult to use as a maintenance drug. The most frequently encountered problem is the extremely variable half-life in newborns. It is not predictable, and frequent blood level determinations are necessary to estimate a useful half-life for the individual baby. Not uncommonly, repeated loading doses must be used several times a day to maintain an adequate blood level. This pharmacokinetic problem is dramatically compounded by oral administration. It is reasonable to avoid the oral use of phenytoin in the newborn altogether.

A second problem is the variability in binding phenytoin to albumin in blood. The binding is

TABLE 20-7

Antiepileptic Drugs

DRUG	DOSE	COMMENTS
Phenobarbital (drug of choice for neonatal seizures)	Loading: 10-20 mg/kg IV to maximum of 40 mg/kg Maintenance: 5-7 mg/kg in 2 divided doses beginning 12 hr after last loading dose	Therapeutic level: 20-25 μg/ml (obtain levels any time 1 hr after dose); respiratory depressant; incompatible with other drugs in solution
Phenytoin (added if seizures not controlled by phenobarbital alone)	Loading: 10-20 mg/kg IV (no more rapidly than 10-20 mg/min) Maintenance: 5-7 mg/kg in 1-2 doses/day beginning 12 hr after last loading dose	Therapeutic level: 15-20 μg/ml (obtain levels 1-10 hr after last loading or maintenance dose; incompatible with all other drugs, glucose, and pH <11.5; give slowly directly into vein; too-rapid administration causes arrhythmias, bradycardia, hypotension, cardiovascular collapse, and/or respiratory distress
Paraldehyde (CNS depressant)	0.15 mg/kg PO, PR, or IM q.4-6h. p.r.n.; mix PR 1:1 with mineral oil	Dissolves plastic—use glass syringes and rubber catheter; protect from light; PR route of choice as a retention enema
Diazepam	0.3 mg/kg IV (0.1-0.3 mg/kg/dose)	Sodium benzoate competes with bilirubin for albumin binding sites—potentiates jaundice, so kernicterus is possible at lower serum bilirubin levels
Pyridoxine	50-100 mg IV bolus	Pyridoxine (vitamin B$_6$) deficiency as etiology of neonatal seizures is rare; seizures will cease within 5 minutes after vitamin B$_6$ injection if deficient
Lorazepam (Ativan)	0.05 mg/kg/dose IV over 2-5 min	Use justified in severely ill newborns with seizures nonresponsive to other drugs
Primidone	Loading: 15-20 mg Maintenance: 12-20 mg/kg/day	Use justified for refractory seizures; close monitoring of phenobarbital levels is necessary, since levels rise after primidone loading and fall precipitously with phenobarbital discontinuance
Valproic acid	Initial dose: 10-15 mg/kg/day PO Maintenance: 10-60 mg/kg/day PO q.12h.	Anticonvulsant for refractory neonatal seizures

affected by the amount of albumin, concurrent drugs, and other poorly understood factors. Since changes in binding alter the amount of drug available to enter the brain, there is often little control over the true "level." Whenever the unbound level of phenytoin can be measured, it is more useful than the total level. Using the unbound level does not make the calculation of an appropriate dosage any simpler, but it does give information that can help avoid needless toxicity.

Maintenance doses of phenobarbital (5 to 20 mg/kg) should be given after blood level determinations indicate that the level is dropping.[5,6] Phenytoin maintenance doses are difficult to predict. Frequent blood levels may be necessary to understand the way in which a given infant metabolizes phenytoin.

If unbound levels of phenytoin are available, these are often easier to use to ensure that a therapeutic range is maintained. Since the characteristic signs of phenytoin toxicity are cerebellar, they are ordinarily not recognized in the newborn. One must rely on the accurate determination of blood levels to safeguard against excessive administration. Maintenance doses for phenytoin as for phenobarbital range from 5 to 20 mg/kg.[1]

Other antiepileptic agents such as primidone, carbamazepine, and valproic acid are used less frequently. Data about safety, effectiveness, and dosage are less available than for phenobarbital and phenytoin.

MINIMIZATION

The fourth goal is minimization of the side effects of antiepileptic drug therapy. In the attempt to control seizures, the potential of antiepileptic drugs to produce side effects must not be ignored. Drug-induced encephalopathy may mimic the clinical changes seen in hypoxic-ischemic encephalopathy or numerous metabolic derangements. The possibility that the pharmaceutical agent may be causing some of the findings being attributed to the underlying disorder always exists. Likewise, improvement in the underlying disor-

der may be masked by induced changes from the drug.

More significant side effects such as pneumonitis or pulmonary vascular thrombosis produced by paraldehyde, hepatotoxic changes induced by valproic acid, or hyperbilirubinemia intensified by diazepam are rare but worthy of recognition.

The issue of long-term side effects of the antiepileptic drugs is far from being settled. Virtually all of the drugs used have been shown in animal or tissue culture studies to have detrimental effects on the growth or development of the brain. The extent to which any of this information can be transferred to the human situation remains the subject of extensive investigation.

Complications and outcome

The evidence for long-term clinical complications that can be directly related to the presence of neonatal seizures is limited and controversial. This should not be surprising, since most neonatal seizures occur in the course of significant insults to the developing brain (hypoxia, ischemia, infection, and malformation).

Studies to date have been unable to separate satisfactorily the effect of the seizures from the effect of the cause of the seizures. Hypoglycemia is a good example. Infants with significant hypoglycemia are likely to have identifiable problems, whether or not they actually had neonatal hypoglycemic seizures.

Another curious example is the syndrome of benign familial neonatal seizures. In this condition even the day of life in which the seizures occur may be characteristic. No sequelae occur in this condition, which suggests that seizures alone can occur without resultant damage to the brain.

Early hypocalcemia (often seen in stressed newborns) is another example of a relatively benign cause of neonatal seizures. These infants have an excellent chance of recovery without complications. It is wise not to be overaggressive in the correction of low calcium levels.

Separate from any discussion of the direct effect of seizures on the developing brain is the question of whether seizures in the newborn period predispose to later seizures. Again, cause seems to be the most important factor. Those seizures caused by transient metabolic changes that do not cause other permanent neurologic dysfunction are themselves likely to be transient and not occur outside the neonatal period. Seizures caused by congenital anomalies or those accompanied by obvious permanent brain damage are likely to persist.

Persistent seizures with structural brain damage are among those seizures that even later in life are hardest to control. Children who develop infantile spasms or the Lennox-Gastaut syndrome frequently have significant problems including seizures in the neonatal period.

Important prognostic findings and signs can be grouped to provide a general guide to assess newborns with seizures. Factors favoring a good prognosis include transient metabolic causes (hypocalcemia, hypomagnesemia), normal neurologic examination, normal EEG findings, and benign familial neonatal seizures.

Factors favoring a poorer prognosis include the presence of a congenital malformation, seizures persisting for more than several days, severe birth asphyxia as the cause, presence of a major intraventricular hemorrhage, severely abnormal EEG findings (burst suppression, extremely low voltage, or isoelectric), or major signs on neurologic examination (hemi-syndrome, multiple brainstem signs, and severe hypotonia with unresponsiveness).

Factors not carrying any particular prognostic significance include duration of individual seizures (other than status epilepticus), total number of seizures in the first few days of life, initial response to antiepileptic drug therapy, and presence of epilepsy in the patient's family.

Parent teaching

At times the desire to "do something" becomes overwhelming for parents and professionals alike. In neurologic medicine this is particularly true for seizures. In the neonate and in older children, parents often perceive seizures as traumatic events that should be stopped at all costs. For this reason parent education becomes important when the first seizures appear.

Careful explanations given to parents of neonates with seizures should address the issues of causes and significance. Attention should be given to an understanding of a seizure as another of the ways in which a dysfunctional brain can behave (things are not working as they should be), like other signs (apnea, lethargy, or hypotonia) the baby may be showing. It should be explained that identification of the cause of the seizures is extremely important and will help decide how much of a problem the seizures represent.

If repeated seizures are experienced, the parents should become familiar with the terminology used by the professionals involved with the baby. The names given to the types of seizures, the medications used (along with the side effects), and the tests that will be monitored should all be understood by the parents.

INTRAVENTRICULAR HEMORRHAGE
Physiology

The problem of bleeding into and around the ventricular system has received more attention in the last decade than any other neurologic problem in the neonate. In large measure, this relates to the frequency with which the problem develops, generally estimated to be 30% to 50% in premature infants under 32 weeks gestational age or less than 1500 g. The growth of routine cranial ultrasound examination in premature infants is directly due to this common problem. Recently, the incidence of these hemorrhages has appeared to be decreasing. With the advent of CT and ultrasound scanning, a large number of infants have been recognized who were not suspected of having an intraventricular bleed but who were diagnosed on scans.

Although the bleeding is regularly spoken of as intraventricular and intracranial hemorrhage, these terms do not accurately reflect its etiology. Highly vascularized areas, with relatively fragile and poorly supported blood vessels, are the source of bleeding.

In term infants the choroid plexus of the lateral ventricles is the most common site in which bleeding originates. In premature infants the germinal matrix, in the subependymal area adjacent to the caudate nucleus, is the primary site of bleeding. Both of these are areas of high arterial and capillary blood flow; in addition, they use an anatomically awkward venous drainage system, eventually draining into the internal cerebral vein (Figure 20-1).

The extent of bleeding generally predicts the likelihood of complications and residua. Bleeding may be confined to the germinal matrix or the choroid plexus, or it may enter the ventricular system. When filled under pressure, the ventricular system may dilate. Blood may also extravasate out into the brain parenchyma (more likely with germinal matrix bleeding than with choroid plexus bleeding).

Several classification schemes have been used, each trying to assess the degree of bleeding or amount of blood present. Ideally, a classification should relate to pathophysiology, treatment, or outcome, but with present knowledge this is not possible.

A classification based on the extent of hemorrhage seen on the CT scan grades germinal matrix hemorrhages as (Figure 20-2):

0—No bleeding

I—Germinal matrix only

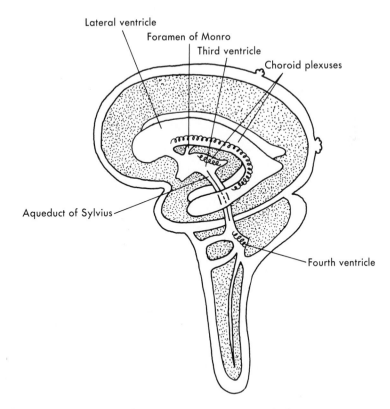

Figure 20-1. Central nervous system/ventricular system.

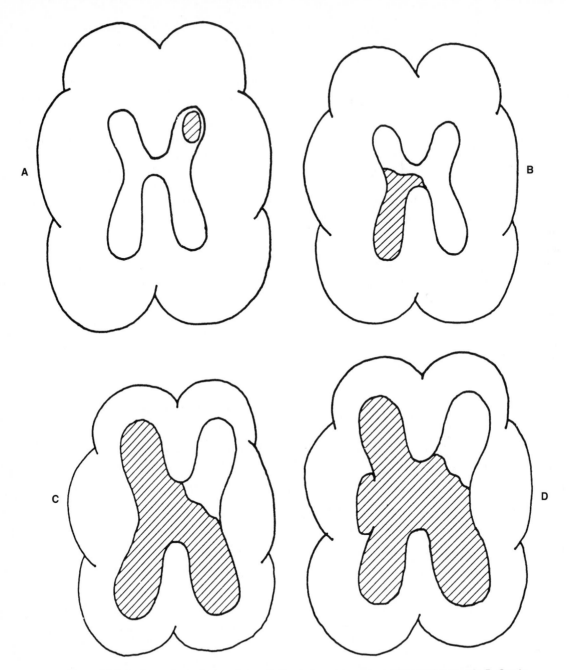

Figure 20-2. Intraventricular hemorrhage. **A,** Grade I—subependymal hemorrhage only. **B,** Grade II—intraventricular hemorrhage without ventricular dilation. **C,** Grade III—intraventricular hemorrhage with ventricular dilation. **D,** Grade IV—intraventricular hemorrhage with parenchymal hemorrhage.

II—Germinal matrix with blood in the ventricles

III—Germinal matrix with blood in the ventricles and hydrocephalus

IV—Intraventricular and parenchymal bleeding (other than germinal matrix)

Etiology

The factors identified in infants who have experienced intraventricular hemorrhage are multiple. Specific factors thought to cause bleeding have included hypernatremia, shock, acidosis, blood transfusions, seizures, and rapid volume expansion. What appears to be the common factor underlying the pathology is a fluctuation in cerebral blood flow.[13]

At times, this may have a systemic counterpart, such as in shock. At other times, changes in brain perfusion occur without any reflection in systemic blood pressure, pulse, or respiration. The fragility of the germinal matrix and choroid plexus seem to allow for the disruption of capillary or small blood vessel integrity with resultant bleeding.

Intraventricular bleeding tends to occur in the first few hours or days of life. The profound physiologic changes normally seen following birth are coupled with the multiple problems (primarily cardiorespiratory) experienced by the typically premature infant to make intraventricular bleeding common. The degree to which the aggressive management of premature newborns has a role in the development of bleeding cannot be accurately assessed. In general, although not exclusively, it is the sicker infants who both require more intervention and have a greater likelihood of bleeding. The preliminary reports of decreased incidence of intraventricular bleeding with antenatal (but not with neonatal) phenobarbital administration suggest a role for prenatal and intrapartum events in the etiology of intraventricular bleeding.

Data collection

As has been suggested previously, the historical information is somewhat varied. Some infants, generally those who are at term, will have intraventricular hemorrhages associated with severe asphyxia.

Premature infants often show one or more of the following: birth weight less than 1500 g, gestational age less than 34 weeks, shock, hyaline membrane disease, need for blood transfusions, coagulopathy, hyperviscosity, hypoxia, and birth asphyxia.

Since premature infants, particularly those weighing less than 1500 g, tend to have multiple problems, it is not surprising that the clinical presentation of germinal matrix hemorrhage may range from subtle (or even undetectable) to catastrophic. Deterioration in clinical condition followed by apnea, flaccid quadriparesis, unresponsiveness, and death from circulatory collapse is a recognizable syndrome. Common signs of germinal matrix hemorrhage include apnea, hypotension, drop in hematocrit, flaccidity, areflexia, full fontanel, tonic posturing, and oculomotor disturbances.

When intracranial bleeding is suspected, appropriate studies of intracranial structures should be performed as soon as possible. In the case of periventricular-intraventricular hemorrhage both ultrasonography and CT scanning are useful tools for defining the presence of bleeding and for following its evolution. Since sonography is the safer procedure and uses no radiation, it should be used for follow-up.

Treatment and intervention

The primary treatment of intraventricular hemorrhage is confined to supportive care. Ventilatory support, maintenance of oxygenation, regulation of acid-base balance, suppression of seizures, and treatment of any attendant coagulopathy are all extremely important in reducing mortality and morbidity. The role that successful management has in the amelioration or prevention of complications is unclear.

Many therapies have been proposed or used but remain unproved. These are listed here not to recommend them for general clinical use, but to suggest the ways in which the problem has been approached.

When the hemorrhage is confined to the germinal matrix, little can be done even from a theoretic standpoint.

The removal of blood from the ventricular system has been used for many years as a treatment for intraventricular hemorrhage. Many studies have shown it to have limited effectiveness. The rationale for removing blood is twofold: (1) to remove an irritating substance from the ventricular system, at the same time reducing clot formation, and (2) to remove protein in the hope of preventing hydrocephalus. Yet, because of high spinal fluid protein levels and the potential for a block in the flow of fluid, there is a concern that repeated lumbar punctures may be ineffective in clearing blood from the ventricles. There are vociferous opponents and proponents to this procedure. A clear answer is not possible at this time.

Lumbar puncture has much less chance of morbidity and is the preferred procedure. Ventricular taps can be used but are rarely recommended.

Care must be given to reduce the risk for continued bleeding, working to maintain perfusion of the brain, reduce wide fluctuations in blood pressure, oxygenation, and pH.

Another theoretical (and unproved) objection to these methods suggests that removing blood will allow for further bleeding by reducing the pressure in the ventricles and therefore upsetting the homeostatic balance.

Medications to reduce intracranial pressure and therefore treat secondary effects of the bleeding include furosemide, acetazolamide, and steroid agents. Mannitol and glycerol have also been used. The same unproved argument concerning upsetting the homeostatic balance may be applied here.

Apparently, the best recommendation for the treatment of intraventricular hemorrhage is to continue the management of ensuing problems without undue attention to the intracranial bleeding.

Complications

The complications from intraventricular hemorrhage relate to the underlying causes and the extent of bleeding. Massive bleeding with dilation of the ventricular system is much more likely to cause an acute change in brain function, with increased intracranial pressure, brainstem findings, and apnea. Milder degrees of hemorrhage may be asymptomatic or associated with seizurelike events, changes in muscle tone, or apnea.

When bleeding extends into the parenchyma, porencephaly may result from liquefactive necrosis or ischemic-induced encephalomalacia. Follow-up structural brain studies may show hypodense areas where blood was present; later they may show areas of porencephaly.

The most common complication is posthemorrhagic hydrocephalus. The possibility of this developing is directly related to the severity of the hemorrhage, with up to 10% of survivors of mild intraventricular hemorrhage and 65% to 100% of survivors of severe intraventricular hemorrhage showing progressive ventricular dilation. Posthemorrhagic hydrocephalus should be looked for in all survivors of germinal matrix hemorrhage. CT scanning or ultrasonography to assess ventricular size should be used. Clinical signs alone are not reliable.

With the hope of avoiding a shunt, some attempts at control of the hydrocephalus have been attempted. Osmotic and diuretic agents, including furosemide, isosorbide, and acetazolamide, have been used to reduce the formation of cerebrospinal fluid. Some clinicians have been enthusiastic about this approach, but it has not gained widespread acceptance. As referred to previously, lumbar and intraventricular taps are sometimes used in an attempt to avoid shunting. This approach holds anecdotal promise but has not been adequately proved. In some small premature infants, ventricular drainage without a full shunt (to the peritoneal cavity) is used.

Outcome studies have been difficult to assess. Clearly, the sickest infants tend to do poorly. They also tend to have more complications, including CNS complications. There is a clear correlation between the grade of bleed and the likelihood of significant neurologic residua, but the correlation is far from perfect. The influence of other factors on neurologic outcome may be more significant than the actual bleed itself. Hypoxia, hypoperfusion, and other conditions known to damage the developing nervous system cannot easily be separated as individual factors in outcome.[11]

Parent teaching

The infant with intraventricular hemorrhage will have varying degrees of problems. Often the acute situation resolves without ongoing problems. In these cases parents should understand the possible complications such as hydrocephalus that may occur in the short term. Teaching the parents to measure head circumference and alerting them to the signs of increased intracranial pressure such as poor feeding, posturing, eye movement difficulties, full fontanel, and lethargy will enable them to participate more fully in the medical follow-up.

Parents must understand the risk for long-term neurologic sequelae. Even though these sequelae are difficult to predict with any degree of certainty, parents should understand that mental and motor handicaps, delays in the acquisition of milestones, seizures, and problems associated with hydrocephalus and potential shunt placement may occur. Specific preparation for these potential problems should begin in the nursery but will be increased during follow-up visits if the possibility for such problems seems greater.

INFANT STIMULATION

Beyond the technologically advanced care given to critically ill newborns, interest in providing continuing care to maximize the neurologic potential of the individual infant has been increasing. Along with advances in the understanding of the developing nervous system and current popular interest in the "wellness" movement, a proliferation in early intervention programs has been developed.

Often a scientific basis for such programs is lacking. Most parents are not likely to make a critical evaluation of the wide variety of programs offered. The obvious desire of parents to do whatever is possible to help their children makes them easy victims for promoters of unproved therapies. Neurologic difficulties arising out of the newborn period are most often persistent. Medical caretakers are required to be aware of the relative benefits and risks of available therapies, both scientific and unscientific, if they are to make meaningful recommendations for families in their care.[8]

Assessment of programs

Emphasis has been given to therapeutic and prophylactic programs. Therapeutic programs have been available for many years and are more familiar to clinicians. Therapeutic programs often have specific goals that are easily understood by everyone. Often parents will have numerous choices of programs offering similar if not identical approaches. Therapeutic programs are best used for specific, identified problems in which the prescribed therapy is likely to cause a significant improvement in function. Progress should be easily identifiable by parents and therapists alike.

Generalized developmental stimulation (prophylactic programs) is a newer approach. Often infants recommended for such programs are merely identified as "at risk" or show nonspecific delays. The programs are often designed to give broad developmental stimulation by a variety of therapists. Frequently parents are led to believe that these programs are "necessary" and that comparable "stimulation" cannot be done independently at home. This subtle pressure is again evidenced by the program providers' lack of desire to become involved in controlled studies designed to show whether or not such programs are of any value.

Even though there is a generally positive sentiment toward early intervention programs, the parents must remember that these programs are unproved treatment modalities. Therefore it is necessary for care providers to educate parents in the appropriate assessment of such programs. Similarly, the medical community should demand the same measures of safety and efficacy that would be demanded of any new therapy before general approval is given to such programs.

In many programs the measures of success are complex reports listing reflex patterns or measures of sensory integration or age scores on tests that have little relationship to what the parents can observe.

It is clear that sophisticated and detailed neurologic and neuropsychologic testing can reveal abnormalities (weaknesses) that do not cause significant compromise of functional ability. Therefore it is inappropriate to design therapy programs on the basis of test results or to make judgments about the success of a program based on changes in test results. Frequently improvements on test results are merely the result of expected maturation and not any specific intervention.

Often the personal involvement of the clinicians and the therapists in a program causes conflict in the smooth administration of family life. No therapeutic program is destroyed by a missed or cancelled visit. A lack of interest in the therapist's suggestion that therapy time should be increased should not prompt a referral to the social worker to investigate the emotional difficulties of the parents. Most parents will investigate alternate programs and consider changing to them. Responsible clinicians will even encourage this activity in parents as a means to prevent later dissatisfaction and "program shopping."

Prejudgment of parents' motives, unfair demands on their loyalty, and overinterpretation of their actions such as missed or late appointments or acquiring second opinions is unfair, presumptive, and indicates a lack of objectivity and professionalism among those responsible for the program.

It is unwise to underestimate the effect of all experiences in the stimulation of developmental progress. Without an awareness of the total input to the infant from all sources, the significance of formal "therapy time" will not be kept in perspective.

Unproved therapies tend to be self-justifying. If a child improves during the course of therapy, the improvement is attributed to the program and the therapy continues. If improvement is not seen, the therapy is increased. Rarely will it be suggested that the program be terminated.

Parents must also be careful about programs in which all patients show success. Either the program was unnecessary to begin with, or goals are set far too low. An appropriate goal is a reasonable measure of progress beyond what would be expected to occur without the program.

A program should not pressure a family to participate. Parents should never hear, "You do want what is best for your child, don't you?" Although this may be overstated, it also reemphasizes the need to be sensitive to all the issues in a family's life to avoid adding new problems to those already being experienced.

Therapeutic programs with specific goals include physical therapy for reduction of contractures, physical therapy for gait training, speech therapy for significant disarticulation, alternative communication for the deaf, occupational therapy for activities of daily living, and occupational therapy for feeding skills. Expectations in a well-designed therapeutic program include specific goals, ease in recognition of progress, a clear time frame for results to be seen, and reassessment of the program if goals are not met.

General guidelines (for parents and clinicians) for the assessment of early intervention and infant stimulation programs include:

1. A clear understanding of the goals of the program

2. Familiarity with the techniques and therapies used
3. Assurance that specific therapeutic programs (physical therapy, occupational therapy, and speech therapy) are carried out by qualified personnel
4. A plan for intervention that is individualized and relevant to the patient's needs (programs in which most children receive a very similar program should be avoided)
5. A means for regular, standardized assessment (at least twice yearly) of the infant's progress in all areas
6. A reliance on functional improvement rather than improvement on tests administered by the therapists delivering the therapy
7. A willingness for an outside individual to do an independent assessment
8. An avoidance of the "talk to Mrs. Jones and see how satisfied she was" approach
9. A willingness to be objective about the success or failure of the program

Parents must understand the time commitment involved and be counseled about potential disruption of family life; parents must have the right to choose and decide. One cannot require a family to participate in an "ideal program" at whatever the cost to the parents might be, any more than one can dictate that the child attend only the best college at whatever cost. Families must be given help in setting priorities for their time and resources. An emphasis on an adjunct home program is important. Only a small portion of the infant's time will actually be spent with the therapists. A program for a developing infant or child needs to be developed within the total perspective of family life and needs, not in isolation.

Assessment of high-risk infants

Two groups of infants deserve more than usual follow-up and might appropriately be considered for early intervention programs or specific therapy. The first group includes those who because of obvious neurologic deficits in the newborn period will need early intervention. The second group consists of those at significant risk for neurodevelopmental problems. These infants may appear normal at discharge from the nursery only to develop obvious neurologic problems at a later date. Also included in this group are those infants for whom adequate parental supervision seems doubtful. Common risk factors for abnormal neurologic development are:

1. Abnormal obstetric history
2. Asphyxia
3. Hypoglycemia
4. Polycythemia
5. Seizures
6. Inappropriate size for gestational age
7. Prematurity
8. CNS hemorrhage
9. Birth trauma
10. Maternal drug abuse
11. Siblings with congenital malformations

Several distinct means for evaluating neurologic function are available and should be used in the assessment of the high-risk infant. No single means of evaluation is likely to provide all the necessary information for this assessment, but a list of necessary conditions for ideal neurologic, neurodevelopmental, and neurobehavioral assessment follows:

1. No acute illnesses present
2. Quiet surroundings
3. Dimly lit room
4. No distractions
5. Normothermia maintained
6. Unrestrained activity
7. Awake, having recently slept
8. At least 1 hour before or after feeding
9. No recent noxious procedures such as blood samples drawn, pulmonary toilet, eye examination, hearing test, medication, or range-of-motion exercises

The formal neurologic examination must be performed by a trained examiner familiar with the wide variations in normal behavior seen at very young ages. The importance of sequential examinations cannot be overemphasized, since subtle findings may be masked by transient environmental conditions. Tendon stretch reflexes and the "primitive" reflexes characteristic of newborns are all dramatically influenced by feeding, sleep, medication, and head position.

Gestational age assessment and neurodevelopmental and neurobehavioral assessments are useful in identifying the high-risk infant (see Chapter 4).

Early identification of at-risk infants can result in improved observation of such infants throughout their early developmental life. As specific problems are identified, appropriate programs can be used to minimize deficits, promote continued acquisition of developmental skills, and reduce long-term morbidity.

Over the last several years the heightened interest in the field of neonatal neurology has been demonstrated by the publication of several textbooks devoted entirely to this topic. Several are listed in the selected readings as resources for further study of topics covered in this chapter and for those topics not covered here.

The incidence of neurologic problems in the neonate requiring specialized care is high. An awareness of the scope of the problems involved, the availability of appropriate diagnostic equipment, the methods of treatment currently in use, and the possible complications of these disorders may lead to decreased neurologic residua.

REFERENCES

1. Bourgeois BFD and Dodson WE: Phenytoin elimination in newborns, Neurology 33:173, 1983.
2. Camfield PR and Camfield CS: Neonatal seizures: a commentary on selected aspects, J Child Neurol 2:244, 1987.
3. Clancy R et al: Focal motor seizures heralding stroke in full-term infants, Am J Dis Child 139:601, 1985.
4. Edwards MSB: Fetal hydrocephalus, Int Pediatr 2:89, 1987.
5. Fischer JH et al: Phenobarbital maintenance dose requirements in treating neonatal seizures, Neurology 31:1042, 1981.
6. Gal P et al: Efficacy of phenobarbital monotherapy in treatment of neonatal seizures: relationship to blood levels, Neurology 32:1401, 1982.
7. Gilles FH et al, editors: The developing human brain, Boston, 1983, John Wright/PSG, Inc.
8. Haskins R, Finkelstein NW, and Stedman DJ: Infant stimulation programs and their effects, Pediatr Ann 7:123, 1978.
9. Lemire RJ et al: Normal and abnormal development of the nervous system, New York, 1975, Harper & Row, Publishers, Inc.
10. Sarnat HB: Disturbances of late neuronal migrations in the perinatal period, Am J Dis Child 141:969, 1987.
11. Shinnar S et al: Intraventricular hemorrhage in the premature infant: a changing outlook, N Engl J Med 306:1464, 1982.
12. Smith BT and Masotti RE: Intravenous diazepam in the treatment of prolonged seizure activity in neonates and infants, Dev Med Child Neurol 13:630, 1971.
13. Volpe JJ: Neonatal intracranial hemorrhage: pathophysiology, neuropathology and clinical features, Clin Perinatol 4:77, 1977.
14. Volpe JJ: Normal and abnormal human brain development, Clin Perinatol 4:3, 1977.

SELECTED READINGS

Allan W and Volpe JJ: Periventricular-intraventricular hemorrhage, Pediatr Clin North Am 36:47, 1986.

Brazelton TB: Neonatal behavioral assessment scale. Clinics in developmental medicine, No 50, Philadelphia, 1973, JB Lippincott Co.

Cunningham M: Intraventricular hemorrhage of the newborn, Dimens Crit Care 6:1, 1987.

Fenichel GM: Neonatal neurology, New York, 1980, Churchill Livingstone, Inc.

Hellman J and Vannucci R: Intraventricular hemorrhage in premature infants, Semin Perinatol 6:42, 1982.

Korobkin R and Guilleminault C, editors: Advances in perinatal neurology, vol 1, New York, 1979, Spectrum Books.

Kuban K and Teale R: Rationale for grading intracranial hemorrhage in premature infants, Pediatrics 74:358, 1984.

MacDonald M et al: Timing and antecedents of intracranial hemorrhage in the newborn, Pediatrics 74:32, 1984.

McLone DG et al: An introduction to hydrocephalus, Chicago, 1982, Children's Memorial Hospital.

Morselli PL et al, editors: Antiepileptic drug therapy in pediatrics, New York, 1983, Raven Press.

Painter MJ, Berman I, and Crumrine P: Neonatal seizures, Pediatr Clin North Am 33:91, 1986.

Powell MJ, Painter MJ, and Pippenger CE: Primidine therapy in refractory neonatal seizures, J Pediatr 105:651, 1984.

Swaiman KF and Wright FS, editors: The practice of pediatric neurology, ed 2, St Louis, 1982, The CV Mosby Co.

Torrence C: Neonatal seizures. I. A developmental and clinical understanding, Neonatal Network 4:9, 1985.

Torrence C: Neonatal seizures. II. Recognition, treatment, and progress, Neonatal Network 4:21, 1985.

Volpe JJ: Neurology of the newborn, ed 2, Philadelphia, 1987, WB Saunders Co.

CHAPTER 21

Pediatric surgery

LINDA POWERS · JOHN BURRINGTON · SANDRA L. GARDNER ·
GERALD B. MERENSTEIN

Surgical problems in the neonate are usually quite obvious and often spectacular in their presentation. However, most problems are surgically correctable with a very high success rate. Modern diagnostic techniques such as ultrasound examination make prenatal diagnosis possible. For the child facing a major surgical procedure in the first hours or days of life, the general precepts of supportive care are extremely important in aiding the infant through the stress of surgery (see Chapters 5, 6, 8, 10, and 11).

MALROTATION AND VOLVULUS
Physiology and etiology

Between the tenth and twelfth weeks of gestation the bowel, which has prolapsed into the base of the umbilical cord, should return to the abdomen. As it returns, it undergoes a characteristic rotation, with the stomach rotating 90 degrees to the right, so that the duodenum comes to rest in the right gutter. The third and fourth portions of the duodenum then migrate under the superior mesenteric artery and form the retroperitoneal portion of the duodenum. The bowel then becomes intraperitoneal again at Trietz' ligament, well to the left of the midline. The colon rotation then follows with the cecum passing anterior to the superior mesenteric vessels and becoming attached in the right lower quadrant. In this position the entire right and left colon should become retroperitoneal. The transverse colon and cecum remain suspended on a long mesentery. In anomalies such as omphalocele, gastroschisis, and congenital diaphragmatic hernia the bowel is mal-

positioned at the time fixation should take place. Consequently all infants affected by such anomalies have nonfixation and nonrotation of the bowel. Fixation and rotation anomalies, however, frequently occur in the absence of other major abnormalities.

The most common form of malrotation involves total failure of rotation and fixation of both the large and small bowels. This results in the failure of the third and fourth portions of the duodenum to rotate beneath the mesenteric vessels, and as a result all of the small bowel is on the right side of the abdomen. The colon also fails to rotate, so that the colon is mainly on the left side of the abdomen and the cecum is abnormally placed. When this occurs, the root of the mesentery does not become attached to the retroperitoneum; consequently, virtually the entire gastrointestinal tract is suspended by a single, thin attachment in the form of the superior mesenteric artery and vein. This long pedicle is prone to twisting and thereby causes a volvulus. In virtually all cases the volvulus involves a counterclockwise rotation as if the cecum had attempted to pass beneath the superior mesenteric vessels rather than anterior to them. Once this occurs, there can be infarction of the entire large and small bowels by obstruction to the superior mesenteric artery and vein.

The cause for malrotation and nonrotation in most cases is totally unexplained. Many people lead a normal life with a nonfixed and rotated bowel. Many, however, have severe symptoms in infancy.

Data collection
HISTORY

Typically the problems with malrotation are divided into two general groups. The first is volvulus with compromise of the blood supply to the entire bowel. The second set of symptoms involves abnormal attachments between the right colon and the duodenum, referred to as Ladd's bands.

Typically infants are healthy for the first several days of life and develop symptoms between 3 days and 3 weeks after birth. Presumably the dilation of the bowel by food and gas is part of the precipitating cause of symptoms.

An infant with volvulus experiences a rather cataclysmic onset of illness. The infant becomes rapidly distended, lethargic, mottled, and dehydrated and may pass some bloody stools per rectum. The symptoms of the infant with Ladd's bands are similar to those of an infant with duodenal stenosis or atresia. The infant also vomits bile.

LABORATORY DATA

The x-ray film may show a variety of patterns that are not pathognomonic for volvulus. However, an infant with a sudden onset of abdominal distention and lethargy who passes blood per rectum should have an emergency barium enema (Figure 21-1). This study will show the occlusion of the colon where it has become twisted around the mesenteric vessels.

On x-ray film the infant with Ladd's bands has a dilated stomach and duodenum with very little gas distally. The diagnosis can be confirmed by an upper gastrointestinal series that shows either the point of obstruction or that Trietz' ligament is abnormally formed.

Treatment
PREOPERATIVE CARE

Initial therapy consists of passing an orogastric tube for decompression, vigorously rehydrating the infants with 20 or 30 ml/kg of Ringer's lactate, correcting any existing acid-base defi-

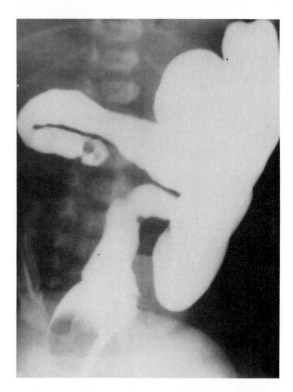

Figure 21-1. Midgut volvulus in 2-day-old male infant who vomited bile-stained fluid for 12 to 24 hours before surgery. Barium enema shows high-lying cecum curved on itself in right upper quadrant.

cit, and administering broad-spectrum antibiotic agents.

OPERATIVE INTERVENTION

Emergency surgery is required for the infant with volvulus, since the bowel can infarct completely within 4 hours.

In infants with Ladd's bands the band must be carefully divided so that the obstruction to the duodenum is relieved. The entire small bowel is placed in the right side of the abdomen, and the colon is placed to the left.

Some advocate doing an appendectomy in all infants explored for any rotation anomaly, since the appendix will be in an abnormal position.

However, most feel that the appendectomy is not indicated and indeed creates a source of possible contamination into an otherwise clean wound.

POSTOPERATIVE CARE

If a significant amount of the small bowel is removed, the infants will require long-term hyperalimentation. In these situations a Broviac catheter (see Chapter 13) or other central line should be inserted.

Complications and prognosis

If promptly diagnosed and treated, about half the cases of volvulus can be reduced without losing bowel. In the remaining half a variable amount of bowel is lost because of necrosis. In most in-

stances 30 to 40 cm of small bowel are required if the ileocecal valve has been removed. If the ileocecal valve is intact, as little as 20 cm of bowel as measured from Trietz' ligament is required for survival. In extreme cases the entire large and small bowels are necrotic, and the infant dies.

OMPHALOCELE
Physiology and etiology

Other than the high association with some of the trisomy syndromes, there is no known cause. Most of the cases are sporadic, although there are several families with two or more affected members.

An omphalocele is a defect above or below the navel that involves the umbilical cord. The defect

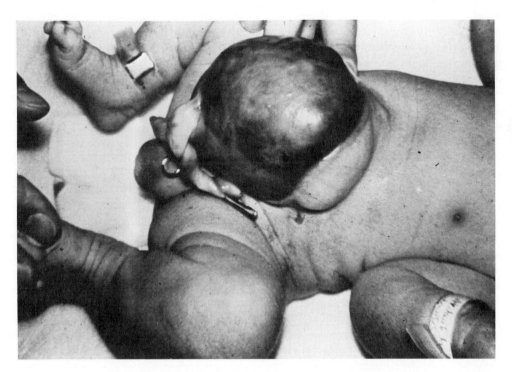

Figure 21-2. Omphalocele: large umbilical defect with viscera protruding from abdominal cavity into transparent moist sac.

is comprised of a large opening in the abdominal wall with viscera protruding into it. The viscera are covered with a transparent sac that is moist to the touch but easily dried out (Figure 21-2).

All infants with an omphalocele have nonrotation of the intestine. Obviously, if the intestine is protruding through a defect in the abdominal wall, it cannot be normally fixed and rotated within the abdomen.

Data collection
HISTORY

Examination by ultrasound may diagnose omphalocele in utero, so that plans for intervention in the neonate may be made before delivery.

PHYSICAL EXAMINATION AND ASSOCIATED ANOMALIES

On examination it should be noted whether the defect is mainly above the navel, centered under the navel, or mainly below the navel. These distinctions are important because there are a variety of defects associated with the different anatomic positions of the omphalocele.

The most common type of omphalocele is centered beneath the umbilical cord. The cord appears to exit from the apex of the sac, and there is a variable amount of the small bowel visible through the transparent sac. Typically, there is no associated protrusion of liver or other organs into the sac.

Usually defects above the navel mainly contain the liver and a few loops of bowel. Frequently a defect in the sternum, a defect in the diaphragm, and congenital heart disease occur. These high defects are frequently associated with multiple congenital defects and syndromes such as the trisomy syndromes.

The lower abdominal wall defects are associated with abnormalities of the bladder, rectum, and lower spine in the form of myelomeningocele. Frequently there is also an associated imperforate anus.

Treatment
PREOPERATIVE CARE

The initial management of all infants with an omphalocele involves preservation of body heat, decompression of the stomach, and protection against infection.

The wet omphalocele sac loses heat rapidly. The highly vascular bowel loops situated below the damp membrane have a very large blood flow, and the blood is cooled rapidly as it passes beneath this thin membrane. The membrane is also permeable to bacteria, so infection is an immediate threat to the infant.

The stomach of infants with an omphalocele often contains a great deal of swallowed amniotic fluid. The stomach and distal bowel may become distended with swallowed air, making the ultimate repair considerably more difficult.

Placing an orogastric tube and aspirating the stomach contents prevents aspiration. The tube also prevents distention from swallowed air. After the sac is gently cleansed with povidone-iodine (Betadine) or some similar bactericidal solution, it should be covered with plastic food wrap or a plastic sheet. If neither of these is available, a saline-soaked sponge covered with a bulky, dry dressing will serve the same purpose. Covering the sac prevents evaporation of water from within the sac and therefore impedes cooling.

An intravenous (IV) route should be established in the upper extremity for infusion of glucose and fluids, and the administration of systemic antibiotic agents should be started immediately. An intravenous route in the foot or leg can be used for the initial resuscitation, but during the operative procedure, increased intraabdominal pressure may render it valueless.

With these early precautions the infant with even the largest omphalocele is quite stable and can be transported or prepared for surgery without great urgency.

In the rare instance where the infant is too ill to undergo immediate operative correction, the sac can be treated periodically with an escharotic agent such as alcohol or 0.5% silver nitrate. These substances are bactericidal and minimize the chance of infection. Ultimately the sac will close spontaneously, but this may take several months. This type of procedure is to be used only when severe associated heart disease or other anomalies make surgery undesirable.

OPERATIVE INTERVENTION

The surgical correction consists of primary repair of all muscle layers when possible. In a significant number of the omphaloceles that are high in the abdomen and contain all or most of the liver, it is not possible to close the muscle layers completely. In such instances skin is dissected and closed over the bowel, leaving the patient with a large hernia defect. This defect can be closed at a later date.

In some large omphaloceles even skin closure is not possible. In such cases a pouch of silicone-coated mesh is constructed and sutured to the edges of the defect (Figure 21-3). This produces an impermeable membrane so that the sac can be reduced in size daily. Within 7 to 10 days the sac usually begins to pull away from the abdominal wall, but by this time it is usually possible to close the skin.

Complications

If the omphalocele is closed with too much tension, the wound can disrupt. More commonly the contained bowel is rendered ischemic and may develop areas of necrosis. The greatly increased intraabdominal pressure will also cause extensive edema of the legs and perhaps oliguria from direct compression of the kidneys and the inferior vena cava. Most important, too much intraabdominal pressure will cause the diaphragm to rise and be held in a high-fixed position. This may greatly compromise the infant's ability to breathe. Late bowel obstructions are relatively common as a result of adhesions.

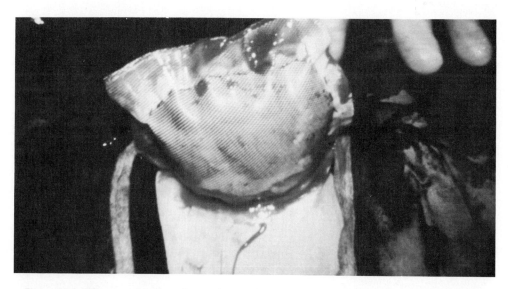

Figure 21-3. Silicone-coated mesh pouch containing abdominal contents that will be reduced daily into abdominal cavity as top is sewn down.

GASTROSCHISIS
Physiology and etiology

Gastroschisis has often been referred to as a "ruptured omphalocele." Embryologically the two conditions are similar, but they occur in different parts of the navel and at different stages of gestation. As in infants with omphaloceles, all infants with gastroschisis have nonrotation of the intestine. However, gastroschisis is not highly associated with the trisomy syndromes or other syndromes; in fact, anomalies are rarely associated with gastroschisis.

For unknown reasons gastroschisis has become increasingly common in the last 10 to 15 years. Once an unusual anomaly, it is now more common than omphalocele in most nurseries, and yet the cause is unknown.

Data collection

The infant with a gastroschisis has no sac or remnant of sac visible (Figure 21-4). The defect is always to the right of the midline, and often a bridge of skin is intact between the defect and the umbilical vessels. Infants with a gastroschisis tend to be very small-for-gestational-age (SGA) and are often premature.

Treatment
PREOPERATIVE CARE

The initial considerations for treating a gastroschisis are identical to those for treating an omphalocele. The bowel should be cleansed gently and then covered with a plastic sac, layer of plastic food wrap, or saline-soaked sponges covered with a bulky dressing. An orogastric

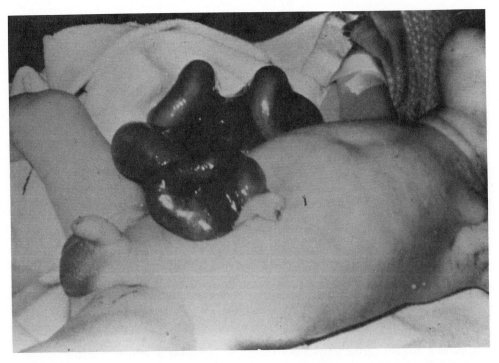

Figure 21-4. Gastroschisis. Abdominal wall defect to right of midline, without sac or sac remnant.

tube should be passed immediately and administration of broad-spectrum antibiotic agents begun. It is also important to place the child on his side so that the bowel can rest on a solid surface without acute angulation as it exits from the abdominal wall defect.

OPERATIVE INTERVENTION

At surgery it is usually necessary to enlarge the defect so that the bowel can be returned as completely as possible to the abdominal cavity. The bowel itself is markedly thickened and has a thick coat of fibrin on its surface. The bowel must be handled gently to prevent rupture or serious damage.

In approximately 80% of cases the abdominal wall can be closed completely. In an additional 10% skin can be closed, and in a final 10% a pouch must be created using mesh coated with silicone rubber.

POSTOPERATIVE CARE

When the pouch is in place, it should be dressed daily after a portion of the contents has been returned to the abdomen. This is accomplished by gently squeezing the outer margin of the pouch and making interrupted sutures through the pouch, effectively reducing the pouch's capacity. Dressings can consist of silver sulfadiazine (Silvadene), povidone-iodine, or any similar substance.

Most infants with a gastroschisis require a period of hyperalimentation (see Chapter 13). A Broviac catheter is inserted 2 days after the initial procedure.

Broad-spectrum antibiotic agents, ventilatory assistance as required, and nutritional support are the basics of postoperative care.

Complications

Infection and increased intraabdominal pressure are the major problems in the postoperative period.

DIAPHRAGMATIC HERNIA
Physiology and etiology

Diaphragmatic hernia occurs very early in gestation before the bowel has normally returned from the umbilical cord to the abdomen; therefore there is always an associated nonrotation and nonfixation of the bowel. The most common defects are in the posterior portion of the diaphragm through Bochdalek's foramen.

In utero the bowel develops in the chest and compresses the left lung. This leads to a pulmonary hypoplasia that involves both the size of the lung and the number of alveoli. Typically, infants affected by pulmonary hypoplasia have only about half the normal lung volume at the time of birth. In utero this does not interfere with development, so the infants are usually born at term and have weights appropriate for gestational age. Once the umbilical cord is clamped, however, the pulmonary hypoplasia becomes a serious problem.

Data collection
HISTORY

An infant with a diaphragmatic defect usually develops respiratory distress very soon after delivery. As respiration progresses, the negative intrathoracic pressure draws increasingly more bowel through the defect up into the chest. Also, if the neonate cries and begins to swallow air, the bowel loops within the chest become more distended and further compress the heart and lungs.

PHYSICAL EXAMINATION

On physical examination infants with diaphragmatic hernia usually have a markedly scaphoid appearance, since most of the bowel is up in the chest. Also, the cardiac impulse is displaced away from the side of the hernia. Since most of the hernias occur on the left, the apex beat is usually displaced into the right chest. The combination of a cardiac impulse in the right chest, severe cyanosis, and respiratory distress is often misinterpreted as dextrocardia associated with heart disease.

LABORATORY DATA

A chest x-ray examination shows the typical pattern of bowel gas in the chest with displacement of the heart shadow to the contralateral side (Figure 21-5).

Treatment
PREOPERATIVE CARE

As soon as diaphragmatic hernia is suspected, an orogastric tube should be passed to prevent further distention of the bowel with gas. The infant may also require endotracheal intubation and positive-pressure ventilation to maintain adequate blood gases. It is usually advisable to insert an umbilical artery catheter as soon as possible for monitoring blood gases. A preductally placed transcutaneous monitor will help detect persistent pulmonary hypertension that frequently accompanies a diaphragmatic hernia.

OPERATIVE INTERVENTION

Congenital diaphragmatic hernia is a surgical emergency for the neonate. The sooner the bowel is returned to the abdomen, the sooner the lung function can be improved.

The infant is explored through a subcostal incision on the side of the hernia. The bowel is then reduced from the chest down into the abdomen, and the diaphragmatic defect is closed. In most cases sufficient diaphragm remains to permit primary closure, and only rarely is mesh or other prosthetic material required. Closing the abdomen is sometimes difficult because the bowel has developed in the chest and the abdominal cavity is smaller than normal. In such cases it is occasionally necessary to close only skin, leaving the infant with a large ventral hernia that can be closed at a later date. A chest tube is left on the affected side drained only to water seal.

POSTOPERATIVE CARE

Suction on the chest tube is contraindicated because it imposes a marked shift in the mediastinum that may further complicate pulmo-

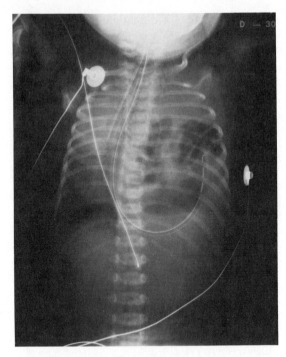

Figure 21-5. Diaphragmatic hernia in newborn girl with respiratory distress. Note nasogastric tube that is below diaphragm, then curves upward into left hemithorax. Note loops of bowel in left chest. Endotracheal tube is in right mainstem bronchus, accounting for increased atelectasis of right upper lobe.

nary and cardiac function. By having the chest tube to water seal, the mediastinum can slowly come back to a more normal position; more importantly, any fluid that is secreted in the chest can be drained.

In most instances the infants are ventilated for a minimum of 24 hours postoperatively. Paralysis is usually desirable to facilitate ventilation. Initial ventilator levels should be set with a rapid rate (>60 breaths/min) and the lowest possible pressures that can be used and still maintain adequate blood gases. Monitoring the oxygen above and below the ductus arteriosus is desirable, since the marked pulmonary hypoplasia often leads to pulmonary hypertension and a right-to-left shunt through the ductus arteriosus (see Chapters 17 and 18).

Infants with diaphragmatic hernia are treated with a rather complex pharmacologic regimen. If cardiac output is diminished, a dopamine drip (5 to 10 μg/min) is begun. Then a minimum of 10 ml/kg of colloid is given; if this does not improve function and perfusion, a tolazoline drip is administered.

By the third postoperative day the pulmonary function usually begins to improve, and the medications can be slowly tapered. Weaning from the respirator usually takes an additional day or two.

Complications and prognosis

The overall mortality of infants with congenital diaphragmatic hernia has improved over the last 10 years. Survival is now between 60% and 80% if no complicating problems exist. The presence of congenital heart disease or a birth weight of less than 1800 g increases the mortality to nearly 100%.

Once infants are weaned from the respirator, they usually lead a normal life. The infant lung has an incredible ability to develop and grow, so that by the end of the first year most of the infants have perfectly normal lung function.

Early diagnosis, immediate resuscitation and stabilization, and urgent surgical repair are of prime importance in salvaging these desperately ill infants.

ESOPHAGEAL ANOMALIES
Physiology and etiology

Esophageal atresia and tracheoesophageal fistula are quite common anomalies, and they are usually associated. In the most common type of tracheoesophageal fistula the upper esophagus ends blindly at roughly the level of the second thoracic vertebra (Figure 21-6, C). The distal esophagus has an abnormal communication to the back of the trachea just cephalad to the carina. This accounts for about 75% of the esophageal anomalies present at birth.

The second most common anomaly involves a single atresia in the middle portion of the esophagus (Figure 21-6, A). In this instance the upper esophagus ends blindly at the level of the second thoracic vertebra, and the lower esophagus is only several centimeters long. There are in addition a variety of combinations of fistulas from the upper

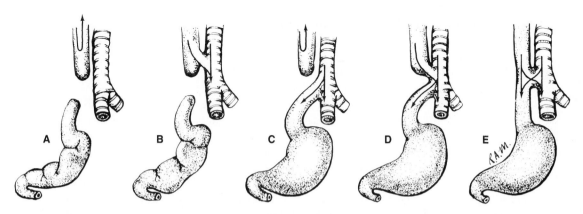

Figure 21-6. Most common types of esophageal atresia and tracheoesophageal fistula. (From Whaley LF and Wong DL: Nursing care of infants and children, ed 3, St Louis, 1987, The CV Mosby Co.)

and lower pouches and an "H" fistula[9] (Figure 21-6, *E*). In this instance the esophagus and trachea are normally formed, but there is an abnormal communication between them at approximately the middle of the esophagus.

The cause of these defects is unknown, although the entire pulmonary system is derived from the foregut of the primitive embryo and develops as a bud from what will ultimately become the esophagus. Most cases of esophageal atresia are sporadic; however, it must be noted that cases have been reported of twins, two or more siblings, and two or more generations being involved.

Data collection
HISTORY

Frequently there is a history of maternal polyhydramnios. This is presumably a result of the fetus being unable to swallow amniotic fluid normally. Soon after birth, copious secretions are noticeable, since the infant is unable to swallow saliva.

PHYSICAL EXAMINATION AND ASSOCIATED ANOMALIES

The infant with esophageal atresia will have great difficulty with feedings. Typically the infant will take one or two sucks and then begin to cough and regurgitate the unchanged formula. An attempt at passing a catheter into the stomach will indicate an obstruction about 8 to 10 cm from the mouth.

Approximately 25% of infants with esophageal anomalies have associated heart disease or abnormalities of the aortic arch, and about 20% have an associated imperforate anus. These infants may have the symptom complex referred to as VACTERL, which is a combination of anomalies affecting the vertebrae, anus, heart (cardiac), trachea, esophagus, urinary tract (renal), and limbs. Infants suffering from VACTERL require prolonged hospitalization to manage their many defects.

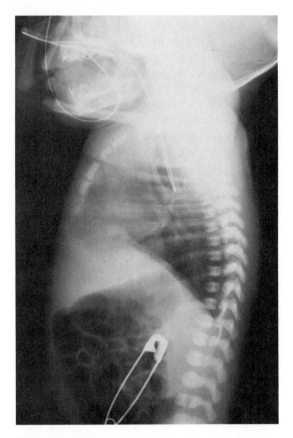

Figure 21-7. Esophageal atresia with tracheoesophageal fistula. Lateral x-ray film shows gastric tube in esophageal pouch and air in gastrointestinal tract, consistent with esophageal atresia with tracheoesophageal fistula.

LABORATORY DATA

If obstruction is suspected, the tube should be taped in place, and the infant should have abdominal and chest x-ray examinations. In the common type of esophageal atresia with distal fistula, the tip of the tube is visible at the interspace between the second and third thoracic vertebrae. Also, gas accumulates in the bowel below the diaphragm, since crying forces air from the trachea through the fistula down into

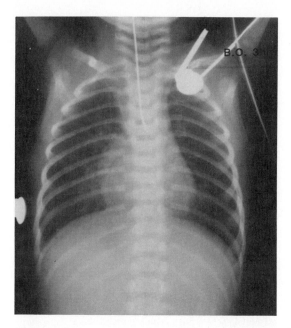

Figure 21-8. Esophageal atresia without tracheoesophageal fistula in 3-hour-old, 36-week infant with feeding difficulty and inability to pass nasogastric tube. Note nasogastric tube in esophagus and gasless abdomen suggestive of no distal fistula.

the stomach (Figure 21-7). If no gas is in the bowel below the diaphragm, there is probably no distal fistula (Figure 21-8).

Treatment
PREOPERATIVE CARE

Once the diagnosis is confirmed, the tube in the upper pouch should be attached to suction so that the infant does not aspirate saliva or secretions from above. The infant should also be placed in the head-up position to minimize the chance of gastric juice refluxing through the distal esophagus and its fistula into the airway. When no distal fistula is thought to be present, the infant can be placed flat or with the head slightly down so that gravity aids in emptying the upper pouch.

An IV line should be started for hydration and glucose administration. Broad-spectrum antibiotic agents should also be administered to protect the infant against aspiration pneumonia and to prepare the infant for surgery.

OPERATIVE INTERVENTION

The surgical repair of esophageal atresia is not an emergency procedure but should be done as soon as possible. The esophagus is approached through a right retropleural incision, and the distal esophagus is divided from the back wall of the trachea. The ends of the esophagus are then sutured together primarily. Occasionally the gap between the two ends of the esophagus is too great; in that instance the distal esophagus is oversewn and sutured to the highest rib possible. Six weeks later there is often enough growth in the distal esophagus to permit an anastomosis.

Gastrostomy tubes are often used to decompress the stomach and to facilitate feeding in the postoperative period. However, not all babies with esophageal atresia require gastrostomy, and its placement is based on the judgment of the surgeon.

Infants with esophageal atresia that is not complicated with a tracheoesophageal fistula are most often treated initially with a gastrostomy tube. The infant can be fed through the gastrostomy tube, and the distal esophagus allowed to grow. Primary repair is attempted at about 6 weeks of age.

POSTOPERATIVE CARE

Postoperative oropharyngeal suctioning should be permitted only to a distance of 8 cm. If this is scrupulously observed, the catheter will never reach quite to the level of the anastomosis. Also, if an endotracheal tube is in place, the suctioning should be limited to the length of the endotracheal tube; the tip of the catheter should not be allowed to protrude beyond the endotracheal tube. Otherwise damage to the recently closed fistula may result. The gastrostomy if in place is drained to gravity. Pacifiers are forbidden because sucking increases secretions.

The retropleural tube is drained to gravity. Antibiotic agents are continued for 3 to 5 days postoperatively.

The first feeding is permitted on the fifth day after surgery if the infant is swallowing secretions without difficulty. Some centers prefer to obtain a contrast study of the esophagus before commencing feeding, but in most cases a leak is painfully obvious because of saliva draining from the chest tube, fever, and tachypnea. Initial feedings should be taken slowly and the infant placed in the chalasia position for at least an hour after feeding.[6,7] Most infants with esophageal atresia have severe gastroesophageal reflux, so from the beginning they should be treated as if it were present.

Problems of esophageal abnormal motility are usually self-limited, but they can be very troublesome in the early postoperative course. The problem is one of poor propagation of the esophageal peristalsis, so that the infant frequently coughs and sputters while eating. Occasionally a gastrostomy tube is required until better esophageal coordination develops. In most cases, however, the infant simply learns to cope with abnormal motility. Most infants with esophageal atresia have some degree of abnormal motility even though they are totally asymptomatic.

Complications and prognosis

The major postoperative problems are stricture, abnormal esophageal motility, and a leak at the anastomotic site. A leak at the anastomotic site is not nearly as dire a complication as it has been in the past. Modern broad-spectrum antibiotic agents have tremendously reduced the mortality and morbidity of this complication. Likewise, the retropleural approach and placement of a retropleural tube prevent empyema or local collection of saliva. In no case should these leaks be explored surgically unless the infant is moribund. In that instance the safest procedure is to exteriorize the

upper pouch in the neck as a cervical esophagostomy and tie off the distal esophagus. This commits the patient to an esophageal replacement at a later date.

Strictures are much less common now than in the past, although they are often associated with a local anastomotic leak. Treatment is usually in the form of repeated esophageal dilations. If marked esophageal reflux is complicated by a recurrent stricture at the anastomotic site, it may be necessary to perform Nissen's fundoplication or a similar antireflux procedure. This often will prevent further stricture formation.

Although primary repair of the esophageal atresia has been undertaken only in the past 30 years, the survival rate is in excess of 95% and approaches 100% in term infants who do not have complicating associated anomalies.

BOWEL ATRESIA AND STENOSIS
Physiology and etiology

Any segment of the bowel may be narrow or discontinuous, although certain areas have high predilection for these abnormalities. The duodenum at the level of the entrance of the common duct is the most common site for atresia or stenosis. Jejunal, ileal, and colon atresia also occur.

Experimental evidence and gross observation show that most bowel atresias are related to a vascular insult to the bowel. The insult can be in the form of occlusion of a major blood vessel supplying the bowel, an intrauterine volvulus, or an intrauterine intussusception.

A rare form of jejunal atresia is called "apple peel mesentery." This results from infarction or absence of the entire superior mesenteric artery. Surprisingly, this defect has a fairly strong hereditary component, and many cases have been reported in siblings. The remainder of the atresias appear to be sporadic.

Data collection
HISTORY

Typically the mother has polyhydramnios, and the infant is SGA. In all cases infants have difficulty feeding from birth and often have obvious abdominal distention soon after birth.

PHYSICAL EXAMINATION AND ASSOCIATED ANOMALIES

If the atresia or stenosis is just beyond the entrance of the common duct, bile-stained vomiting occurs. If the stenosis is just above the entrance of the common duct, the vomiting will consist of saliva or undigested milk and not bile.

Both duodenal atresia and stenosis have a high association with Down's syndrome.

Some infants with bowel atresia will pass a small amount of material per rectum that is incorrectly called meconium. Typically it is much lighter in color and scant in amount. Infants with duodenal atresia or stenosis frequently are deeply jaundiced by the second or third day of life. This is less of a problem with more distal atresias.

LABORATORY DATA

Abdominal x-ray films taken in the upright position show a typical "double bubble" in duodenal atresia (Figure 21-9). The two bubbles are formed by air/fluid levels in the fundus of the stomach and in the markedly dilated first portion of the duodenum. In a case of duodenal atresia no gas accumulates in the distal bowel. If there is merely stenosis or narrowing of the duodenum, a small amount of gas is observed in the distal bowel.

Treatment
PREOPERATIVE CARE

Initial therapy consists of passage of an orogastric tube to decompress the stomach and proximal bowel and to minimize the chance of vomiting and aspiration. Intravenous hydration and replacement of electrolytes is essential.

OPERATIVE INTERVENTION

Surgical repair of duodenal atresia or stenosis usually involves a side-to-side anastomosis, since the common duct enters nearby and is easily injured. It is usually advisable to place a gastrostomy tube during the operation to facilitate proximal decompression in the postoperative period and also to help with early, frequent, small feedings that are required as the bowel is beginning to function. More distal atresias can usually be repaired with an end-to-end anastomosis, although occasionally the size disparity is such that an end-to-end anastomosis is not possible. In these instances it is usually preferable to bring out an ostomy and a nearby mucous fistula. When the proximal bowel has diminished in size to a more normal caliber and the distal bowel has had a chance to grow, the two ends can be anastomosed. Such infants frequently require hyperalimentation and insertion of a Broviac catheter.

POSTOPERATIVE CARE

In the immediate postoperative period the bowel requires continual decompression from above with either an orogastric tube or a gastrostomy tube. Initial care of the ileostomy or jejunostomy is to cover the exposed mucosa with a saline-soaked sponge. Once the stoma begins to function, it is advisable to attach an appliance as soon as possible. A small square of Stomadhesive with the opening cut to accurately fit the stoma is placed next to the skin. A bag is then attached directly to the Stomahesive. The volume of ostomy drainage should be monitored carefully and IV hydration altered accordingly. Sodium and bicarbonate losses from jejunostomies are very high, and in most cases the infant requires continual replacement of these electrolytes.

Complications and prognosis

The major complications in the immediate postoperative period involve infection and prolapse of the ostomy. Surgical techniques are available to minimize the incidence of prolapse, making it much less common than it has been in the past.

Long-term complications are usually related to adhesion formation or poor function of the bowel distal to the anastomosis. Most of these are self-limited, however, and a surprising number of

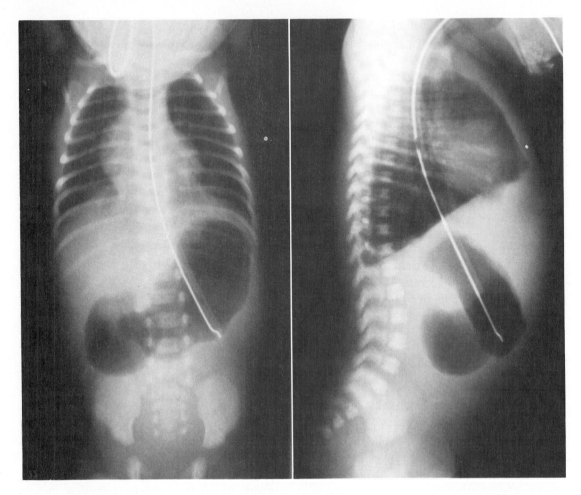

Figure 21-9. Duodenal atresia in 2-day-old, 36-week, SGA preterm infant who was unable to tolerate feedings. Classic double bubble sign of gastric and duodenal dilation secondary to duodenal atresia is noted on both x-ray films. Note airless abdomen; no bowel gas extends beyond duodenum.

these children have no further gastrointestinal problems.

IMPERFORATE ANUS
Physiology and etiology

The general term *imperforate anus* encompasses a large variety of anomalies that are embryologically and clinically quite different. There are approximately 34 major categories. The discussion that follows is somewhat simplified but covers at least 95% of the cases of imperforate anus that are encountered.

The male infant with imperforate anus characteristically has a higher lesion than does the female infant. In the male infant the rectum usually ends above the levator muscles and communicates to the membranous urethra with a long fistula. Fistulas into the bladder are quite rare.

In the female infant, the anorectal anomalies are usually much lower and associated with a fistula somewhere between the posterior fourchette and the normal position of the rectum. The implications of these anatomic differences are rather profound.

Data collection
PHYSICAL EXAMINATION

Most of the anomalies are quite obvious on physical examination. No opening appears where the anus should be, and possibly meconium is in the urine of the male infant or in the vagina of the female infant. A strong association exists between esophageal atresia and imperforate anus, so an infant with either anomaly should be carefully checked for the other.

Careful examination of the buttocks and perineum for contour and sensation are important. If the buttocks are poorly formed and little or no indentation can be observed between the buttocks, there is usually deficient musculature and innervation, so that the operative outcome is likely to be very poor.

Rectal stenosis does occur but is relatively rare. In most cases the ability to pass a soft rectal probe such as a feeding tube or suction catheter rules out any significant anorectal anomaly. A thermometer should not be used, since rectal perforation may occur.

LABORATORY DATA

X-ray examinations are not of a great deal of value in this condition. Rice-Wangensteen x-ray examinations were popular at one time. This involved holding the infant head-down for 5 minutes and then obtaining an x-ray film of the pelvis. In this manner the gas in the intestine would frequently pass to the level of obstruction and no further. In many cases, however, these x-ray films were not accurate, and they have been largely abandoned.

Ultrasound examination can be useful in establishing the exact level of the obstruction and outlining the fistula if one is present.

To look for associated anomalies, x-ray films should be taken of the lumbosacral spine. The absence of one or more vertebra or multiple hemivertebra often means that the infant does not have normal innervation in the perianal region and will be incontinent.

Treatment
PREOPERATIVE CARE

After the diagnosis is made, the infant should not drink anything until some opening has been established for evacuating the meconium. If no meconium has appeared in the urine or in the vagina within 24 hours and no fistula is apparent on the skin, a colostomy should be considered.

OPERATIVE INTERVENTION

Most male infants require a colostomy at birth if no fistula is observed on the perineum. At about 1 year of age they undergo an abdominoperineal or occasionally sacroperineal pull-through operation. This creates a new anus and divides the fistula to the urinary tract. About 1 month after that, the colostomy is closed. With this form of therapy approximately 50% of male infants are completely continent. Another 25% are nearly continent, and a final 25% are totally incontinent.

By contrast, in the female infant most of the anorectal anomalies can be handled at birth with a perineal anoplasty. Only when the fistula is not visible or empties high on the posterior vaginal wall is a colostomy required. In this instance the staged procedures are essentially the same as those for the male infant. At any level of involvement, however, the incidence is much higher in male infants than in female infants.

A high sigmoid colostomy is usually preferable, since it enables the infant to pass relatively formed stools and therefore have fewer skin problems.

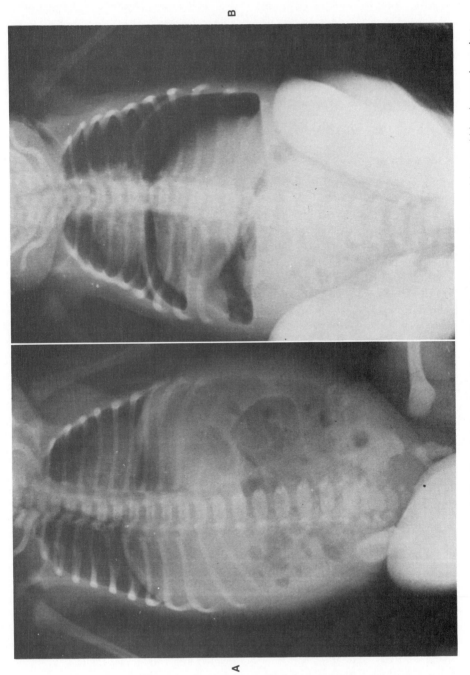

Figure 21-10. Perforated ulcer. **A,** Flat film of abdomen in infant with abdominal distention, vomiting, and bloody gastric aspirate. **B,** Upright film of abdomen. Free air rises and is easily seen in abdomen.

POSTOPERATIVE CARE

Once created, the colostomy usually drains copious meconium within a matter of hours. Therefore it is usually desirable to attach the colostomy appliance in the operating room or soon thereafter. The following day the infant can be started on a regular newborn feeding regimen. An ultrasound examination of the kidneys or an IV pyelogram to establish the presence of both kidneys should be performed.

Complications and prognosis

Infants with imperforate anus have lifelong problems with constipation after the pull-through is complete. They must be followed carefully and kept on a high-residue diet with as much bran and fiber as possible. Even then they may require occasional enemas or suppositories.

IDIOPATHIC GASTRIC PERFORATION
Physiology, etiology, and data collection

Occasionally a healthy term infant will develop sudden abdominal distention, pallor, and peritonitis. X-ray examination will show free air in the abdomen (Figure 21-10). Gastric aspirate will return some blood-stained material. This symptom complex is fairly typical of an idiopathic gastric perforation. The cause of these perforations is unknown, but they almost certainly are not peptic in origin. The cause remains obscure.

Treatment
PREOPERATIVE CARE

As with any infant who has free air in the abdomen, an orogastric tube should be passed promptly and placed to suction. The infant should have a large-bore and reliable IV tube placed and should be resuscitated vigorously with Ringer's lactate solution and colloid if necessary. He should also be started immediately on broad-spectrum antibiotic agents. Occasionally the abdomen is so distended that it must be aspirated with a needle to relieve the respiratory pressure on the diaphragm.

OPERATIVE INTERVENTION

Obviously an exploratory operation should be performed as soon as the infant has been sufficiently resuscitated to withstand an anesthetic. The hole is easily located and must be oversewn in two layers.

Complications and prognosis

The convalescence is usually uneventful, and the infants do not seem to have any increased predisposition to ulcer disease or other digestive problems.

HIRSCHSPRUNG'S DISEASE
Physiology and etiology

Hirschsprung's disease is caused by an absence of ganglia in the wall of the bowel. The defect always begins in the anus and extends proximally for a variable distance. In 85% of cases the transition zone from abnormal bowel is in the region of the sigmoid colon. In about 5% of cases the entire colon is aganglionic, and in rare cases even an extensive length of the small bowel is involved. The absence of ganglia leaves the involved bowel in contraction or spasm most of the time, causing a functional bowel obstruction. The condition is at least 10 times more common in male infants than in female infants, and most children with Hirschsprung's disease are symptomatic from birth.

Data collection
HISTORY

Most infants with Hirschsprung's disease initially have abdominal distention and failure to stool in the first 48 hours. If the obstruction is not relieved by dilation or rectal stimulation, these infants begin to vomit. Rectal examination, however, frequently produces a stool, and thus many infants leave the nursery without the diagnosis being suspected. Over the subsequent weeks or months infants with Hirschsprung's disease have increasing difficulty with passage of stools, poor weight gain, and progressive abdominal distention.

A small percentage of infants with Hirschsprung's disease have life-threatening colitis. These infants are characteristically obtunded, severely dehydrated, acidotic, and frequently have a positive blood culture.

PHYSICAL EXAMINATION AND ASSOCIATED ANOMALIES

Infants with functional or habit constipation usually have firm stools, and the rectal ampulla is full of stool at the time of rectal examination. When these infants have a stool, it is very large. Infants with Hirschsprung's disease usually have an empty rectal ampulla, but a vigorous rectal examination stimulates a small diarrhea stool expelled under considerable pressure. This physical finding is diagnostic of Hirschsprung's disease.

The disease has a strong genetic background with siblings and several generations very commonly involved. Children with Down's syndrome have a 2% to 5% incidence of Hirschsprung's disease.

LABORATORY DATA

Abdominal x-ray films show a pattern of bowel obstruction with numerous visible air/fluid levels on the upright x-ray films. If the infant is highly suspected of having Hirschsprung's disease, a barium enema is the next diagnostic test performed. A lateral projection of the pelvis is particularly important during the early phase of the enema. This shows the abnormality in the opening of the rectal ampulla and the irregularity and spasticity in the rectum. In infants over several weeks old there is usually a very marked transition zone where the proximal normal bowel has become dilated and funnels rapidly down into the narrow spastic-involved segment. When this situation is observed radiographically, the infant should have a rectal biopsy to confirm the diagnosis.

Once the infant with colitis is resuscitated, a limited barium enema to look for the typical findings should be performed.

Treatment
PREOPERATIVE CARE

In infants with colitis immediate resuscitation consists of passage of an orogastric tube, 20 to 30 ml of crystalloid/kg given rapidly IV, administration of broad-spectrum antibiotic agents, and correction of any acid-base deficits that may exist. Rectal biopsy is then performed and submitted for frozen section. In infants without colitis the rectal biopsy can be processed normally.

OPERATIVE INTERVENTION

If ganglia are absent in the infant with colitis, the infant should have an immediate colostomy. In infants without colitis the colostomy can be performed electively.

In centers that have full-time pathology coverage, the ideal place to perform the colostomy is just proximal to the transition zone. This gives the infant a maximal length of functioning bowel and enables the passage of relatively formed stools. The position of the colostomy must always be checked by frozen section biopsy to be sure that ganglia are present at the colostomy site. A colostomy performed even several centimeters into the aganglionic bowel will fail to function, and the infant will remain functionally obstructed.

POSTOPERATIVE CARE

A colostomy appliance should be applied early. Once the colostomy is functioning, the infant may be fed normally and should thrive.

The definitive pull-through procedure that removes the aganglionic bowel and pulls normal bowel down to the anus is usually deferred until about 1 year of age. This permits the infant to be in an optimal nutritional state and also enables the dilated proximal colon to shrink back to a normal size.

Complications and prognosis

Once the pull-through procedure has been completed and the colostomy closed, most of the patients lead a perfectly normal life. Some of the children do require occasional anal dilations, and some require stool softeners or high-fiber diets.

MECONIUM ILEUS
Physiology and etiology

Meconium ileus is caused by very sticky, inspissated meconium obstructing the terminal ileum. At least 95% of cases occur in children with cystic fibrosis. As part of the cystic fibrosis, pancreatic enzymes are lacking. Therefore the proteins that are swallowed from the amniotic fluid are not normally digested and form a sticky plug in the terminal ileum.

Data collection

Since cystic fibrosis is inherited as an autosomal recessive disease, a family history of cystic fibrosis often exists.

In many cases the thickened meconium can be felt through the abdominal wall as a dilated, ropy loop of bowel. Plain x-ray films show several dilated bowel loops with air/fluid levels, and frequently there is a soap bubble appearance in the right lower quadrant. Apparently, this type of x-ray picture is produced by the inspissated meconium. A barium enema shows a tiny microcolon and frequently outlines pellets of highly inspissated meconium in either the right side of the colon or the terminal ileum. The contrast material will then frequently flow into the large, dilated loop of bowel, demonstrating that no atresia is present but rather that a mechanical plug of meconium has formed.

Treatment
PREOPERATIVE CARE

An enema performed with half-strength Gastrografin frequently permits the infant to pass the inspissated meconium. The Gastrografin is hyperosmolar and draws some of the water from the bowel wall. This effectively creates a thin layer of water between the sticky meconium and the bowel wall so that the meconium can be more easily passed. Before the Gastrografin enema an IV line should be placed and the infant should be well hydrated. The fluid drawn in by the Gastrografin enema is lost from the circulation, and the infant may become markedly hypovolemic if not properly hydrated.

Pancreative enzymes can also be instilled from above. One tablet or capsule is dissolved in 60 ml of saline, and 15 ml of this mixture is instilled through an orogastric tube. The tube is clamped for 1 hour and then returned to suction. Using this combined regimen of Gastrografin enema and pancreative enzymes, most infants can be totally unobstructed within 3 days. If the obstruction is still present after 3 days, the infant should be seriously considered for exploratory surgery, since there is most likely an associated mechanical obstruction.

OPERATIVE INTERVENTION

The operation usually consists of creating an ileostomy to establish normal bowel function and enable the patient to grow normally.

POSTOPERATIVE CARE

When the child begins to feed, it is advisable to use an elemental formula that does not require pancreatic enzymes. If breastfeeding is contemplated, pancreative enzyme should be added as necessary to prevent the appearance of protein or sugar in the stool.

Complications and prognosis

All infants with meconium ileus should be evaluated for cystic fibrosis. Their prognosis is related to the severity of the cystic fibrosis.

PYLORIC STENOSIS
Physiology and etiology

Pyloric stenosis is often referred to as congenital hypertrophic pyloric stenosis, although many of the cases are not congenital. Many cases have been recorded where the newborn underwent exploratory surgery, and the duodenum was noted to be normal. By 4 weeks of age the same infant had developed the signs and symptoms of pyloric stenosis. The condition is much more common in male infants and specifically firstborn male infants. There is a definite hereditary component, since about 5% of the offspring of affected men have pyloric stenosis and about 20% of the offspring of affected women have pyloric stenosis.

The abnormality involves a marked hypertrophy of the muscles in the region of the normal pylorus. The muscle cells are normal, and ganglia appear to be appropriate in number and function. There is an increase in extracellular ground substance seen microscopically, and the result is a stiff napkin ring type of deformity at the outlet of the stomach. At one time elevated gastrin levels in the mother and infant were implicated in the development of pyloric stenosis, but subsequent studies have shown the association to be invalid.

Data collection
HISTORY

Typically the infant is in normal health until the age of 2 or 3 weeks. The neonate then begins episodes of vomiting that become more frequent and more forceful. Ultimately the infant develops "projectile" vomiting. The vomit does not contain bile and usually occurs after feeding. The infant is then immediately hungry and will refeed if offered a bottle. If pyloric stenosis is not treated at this time, the infant will begin to lose weight and become increasingly irritable.

PHYSICAL EXAMINATION

The diagnosis can usually be confirmed on physical examination where the typical olive-sized lump is palpable under the liver on the right side. In extreme cases the stomach becomes so hypertrophic in response to its outlet obstruction that visible gastric waves can be seen progressing from the left upper quadrant toward the right lower quadrant. Also, about 5% of infants become significantly jaundiced for unknown reasons. The jaundice disappears promptly after the pyloric stenosis has been removed.

LABORATORY DATA

If the diagnosis is suspected but the "olive" cannot be felt, an upper gastrointestinal series is performed with barium and is diagnostic. The markedly narrow pyloric channel is reduced to a string size, and the pylorus never opens out normally. The "olive" may also be identified by ultrasound examination.

Projectile vomiting can also accompany severe chalasia, so that either a palpable olive-sized mass in the right upper quadrant or a barium study outlining the pylorus is essential before surgery is contemplated.

The hyperbilirubinemia affects only the indirect portion when present. There is also a characteristic metabolic abnormality in neonates with pyloric stenosis; because of the vomiting, they deplete chloride in the form of hydrochloric acid from their stomach. Therefore they become hypochloremic, alkalotic, and ultimately hypokalemic. When the infant is alkalotic, there is a paradoxical acid urine as the kidney tubule exchanges hydrogen ion for potassium.

Treatment
PREOPERATIVE CARE

Initial resuscitation consists of correcting dehydration and metabolic abnormalities and passing an orogastric tube to decompress the stomach (see Chapters 8 and 11). Although many formulas have been developed for repairing the existing deficits, the easiest is as follows:

1. Fifty percent normal saline in 5% dextrose, 100 ml/kg every 8 hours
2. Potassium chloride added to the above solution to produce 40 mEq/L

Within 16 to 24 hours the metabolic alkalosis

and hypokalemia are corrected. The additional fluid corrects the dehydration. When serum electrolytes have returned to normal and arterial pH is equal to or less than 7.35, fluids can be cut back to normal maintenance and the child taken to surgery.

OPERATIVE INTERVENTION

The operation consists of a simple longitudinal splitting of the dense muscular ring at the pylorus. The mucosa and submucosa are left intact so that the lumen of the duodenum is not entered.

POSTOPERATIVE CARE

Feedings with glucose water may be commenced within 12 hours of surgery, and most infants are ready for discharge on the second postoperative day.

Complications and prognosis

In the past, medical treatment of pyloric stenosis has been attempted and is occasionally successful. However, the hospitalization is prolonged and the expense considerable. With present surgical and anesthetic techniques, surgical treatment is preferred.

CHALASIA
Physiology and etiology

Although the normal adult and older child have a competent one-way valve between the distal esophagus and proximal stomach, in many infants this valve is not well developed. Although all the components of this rather remarkable valve system are not known, important factors include (1) the angle of His where the esophagus joins the stomach; (2) a circular sphincter muscle in the distal esophagus, referred to as the lower esophageal sphincter; and (3) a significant length of intraabdominal esophagus. At birth any or all of these components may be deficient, leading to free reflux of gastric juice backup into the esophagus. In most infants this mechanism becomes completely competent by the age of 6 months or

so. In some otherwise normal infants, however, this does not mature normally, and they continue to have reflux of gastric contents up into the esophagus. Likewise, infants born with high bowel obstruction such as duodenal stenosis, duodenal atresia, ileal stenosis, or ileal atresia have delay in maturation of the valve mechanism. Apparently, the in utero regurgitation of the gastric contents has stretched or in some other way altered the normal mechanism. Thus all infants with high small bowel obstructions should be treated in the immediate postoperative period if they have chalasia.

Data collection
HISTORY

Chalasia may be characterized by a variety of symptoms. In very severe cases the amount of food vomited is so great that the neonate cannot gain weight normally and therefore fails to thrive. A second common symptom is aspiration pneumonitis caused by aspirating gastric juice repeatedly into the airway. A less common but more frightening symptom is that of apnea and, occasionally, sudden infant death syndrome. The apnea and death are not caused by massive aspiration but appear to be reflexes triggered by even a small amount of gastric contents in or around the larynx. Infants who develop esophagitis are often very fretful, especially when lying supine.

LABORATORY DATA

The frequency and magnitude of reflux should be evaluated with a barium swallow. The radiologist should also note evidence of esophagitis. If doubt remains, a small pH probe on a fine-wire mesh can be passed through the nose down into the distal esophagus, and an 8- or 24-hour recording obtained. This will demonstrate the frequency of reflux episodes and the duration of the period during which the lower esophagus has a strongly acid pH.

Chalasia is often seen with iron deficiency

anemia and occult blood in the stool from the open ulceration in the distal esophagus.

Treatment
PREOPERATIVE CARE

Treatment consists of giving frequent, small feedings thickened with rice cereal, keeping the infant in the prone position with a 30- to 45-degree angle elevation of the head of the bed[6,7] and adding cimetidine or ranitidine to reduce gastric acid. The prone position, rather than the upright position in the infant seat, decreases the number and length of reflux episodes.[6,7]

If episodes of apnea have been noted, an apnea alarm should be available in the home for monitoring during the night and naptime (see Chapter 17).

OPERATIVE INTERVENTION

Indications for operative intervention include recurrent apnea episodes, persistent failure to thrive, repeated episodes of aspiration pneumonitis, and persistent esophagitis or stricture formation.

Although a variety of operations have been devised to prevent reflux, the most widely used is Nissen's fundoplication. In this procedure the proximal stomach is reflected up onto the wall of the esophagus and sutured in place. This creates an inkwell type of junction with the stomach and esophagus and has been very effective in preventing reflux.

Complications and prognosis

Most infants require a temporary gastrostomy after Nissen's fundoplication because initially they are unable to burp. The tube permits venting of any swallowed gas and minimizes problems with colic and bloating. The tube can usually be removed within 3 to 6 weeks of the procedure.

For reasons that are not clear, some infants also have diarrhea for 3 to 5 days after bowel function returns. Damage to the vagus nerves has been implicated, but the diarrhea is so short lived that probably other factors are involved.

BILIARY ATRESIA
Physiology and etiology

A variety of congenital anomalies of the drainage system of the liver are grouped as "biliary atresia." The most common form and unfortunately the most difficult to manage involves the failure of the extrahepatic duct system to form. The result is an accumulation of bile within the liver substance that leads to progressive jaundice, cirrhosis, and ultimately death. The cause is unknown, but in some instances biliary atresia appears to follow a viral infection.

Data collection
HISTORY AND PHYSICAL EXAMINATION

Typically infants with biliary atresia are normal at birth and are discharged from the nursery as healthy infants. They eat and grow normally, even after the onset of jaundice. At about 1 month of age scleral icterus becomes apparent, and the stools are typically clay colored or very light brown.

LABORATORY DATA

Liver function studies show a bilirubin level of about 8 to 10 mg/dl, marked elevation of the alkaline phosphatase, and less marked elevation of the serum glutamic-oxaloacetic transaminase.

Screening tests should include hepatitis screen, alpha-1-antitrypsin levels, and urinalysis for reducing substances. If these studies are normal, the neonate should be evaluated with an isotope study of liver drainage. A compound containing radioactive technetium is injected intravenously, and the liver and abdomen are scanned. The isotope concentrates in the liver. If there is bile drainage, the radioactivity can be detected in the small bowel within several hours. If no radioactivity is seen in the small

bowel within about 4 hours, there is most likely obstruction to bile flow. Aspiration of duodenal contents that are free of bile for 24 hours also suggests obstruction.

Treatment

Liver biopsy and exploration of the hepatic ducts are indicated if obstruction to bile flow is found. Giant cell hepatitis characteristically has large numbers of giant cells within the liver substance and normally developed microscopic ducts. In biliary atresia, there are few or no giant cells, and there is marked proliferation of the small interhepatic ducts. Exploration of the porta hepatis will demonstrate whether bile ducts are present. A cholangiogram can be performed through the gallbladder.

If no ducts are found and the biopsy is consistent with biliary atresia, the only hope for the child is the Kasai procedure. This involves cutting across the porta hepatis where the ducts normally occur and bringing a loop of bowel up to this area, permitting bile to drain from the raw surface of the liver into the gastrointestinal tract. Although this procedure is not technically difficult and infants tolerate it very well, the results are marginal at best.

Complications

Most of the infants have repeated bouts of cholangitis and slowly deteriorating liver; therefore a liver transplant is an important consideration.

NECROTIZING ENTEROCOLITIS
Physiology and etiology

Necrotizing enterocolitis (NEC) is usually a disease of premature infants but may be seen in term infants. Although the exact cause(s) of NEC is not known, the common pathway appears to be mucosal injury. This injury may be a result of perinatal asphyxia, polycythemia, hyperosmolar feedings, gastrointestinal infection (bacterial or viral), exchange transfusion, or severe cardiopulmonary disease. Once the mucosal injury has occurred,

bacterial invasion and gas formation are common findings.

Prevention

Avoidance of the high-risk factors listed previously is the best preventive measure. Proper obstetric monitoring and intervention will minimize perinatal asphyxia. When perinatal asphyxia is unavoidable, delaying feedings for several days may be beneficial. Treatment of polycythemia with exchange transfusion may help prevent NEC. The incidence of NEC is lower in breastfed infants than in artificially fed infants. The mechanism for protection with breast-feeding is not known.

Data collection
HISTORY

There is usually a history of a complicated pregnancy resulting in a premature birth. Frequently perinatal asphyxia has been noted. Respiratory distress syndrome or other serious illness may also be present. Although the infant had been feeding well, the infant may develop vomiting or increased residual.

SIGNS AND SYMPTOMS

Nonspecific signs and symptoms include apnea, temperature instability, and jaundice. Abdominal distention followed by increased residuals or vomiting is noted. Blood may be seen in the stool. In severe cases localized abdominal wall erythema and induration can be seen.

LABORATORY DATA

Occult blood and positive (2+ or higher) Clinitest results (reducing substances) are early laboratory findings. There is frequently an associated thrombocytopenia. Blood cultures may be positive. X-ray examination of the abdomen is important in the diagnostic evaluation. In the beginning stages diffuse dilation of the bowel compatible with a functional ileus may develop. Pneumatosis, intramural air, is pathognomonic

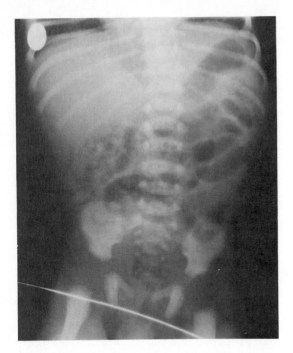

Figure 21-11. Necrotizing enterocolitis in 3-day-old infant with bloody diarrhea and abdominal tenderness. There is extensive pneumatosis intestinalis in left upper quadrant, right midabdomen, and probably near rectum.

(Figure 21-11). Portal vein air may be seen. Pneumoperitoneum indicates a perforation.

Treatment
PREOPERATIVE CARE

Medical management will usually be sufficient treatment. Early recognition and prompt treatment increase the chances for successful medical management. All feedings should be discontinued and an orogastric tube placed for decompression. Parenteral antibiotic agents should be started. Intravenous fluids should be given to maintain circulating blood volume and peripheral parenteral nutrition. Clinical and x-ray findings should be frequently evaluated (at least every 4 to 6 hours).

Indications for surgical intervention include intestinal perforation or evidence of necrotic bowel. Surgical intervention should be considered when induration and erythema of the abdominal wall, a tender abdominal mass, or x-ray evidence of a persistent dilated loop of bowel or free air is noted.

OPERATIVE INTERVENTION

The type of surgical procedure performed depends on the findings. Only grossly necrotic bowel or areas of perforation should be resected. Questionable bowel should be left in place and evaluated at a second laparotomy in 24 hours if necessary. Every effort should be made to preserve the ileocecal valve. In severe cases multiple ostomies may be needed.

POSTOPERATIVE CARE

Initial postoperative care consists of general supportive care and parenteral nutrition. When the infant has recovered sufficiently, low osmotic feedings should be started gradually.

Complications

Early complications include abscess, fistula, or obstruction. Stricture may be seen as a late complication of medically or surgically treated infants. Loss of large amounts of small bowel or of the ileocecal valve place the infant at significant risk for problems of the short bowel syndrome.

PAIN AND PAIN RELIEF
Physiology/Pathophysiology

In the past, neonates have not been given anesthesia and/or analgesia for surgery because of the controversy over whether or not they felt pain and whether or not they were physiologically stable enough to tolerate the effects of these drugs. The rationale for withholding anesthetics and analgesics included the belief that:

1. Neonates have an immature CNS with non-myelinated pain fibers and are thus incapable of perceiving pain. Neonates have no memory of pain.

2. Pain is a highly subjective experience that is difficult to objectively assess in nonverbal neonates.
3. Anesthetics and analgesics are dangerous when administered to neonates, and neonates are safer being unmedicated.

There is increasing evidence from recent research that neonates, including preterm infants, have a CNS that is much more mature than previously thought.[1,2] Pain pathways are myelinated in the fetus during the second and third trimesters, so that they are completely myelinated by 30 to 37 weeks gestation. Even thinly or nonmyelinated fibers carry pain stimuli. Incomplete myelination only implies a slower transmission, which is offset in the neonate by the shorter distance the impulse must travel.[2]

Even though pain is not expressed verbally in semiconscious patients, nonverbal adults (intubated, mute), and infants, this does not negate their experience of pain. Objective parameters for the assessment of pain have been developed. In response to the question of whether the neonate's responses are reflexive or a perception of pain, research has focused on measuring the infant's pain experience. The infant's capacity for memory is far greater than previously thought.[1]

Concern has been expressed that adding potent medications to an already critically ill infant might be dangerous. Local and systemic drugs now available, as well as new techniques and devices for monitoring, enable neonates (including preterm infants) to be safely anesthetized and maintained in a stable condition like any other patient.[2] Neonates, including preterm infants, exhibit physiologic responses to surgical procedures that are similar to adult responses.[2] Pain relief benefits the neonate by decreasing physiologic instability, hormonal and metabolic stress, and the behavioral reactions accompanying painful procedures (Table 21-1). The Committee on Fetus and Newborn of the American Academy of Pediatrics has recommended the administration of local and/or systemic drugs for anesthesia or analgesia to neonates undergoing surgical procedures.[2] They further state that any decision to withhold these drugs should not be based solely on the infant's age or perceived degree of cortical maturity, but should be based on the same criteria used in older patients.[2]

Etiology

Pain is produced with any surgical procedure, as a sequela to surgery, and with invasive procedures such as chest tube insertion and cutdowns.

Prevention

Since the myth that neonates do not feel pain has been proved incorrect and since safe anesthetics and analgesics do exist, care providers should anticipate and assess pain so as to provide prompt, safe, and adequate pain relief.

Comfort measures (e.g., pacifiers, position changes, swaddling, minimizing stimulation, holding/rocking, or gentle tactile stimulation) have been used as interventions for infants assessed as having pain.[5] Although comfort measures may prevent the intensification of pain (e.g., guarding an abdominal incision by positioning will be less painful than four-point restraint), they may not relieve moderate to severe pain. Comfort measures are helpful but inadequate by themselves, considering the intensity of the noxious stimuli causing the pain.

Data collection
HISTORY

The neonate's need for invasive procedures (in the nursery or elsewhere) necessitates the consideration of pain relief during and after the event. Neonatal agitation (e.g., crying, decreased activity, irritability, increased $TcPo_2$, duskiness, cyanosis) secondary to invasive procedures and/or medical problems (e.g., bronchopulmonary dysplasia) may also necessitate a combination of environmental interventions and sedative therapy.[5]

TABLE 21-1

Changes Accompanying Pain (with or without Analgesia/Anesthesia)

WITHOUT ANALGESIA/ANESTHESIA	WITH ANALGESIA/ANESTHESIA
Physiologic changes	
Increased heart rate	
During and after invasive procedure, with tracheal suctioning	Prevents heart rate changes; cardiovascular response abolished by opiate-induced anesthesia
Increased blood pressure	
During and after invasive procedure, with intubation	Prevents blood pressure changes
Palmar sweating	
Increases with painful procedures	Unknown
TcPo$_2$	
Large fluctuations above and below a "safe" range (50-100 mm Hg) occur during surgical procedures, circumcision, and intubations	Prevented with local analgesia
Increased intracranial pressure	
With intubation	Prevented with anesthesia
With tracheal suctioning	
Hormonal/metabolic changes: neonatal stress response	
Increased plasma renin activity (5 min after venipuncture)	
Returns to basal levels after 60 min	Unknown
Increased plasma epinephrine and norepinephrine levels	
In preterm infants with ventilators, chest physiotherapy, and endotracheal suctioning	Less response in sedated infants
Increased cortisol levels	
In neonates during and after circumcision	No change in small number given local anesthetic
Marked release of catecholamines, growth hormone, glucagon, cortisol, and aldosterone, and decrease in insulin with secondary metabolic changes	
In preterm and term neonates undergoing surgery with minimal anesthesia, neonatal stress response was 3-5 times greater than adult response	Use of potent (rather than minimal) anesthesia decreased stress response by halothane anesthesia in term babies; abolished stress response by low-dose fentanyl anesthesia in preterm infants; more were clinically stable with fewer complications
Behavioral changes	
Complex behavioral response	
Circumcision: prolonged periods of non-REM sleep; increased wakefulness and irritability for 1 hr; altered arousal and behavioral states for 22 hr	Circumcision (with local anesthesia): no behavioral change; more attentive to stimuli; better motor responses; less irritability and greater ability to self-quiet

Based on data from Anand KJS and Hickey PR: N Engl J Med 317:1321, 1987.

TABLE 21-1—cont'd

Changes Accompanying Pain (with or without Analgesia/Anesthesia)

WITHOUT ANALGESIA/ANESTHESIA	WITH ANALGESIA/ANESTHESIA
Simple motor responses Diffuse body movements as response to painful stimuli; specific withdrawal from painful stimuli; facial expressions associated with pain	
Crying Crying caused by distress (pain, hunger, etc.) is varied in quality and is able to be reliably distinguished; character of cry is able to be correlated with pain's intensity and can be differentiated by adult listeners; therefore neonate's cry is able to be used as a measure of pain	

SIGNS AND SYMPTOMS

Physiologic changes include increased heart rate, respiratory rate, blood pressure, mean airway pressure, and intracranial pressure. There is an increased oxygen requirement, and PaO_2 may increase or decrease. There may be palmar sweating.

Behavioral changes include crying, grimace or flinch, withdrawal, touch aversion, and asocial gaze. The infant may be difficult to comfort or quiet and may have feeding difficulties. There is increased agitation, irritability, and wakefulness.

Metabolic changes include hyperglycemia, glucosuria, ketonuria, and proteinuria. Urine pH is frequently elevated.

LABORATORY DATA

There are increases in the serum levels of renin, catecholamines, growth hormone, glucagon, cortisol, aldosterone, and amino acids. There are also increases in the serum levels of glucose, lactate, pyruvate, ketones, and non-esterified free fatty acids. There is a decrease in insulin levels and an increase in nitrogen excretion.

Treatment

A combination of comfort measures and judicious use of medications[3,8] (Table 21-2) will provide pain relief. CAUTION: Sedatives are frequently used for agitated babies. If these babies are in pain, sedatives are ineffective in relieving it and may produce irritability and an excessive sensitivity to pain.[4,5] The neonate communicates both subjective and objective data of his painful experience. He relies on the skilled observations, assessments, and interventions of his care providers for prompt, safe, and effective relief.

Complications

The neonate's complex behavioral response to pain has both short- and long-term ramifications. These behavioral changes may disrupt parent-infant interaction and attachment, adaptation to the postnatal environment, and feeding behaviors.[2] Because of the neonate's memory, painful experiences may lead to psychologic sequelae.[2]

Narcotic analgesics may produce respiratory depression severe enough to require mechanical ventilation. Naloxone (0.01 mg/kg IV or IM)

TABLE 21-2

Analgesics and Sedatives for the Neonate

DRUG	DOSAGE	COMMENTS
Analgesics		
Narcotic		
Morphine	0.05-0.2 mg/kg/dose q.2-4h. p.r.n. IV, IM, or SC	CNS and respiratory depressant; easily reversed with naloxone; slower onset but longer duration than fentanyl; increases intracranial pressure; withdrawal symptoms may occur
Meperidine (Demerol)	1-1.5 mg/kg/dose q.4h. p.r.n. IV, IM, SC, or PO	Same as morphine; less respiratory depression with therapeutic dose; less likely to induce sleep/sedation than morphine or fentanyl
Fentanyl (Sublimaze)	1-2 μg/kg/dose q.4-6h. p.r.n. IV or SC Anesthesia: 20-75 μg/kg/dose IV over 5-10 min	Rapid onset of action; decreases motor activity; does not increase intracranial pressure; easily reversed with naloxone; short duration of action; may cause hypotension, apnea, seizures, or rigidity if given too rapidly; withdrawal symptoms may occur
Local		
Lidocaine	0.5%-1% solution (to avoid systemic toxicity, volume should be <0.5 ml/kg of 1% lidocaine solution—5 mg/kg)	Local infiltration anesthesia for invasive procedures
Sedative/hypnotics		
Barbiturate		
Phenobarbital	Loading: 10-20 mg/kg IV to maximum of 40 mg/kg Maintenance: 5-7 mg/kg in 2 divided doses beginning 12 hr after last loading dose	Prolonged sedation possible once therapeutic levels achieved (20-25 μg/ml); depresses CNS—motor and respiratory; slow onset of action; little or no pain relief; not easily reversed; withdrawal symptoms may occur; incompatible with other drugs in solution
Nonbarbiturate		
Chloral hydrate	10-30 mg/kg/dose q.6h. p.r.n. PO to maximum daily dose of 50 mg/kg/day; PR	Gastric irritant—administer with or after feeding; paradoxical excitement; not to be used for analgesia
Diazepam (Valium)	0.02-0.3 mg/kg IV, IM, or PO q.6-8h.	Do not dilute injection; may displace bilirubin; respiratory depression; hypotension; may cause increased agitation; induces sleep; relaxes muscles; withdrawal symptoms may occur; no analgesic effect

Based on data from Bell SG and Ellis LJ: Neonatal Network 6:27, 1987; and Roberts RJ: Drug therapy in infants, Philadelphia, 1984, WB Saunders Co.

is the specific antidote for narcotic potentiation or overdose. An ampule of neonatal naloxone should always be at the bedside with the appropriate dose precalculated on the infant's emergency drug card. The respiratory depression may produce hypoxemia. A pulse oximeter or transcutaneous oxygen monitor should be standard postoperative equipment along with cardiorespiratory monitoring. If available, $TcPCO_2$ monitors should also be used to watch for hypercapnia. All equipment necessary for assisted ventilation should be at the bedside.

Withdrawal symptoms (irritability, increased crying, ravenous sucking, vomiting, tremors, and jitteriness) may occur after the narcotic/sedative is discontinued. Minimal handling and a quiet, darkened environment help decrease external stimuli. A pacifier, swaddling, and holding may provide comfort. A gradual extension of time between doses and/or a gradual decrease in the dose over time will decrease the risk of withdrawal symptoms.

PARENT TEACHING
Preoperative

Parents should be told before surgery about the anesthesia their infant will receive. The need for anesthesia and analgesia should be explained to parents, along with the physiologic and behavioral benefits of pain relief. Comfort measures are ideally provided by parents, who may then actively participate in their infant's care.

Initially parents have a difficult time hearing and understanding what is being said about their baby's condition. Simple, concise explanations are the easiest to comprehend during this stage. In most cases the cause of the baby's anomaly or problem is not known. This may need to be discussed with the parents more than once. Each time, they should be given the opportunity to share their fears and feelings of guilt.

Neonates with obvious or suspected gastrointestinal problems often receive many diagnostic x-ray examinations. Contrast studies must be thoroughly explained to the parents so that they understand the need for and purpose of these procedures.

The surgical procedure and what the baby will look like on return from surgery are explained. It is helpful for both the physician and nurse to meet with the family to discuss the surgery. This provides them with an opportunity to answer questions and to hear how the other has responded to questions. This is especially important for the nurse, who must answer questions and continually explain to and reassure an anxious family when the physician leaves. Parents must receive consistent responses from the health care team.

Since parental fears and fantasies about their infant's problem are frequently worse than reality, parents should see their baby before surgery (see Part V). Infants who are extremely ill should have a picture taken before surgery. In the tragic situation of neonatal death during surgery, these pictures may be very valuable to the family. It may also be helpful for parents to see an infant who has had a similar procedure and has the equipment that has been described (i.e., colostomy, orogastric tube, chest tube). If this is not possible, pictures or drawings are useful in preventing postoperative surprises.

Operative

Accompanying the infant to surgery and seeing the infant as soon as possible after surgery are comforting for the parents. Progress reports, if at all possible during the waiting period of surgery, are always appreciated by an anxious family. After the operation immediate parental contact with the pediatric surgeon for an explanation of the procedure and a progress report on the baby is essential.

Postoperative

After surgery parents need to review the equipment and what it does to help their baby. It is important to help them focus their attention on their infant, rather than merely on the machinery. Early involvement in caretaking helps to personalize the newborn. The parents learn to relate to the infant's normal characteristics and responses and to become familiar with the baby's special needs.

If the infant will be discharged with an ostomy or while receiving total parenteral nutrition, it is helpful to involve the parents in this care as early as possible. They may begin by cleansing the skin around the ostomy or helping to prepare the equipment. Gradually they

---

OSTOMY CARE

Purpose
Alternative stoma pouch system for babies with ileostomy or colostomy

Equipment
1. Soap and water for skin preparation
2. Stomahesive
3. Stomaseal
4. Uri-Drain

Proposed benefits
1. Fewer bag changes, resulting in decreased expense and improved skin integrity
2. Smaller size, resulting in less pull on the bag (thus fewer changes), easily hidden under infant clothes, and easier positioning of the infant on the abdomen
3. Easy to prepare ahead of time, to put on, and to drain

Procedure

To prepare system
1. Cut template of ostomy.
2. Cut Stomahesive using template. Make actual opening for stoma slightly smaller than stoma so that Stomahesive will fit snugly around stoma and decrease leakage of stool onto skin. If cut correctly, the stoma will pop up through the hole in the Stomahesive when applied.
3. Cut circle of Stomaseal approximately ⅛ of an inch wider in diameter than Uri-Drain.
4. Cut out center of Stomaseal so that it is approximately ¼ to ⁵⁄₁₆ of an inch wide.
5. Center Stomaseal ring on top of Stomahesive.
6. Stand Uri-Drain on rim and stretch with fingers to remove wrinkles and thereby prevent stool leakage.
7. Place cork in end of Uri-Drain after deflating air.
8. Steps 1 through 7 can be done ahead of time for a particular baby.

To apply appliance
1. Cleanse skin very well with soap and warm water especially around edge of stoma, since a good seal is important.
2. Let skin dry completely.
3. Apply thin coat of Skin-Prep to skin around ostomy.
4. Wait 60 seconds until Skin-Prep feels tacky.
5. Apply on baby, centering hole over stoma and press so that stoma pops up and Stomahesive seals well.

are able to increase their responsibilities of caretaking as their infant improves. Waiting to teach these special care needs until a few days before discharge does not give parents adequate time for practice and familiarity before being on their own.

The enterostomal therapist, a specialist in educating staff, patients, and families about ostomies, is an important member of the health care team when parents must care for an ostomy at home. Either a prepackaged drainage system or an improved system (see boxed material on p. 560) may be effectively used. The availability of proper equipment and written instructions for home care is essential before discharge. An example of the written instructions on home ostomy care is listed as follows:

1. Keep the infant clean. Sponge bathe daily with soap and water or tub bath.
2. Empty the bag by rolling the infant to the side and emptying the contents into an old container. Rinse the inside of the bag with a cup of cool water. Use toilet or facial tissue to wipe out the inside of the bag.
3. Change only when necessary (1 to 7 days). When stool begins to seep around the edges of the bag, change it.
4. Occasionally the stoma may bleed slightly, but report to the physician a larger amount of bleeding.
5. If you have any problems, call the neonatal intensive care unit.

The possibility of postoperative complications (such as leakage in a tracheoesophageal fistula at the anastomosis site) must always be discussed with parents. Although the development of complications is disappointing, they may be less difficult to handle when the parents are aware of their possibility. In preparation for discharge, parents should know what potential problems might develop and how to recognize them (e.g., late bowel obstruction). Excessive stooling and signs of dehydration should be taught to parents of any infant with an ostomy.

Strict adherence to the special dietary needs of these infants is essential. Dependence on total parenteral nutrition may be a long-term problem. No longer is this form of nutritional support an absolute indication for long-term hospitalization. Total parenteral nutrition may be safely administered at home by properly instructed parents aided by a written procedure (see Chapter 13).

The importance of follow-up care must be stressed to parents. It may be helpful for parents to talk with a "graduate" parent who had an infant with similar problems. Parents should know what resource people, such as visiting nurses, graduate parents, and physicians, are available and how to contact them. It is important for the resource people in the community to know the infant's history and what information the parents have received. Ideally, a written discharge plan should be given to the parents and community resource people.

Discharge is an exciting yet stressful time for parents. Ideally, if they have been actively involved in their infant's care, it will be less stressful.

ACKNOWLEDGMENT

We would like to thank Carol Rumack, M.D., and the Department of Radiology, University of Colorado Health Sciences Center, for the use of material from their teaching files.

REFERENCES

1. American Academy of Pediatrics, Committee on Fetus and Newborn, Committee on Drugs, Section on Anesthesiology and Section on Surgery: Neonatal anesthesia, Pediatrics 80:446, 1987.
2. Anand KJS and Hickey PR: Pain and its effect in the human neonate and fetus, N Engl J Med 317:1321, 1987.
3. Bell SG and Ellis LJ: Use of fentanyl for sedation of mechanically ventilated neonates, Neonatal Network 6:27, 1987.
4. Butler NC: The ethical issues involved in the practice of surgery in unanesthetized infants, AORN J 46:1136, 1987.
5. Franck LS: A national survey of the assessment and treatment of pain and agitation in the NICU, JOGN 16:387, 1987.
6. Orenstein S and Whitington PF: Positioning for prevention of infant gastroesophageal reflux, J Pediatr 103:534, 1983.

7. Orenstein S, Whitington PF, and Orenstein D: The infant seat as treatment for gastroesophageal reflux, N Engl J Med 309:760, 1983.

8. Roberts RJ: Drug therapy in infants, Philadelphia, 1984, WB Saunders Co.

9. Whaley LF and Wong DL: Nursing care of infants and children, ed 3, St Louis, 1987, The CV Mosby Co.

SELECTED READINGS

Chang JHT: Neonatal surgical emergencies. I. Initial care and transport, Perinatol Neonatol 3(3):17, 1979.

Chang JHT: Neonatal surgical emergencies. II. Esophageal atresia and tracheoesophageal fistula, Perinatol Neonatol 3(4):26, 1979.

Chang JHT: Neonatal surgical emergencies. III. Congenital diaphragmatic hernia, Perinatol Neonatol 3(5):22, 1979.

Chang JHT: Neonatal surgical emergencies. IV. Malrotation of the intestine, Perinatol Neonatol 4(1):50, 1980.

Chang JHT: Neonatal surgical emergencies. V. Intestinal obstruction, Perinatol Neonatol 4(2):34, 1980.

Chang JHT: Neonatal surgical emergencies. VI. Necrotizing enterocolitis, Perinatol Neonatol 4(3):51, 1980.

Fletcher AB: Pain in the neonate, N Engl J Med 317:1347, 1987.

Kliegman RM and Walsh MC: Neonatal necrotizing enterocolitis: pathogenesis, classification and spectrum of illness, Curr Prob Pediatr 17:219, 1987.

Lobe TE and Schwartz M, editors: Pediatric surgery, Pediatr Clin North Am 32(5):1101, 1985.

Pain, anesthesia and babies, Lancet 2:543, 1987 (editorial).

Touloukian RJ: What's new in pediatric surgery, Pediatrics 81:692, 1988.

PART V

Psychosocial Aspects of Neonatal Care

CHAPTER 22

Families in crisis: theoretical and practical considerations

ROBERTA SIEGEL · SANDRA L. GARDNER · GERALD B. MERENSTEIN

The technical advances that have characterized newborn care in the last 20 years have resulted in marked improvement in the mortality and morbidity of the high-risk infant.[32] These developments have been accompanied by a heightened appreciation of the psychologic strain and emotional stresses encountered by the family of the sick neonate. Realization of the need for a family-centered approach to perinatal care has emerged out of an enhanced understanding of individual and family functioning and their adaptation to stress.[52] It has become essential for perinatal health care teams to address the psychologic needs of families who are experiencing the painful crisis of the birth of a sick newborn. The purpose of this chapter is to discuss the complex psychosocial needs of families during this stressful period and to offer concrete suggestions for intervention.

NORMAL ATTACHMENT

Emotional investment in the child begins not at birth, but during the pregnancy. The terms *attachment* and *bonding*[30] are used to describe this process of relating between parents and their infant. Attachment behavior is characterized by the same qualities used to describe love: "care, responsibility, respect, and knowledge."[17] The affectionate tie between parents and their newborn is a process of learning and acquaintance that results in "a unique relationship between two people that is specific and endures through time."[31]

The infant's need for the parent is absolute, but the parent's need for the infant is only relative. The neonate is totally dependent, both physically and emotionally, on the caretakers. Recognition of this unique relationship is evidenced cross-culturally by immediate and prolonged contact with no evidence of separation.[26,39] In most animal species the mother engages in "species-specific behaviors"[30] that enable her to become acquainted with and claim the newborn. Interference during this critical period results in rejection by the animal mother and death of the young. Parental attachment and caretaking behaviors are crucial for the infant's physical, psychologic, and emotional health and survival. Ultimately this influence will affect the child's well-being as an adult and a potential parent for a subsequent generation.

Critical and sensitive period

In the immediate period after birth, both mother and infant are physiologically and psychologically ready for "reciprocal interaction."[30] Physiologically, even though labor and birth are tiring, most mothers feel "high" and have an incredible surge of energy after birth. Psychologically, the family is ready to meet and interact with the long-awaited newcomer. Physiologically, the first hour of life is a time of alertness for the newborn. Before the sleep phase the newborn is alert, makes eye-to-eye contact, fixes and follows, and begins to feed. At birth, all five senses are operational, and the infant is ready to cue and shape the environment.

This period of mutual readiness has been compared with the critical period in animals. This human "maternal sensitive period"[30] is the time immediately after birth in which the attachment process is initiated. Called the optimal, but not the sole, period for attachment to develop, the human critical period represents a reciprocal readiness for acquaintance. Klaus and Kennell[28,29,31] and Ringler et al[47,48] have studied the effects of initial separation of mother and infant in these first critical hours after birth and have shown significant differences in caretaking behaviors at 1 month, 1 year, 2 years, and 5 years after birth.

Using the developmental principles of readiness, sustained and early contact between parents and infant completes the process of labor and birth and gives the family the opportunity for interaction. The presence of the baby enables the parents to begin knowing the reality and individuality of their infant. Early parent-infant contact facilitates parent-infant attachment. Unnecessary "routines" and procedures that interfere with initial contact should be deferred until the initial acquaintance process is completed.

Failure to establish immediate contact because of medically indicated interventions necessary to sustain life does not promote attachment, but it also does not undermine the entire process of attachment. Unlike animals, human mothers do not automatically reject their infant if they are unable to interact immediately. Interference or failure to interact during the critical period does not condemn the resilient and adaptable human parent to rejection of or maladaptation to the infant.

Crisis event: pregnancy and parenthood

Pregnancy, birth, and parenthood are almost universally defined as traumatic and a life crisis.[26,34] Parenting is a major adjustment of the prepreg- nancy roles, lifestyle, and relationships. Since previous ideas and coping styles may not be helpful, life crisis situations challenge the individual with the potential for growth as new responses and solutions are used for problem solving. Periods of upheaval, change, and vulnerability provide a time of openness, receptiveness, and readiness for help from significant others (including professionals).

Influences on parenting

Opportunities to experience parenting and to observe others parent within a social setting are essential learning experiences for the development of parenting behaviors. The ability to parent is influenced by a multitude of factors that occur before, during, and after the birth of the baby. Previous life events, including genetic endowment,[30] cultural practices,[26,39] being parented,[22] previous pregnancies,[13] and interpersonal relationships,[22] affect the experience of pregnancy and parenthood. The events of the current pregnancy,[13,30] their significance to the parent, and the availability of support and assistance influence parenting ability. After birth, infant characteristics,[35,49] behavior of health professionals,[14,18,30] separation from the infant,[6,33] and hospital practices[14,18,31,55] may positively or negatively influence parents. Not only the occurrence of these events, but also their meaning to the individual and the type of assistance received influence parenting abilities.

Steps of attachment

Klaus and Kennell[30] have proposed nine steps in the process of attachment.

STEP 1. Planning the pregnancy is the initial step of investment in the life-altering prospect of parenthood. Pregnancies are planned in one of two ways: consciously or unconsciously.

Considering their individual and coupled development, pregnancy may be a joint decision between partners. Or pregnancy may occur as the result of a conscious decision of one rather than both partners.

Pregnancies that are planned on an unconscious level are called "accidents," and they result from no or improper use of contraceptives. Who planned the pregnancy and why this particular time has been chosen are important indicators of the investment of each individual in the decision and in the pregnancy.

Carrying a pregnancy is not assurance that the baby is wanted. It is faulty logic to assume that the mother must want the baby because she has carried the pregnancy and is keeping the child. Although it is a legal option, abortion may not be a cultural, moral, or ethical option for the individual woman. Assuming that if the baby were unwanted, the mother would have had an abortion may be fallacious. Attachment of the mother (or father) to the baby is not assured merely by the mother's remaining pregnant and giving birth.

STEP 2. Confirming the pregnancy occurs after the first and often subtle signs of pregnancy appear. Pregnancy confirmation begins the psychologic acceptance of the pregnancy. Delaying confirmation enables the fact of pregnancy to be denied. Thus denial of the pregnancy abolishes the need to proceed with the acceptance stage.

STEP 3. Accepting the pregnancy usually begins early in the pregnancy. Along with the physical changes of pregnancy come the emotional changes that are characterized by primary narcissism, introversion, and passivity. Being less interested in the outside world and more interested in her own inner world, the mother is able to become attuned to her own needs. Thus she is less interested in the needs of others and more interested in caring for herself. Although she was previously engaged in active, extroverted behaviors, she may, during the pregnancy, contentedly participate in quieter, more introspective activities. The idea of the pregnant woman sitting in a rocking chair "knitting little things" may be more realistic than stereotypical.

At this early stage of pregnancy the fetus is not perceived by the woman as separate from herself, but as an extension of her body. The psychologic changes of pregnancy have survival significance in that caring for herself assures caring for the fetus "as an integral part of herself."[9]

During the early months of pregnancy, the man and woman begin to realize that they will soon be parents. Since parenting requires a major adjustment of prepregnancy roles, lifestyle, and relationships, realization of impending parenthood is associated with ambivalent feelings. The adaptation to parenthood is characterized by upheaval and change, losses and gains. Bombarded with phenomenal lifelong changes, the future parents experience the normal feeling of ambivalence.

STEP 4. Fetal movement is felt by the mother between 16 and 32 weeks of gestation. "Quickening" is the beginning of the acceptance of the fetus as an individual. Fetal movement is the first concrete evidence to the mother of the existence of another person within her. Hearing the baby's heartbeat or seeing the ultrasound readings also confirms the reality of the fetus. Fetal movement is such a significant event that often a pregnancy that began as unplanned and unwanted becomes wanted.

Perception of the first fetal movement is a happy event. When asked, "How did you feel when the baby first moved?" most women respond in a happy tone and with a smile. The mother's speaking of fetal movement in a negative tone is a concern, since the individual (fetus) may already be perceived as an intruder. If fetal movement is seen as bothersome, how will the total dependence of the newborn be perceived?

STEP 5. Accepting the fetus as an individual begins with fetal movement. The fetus has been moving since early pregnancy; however fetal movements have been imperceptible to the mother. The fetus asserts individuality in controlling the movement; the mother can neither start nor stop these movements. With the realization of the concrete evidence of the presence of another person, parents begin the psychologic acceptance and personification of the fetus as a separate individual.

After fetal movement becomes perceptible, mothers (and fathers) experience an opening up of the unconscious. This is experienced as dreams and fantasies about the expected child. Love for the fetus as a separate individual occurs through the parents' investing a personality in the fetus and establishing a relationship with that personality. Fantasies about how the baby looks, the sex, and the wish for a perfect, healthy infant are common.

Outwardly, preparations are made for the acceptance of a baby into the home; baby clothes and furniture are purchased, and a room is prepared. The fetus may be referred to by a nickname or a term of endearment. The baby's name may be chosen. Choosing a name is a highly personal and significant event. The meaning of the name and who chooses it illustrate the power holder and decision-maker within the family. Prenatal questions such as "Do you have a nickname for the baby?" "Do you have a name picked out for the baby?" and "Who picked it out?" may be asked after the birth to elicit information.[4]

Whether the newborn meets parental expectations for "the right sex" may be crucially important in the parent's ability to attach to the infant. "Do you have a sex preference for the baby?" may be asked before or after the birth to elicit this information.[4] Often parents with a strong sex preference have chosen no names for a baby of the "wrong" sex.

"It doesn't matter as long as it's healthy," is often heard and may indicate no conscious sex preference. However, unconsciously the parents may have a strong sex preference. Since dreams and fantasies about the child are not neuter, the unconscious desire for the preferred sex is available. The predominance of dreams about one sex indicates the unconscious preference. If dreams are equally divided between male and female children, there may indeed be no sex preference at the unconscious level.

Most parents are fearful of producing a defective child. This fear is experienced as dreams about dead, deformed, or damaged fetuses and babies, or dreams with a central theme of destruction. These unconscious contents are often expe-

rienced as frightening nightmares that may often be imbued with magical ideas such as, "If I think (or talk about) it, it will come true." Both before and after birth, it is reassuring for parents to know that this is a common and scary phenomenon, that they aren't "crazy," and that the fears are not magical.

Parental expectations of the newborn are established before birth in the personification and relationship with the unseen, unheard fetus. After birth, the developmental task of parenthood is a working out of the discrepancy between the wished for and the actual infant.[53] Before attachment to the actual baby is able to proceed, the fantasized child must be mourned.

STEP 6. Labor is a physiologic, maturational, and psychologic crisis for the family. Birth is the culmination of pregnancy and the reward for the work of labor. Parental attitudes about their labor and birth experiences affect their reactions to the infant. Newton and Newton[41] found mothers more likely to be pleased with their infant at first sight if the mothers were relaxed, calm, and cooperative; had rapport with the attendants; and received personalized, solicitous care.

Paternal participation in labor and birth has been a controversial issue. Professionals saw no benefit to the presence of the father and even wished to exclude him because of imagined "horribles" such as increased infection rate, malpractice suits, and fainting. In study after study these imagined "horribles" have proved to be just that, imagined.[44]

Birth is a powerfully emotional experience, so that those who attend birth are more attached to the baby than those who do not attend.[30] Benefits attributed to a father's participation at labor and birth are outlined as follows*:

1. The mother is less lonely, needs less analgesia, and is less isolated and more supported.

---

*Modified from Phillips C and Anzalone J: Fathering: participation in labor and birth, ed 2, St Louis, 1982, The CV Mosby Co.

2. The father and mother share the emotional experience, deepen their interpersonal relationship, and begin a more active role in parenting.
3. The baby receives more recognition, more claiming behaviors, more interaction, and less analgesia.

The work of labor and the joy of birth is a shared biologic and psychologic event when the father actively participates. Inclusion of the father in perinatal events may "hook" him for inclusion in parenting activities. Rather than merely a social obligation of financially providing, fathering may be perceived as a psychologic necessity for both fathers and children.

Parental behaviors at birth indicate involvement and investment in the baby*:

1. "How does the mother or father *look?*" At the sound of the infant's cry, parents smile and breathe a sigh of relief at this first breath of life. Support, joy, and happiness are positive feelings shared by couples at birth.
2. "What does the mother or father *say?*" By speaking in a positive tone with words of affection and endearment, the parents relate to each other and to the new baby.
3. "What does the mother or father *do?*" When offered the baby, both parents will reach out to take the infant. Spontaneously, parents engage in eye-to-eye contact and touch and explore the infant. Affectionate behaviors such as kissing, fondling, cuddling, and claiming characterize positive parental reactions.

A positive, self-affirming birth experience for the mother "enhances her feelings of self-esteem, thus her self-concept as a woman and mother."[18] A birth experience that does not meet parental expectations may make a negative impact on the self-concept of the mother, her perception of her ability to parent, and her relationship with the

*Reprinted with permission from Child abuse and neglect: the family and the community, Copyright, 1976, Ballinger Publishing Company.

infant.[14,18] In fact, "so intricately are mother and baby entwined in a symbiotic relationship, that what is psychically positive for the mother is positive for the baby. What is psychically negative for the mother will affect the baby."[18] Labor and delivery that have been difficult or prolonged may influence parental overprotection, resentment, or antagonism toward the infant.[1,14]

So powerful is the labor and birth experience that women are unable to proceed with parenting until psychic closure of the experience has been obtained. Even women who experience a normal labor and birth process need to recount the experience to others. Maternal perception of the events are obvious in tone and content of the recounting. "Missing pieces"[1] is the term used to describe the aspects of labor and birth that are forgotten or unavailable to recall. Long labor, short labor, or medicated labor can cause "missing pieces" in the mother's memory of the birth. Labor that did not meet expectations because of difficulty, cesarean section, use of forceps, or episiotomy could also affect the mother.[1] To proceed with parenting, these women need to fill in their knowledge gaps by asking questions or looking at pictures or films of the birth to reconstruct the situation.

STEP 7. Seeing and touching, are the "species-specific" ways in which humans attach to their young.[30]

After birth, parents are intensely interested in seeing the baby's eyes and spend much time encouraging the baby "to look at me." Eye contact between parents and their infants in the initial period after birth may be a positive release of parental feelings of warmth, closeness, and caring. As parents see the reality of the actual newborn, they begin "letting go" of the prenatally fantasized child. As parents see and inspect the newborn, they begin claiming their infant: "He has my eyes; she has your nose." Characteristics of each parent and the family are identified in the baby, and the newborn is claimed as a member of the family.

The term *en face position* is used to describe

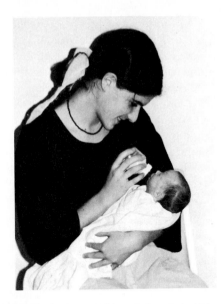

Figure 22-1. En face position: infant is held in close contact (mother's body touching infant's); mother is looking at infant en face; bottle is perpendicular to mouth; and milk is in tip of nipple. (From Klaus MH and Kennell JH: Parent-infant bonding, ed 2, St Louis, 1982, The CV Mosby Co.)

"the mother's (father's) eyes and the baby's eyes positioned in the same vertical plane."[30] This positioning enables the parent and infant to look directly into each other's eyes, to focus, and to regard each other (Figure 22-1).

The importance of the neonate's contribution in the initial attachment period should not be underestimated. Being an active participant in the acquaintance process, the infant cues the mother with eye-to-eye contact. Even "minutes old"[16] newborns see and show a preference for the human face (within 7 to 12 inches from their face). Deterrents to the infant's full participation include removal to the nursery, medication (from analgesia), and eye prophylaxis. Unless medically indicated (necessary for physical survival), newborns should remain with their parents after birth. Since eye prophylaxis irritates and interferes with vision, the "routine" instillation imme-

diately after birth (in the delivery room) can be delayed until after the initial acquaintance process is completed.

The newborn is able to visually follow the parent's face and voice and to signal the parent with facial expressions, movement, and vocalizations. The infant is able to evoke behaviors (smiling, touching, and vocalization) from the care provider. The dyadic interaction, the giving and receiving of interpersonal communication, is begun with the eye-to-eye contact between parents and their baby.

STEP 8. Touching is important to the adult as a means of tactile and sensory knowledge of the baby. To the neonate the "stimulus hunger"[46] is satisfied by parental touch and ministrations.

In exploring the infant, parents systematically use fingertip contact with the infant's extremities. Gradually there is progression to palm contact with the infant's trunk (Figure 22-2). With the healthy term infant, this progression occurs within minutes of the first contact. After gaining confidence and preliminary knowledge, the parent will enfold the infant close to the ventrum of the adult (a cuddling position).

With the preterm infant, this characteristic progression may take hours, days, or several visits (Figure 22-3). Fear of harming the small, fragile preterm infant prevents parents from feeling at ease in touching their infant. Until the parents feel confident that their actions will not harm the infant, they will be reticent to use palm contact with the trunk (vital organs).

Holding and cuddling the baby are significantly different from touching and exploring. Mothers who have only seen and touched their baby still experience "empty arms." The "species-specific" behavior of touch is not completely satisfied until the parent is able "to hold" the baby.

STEP 9. Caretaking, the final step of attachment, is important for psychic closure of the task of bonding. The relationship between the primary caretaker and the infant is described as "a reciprocal relationship."[7] In the caretaking relationship both care provider and infant give and receive

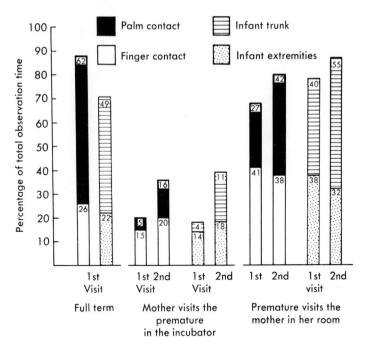

Figure 22-2. Fingertip and palm contact on trunk or extremities in three groups of mothers: (1) 12 mothers of term infants at their first visit, (2) 9 mothers who visited their premature infants in incubators in NICU, and (3) 14 mothers whose premature infants were brought to their maternity rooms and placed in their beds. (From Klaus MH and Kennell JH: Parent-infant bonding, ed 2, St Louis, 1982, The CV Mosby Co.)

from each other. The physical and emotional needs of the helpless infant are satisfied by parental caretaking behaviors such as feeding, soothing, grooming, and playing. Based on the infant's ability to perceive and receive these ministrations, the infant responds to the care provider. Parental expectations of newborn responses include quieting, sucking, clinging and cuddling, looking, smiling, and vocalizing. Parental capability to soothe and satisfy the infant provides emotional satisfaction and positive feedback about the parent's competency as "mother" or "father."

Personal needs for comfort, maintenance of homeostasis, and relief from painful experiences are infant expectations of the relationship with the care provider. Care-eliciting behaviors (crying, visual following, and smiling) are neonatal cues

used to signal the care provider that attention is needed. Relief from discomfort enables the infant to respond positively to the care provider. The infant experiences the world through the caretaker and quickly learns that the environment is either nurturing and loving or hostile and nonresponsive. Consistent, predictable nurturing and caretaking enable the infant to develop a sense of trust in the caretaker, the world, and self.

Care by parents is the ideal neonatal care situation, since the infant learns and reacts to one set of cues or caretaking behaviors. Cared for by one or two people, the infant is able to develop synchrony with expectations of the parents. Single caretaking improves the establishment of biorhythms of the neonate[14,55] for sleep-wake cycles, feeding, and visual attentiveness. Multiple care-

Newborn Center
The Children's Hospital

Born:	Admitted:	Code all phone calls
Birth weight:	Private M.D.:	and visits:
		Ⓜ Mother Ⓕ Father
	MSW:	ⒼⓂ Grandmother
	FCC:	ⒼⒻ Grandfather

Date/time	Called	Visited	Held	Fed	Psychosocial status:	

Figure 22-3. Parent-infant interaction sheet. (Courtesy The Children's Hospital, Denver, Colo.)

taking confuses the infant, increases distress with feeding, causes irritability, and upsets visual attention.[14,55] Care by parents provides for mutual cuing and acquaintance and a natural setting for observation of parent-infant interaction.

BIRTH OF A SICK NEWBORN

The birth of a sick newborn with its consequent family disruption represents to the perinatal health care team a unique crisis, a "dangerous opportunity"[2] within which to practice preventive health care. For the involved individual and family this stressful event results in a period of psychologic disorganization during which their usual problem-solving mechanisms may not be adequate to cope with the events presented to them.[12] In addition to confronting this situational crisis, the individual or family must master the normal developmental process of parenthood.[54]

Parental behavior and responses are determined not only by preexisting personality factors, social and cultural variables, and interactions with significant others[12,29] but also by the immediate situation in which the parents are placed. The situational factors can have an important bearing on the family's ability to cope with the crisis and thus affect the overall outcome.[12,27] These situational factors include[52]:

1. The behaviors and attitudes of the hospital staff (physicians, nurses, and allied health professionals)
2. The sensitivity used in the process of "separation" and transfer of the infant to the intensive care unit or in some cases the referral hospital
3. The flexibility of hospital policy concerning parental and sibling involvement and visitation in the nursery
4. The instruction of parents of their infant's individual behaviors and characteristics (thus facilitating appropriate parent-child interaction and reciprocity)
5. The staff's comprehension and appreciation of the psychosocial functioning of families

and the family's responses and adaptation to stress and crisis
6. The employment of emotionally supportive intervention programs for parents within the nursery setting
7. The development of appropriate discharge planning to provide adequate follow-up care to the infant and family

Families are psychologically vulnerable after the birth of a sick infant. During this period of temporary disorganization, there is a heightened receptivity to accepting help and being responsive to change, because the family is struggling for a way to cope with the crisis. Significant potentialities exist for individual and family emotional growth and development.[11,12,25] The perinatal health team has a rare opportunity to influence how the individual and family adapt to the crisis. By providing appropriate supportive interventions coupled with enlightened policies and attitudes, the team can positively influence the family's coping, thus enhancing the likelihood for a successful resolution of the crisis and ultimately a healthy parent-child relationship.[15,43,52]

As discussed earlier, attachment is a complex developmental process. Attachment occurs over a period of time, in stages, through interactions, and not in one critical period. The family system in which the relationship between the parent and infant occurs is crucial and will affect parental attachment. Recent research studies[10,24] have illustrated that there are many interrelated factors that influence parental behavior and attachment toward the infant. These include the infant, sex of the infant, social class, birth order, parental attitudes and expectations, events of the newborn period and postdischarge period, and level of family functioning.[31,36,52] Very important in any neonatal illness and subsequent hospitalization is the disruption and stress that is frequently created in the nuclear family system.[35] It has been demonstrated that the family's functioning and its adaptation to stress have important consequences on the family's relationship with the infant and the infant's later development. It is a crucial task of the perinatal health care team to intervene in such a way as to facilitate the establishment of a healthy parent-child relationship and to assist families in using the unfortunate event of the birth of their sick infant to maximize their growth, adaptation, and reorganization during this period.[53]

To assist parents through the difficult experience of having a sick infant, it is helpful to identify the psychologic tasks and emotional reactions they experience. This section describes the six psychologic issues facing families; it discusses the clinical and behavioral indicators that parents are struggling with and then suggests interventions that the perinatal health care team can employ to help families. It is extremely important to remember that these are generalizations and that each family or person must be approached individually. Additionally in assessing families' reactions, it is critical to look at how they cope over a period of time. Initially there may be a tremendous amount of upset, disruption, and upheaval within the individual or family system that eventually may lead to improved functioning and a sense of growth and mastery. The key is how the individuals or families reorganize, how able they are to return to a state of equilibrium, the coping strategies they are able to devise, and whether they are adaptive or maladaptive. Attachment and parenthood are complex, normal developmental processes that must evolve and unfold over time.

Psychologic tasks

Kaplan and Mason[27] describe four psychologic tasks that parents of premature infants must deal with:

1. Anticipatory grieving and withdrawal from the relationship established during pregnancy
2. Parental acknowledgment of feelings of guilt and failure
3. Resumption of the relationship with the infant that had been previously disrupted
4. Preparation to take the infant home

Two additional tasks are significant:

5. Crisis events related to labor and delivery
6. Adaptation to the intensive care environment[21]

In general, these six psychologic tasks can be applied to any parent's reaction to a sick infant, with additional specific issues arising depending on whether the infant was premature or born with a congenital anomaly.

LABOR AND DELIVERY

The first psychologic task involves working through the crisis events surrounding the labor and delivery. Medical problems occurring at any point during the pregnancy or delivery that threaten the health or survival of the fetus or the mother can result in the parents' delaying their planning and making an emotional investment in the fetus/infant. Parents psychologically withdraw from the pregnancy as a way of protecting themselves. The parents of an infant born prematurely often do not have the necessary psychologic and physical time to prepare. This deprivation of time may interfere with the parents' ability to complete the final steps of attachment described earlier. Parents who have been concentrating on themselves in a healthy, narcissistic way may not yet be ready to transfer their investment on to the infant because they have been prematurely thrust into the role of parents. There is an overwhelming sense of losing control of the events of the labor and delivery and their timing. Parental wishes to retain the pregnancy can influence their attitude about the delivery and the infant.[56] On the other hand, some parents react oppositely; they may wish to be rid of the pregnancy as a way of dealing with their ambivalent feelings about the infant or their fear of the unknown and the uncertainty facing them. Many mothers of premature infants feel alien to their infants. They do not feel that the infants are really their babies, making it easier to have feelings of rejection toward the baby. In addition to feeling insufficient and inadequate about their ability to deliver an infant at term, they feel empty inside, as if something is missing. This seems to occur because the mother who has been predominantly concerned about herself, her body, and the fetus growing inside is not ready to transfer that emotional investment to someone else outside herself. With a premature birth there is usually a heightened sense of emergency and concern about the health and survival of the infant and at times the mother, who herself may have suffered complications.

In the case of a full-term infant born with a problem despite no complications of pregnancy, there is a sense of overwhelming shock and disappointment. Parents immediately sense the problem; as their apprehension mounts, they frequently imagine and fantasize the worst. Parents of a newborn with a malformation normally experience lowered self-esteem and view this event as an affront to their reproductive capabilities. The mother specifically views it as a failure of her feminine role. Parents often feel that they have failed and that the baby symbolically represents their own defectiveness. Parents not only fear for the infant, they fear for themselves and what this child may mean to their future. The reaction of the parents is based on many factors but most importantly on the specific psychologic, social, and cultural meaning of the defect to the parents and the manner in which the problem is discussed and handled with the parents by the health care team.[30]

The emotional reactions and feelings that parents have at and after the delivery of a sick infant range from shock, fright, and panic to anxiety and helplessness. Parents may be so overwhelmed by the events that initially they may blunt or block any observable emotional response or affect. Staff interventions at this time are extremely important because they lay the foundations for subsequent interactions between parents and health professionals. Early comments and influential statements during this critical time can have lasting impressions in the minds of parents. This is indeed an emotionally difficult time for physicians and nurses also, since they too are struggling with their own feelings of inadequacy, failure, and helplessness. Unconsciously, in an attempt to deal

with their own feelings, staff may withdraw from parents and not be emotionally available to help. This is a normal response, but one that needs to be guarded against because it only perpetuates a breakdown in relationships and communication with parents that are so greatly needed at this time. Many helpful interventions can be employed that are sensitive, supportive, and facilitate the emerging relationship between the parents and their infant.

EARLY COMMUNICATION. In the labor and delivery phase, early communication with both parents is essential. Parents normally are apprehensive and extremely sensitive to explicit or implicit cues such as actual statements by the staff, the atmosphere, looks, or a tone of voice that may indicate how things are progressing. Because of the recent emphasis on prepared childbirth, parents are extremely sophisticated in their knowledge of labor and delivery practices and immediately sense some deviation from what they expected. Prompt, direct explanations presented in a calm manner are very important and reassuring to parents. This explanation of the process of what is or will be happening can have a very helpful effect because it helps to organize the parents at a time when they are extremely vulnerable and feeling out of control. Although it is normal for the staff to be guarded, members of the health care team can comfortably tell the parents the known facts and what actually is being done for their infant without giving any diagnosis, prognosis, or forecast for the future course of the infant. Avoiding or not talking to parents only accelerates parental anxiety and adds to their growing fantasies or distortions. It has been well established and documented that parental fantasies about their infant's problems are usually worse than the reality.[30] Mothers often report that when they actually saw their infant, they were relieved because they had imagined the baby to appear worse.

SUPPORT OF STAFF. It is also important that one of the staff stay with the parents through labor, delivery, and recovery to offer continual support and to reassure parents that communication will continue as soon as more information is known. This is, again, an uncomfortable time for the staff because they may feel helpless and useless and as a result may avoid parents or revert to performing more technical activities. Some parents may need someone to be with them, not only to talk to them, but, more important, to listen; on the other hand, some parents may not be able to talk or verbalize their concerns or fears. Others may wish to be alone with each other or any other significant person in their life. Because of the varying responses and needs of people, it is extremely important to be sensitive to individual differences in approaching parents.

As much as possible, talking to both parents at the same time is helpful when discussing the infant's condition. This decreases their distortions and misconceptions, increases the communication and support between parents, and prevents either parent from feeling excluded. The assumption is commonly made that the father is in a better emotional state to hear about the infant; this misconception leads health professionals to mistakenly exclude or "spare" the mother, which only postpones her ability to begin to cope with the reality of her infant's condition. "Sparing" the mother may cause the parents to be in different stages of their understanding of the baby's medical condition and in their emotional state. Because emotional support between parents is so critical, the staff must avoid "sparing," since it can add to the parents' difficulty in being attuned to each other's needs and create more opportunities for the parents to be out of synchrony with each other.

SEEING THE BABY. The question usually arises about the value of the parents seeing their infant. This is a controversial issue and one that usually gets asked more frequently when a baby is very small and is not likely to survive, or when the baby is profoundly malformed. The general feeling is that it is psychologically better for parents to have had the opportunity to see their infant, but, again, this must be individualized for each family and

newborn. In general, seeing the infant helps to facilitate attachment, decrease exaggerated fantasies, decrease withdrawal from the infant, and enhance the parents' ability to grasp the reality of the situation. Because of the need to respect individual differences in people, the best approach is to give parents the opportunity to decide whether they together or individually want to see the infant.

This decision should be ultimately made by the parents with the support of the health care team. It is not uncommon to find a well-meaning physician, nurse, or social worker advising the parents or taking the decision into their own hands and concluding it would be in the parents' best interests not to see the infant. The argument is given that, "It's better not to get attached," or "It would make them cry or upset them to see the anomaly," or "They could not handle it," or "They would lose control." This decision is for the parents, and not for the professional, to make.

Some parents may know unequivocally what they want to do; others may be ambivalent, unsure, and indecisive. It is the role of the professional to give the parents assistance (information and support) in making the decision. The parents may need time to think about it or may need to discuss their fear and ambivalence first, before being able to decide. They may need some factual information and preparation from the professional, such as concerning the appearance of the baby and a description of the equipment. They may need assurance that someone will stay with them. Although time often is a factor and a decision must be made quickly, it is important to move at the parents' pace. The professional should still follow as much as possible the principle of allowing the parents the option of seeing the infant. If for medical reasons of the mother this is not possible, a self-developing picture can always be taken.[40] If it is medically possible for the parents to touch or hold the infant, the parents should be offered the opportunity. Touching or holding not only facilitates attachment but can provide parents with an emotional experience that is very sustaining and reassuring, helping them proceed through a very critical time of separation.

The parents are very sensitive to the staff's attitude toward the infant as reflected by their comments and the manner in which the staff handle the infant. If the infant is regarded with respect and treated as important, the parent is given the feeling that the infant is seen as valued and worthwhile. This is especially important for parents of an infant with a congenital anomaly; the parents could wonder if their baby is seen as "damaged goods" by society. In describing the infant to the parent, it is important to present a balanced picture of both the normal aspects and the abnormal problematic areas. In discussing the infant with the parents, reference to the infant by name, if they have named the baby, helps personalize the baby and establish the baby's unique identity.

CARETAKING. To reinforce the caretaking needs of parents, it is extremely important to discuss with them their plans to feed their infant. Support and encouragement should be given whether the parents have decided on breastfeeding or bottle-feeding. In many situations breastfeeding a sick infant may be possible. Many mothers are able to pump their breasts with milk that eventually will be given to the infant. There are many psychologic reasons why breastfeeding or pumping may be beneficial for mothers and babies alike. The breastfeeding or pumping experience helps the mother to feel close to her baby and that she has some control over what is happening to her baby; she can uniquely contribute to her infant's care in a way no one else can. Fathers, too, can participate in this activity by their support and interest in the actual breastfeeding or the pumping and milk collection activities. Many mothers are able to successfully pump and eventually put the infant to breast, but others are not, because of emotional stresses, the condition of the baby, the length of time until the infant can feed, and the waning interest of the mother. Regardless of eventual success, the mother should be encouraged to try if she has an interest; then she can feel that she made an attempt to relate to her infant in this way. If a mother does not plan to breastfeed or pump, or if she tries but does not continue, she should not be made to feel guilty or that she failed in her role. She is already vulnerable to these feelings, having had a baby born with problems.

After the delivery when the mother returns to her room "without a healthy baby," she usually experiences a void; "an amputation" has occurred.[30] She and those around her are beginning to grieve. The interventions of the staff should be flexible and sensitive to the individual needs of the family. Empathy, responsiveness, and an ability to listen to the parents are most important at this time.

Encouraging parents to verbalize and express their feelings and concerns (at their own pace), although difficult to do at times, is useful to the parents. Avoiding their grief gives the mother and father the impression that they are "bad parents" for having feelings of sadness, anger, guilt, or loss; this only increases their level of guilt and isolation. Prescribing tranquilizers also gives the message that it is not permissible to talk about what has happened to them and their infant. Tranquilizers only increase the feelings of unreality that normally are experienced. This stifles the parental coping mechanisms at a time when the parents need to begin to come to terms with what has happened.

Room assignments are a very personal matter and one that the mother should decide. Some mothers want to return to the regular maternity ward; for others it is too painful, and they want to be on a separate floor. Flexible visiting regulations for the father and other significant persons are necessary to facilitate support to one another through a very difficult, uncertain period.

In talking to parents, it is important to bear in mind that the parents do not remember much of what has been said; it is very difficult for them to assimilate both cognitively and emotionally all that has happened. It is important for the staff to move at the parents' own pace. If the baby has been transferred or the chances for survival are limited, the mother should be discharged or given a pass as soon as possible. It is also important to acknowledge to the mother (and father) that she is a mother and that she did give birth to a baby. She needs the congratulatory cards, gifts, and attention that she would have normally received.

ANTICIPATORY GRIEVING

After labor and delivery, parents are struggling with the second psychologic task of anticipatory grieving and withdrawal from the relationship established during pregnancy. This task requires that parents acknowledge that their infant's life is endangered or that the newborn might die. Events surrounding the labor, delivery, and post-partum period may have indicated to the parents that their infant's chances for survival are diminished. If this has occurred, parents then can become involved in anticipatory grieving and withdrawal from the relationship established during pregnancy. Studies have shown that the decision to transfer an infant to a newborn intensive care unit alone is likely to initiate an anticipatory grief reaction.[8]

Parents may also be experiencing feelings of grief and sadness over the loss of the expected, idealized child that they had wished for during the pregnancy. For some parents, attaching to a critically ill or malformed infant may be too overwhelming; parents may withdraw from the infant in an attempt to protect themselves from their feelings of hurt, disappointment, and guilt.[21] Some parents may feel ambivalent about the baby; they may feel they could not love or cope with an infant who might die or who would have significant physical or mental problems. Feeling uncertain about whether they want the infant to survive can cause feelings of extreme guilt that may cause the parents to withdraw from the infant as a way of avoiding confronting these difficult, painful feelings.

During this period, parents may find themselves in a very stressful position; they are faced with the task of balancing the painful realities of confronting a possible loss against their hopes for the intact survival of their infant. The emotional withdrawal and grieving that parents experience is normal during the critical time that the infant's life is endangered or when parents are faced with the possibility that their infant may have a lifelong problem. This withdrawal becomes pathologic only if it continues beyond the time the infant demonstrates definite signs (to the parents) of improvement and survival. In the case of a permanently handicapped newborn, parents unable to grieve their idealized infant may maintain this withdrawal, which might lead to attachment difficulties.[43,53]

Parents exhibit many emotional responses and behaviors that indicate they are struggling with the anticipatory grieving and withdrawal. Some parents are very sad and depressed and teary, and others may be highly anxious, at times bordering on panic states; others react by having a flat affect, being withdrawn, and appearing apathetic. Some parents may exhibit very angry, hostile, confrontational behavior as a way of dealing with their distress; others may deny the situation by optimistically feeling that "everything will be OK."

Parents who typically are verbal may ask questions reflecting their concerns about their infant's survival; this is especially true after the child has received medical attention and decisions are being made about treatment for the infant, including transfer to a neonatal intensive care unit (NICU). The questions they ask physicians and nurses are: "Is he going to make it?" "What do you think his chances are?" "He'll be OK, won't he?" "Have you seen other babies with this problem?" "Do other babies make it?" "How long will he be in the hospital?" Parents struggling with their fears may resist seeing, touching, or visiting the baby. If they do visit the infant in the NICU, they may remain distant by having little or no eye contact with the baby, refusing to touch, standing far from the warmer or incubator, and asking few or no questions of the staff. The parents may be reluctant to name the baby; when they do refer to the infant, they say "it," "she," "he," or "the baby."

If the infant has been given a special or treasured family name, they may be reluctant to use it.

A very common phenomenon occurs when parents, being protective of each other, discourage each other's involvement with the infant. This is especially true at the time of transport when the transport nurse may suggest to the father or family members that the baby be shown to the mother before leaving. Many fathers are afraid this will increase the emotional attachment to the infant and thus the feelings of disappointment and loss if the infant should die. The father is usually very apprehensive about how to handle the mother's feelings of grief in addition to his own. This type of behavior also is true with regard to medical information; it is not uncommon for one parent to request that all communication go through that parent. The response is that "my spouse is too upset or anxious and couldn't handle hearing any bad news." Many times it is actually the parent making the request who is most anxious and who is dealing with this anxiety by projecting it onto the other partner. Work and child care responsibilities, transportation difficulties, and financial limitations are all legitimate reasons why parents may not be able to have frequent contact with their infant. However, these factors may also serve as unconscious ways to maintain distance from the infant.

It is important to keep in mind that this withdrawal and grieving is a necessary and natural process. For parents to develop an attachment to and accept the reality of their infant's condition, they must experience their feelings of grief, sadness, anger, guilt, and disappointment over the loss of the expected child.[53] This grieving serves to free the parents' emotional energy so that they can interact with and become attuned to their infant. Grieving enhances the parents' availability to the infant. Availability aids in their feeling competent to handle their infant.[56] The goal, then, of the perinatal health care team's interventions is to help the family realize that their feelings are natural and normal and will be accepted. Parents need permission to have their feelings. It is essential to acknowledge to parents that it is normal to be afraid of attaching to a baby who might die or have a handicap. Giving permission diminishes the guilt that the parents may feel about their behavior being abnormal or about their being bad parents because they are afraid. Simple statements such as, "Many parents tell us they are afraid of getting too close to their baby," or "It's scary to attach when you think the baby may die," are helpful.

It is sometimes useful for parents to verbalize what their fears actually are. They may fear their infant's dying, being retarded, or being paralyzed. Once these fears are clarified in the minds of the parents and either confirmed or refuted by the medical staff, it is usually easier for parents to begin to accept their infant's diagnosis and prognosis and begin relating to the infant. Social workers can provide valuable emotional support to families in helping them deal with their realistic and unrealistic concerns.[42,61]

The role of the physician in communicating medical information is extremely important. There are many schools of thought about how to approach parents, ranging from being extremely cautious and pessimistic ("paint the bleakest picture") to being encouraging and optimistic ("give parents hope"). Although the approach should be individualized for each family, a balanced approach is the most beneficial. Parents need a realistic assessment of the situation that is honest and direct. It is important to acknowledge the baby's condition and possible problems, but not to inundate parents with every potential problem that can arise. Parents who hear "brain damage," "retarded," or "the baby will die" are not likely to forget these statements. These statements can linger in the minds of parents and adversely influence how the parents relate to their newborn. They may believe that some day "brain damage will show up" or that the infant is susceptible and frail and needs to be treated cautiously for fear of a life-threatening condition. Many such children become victims of the vulnerable child syndrome,[23] a condition in which a child is over-protected by his parents and treated as if he or she had a medical problem or is in danger of death when neither are any longer the case. Parents who are told their newborn may die may have trouble attaching or becoming emotionally invested. When talking to parents, physicians and nurses should be very judicious and careful in making dramatic statements of a sensitive nature. Definitive statements should be used only when appropriate and necessary. The long-term emotional implications of such statements need to be weighed.

There are several other rules or guidelines in communicating medical information to parents.[*] As mentioned earlier, parents' perceptions of their infant's condition are extremely important, remain in parents' minds, and can affect their relationship with the infant. Parents easily misperceive information given to them. They may believe that a patent ductus arteriosus indicates open-heart surgery and therefore worry that their baby has a heart condition. Or perhaps they think a bilirubin problem means their baby has liver disease. Therefore in beginning any discussion with parents, it is essential to determine and address their perceptions. A staff member might say, "Could you tell me what you understand about your baby's condition?" This will give the physician or nurse the opportunity to correct any misinformation or misconceptions and to hear about the parents' concerns. A team member might specifically ask about the parents' concerns or worries; "Could you tell me what concerns you have about your baby?" Asking this can make communication between the perinatal health care team and the parents more meaningful and helpful; unless the team deals with the parents' anxiety, discussions become one-sided lectures and only benefit the professional. Discussions need to be a dialogue between parent and professional.

During the course of a discussion and again at the end, it is useful to determine parents' interpretations of what has been said and to modify and clarify as needed. The staff needs to avoid overloading a parent with lengthy explanations that are too technical. It is more productive to move at a pace so that the parent can assimilate the information presented; it is not necessary to describe the entire course of respiratory distress syndrome or bronchopulmonary dysplasia. It is always preferable to use simple language that is understandable to a lay person and to avoid the use of statistics and vivid modifiers. Statistics are confusing because they do not apply to the individual case and can easily be misinterpreted. When asked about the frequency of brain damage with a grade III intraventricular hemorrhage, a team member might say, "A majority of these babies have some neurologic problem, but there are some who do not." Vivid modifiers such as "This is the worst case of sepsis we have ever had" or "Your baby is the sickest baby in the nursery" are of no real benefit to the parents and only accelerate their fantasies and anxieties. Finally, if a referring physician and the nursery team are both communicating with the parents, it is essential to coordinate the particular approach. It is very confusing to parents and decreases their trust level for one to be pessimistic and the other optimistic.

ACKNOWLEDGMENT OF FEELINGS OF GUILT

The third psychologic task parents are dealing with simultaneously with anticipatory grieving and withdrawal is confronting and recognizing their feelings of failure and guilt in not delivering a healthy infant. Most parents struggling with feelings of inadequacy and guilt are likely to search for answers to the causes of their baby's situation. The mother may focus on concrete things such as not eating well, the flu, intercourse, birth control pills, or an unwanted pregnancy. The father may also be concerned about his role in not helping his wife enough, placing too many de-

---

[*]Modified from Taylor PM and Hall BL: Parent-infant bonding: problems and opportunities in a perinatal center, Semin Perinatol 3:73-84, 1979. By permission.

mands on her, an argument he provoked that pre-cipitated labor, or another family member with the same chromosomal abnormality. Parents search for reasons because they need to find a cause for such an event happening to them. It is harder for them to feel out of control and helpless than to feel guilty. Some parents place responsi-bility on themselves, but others shift the blame to others in their external world, such as their spouse, extended family, doctor, nurses, or God. Often both parents are concerned with the disap-pointment that they have caused the other. They may withdraw from each other at a time when they both need acceptance and support. Realistic answers from the medical team are helpful for some parents in diminishing guilt feelings; in other parents the guilt may be so deeply inte-grated in the parents' thinking that it is less easily overcome. For example, some parents may focus on irrational, unrealistic factors such as "This is my punishment for not being a good wife or daughter" or "This is my punishment for running away from home when I was 15." It seems that the more irrational the parental thinking, the harder it is to assuage and resolve the guilt. Many feelings of guilt and failure are normal and expected; the feelings are a problem when the parent does not respond to the infant's progress because the baby may continue to represent the parent's failure.

Parents demonstrate many behaviors that indi-cate they are struggling with guilt and failure. Some parents directly verbalize these feelings and attempt to obtain helpful answers from the staff. Less obvious are the parents who are markedly depressed and remain so despite any improve-ment in the baby. These parents demonstrate the classic signs of depression such as apathy, loss of interest in appearance and self, withdrawal, and loss of self-esteem. They exhibit an overwhelming sense of helplessness because they feel responsi-ble for causing their baby's problem and are help-less to remedy the situation. Their guilt feelings cause them to be very self-deprecating and angry at themselves, a state that often results in depres-sion. Other parents struggling with guilt are

highly anxious about their ability to handle their baby; they feel they have harmed their infant and cannot tolerate facing that infant. Another mani-festation of guilt is hostility and anger that is usually directed toward others, such as the spouse, staff, or God. Instead of focusing their anger on themselves like the depressed parent, they direct it outward to rid themselves of their feelings of responsibility, projecting the guilt feel-ing onto others in their life. They may be angry at the physicians, nurses, or social workers for not making their baby healthy (if the child is prema-ture) or perfect (if the child has a congenital de-fect). They may be hostile toward the social worker for not being able to help them with finan-cial problems. Unconsciously, they are trying to make the staff feel as guilty, helpless, and respon-sible as they do.

To intervene with parents, it is useful to help the parents become aware of and acknowledge their feelings of failure and guilt.[21] By verbalizing their feelings, they can begin to identify the source of the guilt feelings, which may not always be clear to them. The staff can then intervene with appropriate information to modify and clar-ify the perceptions that may be the source of some of the parents' guilt feelings. Many parents di-rectly ask about the causes of their baby's prob-lem, and the medical team should provide them with appropriate information. Other parents are not as direct or verbal; they need to have the subject introduced. A staff member might open the door by saying, "Have you wondered why this has happened?" or "Many parents find themselves feeling responsible for their baby's problem, as if they failed. Have you had these feelings?" As par-ents begin to talk about their feelings, they them-selves are often able to test reality and discover the irrationality in their thinking. Some parents, however, continue to feel guilty even though they have been told they are not to blame. Guilt feel-ings are very complex and may take a long time to resolve; for some they may never be completely resolved, but at least the intensity of the feelings may diminish. If a child recovers from the illness, guilt can be more easily relinquished. If the child has a chronic problem, the parent is daily confronted with feelings of responsibility. The more irrational the source of the guilt, the harder it will be to dispel. Because this persistent guilt can cause problems in the parental relationship to the child, a referral to a perinatal social worker or other mental health professional may be indicated.

To facilitate support between parents, it is useful to ask whether they have shared their feelings of guilt and failure with each other. Often a spouse may assume that one is angry at or disappointed with the other. Discussing this may bring a tremendous sense of relief and reassurance. However, if the parents are blaming each other and relationship problems develop, a referral to a perinatal social worker is appropriate.

In some cases there may be realistic reasons (either intentional or unintentional) why the parent may feel guilty for the infant's problem. Parental drug or alcohol abuse, an accident, or an inherited genetic problem may be real reasons. In these cases the staff must acknowledge to the parent that there is a causal relationship and then give the parents support by allowing them to talk about their feelings. If causes were not intentional, it is helpful to acknowledge that fact; if they were, it is important to be nonjudgmental. A judging attitude only reinforces the feelings parents are already experiencing and further alienates them from the child and the staff. The parents need help with the problem that initially led to the impairment of the fetus. When this type of psychosocial problem arises, the involvement of a perinatal social worker can be of extreme importance.

ADAPTATION TO THE INTENSIVE CARE ENVIRONMENT

The fourth psychologic task involves adaptation to the intensive care environment.[52] All of the reactions of guilt, anxiety, fear, anger, and disappointment become heightened when parents attempt to adapt to this unfamiliar environment. They must learn a new language, establish trust in new relationships, and accept their role in this setting. The intense and sometimes chaotic appearance of a high-risk nursery makes it a frightening experience that serves to increase parental feelings of helplessness and anxiety. Parents need to gain a sense of security in this environment before initiating a care giving role with their infant. There may be cultural adaptations and geographic obstacles for families who live in small, rural communities and must travel to large, unfamiliar cities and become adapted to a large hospital. Locating the hospital and finding accommodations and meals can become overwhelming to parents who have undergone much emotional turmoil. Meeting the infant's caretaker, the competent physician and nurse, can sometimes evoke a mixture of positive and negative feelings. Parents may experience reassurance and gratitude for care being given, yet at the same time a reinforcement of their feelings of uselessness, helplessness, and inadequacy can ensue.[59] The sophistication of the highly technical care and heroic measures provided to attain survival may be met with both awe and uncertainty. Family disruption is exaggerated by distance, especially if the infant was transported and the father must decide whether he is most needed with the infant, wife, or perhaps other children at home. Decisions must be made about work responsibilities as well as child care. The financial concerns related to providing intensive care become an added stress on families and is often compounded by the travel expenditures necessary to visit the infant.

There are a number of nonverbal and verbal signs that indicate parents are struggling to gain a sense of security in the NICU. Some parents appear frightened, overwhelmed, nervous, and withdrawn, asking few questions or being reluctant to call or visit. Others may be highly anxious and unable to focus on their baby and may instead concentrate on other activities or babies in the nursery. Some parents may ask many questions and become very interested in the technical aspects of their infant's treatment, such as respirator settings and laboratory values. Some parents, uneasy with entrusting their child to strangers, may initially feel a need to remain at their infant's side, constantly establishing a vigil. Some may request to read the infant's chart or attempt to read material on their infant's particular condition. Others may get angry or upset at minor things related to the infant's care or the running of the nursery, such as a respiratory setting being a point off or the staff's limiting visitation of friends and relatives.

There are many interventions that can be employed to familiarize and orient families.[52] First, the obstetrician, transport team, or any other personnel who has initial contact with parents can give them preparatory information and a description of intensive care. A booklet that includes basic information and illustrative pictures is extremely useful and should include a discussion of the type of care being provided, normal feelings and reactions parents experience, financial information, a glossary of terms, breastfeeding information, available accommodations and meals, calling and visitation policies, the discharge policy, and a city map. Both at the time of transfer and later in the nursery, a self-developing picture can be taken of the infant for the parents. If the infant is being transported, information should be given as to the approximate length of time of transport, and by whom and when the parents will be contacted after the infant has been admitted and evaluated. A personal phone call from the staff with an introduction, information about the infant and unit, and an inquiry regarding parental visitation plans is useful. Parents feel less anxious when they have an orientation and a name to relate to. The staff can then be prepared to be available when the parents arrive.

Certainly, the first visit to the NICU is stressful, and members of the team should welcome the parents and stay with them to explain the equipment and procedures, answer questions, review the baby's course, give emotional support, and in general orient the parents to this new experience. It is important to be attentive to the mother's physical needs; comfortable chairs or perhaps a wheelchair if the mother has had a cesarean section are helpful. The message needs to be conveyed that parents are welcome and that their visits do make a difference in that they have a useful role to play with their infant. Because many parents are uncertain about what questions to ask, it may be necessary at times to help parents construct questions ("Do you understand why we start IVs in the head?" or "Do you know what blood gases, hood oxygen, and CPAP are?") and to repeat explanations using simple, nontechnical language. Relating to the parents' affect or emotional state seems to establish a relationship with the family and helps them feel that the staff is empathetic and understanding. If parents sense the staff's genuine concern and interest in them and their baby, it is easier for them to leave their infant in the staff's care. A team member might say, "You look frightened or scared," or "This can be an overwhelming situation," or "You look like you want to cry." Facilitating the parents' relationship with the infant is essential and can be done by offering the parents the opportunity to touch or stroke their baby, hold the infant if possible, or at least remove eye patches. Pointing out some of the unique personal characteristics of the infant is helpful. A staff member might say, "Your baby is very active," or "He responds well to touch," or "She seems to prefer lying on her side."

Families coming from out of town should be provided with a list of inexpensive housing and restaurants located near the hospital. In many cities national and local businesses have established nearby homes run by local volunteer organizations for housing parents on a temporary basis. The homes have several sleeping rooms in addition to kitchen and laundry facilities and provide parents with a comfortable, homelike atmosphere at a nominal charge. A natural support system generally emerges among the parents using the home. Apartments and boarding rooms reasonably priced and rented by the day or week can also be made available. To help cover the expenses of traveling, arrangements can often be made, when appropriate, so that parents receive funds from the March of Dimes–Birth Defects Foundation, department of social services, and church groups.

Parents are usually concerned with the cost of their infant's hospitalization. Some parents feel that if they are unable to pay, their child will receive less attention. Parents should be reassured that their infant's care will not depend on their ability to pay. They should, however, be referred to the appropriate funding agencies, such as the Handicapped or Crippled Children's Program or Social Security Disability, that do provide financial assistance.

Since communication is so critical, regular conferences between the family and staff (physician, nurses, and social workers) should be instituted to give consistent medical information and emotional support; this is especially helpful with both extremely critical and long-term babies. Parents should be given the names of the physicians and nurses taking care of their infant, and the personnel's specific role in providing both care to the baby and communication to the family should be outlined. If the physicians and nurses have a rotation system, this also should be explained from the beginning. At the end of a rotation, the transition can be facilitated by the on-coming physician's participation in even a brief conference with the out-going physician, primary nurse, and the parents. Primary nursing, especially for long-term babies, can be very helpful in providing for continuity of care.

For out-of-town families the telephone plays a major role in staff-to-parent communication. The establishment of a telephone calling schedule with families and the use of WATS lines, if available, can be useful. If the family is out of town and unable to visit frequently, the local or referring physician can supplement the communication. That physician often knows the family and can talk with them in person. The physician should, of course, communicate regularly with the nursery team to obtain the current medical information and present a consistent approach to the family.

The use of public health nurses before the infant's discharge is a valuable means of support and teaching.

RESUMPTION OF THE RELATIONSHIP WITH THE INFANT

The fifth psychologic task entails the parents' reestablishing a relationship with their infant and initiating their care-giving role, a process that usually begins when the child's improvement retrieves previous hopes after a disappointing experience. Certain medical events may signal to the parents that it is safe to risk a relationship with the infant. These events may be a regular weight gain, changes in feeding patterns or methods, elimination of life support equipment, the infant's crying for the first time or becoming more active and responsive, or the infant's transfer from the NICU to a level II nursery. The parents may begin to read baby books or pamphlets about their infant's condition, buy clothes, set up the baby's room, send out birth announcements, or name the baby. If the infant has a congenital defect, the parents may become involved with genetic counseling and other parents whose infants have similar deficits.

Parents must begin to shift their level of involvement and activity from that of a passive participant to that of an active primary caretaker. The shift includes their gaining confidence in their ability to care for their infant. The family that has been disrupted must reestablish itself and recover from the crisis in an environment that is sensitive and supportive to this essential task.

Involvement in caretaking lessens the parents' feelings of helplessness and frustration and facilitates their identification with their role as parents. When parents visit, they can help by providing skin care for the infant, putting glycerin on the baby's lips, helping turn the baby even if a respirator is attached, diapering the infant, and feeding the baby if this is possible. If the parents are separated by distance, they can send family pictures that can be posted at the baby's bed; periodic pictures of the infant taken by the staff can be sent back to the family. Parents can send clothing, mobiles, simple toys, and even cassette tapes so that the infant can hear the parents' voices. Some mothers who are pumping send frozen breast milk. All of these reminders help the nursery staff be aware of the real family that is genuinely interested. These personal attempts made by parents that help them feel they are important to their infant's development should be encouraged. Sometimes foster grandparents or volunteers can hold, feed, and talk to babies whose parents cannot visit frequently.

The use of "graduate parents," parents who have had a baby in the NICU and who have successfully dealt with and resolved the crisis of the birth of their infant, can be extremely valuable. They provide support to parents by sharing common feelings, reactions, and experiences about having a hospitalized infant. Graduate parents also visit selected infants whose parents are unable to visit. They can establish written correspondence with the parents and perhaps include a picture of the infant. Graduate parents can provide support and practical assistance for mothers interested in breastfeeding, parents who take their infant home on oxygen, or parents whose baby requires special medical care such as shunt, tracheostomy, or colostomy care, or gavage feedings. Organized graduate parent groups in large tertiary settings have become a very popular means of providing support, but locating one parent or couple to talk with parents in a small community can be just as helpful.

Parent classes can also be offered on a variety of topics such as breastfeeding, infant development, premature baby development, sibling and family reactions, discharge, cardiopulmonary resuscitation, coping with the hospitalization, and special medical needs. These classes provide specific, didactic information combined with group discussions that are mutually supportive in nature. Social workers, nurses, and other related health care professionals (respiratory, occupational, and physical therapists) facilitate the group; graduate parents also participate as a resource group.

A third type of support group is counseling sessions.[37] The purpose of these sessions is to discuss and deal with common issues among parents, arising from the hospitalization of their infant and the effects on their marriage and family life. This type of group has also been helpful for parents whose infant has died. The group is usually short term and is conducted by the perinatal social worker and another staff member such as a physician or chaplain. The focus of the group is not to give specific medical information, but rather to provide parents with an opportunity to verbalize their feelings about their infant's hospitalization and to receive mutual emotional support.

For proper family functioning, support must be given not only to the parents,[3,7,38,51] but also to the siblings of the hospitalized infant. However, siblings are often ignored in comments about family-centered care. By only addressing the problems of the parents and newborn, the impression is made that the infant is always an only child.

Including the other children in the total experience surrounding the birth of a new family member is important for several reasons. From a sibling's viewpoint the anticipated birth of a new baby is a stressful time of noticeable physical and psychologic changes within the family. In preparation for the impending birth, the child is told that the mother will be going to the hospital for a few days and will return with a baby brother or sister. With the birth of a premature or ill infant the mother may go to the hospital unexpectedly, stay "a long time," and not return home with the anticipated playmate. Instead of a celebration of the expected happy event, parents are grieving the loss of the normal newborn and the current crisis of their sick infant.

Parents are often unsure what to tell the other children and whether or not the children should see the baby. The siblings themselves may feel left out, rejected, or worried that they, too, may get sick. They may feel they are to blame and that their jealous feelings about their new rival may have caused this tragedy. Confused by their parents' distress, the other children may speculate that it is related to them and their bad behaviors. They may be disappointed and angry that they did not get the "playmate" they had wanted. Since parents are unsure and confused about how to manage these issues, it is often helpful for the staff to introduce the topic.

Since children will make up an explanation for the baby's illness, it is better to have it based on accurate information. Before explaining the infant's condition to siblings, elicit their ideas and perceptions about "what is the matter." Any fears, fantasies, misconceptions, or proper information is thus used to begin the explanation of "where the baby is." Explanations must be tailored to the individual child's cognitive and developmental level. The child should be told that the baby is sick but in a way that is different from his or her illnesses; the baby's illness is not "catching," and it is not like any of the illnesses the child has experienced. To allay the siblings' fears about medical personnel, they should also be told that the nurses and physicians are trying to help the baby "get better." Because children between 2 and 6 years are involved in magical thinking, they should be told they are not to blame and that they did not cause the baby's problem. If the baby is premature, a team member might say to the child, "The baby came out too early or too soon; he needed more time to grow inside." If the baby has spina bifida a staff member might say, "The baby's spine did not grow right, so he may have trouble lifting his legs or walking."

A child of 3 years or younger usually does not understand much about the coming baby. More important to this age group is the separation from parents who are frequently at the hospital.[3] To ameliorate the separation, child-care arrangements should be structured so that the child is cared for by familiar people in a familiar environment. The most ideal care arrangement would be with a familiar, beloved person in the child's own home; second best would be a familiar, beloved person in the caretaker's home; and third best, an unfamiliar person in the child's own home. Least favorable, of course, would be an unfamiliar person in an unfamiliar setting. Many hospitals have a child-care facility run by volunteers that allows the child the opportunity to go to the hospital to "see where Mommy and Daddy are going" yet allows the parents the chance to see their infant without having to care for their other child(ren). Or parents may choose to include the young child in all or selected visits.

Children ages 3 and older have more interest in babies and a better grasp about the physical meaning of life. Sometimes a picture of the baby or a look into the nursery through the windows is helpful to the other children. Many children benefit from visits to the nursery to see their brother or sister. The natural curiosity of the child about "what is going on" in the family is answered when the child actually sees the baby. Behavior problems such as bed-wetting, sleeping and eating difficulties, and difficult separations from parents may be prevented or reduced by the reassurance of a visit that decreases the sibling's worry about the baby.[5] Sibling visitation must be individualized for every family.

The decision to include siblings in the NICU depends to a great extent on the views, beliefs, and attitudes of the hospital staff. Generally, the staff's concerns about and resistance to sibling visitation focus on a fear of an increase in nosocomial infection, disruption of unit routine and order, and potential harm to young children from exposure to the NICU environment. Infection control is the responsibility of parents and professionals. Parents must be educated about the dangers of infection and instructed on how to screen their children for symptoms such as fever, cough, or diarrhea. Professional staff must inquire about the health of visiting siblings, including their exposure to communicable diseases. Both parents and children wash their hands and don cover gowns. Pediatric patient gowns and small stools to help children reach the sink are used. With vigilance, no increased bacterial colonization and no increased incidence of infection occur with sibling visits.[5,57,58,60]

Since sibling visitation may be beneficial, each NICU must evaluate the center's situation and consider instituting a sibling visitation policy. The following general principles may be used in developing this policy:

1. Communication and coordination between staff and family are necessary to promote successful sibling visitation.
2. Children must be prepared, according to their age and development, for what they will see, hear, and feel in the NICU. Language should be simple and honest; pictures of the baby or other infants are always helpful.
3. Parents and staff screen the visiting sibling for signs of illness that would exclude the child from visiting.
4. Parents and child must scrub and gown.
5. The initial visit should be held at a relatively quiet time in the nursery when a care provider is able to stay with the family. If the infant can be moved to a private room or family room area, this is preferable.

The child is taken to the bedside, introduced to the baby, and seated on a chair or stool at eye level with the infant. The care provider then again explains the equipment the child sees and any of the infant's "interesting" behaviors such as crying because of hunger, sucking on a pacifier, or eyes open "looking at you." Children may even be included in age-appropriate caretaking tasks. Choosing clothes, handing diapers and blankets, holding the bottle, or touching and talking to the infant are all ways "to help." The child may bring a present to the infant such as a simple toy, music box, or handmade picture or photograph of the family. After the visit both parents and staff should be available to talk about the visit or answer any questions. Some children, however, will not discuss the visit or ask questions till some later time. A method for enabling children to express their feelings in a nonverbal way is through play or books. A child who receives a book about physicians and hospitals or a "doctor" or "nurse" doll, may "play out" feelings about the brother or sister and the hospital experience.

Creating a comfortable environment in which children feel free to ask questions is essential when siblings visit. Every question deserves an answer, even "I don't know," when appropriate. Children are often quite unrestrained in their remarks and questions. Comments such as, "He's sure ugly!" or "Is he going to die?" or "Why is she tied up (restrained)?" are common. These may be embarrassing to parents who hesitate to make the same remarks or ask the same questions.

If the baby is hospitalized for a long time, the other children may lose interest or even wish it were all over. This response may upset parents who themselves may be struggling with the same feelings. The longer the infant is hospitalized, the greater the pressure on time and financial resources. Family routines are disrupted by continuing hospitalization, and the disruption may strain family relationships.

Staff and parent response to sibling visitation has been positive in hospitals where the policy has been implemented. Such a policy may facilitate family integrity and promotes mutual support during the stressful time of hospitalization.[5] Another advantage of visitation is that the older siblings do not endure repeated separations caused by parental visits to the hospital but are included as important and special family members. The presence of siblings in a nursery can be a rewarding experience for family and staff alike and perhaps is the ideal example of providing safe yet comprehensive family-centered care.

Although a flexible sibling visitation policy is viewed as the best possible situation, some alternatives must be considered. Staff should be sensitive to the needs of the siblings and understand that the parents must deal with both time and financial constraints.

Psychosocial conferences for staff members to discuss the dynamics of family functioning and

---

HIGH-RISK FACTORS NEEDING SOCIAL WORK INTERVENTION

1. Teenage pregnancy (ages 11 to 18)
2. Single parent
3. Drug or alcohol abuse
4. Psychiatric history of present problem that interferes with appropriate functioning, especially as related to parenting abilities
5. Mother or father with a history of being abused or early deprivation by own family, or history of having abused or neglected own children
6. Battered women
7. Mental retardation, borderline intelligence, or significant physical handicaps
8. History of loss with previous pregnancy or child because of stillbirth, birth defect, prematurity, abortion, custody case, or death
9. Rejection or ambivalence of current pregnancy as manifested by requests for termination of pregnancy, attempted abortion, or relinquishment
10. No prenatal care with previous or current pregnancies
11. Pregnancy exacerbating extreme depression, anxiety, or suicidal thoughts
12. Stressful home or personal situation because of marital or financial problems or lack of support systems
13. Long-term hospitalization during pregnancy requiring intervention in helping family adjust by arranging for younger children at home or for financial assistance
14. Other children with physical or mental handicaps

---

the impact of a seriously ill newborn on the family can be quite useful. These conferences, usually led by perinatal social workers, can give staff the opportunity to discuss and better understand their own feelings and reactions to families, infants, and the many stresses related to working in an NICU. In addition, weekly rounds with the entire multidisciplinary team (physicians, nurses, public health nurse coordinator, social workers, and financial counselors) are an effective vehicle to discuss and develop medical and psychosocial care plans about each infant and family. To complement this approach to family-centered care, a charting system to record the qualitative and quantitative contact (phone calls and visitations) between parents and their infant is recommended (see Figure 22-3). This information can be very helpful in evaluating the frequency and quality of the parent-child interaction and the parent-staff interaction in addition to the parent's individual coping patterns over time. The involvement of perinatal social workers to assess and evaluate the psychosocial functioning of families, to provide support and counseling services, and to coordinate the discharge planning and follow-up care for the infant and family is essential. Social workers need to evaluate all high-risk cases in addition to providing support in complicated medical conditions, including death of the infant (see boxed material above).

Transfer of the infant from a tertiary center back to the referral or local community hospital for convalescent care and discharge is a phenomenon that is occurring more frequently. This can be helpful in facilitating the relationship between the infant and parents, since the infant will be more accessible. Parents generally view the transfer as positive if the hospital is closer to home and if they feel comfortable with the level of care provided. There is always an adjustment period any time a transfer occurs. Parents must adapt to different personalities of medical personnel and different procedures and visiting regulations. Preparing the parents for the transfer, orienting them to the new hospital, and talking to the staff of the referral hospital about the baby and the parents is important to help ease the transition.

PREPARATION TO TAKE THE INFANT HOME

The sixth psychologic task for parents concerns preparations for taking the infant home. Parents must understand their infant's individual needs and personality characteristics in addition to feeling a sense of competency in relating to their infant. Discharge is an anxiety-provoking event and ushers in the "crisis" of homecoming, which parents must face and master. The unsuccessful resolution of the previously discussed five psychologic tasks can contribute to maladaptive parenting and a poor outcome for the infant, including the possibilities of overprotectiveness, failure to thrive, vulnerable child syndrome, emotional deprivation, and battering.[30] To achieve a positive parent-child relationship following the hospitalization and through the transitional period that ensues, provision of appropriate follow-up support through the home adjustment period is crucial.[19,30]

Several behaviors demonstrate that parents are trying to understand the infant's care in preparation for discharge. First, parents may ask questions verbalizing a variety of concerns. For a premature infant they might ask, "Do I need an apnea monitor at home?" or "Can the baby have visitors?" or "Do I need to wash my hands and wear a gown when handling the baby?" For a child with a congenital defect such as spina bifida the parents might ask, "Can I lay the baby on his back?" or "Can I bathe him?" or "Do I need to pump the shunt?" For a child with a heart defect the staff might be asked, "Do I need oxygen?" or "Do I need to handle him differently?" or "What

about going to higher altitudes?" All of these questions on the part of parents are very typical and normal and represent the parents' working through their fears and anxieties.

On the other hand, parents who are highly anxious, extremely overprotective, or very indifferent should be a concern to the health care personnel. The inability to deal with the task of taking the infant home may indicate some unresolved feelings related to the previous psychologic tasks. Although most parents whose infants have been in an NICU do admit to initially treating their infant differently until they "got to know their child," a group of parents who are excessively overprotective does exist. This type of behavior usually stems from parents who are struggling with intense feelings of guilt and failure. These parents either protect their child from everything because they feel so responsible for having caused the infant's initial problem or they demonstrate an indifference or lack of concern for the infant and the infant's welfare. Such parents may have an ambivalent attachment to their infant, who may continue to represent the threat of death or the parents' personal failure. This group of parents should be considered high risk for potential parent-child relationship difficulties and should be evaluated to determine an appropriate intervention.

There are many interventions that the perinatal health care team can employ to assist parents with discharge and through the transitional period that follows. In the hospital adequate teaching of caregiving skills that allow the parent to develop a sense of mastery and competence is of paramount importance. If parents do not feel comfortable with their infant, their anxiety can cause adverse interactions with the baby. The parent needs to know the baby's mannerisms and behaviors; otherwise the parent may feel exhausted and resentful and then guilty. Teaching care-giving skills can often be facilitated in an environment that is less intense and crisis oriented than the NICU. Whenever possible, a baby should be transferred to a setting that is more conducive to the parent's initiating the primary care-giving role; a more conducive setting might be a transitional nursery,[20] a level II unit, or a general pediatric ward.

Adequate discharge planning and follow-up arrangements should include general pediatric care, visiting nurse service, and parenting classes, especially for young or psychosocially high-risk parents. Referrals to county social service departments should be made for single mothers who are eligible for Aid to Families of Dependent Children and Medicaid. For infants with special problems (spina bifida, cerebral palsy, or Down's syndrome) referrals should be made for special programs that provide services for the infants and support groups for parents. Parents whose infants have special medical needs (gavage feedings, tracheostomy or colostomy care, or oxygen) should be evaluated by the medical and nursing personnel to determine helpful community resources (equipment, supplies, or emergency care) and to make appropriate referrals. Home nursing care and homemaker services are sometimes covered by medical insurance and may be necessary to provide actual nursing activities and to relieve parents from the emotional burden inherent in caring for an infant with medical problems. For infants who are developmentally disabled, infant stimulation programs and follow-up programs provided by many hospitals that have NICUs are extremely valuable. Locating babysitters who will care for a child with special problems can be an overwhelming task for parents; cultivating a resource list for parents and suggesting that parents exchange services with each other can also be helpful. Graduate parents and neonatal nurses can provide a useful service to parents in this situation. Lastly, parents should be referred to appropriate funding agencies (Handicapped or Crippled Children's Program, Medicaid, or Social Security Disability) that provide financial assistance.

SUMMARY

It has been emphasized that it is essential for the perinatal health care team to address the psychologic needs of the families who are experiencing the painful crisis of the birth of a premature, sick, or malformed newborn. To effectively assist the parents, the health-care provider must be aware of normal attachment and bonding, the factors that influence them, and the psychologic issues that face the parents of a sick newborn.

Pregnancy and parenthood are life crisis events that are affected by previous and ongoing life events. Normal attachment involves the pregnancy (planning, confirmation, and acceptance), the fetus (movement, recognition as an individual, and birth), and the infant (seeing, touching, and caretaking). The birth of the sick newborn may interfere with normal attachment and provides the perinatal team with a rare opportunity to influence how the family adapts to this crisis.

The parents of a sick newborn will experience difficulty with labor and delivery, as well as adaptation to the intensive care environment. They will undergo anticipatory grieving, withdrawal, and guilt. Appropriate support from the perinatal team, who understand the psychologic issues involved, will permit the parents to resume their relationship with the infant and prepare to take their baby home. Families in crisis because of the birth of a sick or abnormal newborn represent a unique situation within which the knowledgeable perinatal health care provider may practice preventive psychosocial health care.

REFERENCES

1. Affonso D: Missing pieces: a study of post-partum feelings, Birth Fam J 4:159, 1977.
2. Aguilera D and Messick J: Crisis intervention theory and methodology, ed 3, St Louis, 1978, The CV Mosby Co.
3. American Academy of Pediatrics, Committee on Fetus and Newborn: Postpartum (neonatal) sibling visitation, Pediatrics 76:650, 1985.
4. Antepartal questions, Denver, Colo, Colorado General Hospital Pre-natal Clinic.
5. Ballard J et al: Sibling visits to a newborn intensive care unit: implications for siblings, parents and infants, Child Psychiatry Hum Dev 14:203, 1984.
6. Barnett C et al: Neonatal separation: the maternal side of interactional deprivation, Pediatrics 54:197, 1970.
7. Bell RQ: Contributions of human infant to caregiving and social interaction. In Lewis M and Rosenblum L, editors:

The effect of the infant on its caregivers, New York, 1974, John Wiley & Sons, Inc.

8. Benfield DG et al: Grief response of parents after referral of the critically ill newborn to a regional center, N Engl J Med 294:975, 1976.

9. Bibring G et al: A study of the psychological processes in pregnancy and of the earliest mother-child relationship: some propositions and comments, Psychoanal Study Child 16:9, 1961.

10. Campbell S and Taylor P: Bonding and attachment: theoretical issues, Semin Perinatol 3:3, 1979.

11. Caplan G: Patterns of parental response to the crisis of premature birth, Psychiatry 23:365, 1960.

12. Caplan G et al: Four studies of crisis in parents of prematures, Community Ment Health J 1:149, 1965.

13. Cohen RL: Some maladaptive syndromes of pregnancy and the puerperium, Obstet Gynecol 27:562, 1966.

14. deChateau P: The importance of the neonatal period for the development of synchrony in the maternal-infant dyad: a review, Birth Fam J 4:10, 1977.

15. Dixon O: Emotional help for parents of sick neonates, Perinatol Neonatol 4:47, 1980.

16. Fantz RL et al: Early visual selectivity as a function of pattern variables, previous exposure, age from birth and conception and expected cognitive deficit. In Cohen L and Salapatic P, editors: Infant perception, vol 1, New York, 1975, Academic Press, Inc.

17. Fromm E: The art of loving, New York, 1956, Harper & Row, Publishers, Inc.

18. Gardner SL: Mothering: the unconscious conflict between nurses and new mothers, Keep Abreast J 3:192, 1978.

19. Goldberg S: Prematurity: effects on parent-infant interaction, J Pediatr Psychol 3:137, 1978.

20. Goldson E: The family care center: a model for the transitional care of the sick infant and his family, Child Today 10:15, 1981.

21. Grant P and Siegel R: Families in crisis: birth of a sick infant. Presented at the Perinatal Section meeting of the American Academy of Pediatrics, District VIII, Scottsdale, Ariz, April, 1978.

22. Gray J et al: Perinatal assessment of mother-baby interaction. In Helfer R and Kempe CH, editors: Child abuse and neglect: the family and the community, Cambridge, Mass, 1976, Ballinger Publishing Co.

23. Green M and Solnit A: Reactions to the threatened loss of a child: a vulnerable child syndrome, Pediatrics 34:58, 1964.

24. Harmon RJ: The perinatal period: infants and parents. In Spittell JA and Brody E, editors: Clinical medicine, vol 12, Psychiatry, Hagerstown, Md, 1981, Harper & Row, Publishers, Inc.

25. Harmon RJ and Culp AM: The effects of premature birth on family functioning and infant development. In Berling L, editor: Children and our future, Albuquerque, 1981, University of New Mexico Press.

26. Jordan B: Birth in four cultures, St Albans, Vt, 1978, Eden Press.

27. Kaplan DM and Mason EA: Maternal reactions to premature birth viewed as an emotional disorder, Am J Orthopsychiatry 30:539, 1960.

28. Kennell JH et al: Maternal behavior one year after early and extended post-partum contact, Dev Med Child Neurol 16:172, 1974.

29. Klaus MH and Kennell JH: Mothers separated from their newborn infants, Pediatr Clin North Am 17:1015, 1970.

30. Klaus MH and Kennell JH: Parent-infant bonding, ed 2, St Louis, 1982, The CV Mosby Co.

31. Klaus MH et al: Maternal attachment: importance of the first post-partum days, N Engl J Med 286:460, 1972.

32. Koops BL and Harmon RJ: Studies on long-term outcome in newborns with birth weights under 1500 grams. In Camp B, editor: Advances in behavioral pediatrics, Greenwich, Conn, 1980, JAI Press, Inc.

33. Leifer A et al: Effects of mother-infant separation on maternal attachment behavior, Child Dev 43:1203, 1972.

34. LeMasters EE: Parenthood as crisis, Marriage and Family Living 19:352, 1957.

35. Lewis M and Rosenblum L: The effect of the infant on its caregiver, New York, 1974, John Wiley & Sons, Inc.

36. Liederman PH and Seashore MJ: Mother-infant neonatal separation: some delayed consequences. Parent-infant interaction, Ciba Foundation Symposium 33, Amsterdam, 1975, Elsevier.

37. Macnab A et al: Group support for parents of high risk neonates: an interdisciplinary approach, Soc Work Health Care 10:63, 1985.

38. Maloney MJ et al: A prospective controlled study of sibling visits to a newborn intensive care unit, J Am Acad Child Psychiatry 22:565, 1983.

39. Mead M and Newton N: Cultural patterning of perinatal behaviors. In Richardson S and Guttmacher A, editors: Childbearing: its social and psychological aspects, Baltimore, 1967, Williams & Wilkins.

40. Minton C: Uses of photographs in perinatal social work, Health Soc Work 8:123, 1983.

41. Newton N and Newton M: Mothers' reaction to their newborn babies, JAMA 181:206, 1962.

42. Noble DN and Hamilton AK: Families under stress: perinatal social work, Health Soc Work 6:28, 1981.

43. Perrault C et al: Family support in the neonatal intensive care unit, Dimens Health Serv 56:16, 1979.

44. Phillips C and Anzalone J: Fathering: participation in labor and birth, ed 2, St Louis, 1982, The CV Mosby Co.

45. Prugh D: Emotional problems of the premature infant's parents, Nurs Outlook 1:461, 1953.

46. Rice RD: Maternal-infant bonding: the profound long-term benefits of immediate continuous skin and eye contact at birth. In Stewart D and Stewart L, editors: 21st century OB: now, Marble Hill, Mo, 1977, NAPSAC, Inc.

47. Ringler N et al: Mother-to-child speech at two years: effects of early post-natal contact, J Pediatr 86:141, 1975.

48. Ringler N et al: Mother's speech to her two-year-old: its effect on speech and language comprehension at five years, Pediatr Res 10:307, 1976.

49. Rose J et al: The evidence for a syndrome of "mothering disability" consequence to threats to the survival of neonates: a design for hypothesis testing including prevention in a prospective study, Am J Dis Child 100:776, 1960.

50. Sameroff A and Chandler M: Reproductive risk and the continuum of caretaking casualty. In Horowitz F, editor: Review of child development research, Chicago, 1975, University of Chicago Press.

51. Schwab F et al: Sibling visiting in a neonatal intensive care unit, Pediatrics 71:835, 1983.

52. Siegel R: A family-centered program of neonatal intensive care, Health Soc Work 7:50, 1982.

53. Solnit AJ and Stark MH: Mourning and the birth of a defective child, Psychoanal Study Child 16:523, 1961.

54. Solomon MA: A developmental conceptual premise for family therapy, Fam Process 12:179, 1973.

55. Sugarman M: Perinatal influences on maternal-infant attachment, Am J Orthopsychiatry 47:407, 1977.

56. Taylor PM and Hall BL: Parent-infant bonding: problems and opportunities in a perinatal center, Semin Perinatol 3:73, 1979.

57. Turner B, Ellis C, and Merenstein G: Sibling visitation. Presented at the Perinatal Section meeting of the American Academy of Pediatrics, District VIII, Jackson, Wyo, May, 1982.

58. Umphenour JH: Bacterial colonization in neonates with sibling visitation, JOGN Nurs 9:2, 1982.

59. Wilson AL: Neonatal air transport: its stress on families. Presented at Newborn Air Transport Conference, sponsored by Mead Johnson Nutritional Division, Denver, Feb 9-10, 1978.

60. Wranesh BL: The effect of sibling visitation on bacterial colonization rate in neonates, JOGN Nurs 11:211, 1982.

61. Zeanach CH, Conger C, and Jones JD: Clinical approaches to traumatized parents: psychotherapy in the intensive care nursery, Child Psychiatry Hum Dev 14:158, 1984.

SELECTED READINGS

Hatcher D and Lehman K: Baby talk for parents who are getting to know their special care baby, Omaha, 1985, Centering Corp.

Hawkins-Walsh E and Borum S: Kate's premature brother, Omaha, 1985, Centering Corp.

Johnson SH: High risk parenting, Durham, NC, 1979, Duke University Medical Center.

Oehler J: The frogs have a baby, a very small baby (a coloring book for children), Durham, NC, 1979, Duke University Medical Center.

Phillips C: Parental perceptions of children who were hospitalized in neonatal intensive care units, Child Psychiatry Hum Dev 14:76, 1983.

Prugh D: The psychological aspects of pediatrics, Philadelphia, 1983, Lea & Febiger.

Schmitt B: The child protection team handbook, New York, 1978, Garland STPM Press.

Sefert K et al: Perinatal stress: a study of factors linked to the risk of parenting problems, Health Soc Work 8:107, 1983.

Special hospital care for your baby, Columbus, Ohio, 1982, Ross Laboratories.

Your special newborn, Evansville, Ind, 1982, Mead Johnson Nutritional Division.

Zeskin P and Iacino R: Effects of maternal visitation in the neonatal intensive care unit, Child Dev 55:1887, 1984.

CHAPTER 23

Grief and perinatal loss

SANDRA L. GARDNER · GERALD B. MERENSTEIN · AUDREY J. COSTELLO

As a life passage, pregnancy and birth are associated with hopes and expectations, and joy and happiness for the future. Even though pregnancy and birth constitute a developmental crisis and major life changes, expectant parents believe the gains of a healthy, happy child and family life offset any losses. Unfortunately, not all perinatal events have a happy ending. When pregnancy fails to produce a normal, healthy baby, it is a tragedy for the parents whose expectations of childbearing have not been fulfilled. Perinatal loss also affects all of their friends and family (including other children).

Perinatal loss may be the first time the young adult has had the experience of coping with the illness or death of a loved one. Perinatal loss is especially significant because (1) it is sudden and unexpected, the most difficult loss to resolve[8]; (2) it interrupts the significant developmental stage of pregnancy, and the situational crisis of loss is imposed on the normal crisis of pregnancy[8]; (3) it is the loss of a child who did not have the opportunity to live a full life[14,45]; (4) it prevents progression into the next developmental stage of parenting that has been anticipated and rehearsed (at least in fantasy) during the pregnancy.

Unfortunately, loss and grief are often only thought of in relation to death. However, as final and irreversible as death is, it is just one form of separation and loss. Although less obvious, other loss situations may have an equally crucial impact. Loss comes in many forms and during the perinatal period may occur without necessarily resulting in death. Circumstances of perinatal loss are at the same time parallel and different, because they all entail grief and mourning, and yet each has unique dimensions and characteristics.

The process of grief, its stages, and its symptoms are reviewed as a framework for understanding one's own feelings and those of others experiencing a loss. A desire to help and an idea of what is helpful and what is not helpful are presented as a basis for effective intervention by professionals.

DEFINITIONS

Grief, the characteristic response to the loss of a valued object, is not an intellectual and rational response.[15] Rather, it is personally experienced as the deep emotion of profound sadness and sorrow. To the individual, grief feels overwhelming, irrational, out of control, "crazy," and all-consuming. Mourning occurs in phases over time. After acknowledging that the loved object no longer exists, gradual withdrawal of emotion and feeling occurs, so that eventual psychologic investment in a new relationship is possible.

For grief to occur, the object must have been valued by the individual, so that its loss is perceived as significant and meaningful.[2] Since prenatally there is an investment of love in the fetus or newborn, the neonate is a valued object. To the extent the prenatal attachment has occurred, grief should be expected and felt at the loss of the fetus or newborn. Therefore loss at birth is a significant loss of a valued (although as yet only fantasized) person.

Loss, whether real or imagined, or actual or possible, is traumatic. The individual is no longer self-confident or confident about the surroundings, since both have been altered. Mourning and grief are forms of separation reactions. Fears of separation and abandonment are the universal fears of childhood regardless of age or developmental stage. Perhaps loss of a significant other awakens these childhood fears and reminds us of the basic "insecurity of all our attachments."[34]

Life changes are stressful to the individual because they threaten to disrupt continuity and a state of equilibrium.[41] Marked changes in the family configuration, such as accession of a new member, are normally a stressful occasion for family members. Perinatal complication or loss is even more of a stressful event, for which the family has little or no preparation. The results of a crisis may be personal growth, maintaining the status quo, regression, or mental illness.[8,42] Often outcome depends on the type of help received during the crisis.

Decreasing the element of surprise by advance preparation for the situation to be encountered may modulate the impact of the event. Anticipatory grief[33,37,46] functions both to prepare and to protect the individual from the pain of impending loss. Prenatal diagnostic procedures, such as ultrasonography, amniocentesis, and fetoscopy, can now detect a variety of severe or lethal birth defects. When there is forewarning that the pregnancy or newborn is not healthy, the parents may begin a process of anticipatory grief and psychologically prepare for the loss of their child while simultaneously hoping for the neonate's survival.[1]

Parental withdrawal from the relationship established during pregnancy accompanies the intense emotions of anticipatory grief. Detachment protects and defends the parent from further painful feelings associated with the investment of self in a doomed relationship. If anticipatory grief proceeds, the parent may detach to the point of being unable to reattach to the infant should he or she survive. In this situation, the infant survives but the relationship with the parents may be significantly impaired. Maintaining even a remote hope that the fetus or newborn will survive protects the parents from the full experience of grief

and total detachment from the child.

The degree of parental anticipatory grief is correlated with positive feelings about the pregnancy and the mode of delivery, but not with the severity of the infant's illness. The more the parental investment and the higher the expectations for the pregnancy, the more anticipatory grief is associated with the development of a perinatal complication. The relative severity of the medical problem is not associated with the degree of anticipatory grief.

PERINATAL SITUATIONS IN WHICH GRIEF IS EXPECTED

Loss is a fact of life, and not just of death. Every stage of development requires a loss of the privileges of the preceding stage and movement into the unknown of the next stage. Any life event involving change or loss is accompanied by grief work, including[9,41] moving, divorce, separation, death of a spouse or family member, injury or illness, retirement, job change, menopause, and even success. The concept of loss is even applicable to the physiologic and psychologic events of normal pregnancy and birth. Certainly, when pregnancy fails to produce a live, healthy baby, a perinatal loss situation exists (see outline below). These perinatal losses, including stillbirth, loss of the perfect child, and neonatal death are discussed in detail in this chapter.

Perinatal situations in which grief reaction is expected

    I. Pregnancy
   II. Birth
      A. Normal
      B. Cesarean section
      C. Forceps
      D. Episiotomy
      E. Medicated
      F. Prolonged or short labor
      G. Place of birth
  III. Postpartum
      A. "Postpartum blues"
      B. Depression
      C. Psychosis

Stillbirth

Demise of a viable fetus occurs after fetal movement when the infant is invested by the parents with a personality and individuality. Since stillbirth occurs later in pregnancy than most abortions, there are increased parental expectations about the baby and the birth process. Selective abortions for genetic indications often occur in the second trimester of pregnancy and involve the death of what was initially a wanted child. When parents make the decision to terminate a known affected pregnancy, they experience feelings of anxiety, sadness, and anger. The anxieties related to termination procedures that include labor and birth, and the feelings of helplessness, isolation, and depression should be acknowledged and handled as in a stillbirth.

Fetal demise in utero happens either prenatally or in the intrapartum period. For 50% of stillbirths, death was sudden, without warning, and from unexplainable causes.[13] The majority of women whose fetus has died in utero spontaneously begin labor within 2 weeks of fetal demise.[13] Carrying the dead baby and waiting for spontaneous labor or induction is sad and difficult for the woman and her entire family. Feelings such as helplessness, disbelief, and powerlessness characterize this period.[21] There is often an uncontrollable urge to flee and escape the unpleasant situation.[21]

For the family who experiences an intrapartum demise, the joyous expectations of labor and birth suddenly change to fear, anxiety, and dread that the "worst" could have possibly happened to them. The suddenness of fetal demise in labor and birth affects both parents and professionals with feelings of shock, denial, and anxiety. Whether the loss is an early or late fetal loss, the woman and her family maintain hope by believing that the professional has made a mistake and that the baby is still alive.[44] The onset (or continuation) of labor is approached with both hope and dread—hope that the infant may be born alive and dread that the infant's death will soon be a stark reality.

The discomfort of labor and birth is particularly difficult for the woman whose infant has died, since her work will not be rewarded with a healthy baby.[47] Oversolicitous use of drugs at birth is not recommended, because they relegate the experience to unreality and give it a dreamlike quality.[58] Keeping parents together through this crisis is important for mutual support and sharing of the birth.[47,56] The deadening (and deafening) silence of a stillbirth forces the reality of the baby's death on both the parents and the professionals present at birth.[47]

In the past at the birth of a stillborn, the mother was heavily sedated or anesthetized and the baby was hidden and whisked away immediately. These women were often left with fears and fantasies: "Was the baby normal?" "What was the sex?" "What did the baby look like?" Seeing, touching, and holding the baby promote completion of the attachment cycle, confirm the reality of the stillbirth for both parents, and allow grief to begin.[5,44,58] Since it is easier to grieve the reality of a situation than a mystical and dreamlike fantasy, contact with the stillborn enables parents to grieve the baby's reality rather than their most frightening fantasies about the infant.[27,31,32,56]

After confirming the reality of the infant's death, a search for the cause, characterized by the universal question, "Why did the baby die?" begins. Either or both parents may blame themselves or feel guilty about real or imagined acts of omission or commission. An autopsy may determine the cause of death, but most often the cause is unknown, even after an autopsy. Yet it is useful in reducing parental guilt and uncertainty about future pregnancies, as well as in aiding the recovery from the loss.[21,58] The "empty tragedy"[32] of stillbirth forces the mother to deal with both the inner loss of the fetus and the outer loss of the expected newborn.

Loss of the perfect child

Even though pregnancy ends in the birth of a live child, the pregnancy outcome may not be what the parents had anticipated. Birth of a baby who does not meet parental expectations represents the realization of the parents' worst fears: a damaged child. Newborns who are preterm, anomalied, sick, the "wrong" sex, or who ultimately die represent the loss of the fantasized perfect child.

After the birth of such a child, parental reactions include grief and mourning for the loss of the loved object (the perfect child) while simultaneously adapting to the reality and investing love in the defective child.[49,52] This reaction is analogous to parental mourning at the death of a child.[49] However, unlike the finality of death, birth of a living, defective child entails a persistent, constant reminder of the feelings of loss and grief because of parental investment of time, attention, and care for either a short time (preterm or sick newborn) or a lifetime (physically or mentally afflicted child).[49]

The psychic work involved in coping with the reality of the imperfect child and the inner feelings of loss is slow and emotionally painful.[52] The process is gradual and proceeds at an individual pace that cannot be hurried but can be facilitated and supported. Detachment and mourning the loss of their fantasized child is necessary before parents are able to attach to the actual child.

Birth of an imperfect child represents multiple losses for parents. A primary narcissistic injury, a threat to the female's self-concept as a woman and mother and the male's self-concept as a man and a father, occurs when a less than perfect child is born.[11,12,24,29,52] Since the child is an extension of both parents, a less than perfect (i.e., deformed) child is equated with the perceived less than perfect part of the parental self.[52] In the mind of the parent, the imagined inadequate self has failed and caused the birth of the damaged child.[24]

PREMATURITY

Every woman expects to deliver a normal, healthy baby at term. Therefore the onset of premature labor is both physiologically and psychologically unexpected. Premature birth is a crisis and an emergency situation characterized by an increased concern for the survival of the infant and often the mother. Premature labor and birth is accompanied by feelings of helplessness, isolation, failure, emptiness, and no control.[24,49] The negative and dangerous atmosphere surrounding the premature birth experience may influence the relationship with the premature infant, who may also be perceived as dangerous and negative.

Normal adaptations to pregnancy are abruptly terminated by the birth of a premature infant.[24] Prenatal fantasies about the baby and the new roles of mother and father are interrupted by a premature birth. This forces parents who are "not ready to not be pregnant" to grieve the loss of a term infant. Giving birth before term forces premature parenting on individuals not yet ready for the experience.

As discussed in Chapter 22, anticipatory grief is one of the normal psychologic tasks accompanying premature birth. Anticipatory grief may be decreased by early contact between parents and infant and conversely increased by separation of parents from preterm infants.[24] Prolonging anticipatory grief with failure to progress through the other tasks results in altered relationships with the parents if the preterm infant survives.

DEFORMED OR ANOMALIED INFANTS

In approximately 2 of every 100 births,[24] a baby is born with a birth defect. Since society values physical beauty, intelligence, and success, the birth of a physically or mentally defective child is seen as a catastrophe in our culture.[52,57]

Recent medical advances now make it possible to identify potential fetal problems in utero. As parents receive the information antenatally, they begin the process of anticipatory grief. They experience feelings of shock, anger, guilt, and hope. At the birth of their baby, there usually is the confirmation of the anomaly, and parents must deal with the reality of the situation. Whether anticipated or not, however, the birth of a child with a congenital defect is accompanied by ambivalent feelings for all concerned (parents, relatives, friends, and professionals). The first reactions to the reality of the situation are feelings of disbelief and shock. Feelings of shame, revulsion, and embarrassment at creating a damaged and devalued child are common.[57] Guilt, self-blame, and a search for a cause or reason for the tragedy are intermixed with feelings of anger.

The severity of loss and feelings of disappointment heavily burden the parents, a burden they feel no one else has experienced.[24] Their loneliness and isolation may be intensified by their self-imposed withdrawal from others. Unlike the birth of a healthy baby, the birth of an anomalied or sick child is not celebrated by society with announcements, visits, and gifts from friends and family. The negative responses of society's representatives (family, friends, acquaintances, and professionals) may increase the parent's negative feelings for a defective child.[57]

The extent of the baby's anomaly cannot be used as a criterion for the degree of parental grief reaction,[29] although a gross, visible anomaly may elicit more emotional reaction than a hidden or more minor one.[24] A seemingly "minor" anomaly as defined by the professional may represent a severe impairment to individual parents. The professional, who has had more contact with infants with a wide range of anomalies, views the individual infant's anomaly in a different context than the parents, who may have limited or no previous experience with a deformed child or adult. The professional also views the infant's defect from a less personal, more objective, and less narcissistic position than the new parents.

When the newborn is sick, the degree of mourning and parental feelings of grief and loss are not equated with the severity of the neonate's illness.[1] Even seemingly "minor" illnesses such as jaundice or respiratory difficulty requiring phototherapy or minimal oxygen supplementation are associated with parental concern for survival and feelings of grief and loss. These feelings are often not acknowledged by the parents or caretakers because of the nonserious medical nature of the condition. In the mind of the caretaker, self-limiting and treatable conditions are compared with more serious and often fatal neonatal illnesses. The caretaker feels relieved about the "minor" nature of the neonate's condition and conveys this to the parents. "This is an easy condition to remedy. You don't have anything to worry about. The baby will go home in a few days."

Thus only the medical aspects of the newborn's illness are dealt with, whereas parental feelings remain unspoken and unresolved. In an altruistic attempt to reassure and comfort the family about the newborn's complete recovery, the professional unwittingly may discount the parents' real feelings. If the caretaker is not concerned, parents may feel that they, too, should not be concerned and thus distrust and discount their own feelings.

NEONATAL DEATHS

The reactions accompanying neonatal illness are similar to the grief reactions experienced by parents whose infant dies.[1] Failure to acknowledge (even minor) neonatal illness as a loss situation and to work through the associated grief prevents parents from detaching from the image of the perfect child and taking on the sick newborn as a person to love. This may result in an aberrant parent-infant attachment. The liveborn infant who is critically ill or has a severe anomaly represents a "painful time of waiting"[5] for the family. They must deal with the uncertainty of whether their child will live and be healthy, live and continue to need extensive medical or special care, or die.

More deaths occur in the first 24 hours of life

than in any other period of life. Yet death of a newborn is not the expected outcome of pregnancy. The majority of neonatal losses are caused by prematurity (80% to 90%) and congenital anomalies that are incompatible with life (15% to 20%). Regardless of the cause of death, even babies who live only a short time are mourned by their parents.[23] Prenatal attachment and investment of love in the newborn result in a classic grief reaction at the newborn's death.[25]

Even a short period of life between birth and death gives parents an opportunity to know their child. Completion of the attachment process enables parents to psychically begin the next process of detachment. Attachment to the child's reality encourages detachment from that reality, rather than from the parents' most dreaded fears and fantasies about their baby. Parental contact with the child before death enables them to share life for a brief time.

In the case of multiple births when one (or more) child dies and the other(s) lives, parents simultaneously grieve the loss of the dead baby(ies) while attaching to the survivor(s). In many situations of multiple birth, the surviving baby(ies) is in an intensive care nursery. The diametrically opposite feelings of love and attachment and grief and detachment, as well as the anxiety associated with the care and well-being of the surviving baby(ies) are emotionally draining for new parents. The process of grief may slow the parents' ability to become intimately involved with their surviving baby(ies).[54] They may have ambivalent feelings toward the baby(ies) who survives or toward the baby(ies) who dies.

Generally, death of the newborn occurs despite everything done to prevent it. This provides parents with some measure of comfort in knowing "that we did everything that could have been done." Yet when the neonate is so severely ill or deformed that a decision about initiating or continuing life support is necessary, the parents have an extra burden. The situation may involve conflicts between physicians, nurses, and family wishes, causing significant personal anguish. As part of the Federal Baby Doe regulations, most hospitals now have ethics committees that address the medical, legal, and ethical controversies (see Chapter 25). Regardless of who makes this decision, it is first and foremost the parents who will live with the ramifications of that decision. When parents are involved in the decision-making process, they wonder if theirs was the right decision regardless of what the decision is. If the child lives or dies, they wonder how a different decision would have changed their lives.

STAGES OF GRIEF

The experience of grief is a staged process that occurs over time. To detach both externally and internally from the lost loved object, emotional investment is withdrawn so that it may be invested in new love relationships.[33] Each stage of grief represents a psychologic defense mechanism used to help the individual to adapt slowly to the crisis. This slow adaptation is purposeful, since it prevents the individual psyche from being overwhelmed by the pain and anguish of loss.[35,39]

Although the stage of grief is recognizable, the process of grief is dynamic and fluid rather than static and rigid. Parents, families, and professionals progress cyclically through the stages of grief rather than in an orderly progression from beginning to end. However, each person experiences the process of grief uniquely and at an individual rate. Knowledge of each stage is necessary to assess where an individual family member, the family as a unit, and the staff are in their grief process. This information is then used to support individuals when they are in their particular stage of grief (rather than attempting to maneuver them from stage to stage), contributing to the defense, or stripping the individuals of their defenses. Regardless of the type of perinatal loss, the experience of that loss through staged grief work closely parallels the grief stages of Elisabeth Kübler-Ross.[28]

The feelings of disbelief and rejection of the news are reflected in the responses "No! This couldn't happen to me!" "It isn't true! They've made a mistake!" This immediate response protects the individual from the shocking reality of loss by postponing the full impact of reality until the psyche is able to handle it.[44] By holding on to the fantasy of a positive outcome (i.e., the loss of the heartbeat is only temporary or the dead baby belongs to someone else), facing the awful truth and the grief associated with it is delayed at least temporarily.[35,44,47]

The initial stage of grief is characterized by overwhelming feelings of being stunned and surprised—often seen as emotional numbness, flat affect, or immobility.[5,57] Emotional detachment is often expressed as an inability to cope or respond with activities of daily living, an inability to remember what others have said, and a tendency to repeat the same questions.[15,24,28,35,57] For the tragedy to be handled in manageable pieces without overwhelming the individual, the mind may acknowledge the event only intellectually, and there is a corresponding lack of emotional reaction.[35,57] Or the event may be compartmentalized so that only a part of the situation rather than the whole becomes the focal point of attention.

Anger is the result of a gradually developing awareness of the situation's reality. As the significance of their perinatal loss begins to dawn on them, parents (and significant others) experience the diffuse emotions of anxiety and anger.[28] With the full impact of their loss comes more focused feelings of bitterness, resentment, blame, rage, and envy of those with normal pregnancy outcomes.[28]

Social prohibitions against the expression of anger, especially for women, encourage this powerful emotion to be turned inward toward the self. Anger directed inward results in depression and a deepening sense of guilt. "Why?" "What did I do wrong or not do right to have caused this to happen?" are the hallmarks of the self-examination and self-blame that accompany perinatal loss.[24,35,57] Answers are often irrational and have no cause-and-effect relationship with the reality of the circumstances. Irrational causation includes sexual intercourse (common worry of both

men and women), career (of the mother) outside the home, dietary habits, or lifting of heavy objects.[58] Ideas of punishment (for past wrongs, for negative or ambivalent feelings, or for an unwanted pregnancy)[3,52] are often thought to be the reason for the failed outcome. The search for a reason to answer the question "Why me?" requires correct information to dispel unrealistic fantasies of causation. However, the question does not require a literal answer (often no concrete answer exists) but is merely a wish for a change in the situation.[3]

Anger directed outward is usually expressed as overt hostility to those in the immediate environment (family, children, care providers, and infant)[30,35,57] or toward God.[30,39] Blame and anger may be a destructive force in the relationships among family members and prevent these relationships from being a source of comfort and support.[35] Ventilation of angry feelings toward professional care providers protects these family relationships for more positive interactions. Anger moves the grieving process along, but persistence of anger may prevent grief work from progressing to subsequent stages.

Bargaining may occur concomitantly with denial and shock as an attempt to prevent or at least delay the loss.[38,47] Bargaining usually occurs with whomever the parents (family or staff) believe the supreme being to be. The "Yes, but" of this stage is a form of "conditional acceptance," while still attempting to make the reality other than what it is.[3,28] With the defective child, bargaining may take the form of shopping for a physician or searching for the magic cure.[57]

The onset of depression and withdrawal marks the stage of a greater level of acceptance of the tragedy. With the true realization of the impact of the loss, the individual acknowledges that indeed there is a reason to be sad. The predominant feelings of this stage are overwhelming sorrow and sadness[35] evidenced by tearfulness, crying, and weeping.[44,47] Feelings of helplessness, worthlessness, and powerlessness contribute to the sense that life is empty and futile. Withdrawal may be evidenced by requests to be left alone, by decreased or complete cessation of visits to the infant, and by silence.[28,38] The degree of withdrawal may be indicative of the depth of depression and the extent to which there is guilt and self-blame.[44]

Acceptance is the resolution stage of the grief process that is heralded by resumption of usual daily activities and a noticeable decrease in preoccupation with the image of the lost infant.[33] This stage most often is not witnessed by the perinatal professionals. The acceptance stage is characterized by emotional detachment of life's meaning from the lost relationship and reestablishing it independent of the lost object.[28,34] The lost relationship is seen in a new light—as giving meaning to the present.[34] The aggrieved person relinquishes that part of himself or herself that was defined in the lost relationship and establishes a new identity that is emotionally free to attach in another relationship.

For the family of a deformed child, acceptance is not an all-or-nothing proposition, but rather a daily adaptation and coping with the child and the defect. For the family, periods of frustration and sorrow alternate with periods of delight and enjoyment of the child.[30] Because of the chronic sorrow experienced throughout the life of a defective child, the final stage of resolution of the family's grief is only possible after the child's death.[37,57]

The acceptance stage represents the ability to remember both the joys and sorrows of the lost relationship without undue discomfort.[15] With gradual integration of the loss, there are progressively fewer attacks of acute, all-consuming pain.[34] When recalling the lost infant, there are fewer feelings of devastation and more a feeling of sadness. The ability to "celebrate the loss" also identifies grief resolution. Celebration of the loss does not mean recall without sadness and sorrow but with an ability to find some meaning, some good, and some positive aspects in the situation (e.g., "At least we had our child for a time, even though it was a short time.").

SYMPTOMATOLOGY OF GRIEF

Although each person copes with grief in individual ways, there are expected reactions to loss situations. Knowledge of the differences and commonalities of the grief experience enables care providers to understand their own reactions as well as to share their thoughts and feelings with the grieving family. The caretaker must learn to "hear" what the family says about how and where each member is in the process of grief resolution. Often the "message" is not a direct reference to the loss or one's feelings, but rather nonverbal communication. The professional must learn to recognize that individuals often communicate more by what they do and what they omit than by what they say.

The signs and symptoms of acute grief have been well described and include both somatic and behavioral manifestations of the emotional experience of the loss (see outline below). The behavior of the bereaved is characterized as ambivalent.[34] In perinatal situations parents simultaneously hope that the child will live and wish for the infant to die; they want to love and care for the child while at the same time wish to reject the child.[24,30] These feelings are frightening and socially unacceptable, and therefore often remain unspoken.

Signs and symptoms of grief*

I. Somatic (physiologic)
   A. Gastrointestinal system
      1. Anorexia and weight loss
      2. Overeating
      3. Nausea or vomiting
      4. Abdominal pains or feelings of emptiness
      5. Diarrhea or constipation
   B. Respiratory system
      1. Sighing respiration
      2. Choking or coughing

*Modified from Lindemann E: The American Journal of Psychiatry 101:144-146, 1944. Copyright, 1944, the American Psychiatric Association; Marris P: Loss and change, New York, 1974, Pantheon Books, Inc; and Colgrove M: How to survive the loss of a love, New York, 1976, Lion Publishing Corp.

3. Shortness of breath
4. Hyperventilation
C. Cardiovascular system
   1. Cardiac palpitations or "fluttering" in chest
   2. "Heavy" feeling in chest
D. Neuromuscular system
   1. Headaches
   2. Vertigo
   3. Syncope
   4. Brisaud's disease (tics)
   5. Muscular weakness or loss of strength
II. Behavioral (psychologic)
A. Feelings of
   1. Guilt
   2. Sadness
   3. Anger and hostility
   4. Emptiness and apathy
   5. Helplessness
   6. Pain, desperation, and pessimism
   7. Shame
   8. Loneliness
B. Preoccupation with image of the lost infant
   1. Daydreams and fantasies
   2. Nightmares
   3. Longing
C. Disturbed interpersonal relationships
   1. Increased irritability and restlessness
   2. Decreased sexual interest and drive
   3. Withdrawal
D. Crying
E. Inability to return to normal activities
   1. Fatigue and exhaustion or aimless overactivity
   2. Insomnia or oversleeping
   3. Short attention span
   4. Slow speech movement and thought process
   5. Loss of concentration and motivation

Often the intensity of grief is greater when the relationship and feelings for the lost person are ambivalent.[34] Even with the most positive of pregnancy outcomes, taking a new baby into the family results in ambivalent feelings for all family members. The degree of disruption that a perinatal loss brings to the family is equated with the severity of grief, especially since reproduction and a healthy perinatal outcome are highly valued in our society.[34]

Male-female differences

Although members of both sexes have the same grief reactions, women express more symptoms (crying, sadness, anger, guilt, and use of medications)[1,11,12] than men. This difference in symptomatology does not represent a different experience of grief, but merely a different expression of it. Understanding these differences and the reasons for them are crucial for care providers working with parents at the time of perinatal loss.

The father's degree of investment in the pregnancy, impending parenthood, and the circumstances of birth all affect his feelings of loss. Since the father's body does not directly experience the changes of pregnancy, the pregnancy may initially be less of a reality to him than to the pregnant woman. This lag in the physiologic reality contributes to a lag in the psychologic investment of the father in the child. Fathers often comment that the baby became real when he felt the fetus move in the mother or at first sight of the new baby. Fathers who form an early attachment to the child feel sadness, disappointment, and often anger at being denied the expected son or daughter.[47] Conversely, fathers who have been normally ambivalent or overtly negative about the pregnancy may feel guilt and responsibility for the failed outcome.[47]

Participation of the father in the events of labor and birth also influence his attachment and ultimately his feelings of loss. Exclusion decreases his involvement in these life-crisis events, whereas inclusion has many advantages for the mother, baby, and self (see Chapter 22). If the baby is ill, the father may initially have more and closer contact than the mother.[1,38] In the birth place, the father may see, touch, or hold the baby before the mother. The father observes the initial resuscitation and stabilization and may accompany the baby to the nursery and on transport to a regional center. Often the father receives the first information about the infant's condition and returns to the hospitalized mother with the news. This early, prolonged contact coupled with the father's increased responsibility often contributes to the development of a closer and earlier bond between father and child than between mother and child. The initial lag in prenatal investment may be off-set after birth by concentrated contact between the father and child, so that a loss is highly signifi-cant to the father.

Societal expectations about masculinity and femininity markedly influence the expression of grief. Society's message to men starts early in life: "Big boys don't cry." "Don't cry, you'll be a sissy (i.e., girl)." The preferred male image in our so-ciety is the autonomous, independent achiever who is always strong and in control, even in the face of disaster.[18] In keeping with this image, the father may feel that he must make all the deci-sions and have all information filtered through him to protect the mother. However, this altruistic gesture prevents full disclosure and involvement of the mother. Assuming the role of strong protec-tor also involves a heavy price for the father in suppression of his own feelings and delay of his own grief work. The role of "tower of strength" often engenders feelings of resentment from the mother. While he attempts to live up to his (and society's) expectations of himself, the woman views his lack of feelings and emotions, especially crying, as "He doesn't care."

Many men have difficulty dealing with irra-tional behaviors as well as with the normal ambi-guity and conflict of life.[18] This difficulty makes the emotional response of grief and its accom-panying ambivalent feelings and conflicts produce discomfort and anxiety in many men. The expres-sion of appropriate human emotions becomes threatening and makes them feel vulnerable.[18] To decrease the anxiety associated with grief and its expression, men often deal with feelings by deny-ing them, increasing their work load, or with-drawing from the situation and refusing to discuss it.[24,33]

The father's attitude and ability to communi-cate about the loss may help or impede the moth-er's grief work.[44] Lack of communication between a couple may contribute to intense mourning, psychiatric disturbances, and severe family dis-ruption.[10,23] Synchrony of grieving between the mother and father is important in an ultimate healthy resolution for the family. If the father denies and suppresses his own feelings of loss and grief, he may react to the normal signs and symp-toms of grief in his partner as if they were abnor-mal. Often the father is able to resolve his grief faster than the mother, and he may become impa-tient with her continual "dwelling" on the loss. Sometimes fearing the woman's prolonged grief, the man decides to "spare her" from his feelings and does not discuss them with her. Instead of being comforting as intended, failure to share grief leads to isolation and alienation within the relationship.[24]

In some situations, the man may experience intense emotions, not unlike those his partner experienced at the time of the crisis, several months after the death. Because these intense emotions occur so long after the crisis, he may not even associate them with the death.[3,24]

TIMING

Emotional recovery from the pain of perinatal loss occurs with time. There is not complete agree-ment on the length of time necessary for the individual to resolve grief. Indeed, a specific time-table for mourning may be impossible to estab-lish.[3,10] However, some general time frames are available for the duration of a normal grief reac-tion.

Acute grief reactions are the most intense dur-ing the first 4 to 6 weeks after the loss,[33,34,39] with some improvement noted 6 to 10 weeks later. Normal grief reactions may be expected to last from 6 months to 1 year[15,24,39] or 2 years.[34] In-deed, significant losses of a spouse or child may never be completely resolved[35]: "I'll never get over it."

One parameter for differentiating normal from pathologic grief has been the length of time for grief to be resolved. Grief work may still be cate-gorized as normal even if it lasts longer than 1 year, especially if the person is working through unresolved grief from the past. Grief work is normally energy draining. Dealing with more than one grief or loss situation compounds the intensity of mourning and may prolong the grief reaction. Since perinatal loss represents more than the loss of the child (loss of the perfect child, loss of plans for the future, and loss of self-esteem), feelings of sadness and depression may still be evident for a year or longer.[24,58]

Sorrow and grief may even last a lifetime. For families of defective children, "chronic sorrow"[37,49] is experienced as long as the child lives. These parents live with the constant reminder of what is not and what the child will never be and can never do. The grief of death is final—parents do the work and go on; chronic sorrow is grieving on a daily basis. Expecting the parents to "adjust" or "accept" their child's defect without any elements of lingering sadness is unrealistic. Chronic sorrow is a justifiable reaction to the daily stresses and coping necessary when a child is defective. The final stage of grief resolution is only possible with the finality of the death of the child.

Even when grief has been resolved, anniversary grief reactions are normal. Renewal of sadness, crying, and normal grieving behaviors may be reactivated at certain times. These anniversary reactions may not be limited to the infant's date of death but may also be felt on the expected date of confinement, the actual birthday, or when seeing an infant of the same age and sex as the lost child. Holidays may also reactivate grieving behaviors, especially those that bring together family and friends and recall memories of joy and happiness.

STAFF

Those sharing a crisis (complication, illness, or death) often become closely attached, so that the loss is felt not only by the family but also by the professional care providers.[16] Repeatedly dealing with death and deformity increases the professional's exposure to personal feelings of grief and loss. This may be perceived either as a threat or a personal opportunity for growth.

The critical variable in the ability to face or assist others in handling loss is the manner in which the caretakers have been able to resolve their own personal losses.[55,56] Unless the care providers are able to cope with personal feelings of loss and grief, they may not be able to give of the "self" to others. Care given without genuine involvement and responsiveness to the family's feelings does not facilitate and may actually impede the mourning process. Professionals who are able to deal honestly with their own feelings will be able to help others cope with theirs.

Helping parents deal with their grief may be difficult for professionals because of their attitudes and feelings about perinatal loss. For professionals trained to preserve life, loss of the best pregnancy outcome or death itself represents both a personal and professional failure.[24] When success is equated with life, the failure of death (or loss) is associated with feelings of guilt, anger, depression, and hostility.[35,50,58] Just when professionals are expected to be supportive and therapeutic, they may be overwhelmed with their own feelings. Professionally, the care providers may feel helpless when all efforts inevitably result in no change in the outcome.

The feelings and stages of grief experienced by the family are the same ones felt by the staff who are attached to the parents and their newborn. Many professionals working in perinatal care are of childbearing age, so that identifying with the parents and their plight is relatively easy. Because the sick, deformed, or dead baby could easily be that of the staff, they share with the parents the special stress of the loss of a child. The care provider often experiences the same fantasies of blame as the parents. "What did I do (or not do) to cause this?"

Repetitive contact with loss situations and death exposes the staff to recurring feelings of frustration, guilt, self-doubt, depression, anger, and classic grief reactions. Such uncomfortable feelings often lead to behaviors of avoidance and withdrawal as a means of self-protection.[10,16,17] Adequate medical care may be given, but psychologic care of the family may be neglected. Or the involved primary care providers may decrease their attachment to both parents and baby when an unfavorable outcome is inevitable. Withdrawing emotional support and involvement may spare the professional but only adds to parental feelings of isolation, inadequacy, and worthlessness. Professionals who have risked family attachment and shared grief work may be more cautious in future involvements to protect themselves from the pain of loss.

Asynchrony and individual differences in handling grief reactions may also cause problems among the professional staff. Constant exposure to perinatal loss may desensitize some individuals until they are blasé or even callous about the crisis, whereas others have grief reactions that parallel the family's reaction. Some staff members may have reached the stage of acceptance, while others who are unable to let the infant go persist in the idea of a magical cure,[10] a characteristic of denial. The rationale of prolonging the child's life may in reality be prolonging death, and inevitably one needs to accept death's finality.

The staff cannot offer support to families experiencing loss unless they receive support in dealing with their own grief reactions. Those who receive support learn about their feelings and how to handle them, and so have no need to displace their pain to others. Various formats are available for meeting staff needs, such as mutual support of colleagues or group sessions involving peer counseling on a long-term or short-term basis.[24,36,55] Group meetings provide a vehicle for support and for sharing information and feelings among staff members.[16,24,55] Facilitated by an objective person with expertise in group process and the concepts of grief, the goal is to help the staff deal with their reactions so they will be better equipped to help the parents. Group sessions also serve to decrease stress, increase job satisfaction, and ultimately to help prevent burnout. Staff members are encouraged to retain their humanity when an environment is created in which emotions are valued and their healthy expression facilitated, both at the time of loss and in its resolution.[22]

Sharing grief work with a family gives the care provider a chance for personal growth, to review past personal losses, and to evaluate the adequacy of their resolution. Helping others with loss or grief provides the professional with the opportunity to contemplate present and future losses, including one's own mortality. By working with those who have suffered a significant loss or death, a health care provider may gain a deeper perspective about life.

INTERVENTION

During a crisis there is an openness to help and assistance from others, so that those in the crisis merge either stronger or weaker depending on the help they receive.[6,42] This increased openness also makes those in a crisis more vulnerable to the reactions of others—to their facial expression, tone of voice, and choice of words. Helpful professional interventions provide psychologic assistance during a highly vulnerable period of personal development. The goal of intervention is to maintain the precrisis level of functioning and improve coping and problem-solving skills beyond the precrisis level (i.e., to facilitate personal growth). Effective intervention is characterized by helping grief work get started, by supporting those who are grieving adaptively, and by intervening with individuals who display maladaptive reactions.

Nonhelpful interventions

Caring for pregnant women and their babies is supposed to be a "happy" job. Birthing and babies are supposed to be times of joy and celebration. Since no one expects death or loss to occur in maternity or nursery areas, when it does, both staff and families are shocked. To protect themselves from the reality of the situation or to "spare" the family, professionals may engage in interventions that do not help themselves or their patients. Such interventions may be meant altruistically, but do not have the characteristics of effective intervention.

Maintaining the state of denial arrests grief work by preventing or delaying the acceptance of the reality of the loss situation. Progress toward resolution is not begun until the stage of disbelief is relinquished. Using drugs, not talking or crying about the loss, and using distraction all contribute to maladaptive reactions by maintaining the state of denial. The use of tranquilizers, sedatives, and other drugs does not help the recipient, but rather the giver. Excessive use of these medications prolongs the denial stage by making the feelings and emotions foggy and dreamlike.[6,17,23,24] The energy needed to begin the grief work is dissipated by the effect of the medications. Avoiding the reality of the situation becomes easier when mind-altering drugs make the tragedy even more unbelievable.

Not talking about the loss is a powerful way of denying that it ever existed. The inability of professionals to acknowledge that the loss has occurred and that the family is in pain maintains denial and repression.[27,35,56] Not discussing the loss prevents parents from learning the facts and facing its reality. Since a fantasy will be created to substitute for the unknown, the fantasy of what happened and why will be worse than the reality. By receiving truthful, honest communication, parents are not left to spend energy dealing with frightened fantasies.

Professional avoidance and unwillingness to talk with parents after a loss communicates other powerful messages that impede grief work. If the loss is not important enough to discuss, then perhaps it is not important at all. Not talking about the loss serves to reduce it and communicates to the parents, "I don't care; therefore neither should you." Avoidance of the topic or a hurried, businesslike or social communication that skirts the issue tells the parent that grief work is dangerous, that grief emotions are dangerous, and that others are afraid of grief and those experiencing it. In essence, not discussing the loss gives a loud and clear nonverbal message "to not grieve."

An inability to cry in response to a significant loss is not helpful and impedes grief work. The prohibition against crying may have been learned early in life or may be the result of unresolved

grief work. Parents may feel the need to be strong for each other, their family, or the staff and thus do not cry. Sometimes role reversal occurs, so that the grieving person feels the need to support others rather than be the recipient of support. Often the significance of parental loss is neither recognized nor acknowledged by the professional for fear that "She or he will cry." Rather than talking about the loss as a technique to facilitate tears, no one says anything so no one will cry, and no one's grief progresses through the grief stages.

Distraction is another way of denying the loss or its significance. Professionals, a spouse, or other family members try to distract parents from the feelings and emotions of acute grief by engaging in light, social conversation or by keeping them busy with work or recreation. Dealing only with the physical care and not the need for psychologic care after birth is a form of distraction used by care providers. Parents are preoccupied with their shattered expectations of the past and the stark reality of the present, and they are not interested in distractions.

After an unfavorable perinatal outcome, there is often confusion by the couple about their status: "Am I a mother or father . . . or not?" Failure to acknowledge the newly acquired role of mother or father (even if the fetus or newborn dies) discounts their psychologic investment in the pregnancy, fetus, and newborn. Quickly removing the baby from the maternity or nursery areas or removing all the baby items from the home negates the baby's existence.[24] This is not helpful to grief resolution and prevents parents from making choices and decisions and thus maintaining control over the reality of the situation.

Isolation of the grieving family prevents the development of dependent relationships with others that might potentially provide support and comfort. Without others, parents are unable to share their grief and may thus increase their feelings of guilt, anger, blame, and lack of self-worth at their failed pregnancy. Those directly experiencing a perinatal loss may be isolated from the rest of society, including their families who do not view loss of a pregnancy or neonate as significant.[5,24] Empathy with the parents' definition of the loss as important is necessary for society to be supportive. The goal of recent research, professional literature, and education has been to sensitize the care provider to the impact of perinatal loss. Only recently have books specifically about perinatal loss become available to give information and assistance to parents.

To decrease contact with the grieving mother, the staff may neglect her or perform cursory physical care. Or there may be overconcern for providing physical care.[35] Assigning a room at the end of the hall, not going into the room, delay in answering requests, or placing the mother on another floor are ways of avoiding families. Use of private rooms and room assignments off the maternity floor may be helpful but may be used by staff to remove the unpleasant and uncomfortable situation. Early discharge to a supportive environment may be helpful, but without plans for follow-up may merely be a way to remove the constant, painful reminder.

Keeping the childbearing couple together throughout the perinatal events facilitates a shared experience of the reality of the situation.[27,56] Separation of the mother and father or of the couple from friends, family, and other children is not helpful. Exclusion of family members from the experience also excludes them from providing support for the mother and the couple. Relaxed visiting policies and as much contact as possible between the hospitalized mother and father (and other family members) are important.[56]

Prohibiting contact between the parents and the baby allows for fearful fantasies of the truth that are always more frightening than the reality of the situation. Delayed contact prolongs the state of disbelief and denial. Restrictive visiting policies in the nursery, institutionalizing a baby without looking at all alternatives, or any other policy that separates parents from their baby does not facilitate grief. Especially in the case of a deformed, stillborn, or dead baby, the message of delayed or no contact is that the baby is too hor-

rible and too unacceptable to be seen or touched. Since parental egos are so symbiotically attached to their offspring, an unacceptable child is equated with an unacceptable and unworthy self. The fantasy that the damaged or dead child is representative of the damaged and defective self is borne out in the behavior and separation policies of the care providers.

In an attempt to offer the grieving family comfort, friends, relatives, and even professionals often make comments that are nonsupportive and nonhelpful[21,24,50]:

- "Well, you're young. You can have more babies."
- "Just have another baby right away."
- "Well, at least you have others at home."
- "It's better to lose her now when she's a baby than when she's 4 years old."
- "He never would have been totally normal anyway."
- "He was born dead. You didn't get a chance to know or get attached to him anyway."
- "It's God's will."

Cliches and platitudes such as these do not help because of the message they give about the parents and the baby.[36,44] These comments at best reduce and at worst negate the impact of prenatal attachment to the fetus. The importance of psychologic investment and attachment by the parents to this fetus or newborn is said to be basically unimportant and essentially nonexistent.[21] Because babies are viewed as an extension of the parents' self, "by a not very subtle process of identification, the parents see a part of themselves in the baby, and nobody likes to be told that part of them is better off dead."[44] Also, comforting parents whose baby has died with the information that the child was not perfect and never would have been normal and healthy reinforces their belief that they are as defective and unsatisfactory as their dead child.[24]

Such comments also convey a message about the importance of an individual life.[27] Essentially, they say that one fetus or newborn is fairly interchangeable with another. They negate the importance of and indeed the existence of the baby for the parents, siblings, family, and society. The life of the individual is devalued, since he or she is easily replaced by "another baby." Comparing one baby's illness or deformity with another's is not helpful for parents whose own baby's deformity is certainly more important than any other baby's problem.[36]

The power of words to help during grief is outweighed only by their power to not help. Since parents are increasingly open during a perinatal crisis, they are sensitive not only to what is said and how it is said, but also to the nonverbal message. Giving premature or false reassurance may be more for relief of the professionals than for the parents.[6,21,36] Comments such as "It's okay" and "Everything's going to be all right" must be genuine and timed appropriately for the parent. Telling parents that they have a child with Down's syndrome and then saying, "But everything will be all right" is hardly helpful. Giving reassurance that subsequent pregnancies and babies will be all right or unaffected is not helpful before the parents are ready to think about and project into the future.

The basic terminology accompanying perinatal grief situations may be upsetting to parents. Instead of "dead," professionals substitute less frightening and less final words. The use of "loss" when "death" is appropriate may be misinterpreted (especially by children). The terms "lose, loss, and lost" connote misplacing, so that comments such as "I'm sorry you lost your baby" may be responded to by "I didn't lose (misplace) my baby. My child died." Medical professionals skirt the use of the words "dead, died, and die." Care providers are taught as students to use the word "expired" when referring to a patient who has died. Meant to soften the impact of "dead," the word "expired" may have its own impact, as a mother whose baby son died wrote in a poem: "The baby expired they said, as if you were a credit card."[51]

Other situations that do not facilitate grief work include dealing with multiple losses or stresses and ambivalence or mental illness.[58] The reaction to the loss of a significant relationship is intensified in the context of multiple losses, stresses, and problems.[2,58] Since perinatal losses represent not only a loss of the wished-for perfect child, but a threat to the parental self, self-concept, and self-worth, they represent situations of multiple loss.

Helpful interventions

Professionals have an opportunity to make a significant difference in the outcome following the crisis of perinatal loss for the individual, the couple, and the family unit. A care provider who is knowledgeable about the grief process and comfortable in sharing another's grief is equipped to assist the family and its members toward a long-term healthy adjustment rather than a dysfunctional and pathologic one. Interventions that are helpful for family members also assist staff members in their own grief work.

Factors that influence an individual's personal experience of grief (and ultimately appropriate interventions) are outlined below. Care for the grieving is individualized through assessing these factors, planning, and continually evaluating the individual. Eliciting such personal information may not be so difficult as it first seems. Those in crisis often spontaneously share crucial data with little prompting. The importance of active listening to questions and comments or a more formalized therapeutic interview process may provide the needed encouragement and permission to begin communication.

Factors to evaluate in individualizing grief interventions

I. Previous losses
   A. Type
      1. Separation
      2. Divorce
      3. Death
      4. Spontaneous abortion (miscarriage)
      5. Elective or selective abortion
      6. Period of infertility
      7. Relinquishment of child
      8. Perinatal loss

B. Timing in the life cycle
1. Distant
2. Recent
C. Coping styles (of each individual and the family as a unit)
D. Grief work
1. Resolved
2. Unresolved
II. Prenatal attachment
A. Degree of psychologic investment in relationship with fetus or newborn
B. Decision making about pregnancy and baby
1. Planned or unplanned
2. Wanted or unwanted
C. Meaning of pregnancy and baby to individual and family
D. Parental expectation about childbearing
III. Nature of the current loss
A. Timing
1. Sudden and unexpected
2. Anticipatory grief
B. Definition and meaning of the event (death, deformity) to individual members of the family
C. Multiple losses
1. Self
2. Perfect child
D. Nature and severity
1. Of loss
2. Of defect
IV. Cultural influences
A. On experience and the expression of grief
B. Societal expectations dictate acceptable and unacceptable behaviors of mourning
V. Strengths (individual and family)
A. Support system (family, friends, religious, community, or social agencies) mobilized when necessary
B. Stable relationships—couple supportive of each other
C. Financial stability
D. Coping abilities—can evaluate, plan, and adjust to novel situations
E. Good health
F. Receptive and intelligent
G. Realistic expectations about childbearing and child rearing

A history of previous losses and their type and timing in the life cycle are important data for the care provider dealing with the current loss. Past experiences with a crisis or loss influence an individual's behavioral and coping style with current problems. Dealing with problems alone, with help and support from others, or withdrawing altogether are possibilities of coping with the loss.

The degree of attachment and the meaning of the pregnancy and impending parenthood to the family define their expectations and influence their reaction if an optimal outcome does not occur. The experience of grief depends on whether the loss situation was sudden and unexpected or if there was forewarning about a problem or complication. The definition and meaning of the crisis (i.e., the nature and severity of a deformity, the finality of death, or the chronic sorrow of a defective baby) reflects the individual's and family's value system and previous crisis experience. The process of grief is affected by the event itself, the previous and current coping mechanisms, and the family's definition of the event.[20] Consideration of all these factors is crucial in instituting appropriate intervention.

ENVIRONMENT

The first step in facilitating grief work is to create an environment that is supportive, permissive, and conducive to the expression of feelings. This type of environment is not dependent on physical surroundings but rather is created and maintained by a warm, receptive, accepting, and caring staff. Such an environment centers its concern more on the people giving and receiving care than on the tasks of care.[24] This type of environment is nonjudgmental and is characterized by an attitude of openness and freedom.[44] People feel safe enough to ventilate a full range of feelings—sadness, anger, despair, and even humor—without the fear of condemnation or rejection. The staff become role models of open communication, facing grief, and feeling comfortable in an uncomfortable situation. The safety of such an environment generates feelings of acceptance and understanding so that grieving and healing may proceed.

Professional presence and support is essential to families in crisis because of the increased dependency needs that accompany grief and loss. Yet certain aspects of a conducive environment such as privacy, quiet, and comfort may be difficult to obtain in a noisy and busy perinatal setting. The recommendation to never leave the family alone must be balanced with their need for privacy and personal time alone with their baby (i.e., stillborn, ill, or dying).[56] Simply saying, "I will stay with you unless you ask me to leave so that you can have some private time alone with your child" or "Would you like me to leave for a while so that you can be alone with your baby?" offers both support and privacy. Many parents later regret not having time alone and not thinking to ask to be alone with their baby.

A quiet place away from the hustle and bustle of the routine may facilitate both attachment and detachment. The mother of a stillborn child who is quickly shown her baby in the delivery room as her episiotomy is being repaired is not in an optimal physical (or psychologic) environment. Attaching to and saying good-bye to her baby is better accomplished in a quieter and more private setting with significant others present. Active participation of parents at the death of their newborn may not optimally occur in a busy intensive care unit. Rather, adaptation of hospice concepts to neonatal care provides a private, homelike room and more palliative care than cure to the dying newborn and the family.[53]

SUPPORTIVE, TRUSTING RELATIONSHIPS

A relationship with a caring individual who offers consistency and support is the foundation of a therapeutic environment. During periods of crisis when there is a temporary increase in dependency needs and feelings of loneliness, it is an adaptive behavior to seek emotional support from family, friends, and professionals.[34,35] Even the crisis of normal childbearing prompts many cultures to provide a "doula"[43] to teach the new mother and give her emotional support. For the mourning family, the relationships established with helpful professionals are more important than the physical care given.[16]

Support, "sharing one's ego strength with another in a time of need,"[19] is particularly helpful in perinatal loss because of the threat to self-concept and self-esteem suffered by parents. Support may be as simple as remaining with the parents. "Being there" indicates not merely physical presence, but an emotional availability and willingness to share their experience of loss. Often professionals, family, and friends are hampered by "not knowing what to say." Usually words are initially unnecessary or do not adequately describe the moment, and silent "thereness" may better convey the message. Often it is not what is said but the mere presence of loving others that conveys empathy and support to parents and colleagues. Yet presence is not enough; meaningful interaction between parents and professionals is also necessary for a trusting relationship to develop.

The initial meeting with the professionals, including verbal and nonverbal cues, leaves a lasting impression on the family. Addressing family members by name personalizes the encounter, and a brief touch or handshake represents an extension of self, a gesture of warmth, concern, and acceptance from professional to parents. An introduction that includes a brief explanation of the professional's role in relation to them and their baby helps to orient them: "Good morning, Mr. and Mrs. Black. I'm Sue, your baby's primary nurse. That means that I will be caring for Jason while he is here and working with you." Orientation to the physical surroundings and technical equipment eases the transition to an unfamiliar and often intimidating hospital environment. Providing physical comfort such as rocking chairs, privacy for interaction, and sleeping facilities for parents demonstrates the philosophy of the parents' worth and importance to their infant.

Empathy, an emotional understanding and identification with the plight of another, characterizes a helping relationship. In such a relationship, "How are you?" is asked with the emphasis on *you* and a genuine interest in the answer, unlike a social inquiry in which an automatic "Fine" is expected. Recognition of verbal and nonverbal cues of parental feelings (e.g., "You look tired" and "I hear that you are frustrated") communicates that these emotions are legitimate, understood, and accepted. A willingness to help, listen, console, and give encouragement and positive feedback establishes the professional as a sensitive, responsive person whom parents will trust. Supporting any and all parental involvement, supporting damaged parental egos, and helping parents to succeed in the tasks of attachment and detachment are goals of effective intervention.

The tone of in-hospital perinatal settings is often determined by the nursing staff. Generally, residents, interns, and specialists remain for short periods and the private physician or permanent medical staff are not available on a minute-to-minute basis. Development of a safe, trusting environment depends on viewing parents as essential and not as visitors or "disruptors" of the ward routine. Pleasant and relaxed surroundings convey the message of hospitality and "you are welcome here."

Both professional and nonprofessional support systems are available in the crisis of perinatal loss. Yet relating to many people during crisis is difficult for parents. Primary care (both medical and nursing) provides the same care provider for both the physiologic and psychologic care of the infant and the family. Thus the family is able to relate to as few professionals as possible. This special caring reassures parents that a few special people love, know, and are invested in their baby. Primary care providers share with the parents the joys of even small gains and the sorrows and tears of complications or death. Professionals and parents benefit from primary care systems in the emotional and psychologic satisfaction of such involvement. Yet this involvement is not without a price of vulnerability to an individual's feelings of loss and grief. Peer support on an individual basis or in a group setting is essential in dealing with the stress of continual attachment and loss.

Normal grief reactions may be facilitated by nursing and medical professionals using others (social workers or counselors) when necessary.[1] Collaboration and consultation with these professionals help gain insight into parental and personal behaviors and appropriate intervention strategies. Maladaptive responses (listed below) to perinatal loss are indications for referral for more specialized care.[57] The staff may also benefit from the expertise of a trained counselor in dealing with their own feelings of loss and grief.[36]

Pathologic grief*

Overactivity without a sense of loss

Acquisition of symptoms belonging to the last illness of the deceased

Psychosomatic conditions (ulcerative colitis or asthma)

Altered relationships to friends and relatives

Furious hostility against specific others

Formal manner resembling schizophrenia

Lasting loss of social interaction patterns

Assuming activities detrimental to social and economic existence

Agitated depression

Involvement of clergy and religious organizations is often comforting and supportive to the family. Religious rituals (i.e., baptism, prayer service, or anointing) may be advocated by certain denominations. Often parents in crisis do not think to request infant baptism or calling their priest, minister, or rabbi. Offering to call a clergy member of their choice or the hospital chaplain may be helpful. Primary caretakers who have shared intimately with the parents the experience of their child's life and death may be invited to attend the funeral or memorial service. For both caretakers and parents, this may represent the final act of caring for the infant.

Nonprofessional support systems such as the couple, family, friends, and parent groups are often forgotten as sources of potential help to grieving parents. In our society of isolated, mo-

*From Lindemann E: The American Journal of Psychiatry 101:141, 1944. Copyright, 1944, The American Psychiatric Association.

bile, nuclear families, it may be erroneous to assume that a support system exists. On the other hand, it may be unrecognized because it does not fall into a traditional definition (the next-door neighbor or other friend who may be more supportive [and available] than the grandparents). Biologic kinship is not the only valid criterion for a support system; an emotional kinship is the most important factor.

Because professional availability and involvement with the parents is not lasting, the professional has a responsibility to identify, foster, and facilitate a nonprofessional (social) support system. Simply identifying supportive others and expecting them to automatically help in a perinatal loss situation may not be realistic. Unless those who constitute the support system are as well informed and instructed as the parents about the situation, they will not be able to offer emotional comfort. For example, if the parents wish to talk about their loss but the support system empathically wishes to spare them by not discussing it, no help will be given or received.

Open communication between the parents is essential in preserving and fostering a close relationship by the giving and receiving of mutual support. Sharing the experience presents the couple with the opportunity for personal growth and growth as a couple. Yet the individual experience of grief within the context of a couple is all too often fertile ground for misunderstanding and resentment.

Parental support groups offer their members an opportunity to discuss their feelings with others who have been through similar traumas. Knowing how others who experienced perinatal loss have felt and dealt with similar situations is emotionally comforting and stabilizing to parents experiencing their own loss. Parents provide each other with validation for their feelings and a sense that they are not alone in their pain.

Each individual has different needs, different ways of adapting to crisis, and different ways of giving and receiving support. It is essential that the professional use those techniques that are real and spontaneous and not adopt words or actions that are foreign to one's own self. Interventions must also be gauged to the parent's needs and pace.

INFORMATION

Information aids in intellectually understanding the crisis, thus facilitating a sense of control over it. Actively seeking and using information enables confrontation and mastery of the crisis. Knowledge about a situation strengthens the ego, since it enables "worry work" and psychologic preparation for expected events. Since "the void of the unknown is more frightening than the known; facts are more reassuring than awesome speculations,"[6] a major role of the professional is to provide and clarify facts and information relevant to the perinatal loss situation. In the search for meaning that always accompanies loss, medical facts may help alleviate some parental guilt about causing the tragedy. Repeating to the parents that "Nothing you did or did not do could have caused this problem" is reassuring. Sketchy or no information only serves to contribute to parental denial of the reality or to their fantasies of causation.[36,44] Confronting the crisis and realizing its real element of danger and trouble starts the process of grief by giving permission for the expression of feelings of fear, sadness, and loss.

Since the family as a unit composed of each individual member must deal with perinatal loss, it is important to encourage and support open, interfamily communications. Keeping secrets, especially between the parents, should be discouraged because this eventually undermines trust and promotes asynchronous grief work. When parents are given the same information and talk with each other about their loss and their feelings, more synchronous grief reactions develop.[24,36] Telling parents together with the baby present prevents misunderstanding, misinterpretations, and "shading" of information to one parent.[24] Informed parents are better able to share their experience with each other and to participate in joint decision making with the professional.

The question often arises, "When to tell?" and "How much to tell?" the parents. Parents should be told as soon as possible about perinatal complications or problems.[24,36] Receiving this information at the earliest possible time helps parents establish trust in the care provider, appreciate the reality of the situation, begin the grief process, and mobilize both internal and external support. Information must be given in its entirety, since attempts "to spare" parents by staging the truth only serves to undermine their trust in professional credibility. The couple's relationship may also suffer if one parent colludes with the professional in a conspiracy of silence. This is best illustrated by the following incident:

To spare a diabetic mother from the truth about her baby's congenitally absent limbs, the physician and father decided to tell her about his missing legs, but not the missing arm. On arriving to transport the baby, the nurse asked if the mother had been told. "Yes" was the response, so she took the baby to the mother's room before transport. As she uncovered the baby, the mother gasped and looked at the physician and father and said, "You lied to me. You didn't tell me about his arm, too."

When given the unedited truth, parents are able to face reality and begin the grief process without fear that "something else is the matter that they aren't telling me about."

The individual's stage of grief influences not when or what will be said, but how the information will be given and received. During the initial stage of shock information, if processed, is processed slowly.[24] Often events take on a foggy, dreamlike quality so that sensory information remembered is not believed. Yet to give no information only perpetuates this frightening feeling. Communication to those in shock and denial must proceed simply, slowly, and with much repetition and reinforcement. Giving information once does not ensure it will be either retained or understood. Repetition by the professionals is necessary for gradual acceptance of the reality of the situation. This may be a nuisance for the professional who "has already told her that. Why can't she remember it?" Parents are so shocked they do not hear what is said and information must be patiently repeated.

Even though an early contact with parents almost ensures they will be in a state of shock, the tone and content of the first meeting is not forgotten.[24] Initial information about the baby and his or her condition may have long-term effects on the parents' ability to attach or detach. In the past parents were given a pessimistic outlook with the belief that "It will be easier for them. They won't get so involved." Negative descriptions and initial pessimism only increase the amount of grief and detachment while effectively blocking attachment behaviors. Should the sick or defective baby survive, the parents may have detached to the point of at least emotionally burying the baby. Knowledge of better survival rates and the quality of survival enable a truthfully optimistic outcome for many sick neonates. Therefore information must be given clearly (in English, not medical jargon) with a minimum of possible complications and medical odds.[24,57]

Volunteering information to parents is essential, but encouraging their questions is equally as important. As the normal mechanism for adapting to crisis and gaining mastery over a situation, questions help the professional "to start where the parents are" and to begin communication with their concerns. Questions and comments unrelated to the discussion may indicate either failure to comprehend or failure to send the information clearly.[57] Direct questions deserve direct answers, since they indicate a readiness and desire for information. Indirect questions or comments by the parents may indicate concern about their own baby that cannot be directly expressed. "Baby Stevie (who died yesterday) had severe respiratory distress syndrome, didn't he?" The parents want to be reassured that their baby is not going to die, too.

During the crisis of perinatal loss, interpersonal communication is difficult. Therefore it is important that as few professionals as possible relay information to the parents. Primary care providers (nurse and physician) should coordinate and provide continuity in giving information to parents because individual care providers will supply information about the same topic in different ways. The use of varied terms, inflections, and attitudes by a multitude of professionals becomes a monumental source of confusion and anxiety for parents. A trusted relationship with a primary nurse and physician through whom all communication flows minimizes unnecessary anxiety and concern for parents.

It is absolutely essential that the nurse (or primary nurse) be present and assist the physician in communication with the parents. Any anxiety-producing information (poor prognosis, complication, or impending death) may not be heard or understood initially by the parents. The nurse must know exactly what and how parents were given this information. After the physician departs, the nurse must be able to offer clarification, explanation, and support to distraught parents. Nothing is more distressing than finding a crying, upset mother who is unable to relate what the physician said, why she is upset, or even if she understood what was said.

No family or parent should have to wonder and worry about a dreaded or feared outcome without being given the proper information. If the primary care physician is unavailable to speak with the family, then someone from the health care team must assume this responsibility. No mother whose baby is ill, deformed, or dead should awaken from an anesthetized birth to find her physician absent and the nurses unable to answer "How's my baby?" A plan of action for telling individual parents must be decided and agreed on by all care providers.

Parents are interested in the daily (or hourly) progress of their infant, including both positive and negative developments. A crisis or negative development in an infant's condition is important for parents to know about a soon as possible. They are then able to participate and care for their baby through the difficulty and to trust professional communication. Parents should have unlimited access to phone and/or personal contact with the staff in the perinatal care setting. Phone calls into the hospital from concerned parents should be possible any time of the day or night. Being encouraged to call at any hour is often reassuring to parents that access to information and a caring professional is always possible. The knowledge that "everything is the same as 1 hour ago, all is stable" may be enough to comfort parents of a critically ill infant.

ENCOURAGE EXPRESSION OF EMOTIONS

Since grief is an emotional reaction to loss, expression of these emotions is necessary for grief work to begin and proceed. Verbalizing thoughts and feelings provides an outlet for the intense emotions accompanying grief and signifies to others that emotional support is needed.[35] For some the open expression of emotions may be difficult because of influence from culture, sex roles, and social status. Yet the containment of intense feelings uses a great deal of emotional and physical energy that could be more productively used in "moving on" with the grief work. Those who are stoic and noncommunicative have symptoms of grief for a longer period of time than those who freely express their feelings and emotions.[4]

Talking about the loss helps parents to validate and assimilate the experience. Timing and events are clarified, including forgotten details, by discussion with each other and with their care providers. Confronting the reality enables them to work through the shock and disbelief, verbalize their fears and disappointments, and begin to cry and grieve. Expression of feelings gradually permits a clarification of the meaning of the loss to the parents.[6,56] Talking lightens the burden of loss because every time the experience is shared with another, half of the experience and the accompanying emotions are given away. Telling, retelling, reviewing, and reliving the experience are all necessary ways to understand and gain mastery over a frightening and most often unexpected situation.[30,38,47,50]

Verbal and nonverbal cues tell professionals

"where the parents are" in their grief process. To elicit feelings, the professional may verbalize his or her own perceptions and observations:

- "Mrs. Green, you sound tense (upset, tired) today."
- "Mr. Brown, you look worried today."
- "I'm sorry that your baby died."

These statements indicate the listening ear and observing eye of one who cares. They set the stage for communication: "It's okay to talk with me about how you are feeling because I acknowledge your pain."

Feeling scared, alone, and out of control, parents often deny their feelings under direct questioning. Thus "Do you think you did or didn't do something to cause your baby's problem?" may be answered negatively, even though parents are consumed with guilt. Direct questioning places parents in an awkward and vulnerable position of revealing their most personal doubts and fears. Direct questions may be reworded with safer and more indirect statements:

- "Most parents feel overwhelmed and sad when their baby is sick."
- "Many parents wonder if the cause of their baby's death is something they did or didn't do."
- "It is helpful to many parents to talk about their doubts and fears. These feelings are common and normal in such a difficult situation."

The professional gives parents information about the feelings and emotions commonly felt in similar situations. Since there is safety in numbers, if "most" or "many" parents feel this way and it is expected, then it might be safe to share their feelings. Validating parental reactions as appropriate reassures them that they are not crazy. With this type of invitation, the feelings may be free to come spilling forth or the parents may need time to establish a relationship with this professional before they are ready to talk about such personal emotions.

Empathetic actions and comments may open communication pathways with parents. A professional presence that is warm and caring may facilitate more communication than any words. Touching or holding grieving parents may help feelings be expressed. Nonverbal cues such as nodding, direct eye contact, uninterrupted attention, and the physical closeness of pulling up a chair and sitting down gives positive feedback to verbal communication and indicates active listening by the professional.

Crying is the expression of feelings of sadness, sorrow, and intense longing that accompany the pain of loss.[6,33,58] A healthy catharsis, crying should be expected and encouraged in any loss situation. Yet the cultural, sexual, and professional taboo against crying has defined it as an acceptable and inappropriate response, and one that should be suppressed. Since tears are healing and therapeutic, professionals must learn to be comfortable with the crying of others. "Don't cry" is often heard from those attempting to comfort grieving parents (or colleagues). This is an admonition against the behavior rather than an empathetic comment "It's okay to cry" or "Go ahead and cry—let it out" gives permission and acceptance to the behavior and the need for it.

By expecting tears, providing a safe environment for their expression, and encouraging the behavior by words and actions, the professional may facilitate crying in both mothers and fathers. All too often, tears are blocked in a relationship in which one partner (usually the man) is expected to be stoic and in control, while the other's (usually the woman's) tears are defined as too upsetting or difficult. Since the ability to cry is a healthy response, the couple must be encouraged to use this outlet together.

In the past, crying in the presence of patients and their families was not defined as "professional." Yet the cool, controlled exterior defined as "professional" was seen by others as noncaring and nonfeeling. When the professional cries with the parents, it is an acceptable expression of genuine emotion, a demonstration of empathy, and a role model of the appropriateness of tears given the situation. Parents do not define the tears of care providers as weak or unprofessional. Rather, they feel a special bond of love and care with professionals who have been free enough to share their grief. Instead of relearning that crying is acceptable, many parents and care providers must learn for the first time.

Talking and crying about the loss are easier to facilitate than the expression of anger. Because of the social expectations of dependency of the patient role and real or imagined consequences of retaliation (against the baby or against job status), perinatal care settings are not safe environments for the expression of anger. Parents (and colleagues) will only be able to vent anger in an environment free of punishment or retaliation for their behaviors. It is the responsibility of the professionals to create an environment that allows open expression of negative criticism and anger.

SEEING AND TOUCHING

Seeing and touching are as important to the parents of a sick, deformed, or dead baby as they are to the parents of a normal, healthy one. In the past, fear that seeing a deformed or dead baby would intensify grief and be overly upsetting resulted in no contact between parents and their newborn. Despite the fact that many mothers wished to see their babies, the prevailing practice was to discourage and prevent it. Often no information, including sex or physical characteristics, was given to grieving parents, who were left to fantasize about their newborn's problems or cause of death. More recently research and practice indicate that parental contact with the baby does not cause "unduly upsetting immediate reactions or appear to result in pathologic mourning."[23]

The decision to see and touch their baby is ultimately a parental one.[27,58] Making decisions for clients is not the professional's role; making decisions with clients is the professional's role. Each parent must make the decision for him or herself; neither may decide for the other. Altruistic others such as professionals, spouse, or other family members must not usurp the right to individual decision making. Often in an attempt to protect the mother, the father or professional decides that she should not have contact with her baby. They either actually discourage it or do nothing to facilitate it. Mothers who have not seen their babies always know who prohibited it. The couple's relationship may suffer irreparable damage if one decides for the other, even if the motive is altruistic. The professional's role is to facilitate a healthy decision by each parent so that their individual needs to see or not to see the infant are met.

Parents may not realize that seeing and touching their baby is an option.[56] Or they may just be too overwhelmed or afraid to ask if it is possible. "Allow(ing) the mother to see the dead child if she requests it" overlooks the fact that the parent may not know or be unable to ask. Instead of waiting for parents to ask, the professional care provider takes a more active role by offering the possibility to the parents: "Would you like to hold your baby?"

Time is often required to make the decision because initially parents are ambivalent about seeing and holding a deformed or dead baby. Most mothers and fathers want to see their child but fear what they might see and how they may feel.[47] The caretaker may alleviate parental ambivalence by acknowledging that being with the baby will be difficult but that the professional will remain with them unless asked to leave. The emotional support of the physical presence of an empathetic professional may allay the fear of becoming out of control. The professional can reassure the family by explaining what they will see before they hold their baby. Making such a crucial decision in the initial stages of loss is difficult. Giving parents information about the positive aspects of seeing and holding the baby in facilitating their grief process helps make their decision an informed one.[58]

Seeing the baby brings the dreaded impossibility of perinatal loss into stark reality.[36,58] Parents confirm with their own eyes that the baby is alive or dead, or normal or abnormal. Contact enables claiming behaviors and identification of the baby as their own. While holding their infant, parents examine it and begin to recognize familiar family characteristics: "She has my long fingers and her father's red hair." Even small, severely deformed, or macerated babies are able to be recognized and claimed by the parents as part of their family.[27] The normal, endearing characteristics that identify the child as "mine" are remembered.

Parental contact confirms the baby's own reality and eliminates the prenatal fantasy of the expected child. For the parents of an anomalied baby, grief work about the fantasized perfect child may begin, so that the actual child may become the object of love. Early and frequent contact between the parents and the baby encourages a realistic perspective of the infant's problems. The stillborn or aborted fetus may be physically normal rather than the deformed baby imagined by the parents. Seeing the baby allays doubts and fears about the infant's normal state and about the parents' ability to subsequently have a normal child.[31,32,44] Seeing and touching enables parents to grieve the baby's reality rather than a feared and dreaded, thus more frightening, fantasy. It is easier to grieve a real baby than a mystical dream-like fantasy of the infant.[24,27,31,32]

Whether the ultimate decision is to see or not see the infant, the professional must honor and respect that choice.[58] Cultural taboos against viewing dead bodies may preclude some parents from seeing and touching their baby. Yet many such cultures support their members by formalizing the grief process in sanctioned ritual and ceremony. For those parents who decide not to see and touch, it is important for the professional to reassure them of their baby's normal condition (e.g., "He had ten fingers and toes"). Describe the infant in as much detail as necessary to give parents a mental picture. Include sex, size, hair color, skin, weight, and distinguishing characteristics. A simple, realistic description of any anomaly is also helpful, because the fantasy of the defect is worse than its reality.

Adequate preparation for the first encounter with their infant includes a description of everything parents will see, hear, and feel.[27,58] Verbal preparation for viewing a baby with a congenital anomaly includes not only a simple description of the abnormality, but also the baby's normal characteristics. Seeing a picture of the abnormality first may help parents prepare for seeing their baby. Remaining with the parents at the initial visit, the professional describes the anomaly and points out normal findings. Focusing by parents on the normal familial characteristics helps in attaching to the less-than-perfect child. Although parents of a dead, deformed child view the abnormality, they often focus on the normal traits and remember the baby not as "monstrous" but as beautiful.

For those who have never seen a dead body, the mind may invent frightening images and sensations. Certainly, "dead" is associated with the temperature sensation of cold. However, a newborn who has been placed under a radiant warmer or in an incubator (Isolette) may feel warm rather than cold shortly after death. Hence, the statement by a mother, "You couldn't be dead. You feel so warm." The professional must touch the baby and prepare the parents for the tactile sensation of warm or cold: "The baby will feel warm to you because she (or he) has been under the radiant warmer."

To prepare parents for seeing their infant, the professional must observe the child. Color, skin condition, and size must all be described: maceration, "peeling of the skin," peripheral shutdown, "the blue-white discoloration," and the small size, "as long as the length of my hand" are not shocking with adequate preparation. Any equipment that must remain on the body should be described and explained before viewing. Even an umbilical cord clamp may cause concern in a parent who has never seen one. The reason for not removing equipment must also be explained. Respectful care of the baby's body after death shows respect for the person of the baby and for the grieving parents. Attention to details such as wrapping the baby in a blanket rather than a surgical drape or towel, cleaning the baby, and holding the baby in a cuddling position indicate care and concern.

Parents whose infant has died, is deformed, or ill proceed with attachment behaviors of seeing and touching in the same manner as parents of normal, healthy babies.[24,27] Touching is important, but the distinction must be made between touching and holding. Cradling one's baby is quite different from merely touching with a hand. Holding the infant, whether healthy, sick, or dead, for the first time is a momentous event. Touching the infant who has died is not sufficient; parents must be given the opportunity to hold and cuddle the child before, during, and after death. Other parenting behaviors such as bathing and dressing their baby should also be offered parents.

Parents of a dead baby may need more than one chance to see and touch the baby. The first time, they attach to the reality of their baby. Subsequent encounters allow a final chance to see and hold their child. Parents have described the initial encounter as saying "Hello" and the subsequent one as saying "Good-bye." Some parents may be able to accomplish closure with one visit, whereas others who might benefit from a final visit may not ask or think to ask. Offering another contact with their baby leaves the decision with the parents.

The emotional impact of seeing the infant requires support, time, and permission to cry. Attaching is a process that occurs over time. Providing parents sufficient time with their infant takes precedence over paperwork, ward routine, or taking the infant to the morgue. Even infants who have been removed to the morgue may be returned if parents need more time and contact for detachment.

When a baby dies, there are limited opportunities for memories. Professionals have the responsibility of helping parents make memories in order to have a tangible person to mourn. Encouraging parents to name their infant gives the child a separate identity, which helps facilitate the grieving process. Tangible mementos may include photographs, handprints and footprints, a lock of hair, measurements of the baby, identification bands, the blanket the baby was wrapped in, a blessing or baptismal certificate, and birth and death certificates. Even when parents say they do not want mementos, they should be kept in hospital files and parents made aware that they will be available to them in the future if they want them. Taking a picture(s) of the baby, obtaining other mementos, and telling the parents that they will be available to them on request respects their immediate decision not to see or have information on the baby, but also provides a mechanism for them to "know" their baby at a later date if they wish to do so.

Before a baby is transported to a newborn special care unit, a photograph(s) should be taken and given to the parents to promote bonding. If the baby remains hospitalized for a long time or requires surgery, pictures taken at weekly intervals or before and after surgery can help confirm the reality of the child's condition and progress and assist with bonding as well as the grief process. Despite the outcome, parents will appreciate some lasting record of their child's life.

The staff who provides emotional support for parents must also receive support from each other. Expecting the staff to immediately return to work is unrealistic. Such an emotional experience takes time and space for decompression.

OPEN VISITING AND CARETAKING POLICIES

Perinatal care settings with open visiting and caretaking policies foster a shared family experience and support from others. Regardless of the type of perinatal loss, no mother should experience it alone—a spouse, friend, family member, or an identified supportive other should remain with her.[27] Members of the mother's support system will also need an outlet for the expression of their grief.

Women suffering the grief of perinatal loss

should be given a choice about their room assignment. Arbitrary removal from the obstetric unit may deny the mother's maternity: "Am I a mother or not?" It may also escalate her feelings of failure, guilt, and worthlessness as a woman and a mother. Since she did not produce a normal, healthy baby, she may feel punished and banished from the maternity area by isolation on another floor. Her care may be entrusted to those without expertise in the physiologic and psychologic care of the normal postpartum period, much less a postpartum complicated by loss. Placement at the end of the hall far from the nurse's station, with the door closed and no company from staff and family, only increases her feelings of loneliness and isolation. Yet being on a happy maternity floor with normal, healthy infants and their mothers may be an exceedingly difficult and constant reminder of her loss and even complicate her recovery.[23,56] Information about the advantages and disadvantages of staying or leaving the maternity ward should be given by the professional. The mother, knowing what will be helpful, makes the decision.[58]

The alternative to maternal hospitalization is early discharge as soon as medically possible so the mother may join her baby, who has usually been transported to another hospital. Early discharge also facilitates an easier mobilization of supportive others in the familiar surroundings of home. Removal from the constant reminder of one's failure (i.e., other healthy babies) may let the grief work begin.[58] Early discharge is not therapeutic when the professional assumes there is a support system to provide care and no one is available. Without a plan for follow-up care and contact, early discharge merely relocates the problem.

Caretaking is as important for the parents of a sick, deformed, or dead baby as it is for the parents of a normal infant. Open visiting and caretaking policies increase interaction between the parents and their infant by actively involving them in the reality of their child's illness, deformity, or impending death. Even if the child lives only a

short time, parental access and taking care of the baby complete the attachment process and enable them to begin the detachment of grief work. Even minimal caretaking helps parents overcome their sense of helplessness and be comforted by "We did all that we could have done. We cared; we made a difference to our baby." Active parental involvement decreases poor outcomes such as aberrant parenting styles, attachment problems, and unresolved grief.[24]

The loneliness and isolation of death is decreased for both parents and infant when they are together at the time of death. Parents are often comforted and relieved that their fantasy of the agony of the death scene is not borne out in the quiet, peaceful reality of death.[24,55] Having experienced the beginning of life together, experiencing the ending of life as a family symbolizes closure and completion. Parents who are able to share even a brief life with their child and the moment of death are able to face death's finality knowing they did not abandon their child but provided the infant with love and care. Parents who are not present at death may take care of the baby afterward by seeing and holding their infant.

Parents need to be given the opportunity to make final plans for their deceased infant. The planning will help them face the death and facilitate the grief process. For many parents, this is their first experience with death and making final arrangements, and they are not aware of the options. A number of choices are available, including cremation, burial, or hospital disposal.

A funeral may be chosen for religious reasons or as a declaration of the fetus or newborn as a person befitting burial rather than disposal. Burial leaves a specific place of remembrance that this baby lived. Care for the infant after death may include funeral arrangements such as choosing the clothes, bathing, and even dressing the infant.[55] If parents choose not to have a funeral, they may wish to have a memorial service or do something special, such as plant a rosebush or tree, in memory of their infant. Regardless of their decision, the birth and death of their baby is a life event for the family and it is important to recognize it.

AUTOPSY

For parents who experience a stillbirth, spontaneous abortion, or a neonatal death, knowing why the baby was deformed or died eases their recovery from grief.[58] In the search for a cause, all parents blame themselves for doing too much or too little to favorably influence the outcome. Knowing why the baby died or the converse, that not even the "experts" know why the baby died, may help assuage their personal feelings of guilt and failure.

Approaching the family for permission for an autopsy must be done by the primary care providers (physician and nurse) with the utmost of tact and respect for the family's feelings.[55] Too often the permission for autopsy is denied because of the way the subject is broached by professionals. Telling the family about their baby's death in one breath and asking for an autopsy with the next breath is not appropriate. Parents need time to deal with the reality of the death, including seeing and holding their baby and being with each other and supportive others before they are even ready to think about an autopsy. Consideration of the family's feelings and their stage of grief greatly enhances communication with the professional.[55] Reasons for the autopsy, including a possible answer to the question of "Why?" their baby died or was deformed, are important to discuss in a relaxed and unhurried manner. Parents may feel rushed to make a decision without clearly understanding the advantages and disadvantages and resist the emotional topic of a postmortem examination. Time for discussion with an empathetic professional as well as between themselves facilitates an informed parental decision.

The professional who receives permission for an autopsy is then obliged to discuss with the parents all findings.[17,23] This may entail more than one meeting with the parents, since they should be informed of the findings as soon as they are available. Therefore the professional may meet with them within 24 hours of completing the autopsy to discuss gross and preliminary findings and again 6 to 8 weeks later to discuss microscopic results.[24,55] Autopsy data may indicate either a condition that has implications for subsequent pregnancies or one that has little chance of recurrence. The need for genetic counseling for future pregnancies may be evident from autopsy results. Discussing the results with the report in hand and offering parents a copy for future reference is also important.

ANTICIPATORY GUIDANCE

Encounters with parents after the death of their infant give professionals the opportunity for *anticipatory guidance*—information about what to expect from themselves and from others. Reactions to perinatal loss differ markedly, so that family, friends, and acquaintances may not act as parents might expect. Some will be supportive and emotionally empathetic, especially if they have suffered a perinatal loss. Others will be uncomfortable and, not knowing what to say or do, may choose to avoid the couple and never mention the loss, even in future conversations. Those who are unaware of the loss may question the newly nonpregnant parents about the new baby. These inquiries are both awkward and painful.

Knowledge of the universal feelings and behaviors associated with grief gives comfort and relief to parents. What to expect from grief (i.e., how it progresses and how long it takes) is valuable to those who are or will be experiencing it.[24,58] Knowing the stages of grief and that the accompanying behaviors and emotions are normal decreases the feeling of "going crazy." Recovery from the loss takes time and cannot be hurried or ignored. The most difficult time is immediately after birth and the first few months after the loss (2 to 4 months).[48] The emotions of grief begin to lessen toward the end of the first year.

Parents should be encouraged to support and care for each other in their time of loss. Professionals should advocate mutual support by a free expression of feelings and emotions between the parents. Although parents need each other during grief, they also need an identified support system with whom to talk and cry. The ability to reach outside of the nuclear family to friends, extended family, and professionals should be encouraged. Professionals have a responsibility to ask whom parents turn to for help and support in a crisis. If there are no identified supportive others, parents must know whom to call for help in the initial bereavement period.

Anticipatory guidance is also essential at the discharge of an anomalied, preterm, or previously ill newborn.[24] Knowing what to expect when going home with a baby with a defect or a baby who has been hospitalized for months makes the transition from hospital to society easier for parents. Evaluation of the grief process and the attachment level of the parents to a less-than-perfect baby is vital.

LONG-TERM FOLLOW-UP CARE

Follow-up care and contact with professionals are needed by grieving parents.[16] Follow-up meetings function as a catharsis for parents, as well as an opportunity for assessment, counseling, and possibly referral. Primary care providers (physicians, nurses, and social workers) from the perinatal care setting may provide follow-up. For the family, relating to providers with whom a relationship has been established may be easier than establishing a new relationship with a stranger. However, being with those who are associated with the loss event may be uncomfortable for the parents at the height of their grief. For the professional, the ability to continue to be a source of help and comfort to families with whom one has established a relationship may help complete their grief reactions. Maintaining contact with the family may be painful as the professional relives the feelings of grief and loss associated with sharing their tragedy. Although painful, this reexperience of intense feelings gives both parents and professionals another opportunity to work toward grief resolution.

When and where to provide continuing care for families are crucial questions. Contact in the perinatal care setting both at the time of death and daily until discharge provides immediate care. However, when discharged, all too often the family returns home alone to face weeks and months of unsupported and lonely grief. Without feedback about their normal reaction and society's expectation that they will shortly be "back to normal," they are abandoned to their emotions. They suffer in silence and often drift apart in their misery. With their support system withdrawn but still feeling overwhelmed with grief, parents describe the period between 2 and 4 months after the loss as the most difficult time.[23,48,55] Follow-up care from professionals is most meaningful and needed by parents during this period when they feel deserted by previously supportive others. Meeting with families sooner (within weeks of their loss) may alleviate the impact of decreasing support as the months go by.[55] The professional who acknowledges the withdrawal of others but can be relied on to be available provides the parents with the emotional anchor of long-term care and support.

Breaking appointments or continually not being available may be resistance to follow-up contact with the professionals but also represents a reluctance to return to the perinatal care setting with its painful memories. A visit from the professional in the home provides a nonthreatening, familiar environment for follow-up care. The more comfortable home environment enables assessment of family interactions and facilitates communication at the "feeling" level.

Each family member and the family as a unit must be assessed for their place in the grief process:

- "In what stage of grief is each family member?"
- "Is anyone 'stuck' in a stage of grief?"
- "Are behaviors appropriate for normal grief reactions, or do altered behaviors represent pathologic grief reactions?"

- "Do altered behaviors warrant referral for further treatment and evaluation?"
- "Do the caretaking and attachment behaviors of the parents reflect resolution of grief over loss of the perfect child and adoption of the less-than-perfect child as the love object?"

Just because everything was progressing normally at previous encounters does not mean that it should be assumed to still be so. As the flood of initial grief subsides, problems and questions that were not considered suddenly become of great concern. For the first time in months, the regressive behavior of siblings may not only be noticed but be extremely annoying to parents. The beginning of grief resolution may allow future projections such as "When can I have another baby?" or the dread of the painful anniversary of the loss.[55]

Referral to public health nurses or visiting nursing services in the community for follow-up care is appropriate. However, a written referral alone is not enough. Involving them in the hospital care and discharge planning is essential for a smooth transition to home care. Having the new professional meet the family in the hospital with the primary care providers facilitates trust transference from the familiar to the unfamiliar. Traditionally, home care providers have been involved in care of normal mothers and babies in the community. Involvement in perinatal loss situations requires knowledge about the process of grief and willingness to share the grief of the parents. Since these may be new skills for many, continuing education programs that teach the theory and skills of effective intervention help the professional be more comfortable with a perinatal loss situation.

Additional expertise may be warranted when the professional recognizes signs and symptoms of pathologic grief, delayed or absent grief, or concurrent multiple stresses or losses. Parents may not be ready for genetic counseling, infant stimulation programs, or financial programs until months later. Between 3 and 6 months after their loss parents may be ready to reach outside of the nuclear and extended family for help and support

for the first time. Suggesting a local hospital support group or the local chapter of a national support organization may at first be met with resistance. Leaving the name and phone numbers of such organizations ensures that the parents have the information at their disposal when they are ready to use it. Until their own support system has withdrawn, parents may not be ready for a support group of other parents.

Throughout this section, examples of "what to say" and "how to say it" have been used to illustrate helpful interventions for grieving families. It is essential to state that "there are no scripts." Parents do not say one thing and the professionals answer with a parroted response. Each encounter is a unique situation consisting of distinct parental and professional personalities. Each situation must be evaluated separately and individual interventions instituted. It is recommended that the professional learn by observing an experienced colleague work with grieving families and that the professional "practice" with role playing and situation solving before actually attempting to intervene with the parents.

CHILDREN AND GRIEF

Explaining and helping a surviving child to understand the loss of an infant is an enormous task for parents. Facilitating the child's normal feelings of sadness, worry, and anger after a loss may be difficult for parents who fear being flooded with their own emotions. Unresolved grief from the parents' own childhood may prevent the expression of grief by their children.

To maintain the myth of childhood (innocent happiness), children are often shielded from any knowledge about death, even when it is an inevitable event in their lives. Thus children are prevented from full realization, validation, and expression of their feelings and emotions. They are not able to formalize and express their grief over the loss of a significant person.

Even though adults are encouraged to cry, talk, and gradually understand and integrate their feelings of grief, no one helps the child deal with the same frightening feelings. No one discusses the loss with the child, because "He might cry" and because of the adult's inadequacy and lack of understanding of how and what to say. No amount of secrecy or denial of the situation will hide the fact that the child is being excluded from an important family event.

Attempts to protect children from feelings of grief and mourning because of death or other important losses isolate the child. Age and developmentally appropriate explanations include the child in the family's experience, rather than separating and excluding him from "what is going on." Shielding children from the knowledge of death denies them the reality of life and the opportunity for personal growth and mastery of the experience. Like the subject of sex, death is taboo for children.

A child's grief and mourning in response to perinatal loss depends on his cognitive and developmental level, the extent of prenatal attachment and expectation about the baby, and the degree of ambivalent feelings. Because the child's understanding of death differs from that of adults, knowledge of the stages of growing awareness is essential for both parents and professionals working with children experiencing grief.[25,26] Regardless of age or developmental stage, the universal fear of childhood is the fear of separation and abandonment. For the young child (under age 5), the loss of the baby is experienced indirectly through parental grief. The young child reacts to the emotional withdrawal of grieving parents and fears loss of them (and their love).

The infant (less than age 1) who survives the death of a sibling has no cognitive knowledge of the loss. Rather, the loss is experienced through the changes in parental behaviors. Grief-stricken parents may be unable to provide the surviving infant with concern and continuity in caretaking behaviors, or they become overly concerned with the infant because of fear of a recurrent loss.[54]

The naturally self-centered toddler (between ages 1 and 3) has little understanding of cause-and-effect relationships. The toddler reacts to changes in the behavior of the grieving parents and reflects their feelings and anxiety. The preschooler (between ages 3 and 6) views death as a temporary state and not an inevitable occurrence. This stage is characterized by egocentricity, magical thinking, and sibling rivalry. Preschoolers believe they are the center of the world, that they can do anything, and that thinking is doing. Since their thoughts have the power of actions, preschoolers may fear that their negative thoughts or actual death wishes caused the baby to die.

School-age children (between ages 6 and 12) begin to understand death as inevitable and irreversible. The younger members of this group (between ages 6 and 9) personify death in the form of a separate person such as a boogey man, skeleton, or death man. With maturation, the concrete, literal child becomes the more realistic, logical, and abstract child who is able to conceive of death's universality. Preoccupation with thoughts of the child's own death or that of a loved one, particularly parents, characterizes the normal developmental phenomenon of "death phobia" (around 8 years of age). The child now realizes that death occurs not only in older people, but also in adults like their parents, and even in children. The adolescent (over age 12) has a more mature concept of death and one that is similar to the adult idea.

Parents are the primary caretakers for their children dealing with the death of an infant. They may benefit from guidance by the nurse, social worker, or other health professional regarding beneficial approaches to facilitate the child's grief work. The professional serves as a resource, role model, and support system to parents caring for their surviving children. Printed materials are also available to assist parents in helping their other children understand death (see the selected readings at the end of the chapter).

Although children at different developmental stages have their own conceptions of death, adults must provide them with the facts about the situation in language that they are able to understand.

Just as grieving adults need repetition, children need repeated explanations and discussions about the loss. Constantly in a state of developmental flux, the child attempts to view the loss in new ways as a result of increasing maturation. Asking questions (usually at inopportune times) and making comments about the infant are ways the child continues to process the experience, often long after the parents have completed it. These questions and comments may seem endless and resurrect the parent's own grief. The child's inquiries must be encouraged and supported so that he or she knows that talking about the loss or death is acceptable. Exploring the child's feelings for fears of causation, guilt, or the wonder if "death is catching" enables them to be dealt with appropriately. Truthful discussion with the child dispels the worst fears and fantasies and replaces them with reality that is "not too horrible to discuss" with parents. If the cause of the infant's death is known, it is explained to the child in simple, direct terms: "Baby Bobby couldn't breathe by himself because his lungs were sick. His sick lungs only happen to little babies."

A subsequent illness may precipitate worry by the child that he or she, too, will die. Often this fear is not verbalized but acted out by significant behavioral changes such as withdrawal, clinging and whining, or overactivity that are uncharacteristic for the child. Verbal reassurance that the child is not going to die and a reminder that "the baby died of a sickness that only little babies get; big boys and girls can't get it" are helpful.

The normal feelings that accompany grief should be acknowledged and explained to the child. "Mommy and Daddy feel sad that Baby Jean died. Sometimes we will cry because we feel sad. It's okay to cry when you feel sad." Permission for the expression of the child's feelings should also be given verbally: "You might feel sad, too. It's okay for you to cry when you're sad. Then we will talk about how you are feeling." Encouraging children to draw or write their feelings is another way of giving them permission to express their grief.

Using words such as "went away," "expired," "lost," or "went to sleep" is dangerous in describing death to children. Since young children are concrete and literal, they think they might die if they "go to sleep," or that anyone who leaves them is in danger of dying. Children also relate current experiences to past ones and interpret "lost" quite literally. In the mind of the child, if the parent only searched well enough, the misplaced (i.e., "lost") child would be found.

Including children at funeral or memorial services facilitates their grief and prevents exclusion from a significant family event. Consideration of the family value system, age of the child, and religious custom must enter into the decision to include the child. Adequate preparation includes a discussion of everything the child will see, hear, and feel, including the normal adult emotions of crying and sadness. An adult besides the grieving parents should accompany the child to reiterate what is happening and to facilitate the child's physical and psychologic needs. Adult support is necessary so that the child is able to express and deal with his or her feelings.

Helping children with their grief is also therapeutic for parents. Assisting children to master the crisis of loss ultimately augments the parents' self-esteem and restores confidence in their parenting skills.[24] Parents are able to deal in a healthy way with their own grief when they are able to facilitate the grief of their other children.

PATHOLOGIC GRIEF

The absence of grief when it would be expected is not a healthy sign but rather a cause for concern. The emotions of grief and their expression are healing. Early and full expression of grief is associated with an optimal outcome.[24] However, many people in grief-producing situations attempt to avoid the pain of grief and the expression of emotion, the result of which prolongs mourning, delays a return to the previous lifestyle, prevents the creation of new attachments and relationships, and ultimately results in pathologic grief (see list on p. 610).[10,24,33]

Not grieving precludes opportunities for growth and change. No new coping styles will be attempted. No novel alternatives to problem solving and adapting to a crisis will be added to the repertoire of behavior for future use. In other words, those who choose not to do grief work say "no" to their own potential and remain frozen in development.[22] Under the stress of not resolving their grief, some may even regress in their development.

Reproductive loss is a blow to self-concept and self-esteem, as well as loss of the infant. Blocking appropriate feelings of loss, grief, and anger results in a significant decrease in one's sense of self-esteem.[12] After death of their neonates, 33% of mothers suffered severe and tragic outcomes (including psychoses, phobias, anxiety attacks, and deep depression).[10,24,58] Those who are unable to effectively resolve their grief may suffer lifelong emotional damage.[34]

Not working through grief associated with repetitive contact with perinatal loss also affects the staff. To cope with feelings, they may hide behind a "professional" demeanor characterized by decreased spontaneity and withdrawal. Such a provider defends against the repeated pain of loss by emotional dissociation from the situation; the real self does not respond, but the role of the omnipotent, unemotional physician or nurse responds. The result, self-alienation, eventually desensitizes the professional to the experience and ultimately prevents any empathy with the experience of others.[22] Emotions that are unable to be acknowledged or expressed healthily are vented in ways that may be destructive to relationships in personal and professional life.

Unresolved grief does not disappear and is not dissipated. The emotions accompanying grief may never be expressed but are not forgotten by the unconscious mind. Containment of these emotions through repression or suppression takes psychic energy. A conscious, intentional decision to postpone or dismiss grief to meet others' needs or to meet immediate demands of the loss situation (e.g., funeral arrangements) is called delayed

grief.[33,34] For a period of time (days, weeks, or longer), there is little or no grief response when such a reaction would be expected and appropriate. Delayed grief may also be the result of repression, the unconscious contents that seem to have a life and energy of their own that become the sources of later emotional conflict.

Grief that is inhibited and never resolved is called abortive.[34] Those who have aborted their grief work often live bereft of "joie de vivre" with no interest, concern, or enthusiasm for life. Chronic grief is characterized by an indefinite prolonging of the acute stage of depression.[34] Indeed, chronic depression may be traceable to unresolved grief from the past.

Grief that is not resolved remains buried in the psyche, waiting for an opportunity to "rear its ugly head." A current loss may remind the psyche of the unmourned grief from a previous loss or losses.[15,35] As the two (or more) losses become intertwined and are experienced as one and the same, repressed emotions of unresolved grief pour forth.[35,50] Grieving more than one loss or a lifetime of losses is more difficult and emotionally draining than grieving one event at a time.[15] Cumulative grief work may also be occurring when a current loss of seemingly little importance overwhelms the person with intense emotions.[15,34] This flood of emotions seems disproportionate to the current loss and is only peripherally related to it. The unconscious, unresolved grief, is finally uncovered when the individual is flooded with emotions. Thus the emotional components of any grief reaction may be influenced by aspects of unresolved grief from the past.[35]

Grief and loss events of the perinatal period have only been equated for a relatively short time (less than 20 years). Since loss during the perinatal period is a common experience, many childbearing and older women (and men) have never grieved over their spontaneous abortion, stillbirth, or neonatal death, even 10 to 20 years after its occurrence. Parents in a current perinatal loss may also be dealing with unresolved grief from a previous perinatal loss. Unresolved grief (whether from perinatal or other loss events of life) may become available for resolution in subsequent crisis events. A mother who delivers a normal healthy newborn, yet is depressed postpartally, may not have postpartum depression. Instead she may be grieving the unresolved loss of a spontaneous abortion, therapeutic abortion, or other perinatal loss.[47,50] Her depressed mood could also be resulting from unresolved grief from the loss of a parent, spouse, or child. Depressed menopausal women may be experiencing the cumulative effects of a lifetime of unresolved grief. The symptomatology of unresolved grief is listed below.

Symptomatology of unresolved grief*
Vivid memory for the details of the perinatal loss event
Flashback to the event
Anniversary grief (date of birth or expected date of confinement)
Emotions of grief (sadness, anger, or crying) when talking about loss
Intense emotions with subsequent loss or crisis

Recognizing unresolved grief has implications for facilitating grief work in a current loss, episodic care, and health maintenance. The energy to keep unresolved emotions restrained could better be used in personal growth and development, grieving, and maintaining and establishing relationships. The lifelong stress of unresolved grief contributes to both psychologic and physical illness, including increased death rates and an earlier death.[41,55]

Not grieving a perinatal loss affects the individual involved and the relationships with significant others, including present and future children. Asynchronous grief and the absence of grief in one or more family members weakens and strains family relationships.[1,24] The irritability and preoccupation of normal grief may overly disrupt the family. Differences may be magnified to the extent that major rifts and disruptions in the relationship occur, resulting in increased incidence of separation and divorce.[24]

°Modified from Stack J: Spontaneous abortion and grieving, Am Fam Pract 21:99, 1980.

Exclusive dedication to the care of a deformed or ill child to the detriment of other family relationships is symptomatic of a pathologic grief reaction.[24,49,57] The parent who neglects other children, the couple's relationship, and social outlets is so overwhelmed with guilt about having caused the child's defect that nothing else in life matters. This guilty attachment and exclusive dedication are ways of avoiding grief work.[49] Other forms of pathologic reactions include parental rejection and intolerance of the deformed or ill child.[24]

The parent who is emotionally withdrawn and unavailable to the family because of chronic grief and depression is not able to attach and care for present or subsequent children. Aberrant parenting styles (resulting in a vulnerable, battered, or failure to thrive child) may be the result of prolonged separation, unresolved grief, or grief that has progressed beyond the anticipatory phase, so that emotional ties with the infant have been severed.[24] These difficulties with caring and parenting may affect the deformed or ill child and all the children in the family. In turn, these children may grow up unable to parent subsequent generations because of the type of ineffectual parenting they received. Parents who grieve inappropriately may leave their children a legacy of psychosocial problems such as difficulty with separation, independence, control (e.g., school phobia and toilet training), a failure to thrive, and sleep disturbances.

Since detachment is necessary before a healthy attachment may again occur, unresolved grief affects future children. It is necessary to first complete the grief work over the loss of one child to be optimally ready to emotionally invest in a new baby.[24] The replacement child, a well-documented psychiatric syndrome, is associated with unresolved parental grief after the death (or loss) of a child.[7,15,40] Without withdrawing their emotional attachment to the lost child, parents plan, conceive, and bear another to replace their loss and alleviate their grief. Parental hopes, desires, and fantasies invested in the lost child are not relinquished but merely transferred to the replacement child. Planning for a new pregnancy and another child should begin only after the grief process for the lost child is completed.[24,50] Generally, 6 months to 1 year is the earliest that grief will be resolved so that the ego is free to invest in a relationship with another fetus and newborn.

REFERENCES

1. Benfield D et al: Grief response of parents after referral of the critically ill newborn to a regional center, N Engl J Med 294:975, 1976.
2. Benoliel JQ: Assessment of loss and grief, J Thanatology 1:182, 1971.
3. Berezin N: After a loss in pregnancy: help for families affected by a miscarriage, a stillbirth, or the loss of a newborn, New York, 1982, Fireside Books.
4. Bibring GL: The death of an infant: a psychological study, N Engl J Med 283:370, 1970.
5. Borg S and Lasker J: When pregnancy fails: families coping with miscarriage, stillbirth, and infant death, Boston, 1981, Beacon Press.
6. Cadden V: Crisis in the family. In Caplan G, editor: Principles of preventive psychiatry, New York, 1964, Basic Books, Inc, Publishers.
7. Cain A and Cain B: On replacing a child, J Am Acad Child Psychiatry 3:443, 1964.
8. Caplan G: Principles of preventive psychiatry, New York, 1964, Basic Books, Inc, Publishers.
9. Colgrove M et al: How to survive the loss of a love, New York, 1976, Lion Books.
10. Cullberg J: Mental reactions of women to perinatal death. In Morris N, editor: Psychosomatic medicine in obstetrics and gynecology, New York, 1972, S Karger.
11. Cummings ST: The impact of the child's defect on the father, Am J Orthopsychiatry 46:246, 1976.
12. Cummings ST et al: Effects of the child's deficiency on the mother: a study of mothers of mentally retarded, chronically ill, and neurotic children, Am J Orthopsychiatry 36:595, 1966.
13. Danforth DN: Obstetrics and gynecology, New York, 1977, Harper & Row, Publishers, Inc.
14. Eason WM: The dying child, Springfield, Ill, 1970, Charles C Thomas, Publisher.
15. Engel GL: Grief and grieving, Am J Nurs 64:93, 1964.
16. Geis DP: Mothers' perceptions of care given their dying child, Am J Nurs 65:103, 1965.
17. Giles PFH: Reactions of women to perinatal death, Aust NZ J Obstet Gynaecol 10:207, 1970.
18. Goldberg H: The hazards of being male, New York, 1976, Sanford J Greenberger, Assoc, Inc.
19. Gonzalez MT: Nursing support of the family with an abnormal infant, Hosp Top 15:68, 1971.
20. Hill R: Generic features of families under stress. In Parad H, editor: Crisis intervention, New York, 1965, Family Service Association of America.
21. Johnson JM: Stillbirth: a personal experience, Am J Nurs 72:1595, 1972.
22. Jourard S: The transparent self, rev ed, New York, 1971, Van Nostrand Reinhold Co, Inc.
23. Kennell J et al: Mourning response of parents to death of a newborn infant, N Engl J Med 283:344, 1970.
24. Klaus M and Kennell J: Parent-infant bonding, ed 2, St Louis, 1982, The CV Mosby Co.
25. Koocher GP: Children, death, and cognitive development, Dev Psychobiol 9:369, 1973.
26. Koocher GP: Talking to children about death, Am J Orthopsychiatry 44:404, 1974.
27. Kowalski K and Osborn M: Helping mothers of stillborn infants to grieve, Matern Child Nurs J 2:29, 1977.
28. Kübler-Ross E: On death and dying, New York, 1969, Macmillan Publishing Co, Inc.
29. Lax RF: Some aspects of the interaction between mother and impaired child: mother's narcissistic trauma, Int J Psychoanal 53:339, 1972.
30. Lepler M: Having a handicapped child, Matern Child Nurs J 3:32, 1978.
31. Lewis E: The management of stillbirth: coping with an unreality, Lancet 18:619, 1976.
32. Lewis E and Page A: Failure to mourn a stillbirth: an overlooked catastrophe, Br J Med Psychol 51:237, 1978.
33. Lindemann E: Symptomatology and management of acute grief, Am J Psychiatry 101:141, 1944.
34. Marris P: Loss and change, New York, 1974, Pantheon Books, Inc.
35. McCollum A and Schwartz H: Social work and the mourning parent, Social Work 17:25, 1972.
36. Mercer R: Crisis: a baby born with a defect, Nursing '77 7:45, 1977.
37. Ohlshansky S: Chronic sorrow: a response to having a mentally defective child, Social Casework 43:190, 1962.
38. Opirhory GJ: Counseling the parents of a critically ill newborn, JOGN Nurs 8:179, 1979.
39. Parkes CM: Bereavement: studies of grief in adult life, New York, 1972, International Universities Press, Inc.
40. Pozanski E: The replacement child: a saga of unresolved parental grief, J Pediatr 81:1190, 1972.
41. Rahe R et al: Social stress and illness onset, J Psychosom Res 8:35, 1964.
42. Rapaport L: The state of crisis: some theoretical considerations. In Parad H: Crisis intervention, New York, 1965, Family Service Association of America.
43. Raphael D: The tender gift: breastfeeding, New York, 1973, Schoken Books, Inc.
44. Saylor D: Nursing response to mothers of stillborn infants, JOGN Nurs 8:39, 1977.

45. Schoenberg BA et al: Loss and grief: psychological management in medical practice, New York, 1970, Columbia University Press.
46. Schoenberg BA et al: Anticipatory grief, New York, 1974, Columbia University Press.
47. Seitz P and Warrick L: Perinatal death: the grieving mother, Am J Nurs 74:2028, 1974.
48. Siegel R et al: The impact of neonatal loss, Pediatr Res 16:93A, 1982.
49. Solnit A and Stark M: Mourning and the birth of a defective child, Psychoanal Study Child 16:523, 1961.
50. Stack J: Spontaneous abortion and grieving, Am Fam Pract 21:99, 1980.
51. Traxler P: Poem for my son, Blood calender, New York, 1975, William Morrow & Co, Inc.
52. Waechter E: The birth of an exceptional child, Nurs Forum 9:202, 1970.
53. Whitfield J et al: The application of hospice concepts to neonatal care, Am J Dis Child 136:521, 1982.
54. Wilson AL et al: The death of a newborn twin: an analysis of parental bereavement, Pediatrics 70:587, 1982.
55. Wooten B: Death of an infant, Matern Child Nurs J 6:257, 1981.
56. Yates SA: Stillbirth: what staff can do, Am J Nurs 72:1592, 1972.
57. Young RK: Chronic sorrow: parent's response to the birth of a child with a defect, Matern Child Nurs J 2:38, 1977.
58. Zahourek R and Jensen J: Grieving and the loss of the newborn, Am J Nurs 73:836, 1973.

SELECTED READINGS

Berezin N: After a loss in pregnancy: help for families affected by a miscarriage, a stillbirth, or the loss of a newborn, New York, 1982, Fireside Books.
Canadian Pediatric Society, Fetus and Newborn Committee: Support for parents experiencing perinatal loss, Can Med Assoc J 129:335, 1983.
Davidson GW: Understanding mourning, Minneapolis, 1984, Augsburg Publishing House.
Dodge H: Thumpy's story, Springfield, Ill, 1983, Prairie Lark Press.
Eichner S: Dealing with long term problems: a parent's perspective, Neonatal Network 5:45, 1986.
Friedman R and Gradstein P: Surviving pregnancy loss, Boston, 1982, Little, Brown & Co, Inc.
Gardner SL and Merenstein GB: Helping families deal with perinatal loss, Neonatal Network 5:17, 1986.
Gardner SL and Merenstein GB: Perinatal loss: an overview, Neonatal Network 5:7, 1986.
Garland KG: Grief, the transitional process, Neonatal Network 5:27, 1986.
Garland KG: Unresolved grief, Neonatal Network 5:29, 1986.
Gordon A and Klass D: They need to know: how to teach children about death, Englewood Cliffs, NJ, 1979, Prentice-Hall, Inc.
Grollman E: Explaining death to children, Boston, 1967, Beacon Press.
Grollman E: Talking about death (a dialogue between parent-child), Boston, 1970, Beacon Press.
Kirk EP: Psychological effects and management of perinatal loss, Am J Obstet Gynecol 149:46, 1984.
Limbo RK and Wheeler SR: When a baby dies: a handbook for healing and helping, LaCrosse, Wis, 1986, Resolve.
Mills GC: Books to help children understand death, Am J Nurs 72:291, 1979.
Mills GC et al: A guide to death education, Palm Springs, Calif, 1976, ETC Publications.
Oehler J: Coloring books for children: The frogs have a baby, a very small baby; and The frog family's baby dies, Durham, NC, 1979, Duke University Medical Center.
Parad HJ: Crisis intervention, New York, 1965, Family Service Association of America.
Rudolph M: Should children know? (encounters with death in the lives of children), New York, 1978, Schocken Books, Inc.
Schweibert P and Kirk P: When hello means goodbye: a guide for parents whose child dies at birth or shortly after, Portland, Ore, 1981, University of Oregon Health Sciences Center.
Sheer BJ: Help for parents in a difficult job: broaching the subject of death, Matern Child Nurs J 2:320, 1977.
Wilson AL et al: Parental response to perinatal death, Am J Dis Child 139:1235, 1985.
Worden JW: Grief counseling and grief therapy: a handbook for mental health practitioners, New York, 1982, Springer Publishing Co, Inc.

FILM/VIDEOTAPE

Death of a newborn, Cleveland, 1977, Health Sciences Communications Center, Case Western Reserve University.

CHAPTER 24

The neonate and the environment: impact on development

SANDRA L. GARDNER · KELDUYN R. GARLAND · STACY L. MERENSTEIN · GERALD B. MERENSTEIN

For centuries the newborn baby has been considered a "tabula rasa"—a blank slate on which parents and the world "write" to create the individual. In the first half of this century, research emphasized the contributions of the environment in shaping the infant and child. Only recently has the individuality of the infant been recognized as a powerful shaper of the care giver, the care given, and thus the environment.

This chapter deals with the psychosocioemotional development of the term and preterm neonate. Infant development depends on the dynamic relationship between *endowment* and *environment*. Along the continuum of development, development of the infant is the beginning of the child and, ultimately, of adult competence in the world. Understanding the dynamic relationship between endowment and environment is enhanced by a review of the principles of development in Table 24-1.[8,56] First, the developmental tasks of infancy are presented, along with the influences of endowment and environment on mastery. Home and family life, in which most infants are raised, is then contrasted with the experiences of babies in the newborn intensive care unit (NICU). Intervention strategies to normalize the NICU environment are then presented, along with strategies for parent teaching. The developmental and social outcomes of infants exposed to the NICU are then briefly discussed.

DEVELOPMENTAL TASKS OF THE NEONATE AND INFANT

Infancy (birth to 12 months) is a time of emergence from a global egocentric orientation to a recognition of objects and people as separate from one's self.[36,73] Involuntary reflex responses are replaced by planned responses and intentions. Throughout this evolutionary process newborns demonstrate amazing "competence in making sense out of their environment."[115]

Biorhythmic balance: primary developmental task of the newborn

In utero, the fetus is dependent on the mother's physiologic systems to automatically regulate its own. At birth, the neonate's basic physiologic needs (feeding, elimination, cleaning, heat balance, stroking, and communicating) are met in new and different ways. Emerging from a physiologically dependent preonate° into a physiologically independent neonate introduces new variables for both mother and baby in the development of their extrauterine relationship.

Newborns express the impact of their birth experience and initial encounter with their extra-

---

°*Preonate* refers to the infant in utero during the three stages of development (zygote, embryo, fetus) from conception to birth.

TABLE 24-1

Principles of Development

Development is a continuous process from conception to maturation (i.e., development occurs in utero, too).

Growth and development are influenced by genetic makeup and environmental experiences.

Development occurs in an orderly sequence, largely determined by readiness or maturation. The sequence of development is the same in all children; the rate of development is individual.

Development occurs cephalocaudad (head → foot) and from gross to specific (e.g., central → periphery).

The first 5 years of life are marked by a rapid period of growth of all body systems. During this time behavior patterns are developed and are greatly influenced by the environment.

Environmental stimulation provides conceptual development and influences the level of intelligence.

Learning occurs when behavioral change is not due solely to maturation; learning is facilitated by reinforcement of the behavior.

Development of the infant occurs within the framework of interaction with a caretaker and within the family.

Modified from Illingworth RS: The development of the infant and young child, ed 5, Edinburgh, 1972, Churchill Livingstone; and Barnard K and Erikson M: Teaching children with developmental problems, ed 2, St Louis, 1976, The CV Mosby Co.

uterine environment through disstasis* in their circadian rhythms (their sleep/wake cycle, respiratory and heart rates, blood chemistry levels, metabolic processes, body tension/relaxation, and eating patterns).[29,60] The primary task of the newly born is to reestablish the biorhythmic balance by stabilizing the function of these systems. The extent to which this balance needs to be reestablished is determined by the amount of disstasis experienced both in utero and during labor and birth. The Apgar score is an indication of the degree of disstasis a newborn experiences in the birthing process.

*Disstasis refers to imbalance, disharmony, and upset in rhythmic order.

Although biorhythmic balance is internally determined, caretaking interaction between newborn and parent/caretaker either facilitates or disturbs this transition. After birth, balance is facilitated by contact with familiar surroundings (i.e., the mother's body). The mother's auditory, tactile, and visual stimuli reconnect and reorient the baby so that transition and adjustment to novel surroundings is easier.[48,60,98,118] When immediate recontact between the neonate and the mother is not possible (i.e., the mother refuses or is ill; or the neonate is preterm, sick, or anomalied and requires immediate emergency medical intervention or transport), the primary "mothering" role is transferred to professional (medical and nursing) care providers.[47] Interactional dynamics necessary for reestablishing biorhythmic balance and fostering the psychosocioemotional development of the newborn are also transferred into the NICU.

Just as in a home/family setting, the infant's personality and behavioral development are affected by the nature and dynamics of the stimuli and relationships encountered with the staff in a nursery/NICU setting.[51] The level of function or dysfunction in the biorhythmic balance affects the neonate's long-range outcomes and is intrinsically interwoven with the development of a basic trust and a sense of self.

Sense of self

In utero, the fetus has continuous tactile-kinesthetic stimulation that develops and matures the central nervous system (CNS) and establishes kinesthesis as the most natural pathway for growth and development. The interaction between infants and the extrauterine environment is also kinesthetic. The neonate has an inborn "stimulus hunger"[98] for gentle touch, body contact, body positioning, and vestibular stimulation. Tactile contact and vestibular stimulation are essential for (1) the development of a physical identity (body image), (2) organization and sorting of stimuli, (3) coordination of sensory-motor skills, (4) a psychologic and social sense of self, (5) normal neurophysiologic development—mental and cognitive abilities, and (6) emotional stability and temperament.*

Daily caretaking and interaction (feeding, diapering, holding, playing, etc.) with the parent/caretaker provides infants with the stimuli for developing their identity. Through the manner in which the infant is handled, the infant receives messages about how the caretaker feels about him or her. Response cues given by infants affect the caretaker's response to and interaction with them.[2,13,36,46,89] Quieting and soothing by the baby in response to caretaking positively reinforces the parent to continue. Withdrawal, irritability, or continuous crying is perceived by the caretaker as rejection and may result in parental frustration, withdrawal, and decreased interaction. Repeated exposure to the caretaker's style and nonverbal messages thus enables the infant to adopt these patterns of caretaking.[73] The self of the infant is formed through interaction with people and objects within the environment.

Since the nature (amount and kind) of the kinesthetic interaction between infants and caretakers determines how infants develop and mature, lack of appropriate stimulation has long-term consequences. Stimulus deprivation results in impairment, retardation, or deviancy in skill development for productive living. The degree or extent of impairment is dependent on the severity of the restrictions and limitations encountered. Studies have demonstrated that infants who were well cared for physically (fed, diapered, cleaned) either died or were seriously impaired (mentally, emotionally, and socially) because of lack of tactile/kinesthetic stimulation.[13,46,107]

Institutionally reared infants who had minimal contact and no social interaction with their caretakers displayed significant developmental delays.[95] The impact of kinesthetic deprivation was seen in the minimal expression of social skills (cooing, babbling, crying), minimal interest in objects in the environment, increased self-stimula-

tion (rocking), touch aversion, flat or withdrawn affect, and retarded mental and motor development. Environmental deprivation may also affect the physical growth of the infant.[46] Montague[83] believes infants are able to overcome mental and nutritional deprivation as long as they are not deprived of tactile stimulation.

The psychosocial task: trust versus mistrust

Trust versus mistrust in oneself and the environment is developed during infancy.[2,36,118] The response of the environment from the moment of birth is the means by which neonates develop trust in themselves and decide on the reliability of their new environment.[48,98,118] Two major factors influence the development of trust versus mistrust: (1) the infant's ability to communicate needs to the environment and (2) the reliability and constancy of the environment in responding.

In the course of routine caretaking, the infant associates the caretaker with either comfort and trust or with lack of need satisfaction and mistrust. Initially the baby cries as a reflex response to a need stimuli (e.g., "I'm hungry"; "I'm wet"). The caretaker responds to the infant and meets the need—the infant is fed; the infant is changed. Thus the newborn learns to communicate when the need arises again, because the environment/caretaker has and will respond. This contingent response of the caretaker to the infant's need is the necessary reinforcement for the development of trust in self, in others, and ultimately in humankind. The infant develops a sense of mastery over his or her world and a sense that it is okay to have needs and to have them met.[36,115]

Caretaking that ignores or delays need gratification is noncontingent to the infant's cues for care. Need meeting that is externally defined by the caretaker's agenda (e.g., feeding schedule, rigid or inflexible routines, medical/nursing procedures in the NICU) discourages the infant from being aware of and experiencing needs and communicating them. Such infants will eventually detach themselves (emotionally and kinesthetically)

*References 13, 36, 65, 66, 68, 73, 94, 98, 99.

from the sensation of their needs, thus no longer experiencing or communicating them.[15,46]

As a result, these infants conclude that they and their needs (which they perceive as one and the same) are *not* important and that they have no impact on their environment. They do not have a sense of self or of their own existence—physically (where their boundaries end and another's begin) or psychologically (their identity that exists independent of another). Some people with severe mistrust in themselves and their environment do not experience the sensation of hunger when hungry, or express appropriate emotional responses to situations. They also do not kinesthetically feel where their body ends and another's begins when they are hugging—they totally merge and experience the two as one and the same person. Low self-concept and self-esteem and a sense of helplessness about succeeding in life are a result of lack of trust. Behaviorally this is manifested in touch aversion; avoidance of eye contact; flat, withdrawn or depressed affect; and/or hyperactivity, restlessness, low frustration level, demanding behavior and perpetual dissatisfaction, and poor social relationships.[14,68,95,107]

Survival is dependent on the caretaker meeting the newborn's needs. Need meeting is either contingent on the infant's cues or noncontingent on an external agenda. The degree of the mother's emotional investment and connectedness with the newborn will determine the nature and quality of the caretaking.[36,115] Likewise, the temperament and responsiveness of the baby will affect the mother's feelings of competency, success, and emotional connectedness to her infant.[15,46] Parents who relate to the newborn as an individual (i.e., a person with feelings, wants, and needs; a person who knows what these are) will be sensitive and responsive to the infant's needs and interact with the baby during caretaking. This relationship facilitates the development of a good sense of self (esteem, confidence, and emotional security) and mastery of the world. Caretakers who do not perceive infants as individuals do not respond to their need cry or interact with caretaking. This style fosters the development of mistrusting, suspicious, helpless, emotionally insecure, and isolated children and adults.

ENDOWMENT

Babies possess innateness and individuality. Primitive reflexive behaviors, higher cognitive abilities, temperament, and sensory-motor competencies are the *endowment* of the individual baby. Individual variation and utilization of these components of endowment are influenced by the environment of the newborn.

Even before conception, the genetic endowment of the parents and preceding generations affects the fetus/newborn. Everything that the individual will inherit from his parents is determined at the moment of conception. Of the vast number of possible combinations of chromosomes, chance determines which characteristics the individual receives. Thus each individual is genetically and biologically different from every other person. Either a faulty gene (e.g., sickle cell anemia) or an altered number of chromosomes (e.g., Down's syndrome) is responsible for inherited defects.

Even though after the moment of conception, hereditary endowment is never able to be changed, it is influenced by the intrauterine environment. Some birth defects are caused by teratogens—any environmental agent (drugs, virus, chemical, pollutant) that interferes with normal fetal development. The individual's potential for growth and development is limited by his or her genetic endowment. As Montague[82] states, "Genetic endowment determines what we *can* do—environment what we *do* do."

The one exception to individual genetic endowment is identical twins, who share the same heredity. Identical twins have been extensively studied, since it is hypothesized that any differences between them are due to environmental effects. Identical twins raised apart have been found to be more similar in intelligence, temperament, and personality characteristics than are fraternal twins raised together.

Genetic endowment imposes limits on a child's potential. Studies show that children resemble their parents both physically and mentally more than they differ from them. Parental expectations that are unrealistic or beyond the child's capacity may set the child up for disappointment when he or she fails to meet these expectations. All too often abilities and potential are stifled within this environment, so that the child is unable to achieve what is within his or her capability.

The exact influence of genetics for most psychologic traits is unknown. Introverted (timid, shy, withdrawn) and extroverted (active, friendly, and outgoing) personality types may be partially genetically controlled. The degree to which intelligence is inherited is currently unknown, although intelligence of children is most often similar to parental intelligence (i.e., intelligence is more similar between child and biologic mother than child and adopted mother).

Freedman[45] studied newborns of many ethnic groups to see if there were any similarities in disposition within the group and/or differences from other ethnic groups. He found that Chinese-American newborns were more adaptable, less irritable, and easier to console than caucasian-American babies. Maneuvers such as the Moro and covering the face with a cloth elicited very different responses, depending on the newborn's ethnic origin.

The same environmental stimuli elicits very different behavioral responses, which are individual and genetically influenced. These genetically influenced behaviors are also influenced by environment—both internal and external. Thus an individual may be more vulnerable to or more resilient in a specific environment. Therefore we are totally endowment and totally environment (100% endowment + 100% environment = an individual).[45]

Temperament

Parents often notice behavioral differences in their children from the first day. These differences are obvious in motor activity, irritability, and passivity. Some infants are quiet and placid, others are irritable and easily upset, and others are somewhere in between. Thomas et al[113] have delineated nine categories of behavior that describe individual temperament (Table 24-2). These temperamental qualities enable three basic types of infant to be identified:

1. The "easy" child who is seen as regular, pleasant, and easy to care for and love
2. The "difficult" child who is difficult to rear and reacts with protest and withdrawal to strange events or people
3. The "slow to warm" child who reacts with withdrawal or passivity to new events

Neurologic development

Brain growth of the fetus/newborn occurs in two stages.[30]

STAGE I. Stage I occurs from 10 to 18 weeks of pregnancy. During this period the number of nerve cells that the individual will have is developed. Any environmental occurrence (e.g., maternal malnutrition, medications, infections) that affects brain growth during this stage may also affect neonatal behavioral responses.

STAGE II. Stage II occurs from 20 weeks gestation to 2 years of age. This period marks a brain growth spurt and the most vulnerable period of growth of the dendrites of the human cortex.

The maturity of the infant is reflected in his or her behavior. Infants of a younger gestational age have less mature responses than infants of an older gestational age. A neurologic assessment of the newborn includes evaluation of (1) newborn reflexes, (2) neonatal states, (3) psychosocial interaction, and (4) sensory capabilities. The neonate is born with behaviors that are unlearned, instinctual, and of an adaptive and survival nature. They reflect the state of the nervous system and the level of neonatal maturation (see Figure 4-3). Table 24-3 summarizes neonatal reflexive behaviors, their significance, and the time of their integration into voluntary movement. Serial testing of reflexive behavior gives more reliable data than one observation. Observations indicative of

TABLE 24-2

Behavioral Categories Descriptive of Individual Temperament

TEMPERAMENTAL QUALITY	RATING
Activity level	*High*—Increased movement when asleep; increased wiggling and activity when diaper changed
	Low—Decreased movement when dressed or during sleep
Rhythmicity	*Regular*—Established own feeding; sleep and bowel movement pattern is fairly predictable
	Irregular—Amounts of sleep, feeding variable; "no two days are alike"; no pattern established
Approach/withdrawal	*Positive*—Eagerly tries new foods; interested in new surroundings and people
	Negative—Rejects new foods, new toys, and new environments; apprehensive, cries with new people
Adaptability	*Adaptive*—Little resistance to first bath; may enjoy bath
	Nonadaptive—Startles easily; resists diapering, bathing, and other manipulating
Quality of mood	*Positive*—Pleasant, easygoing disposition; easy to comfort; smiles
	Negative—Fussy; cries easily and is not easily comforted by external stimuli; unable to comfort self easily
Intensity of mood	*Intense*—Vigorously cries; rejects food
	Mild—No crying when wet; frets instead of crying when hungry
Sensory threshold (intensity of stimulus necessary to elicit a response)	*Low*—Noise, activity, or other stimuli enough to interrupt infant's behavior
	High—Not startled or interrupted by noise or other stimuli
Distractibility	*Distractible*—Rocking, pacifier, toy, voice, music will decrease fussing
	Nondistractible—No stimulus will decrease distress until need is met—food; stop changing diaper; bath over
Attention span and persistence	*Long*—Repeatedly rejects substitutions for perceived needs (no pacifier till diaper is changed; no water if milk is wanted)
	Short—Cries when awakened but stops immediately; mild objection if needs are not immediately met

Modified from Thomas A, Chess S, and Birch HG: Sci Am 223:102, 1970.

TABLE 24-3

Neonatal Reflexive Behaviors

BEHAVIOR	BEGINS	INTEGRATES
Protection		
Moro	28 weeks	At 6-8 months to allow sitting and protective extension of the hands
Palmar grasp	28 weeks	At 5-6 months to allow voluntary grasping of objects
Plantar grasp	28 weeks	At 7-8 months with foot rubbing on objects; complete at 8-9 months for standing and walking
Babinski	28 weeks	(Same as plantar grasp)
Tonic neck	35 weeks	At 4 months, so rolling over and reaching/grasping may occur
Gag	36 weeks	Protects against aspiration—does *not* disappear
Blink	25 weeks	Does *not* disappear
Crossed extension	28 weeks	Disappears around 2 months of age
Survival		
Rooting	28 weeks	At 3 months; decreased response if baby is sleepy or with satiety
Sucking	26-28 weeks	Not yet synchronized with swallowing
Swallowing	12 weeks	32-34 weeks, stronger synchronization with sucking; perfect by 34-37 weeks

major deviations include asymmetry—total absence or no response on one side or in upper or lower extremities.

Psychologic interaction/neonatal states

For years newborn behavior was thought to be only on a reflexive, instinctual level. Through the work of Brazelton and others, newborns have been shown to have the ability to interact with and shape their environment. The Brazelton Neonatal Behavioral Assessment Scale[18] enables the interactive behavior of the newborn to be observed and scored.

The Brazelton scale enables assessment of the infant's individual capabilities for social relationships. Rather than the average performance, the Brazelton rates the infant on the best performance. Interest in the best performance is based on the belief that the newborn may briefly respond to external stimuli from higher centers of the nervous system (i.e., the cerebrum). The best performance gives more data related to prediction of future developmental outcomes (whether positive or negative) than does the average performance. Several other concepts of neonatal behavior also influence the choice of best, rather than average, performance: habituation, dishabituation, imitation, and learning.

Habituation is the protective mechanism by which the infant decreases responsivity to external stimuli. Habituation represents the cerebral behavior of memory—the infant stores the memory of the stimulus and with repeated presentation learns not to respond. Infants who are able to habituate are able to "tune out" noxious stimuli in the environment and protect themselves from overstimulation. An infant who is unable to habituate will continue to react vigorously to repeated stimuli. Babies who become "bored" with their toys have habituated to them—babies like variety. Dishabituation represents increasing attention to a new stimulus (new mobile, toy, face) after habituation to an old stimulus. The infant thus "recognizes" the novelty of the new stimulus and chooses to respond.

The neonate is able to imitate the facial and manual gestures of adults.[77] Infants as young as 12 days old imitate gestures such as mouth opening and tongue protrusion. Since the neonate has never seen his or her own face, this innate ability to match behaviors to those of another is a remarkable utilization of the cerebral cortex. Imitation may operate as a positive feedback mechanism to care givers; thus it is important in parent-infant reciprocity and represents early learning behaviors.

Learning, a function of the cerebral cortex, occurs with habituation and imitation. Early cognitive development is important to later learning and future cognitive development. Knowledge of the cognitive ability of the neonate enables care providers to provide opportunities for learning. Learning influences structural development; there is increased CNS development during the first 2 years of life.[18,30]

In evaluating the performance of the infant using the Brazelton examination, six categories of abilities are considered in each response:

1. Habituation—infant's ability to decrease responsivity to light, sound, and pinprick—is determined.
2. Orientation to auditory and visual stimuli is determined. Both animate (face and voice) and inanimate (bell, rattle, ball) stimuli are presented to the infant.
3. Motor maturity measures the infant's motor coordination and control.
4. Variations in the rate and amount of change during alert states and between states, color, and activity are measured.
5. Self-quieting abilities of the infant and the caretaker's gradual efforts to quiet the infant are measured. How much, how soon, and how effectively the infant is able to quiet and console himself are scored.
6. Social behaviors of the infant as a response to parental care are determined.

The state of consciousness influences the reactions of the newborn to internal and external stimuli. The infant's state at the time of observation must be considered in interpretation of the findings. Table 24-4 shows the six states of the newborn and specific considerations for care giving in each state.

Clinical application of the Brazelton scale includes evaluation of infant capabilities after illness, prematurity, or maternal medications. The most important application of the Brazelton examination is in anticipatory guidance for parents. Demonstration of parts of the examination for parents enables them to become familiar with their infant's individual patterns of behavior, temperament, and states. Thus parents are able to more accurately assess and interpret their infant's cues for interaction and for distance.

Circadian rhythms

Circadian rhythms are cyclic variations in function that occur daily at about the same time. Humans cycle their bodily functions (i.e., temperature, hormonal changes, blood pressure, urine volume, sleep-wake cycles) in a 24-hour period. These daily fluctuations are innately controlled by the individual's "biologic clock" in the brain. Environment does not cause cyclic variations; they are innate to the individual and persist despite environmental influences.

The term newborn sleeps from 16 to 19 hours a day. As sleep begins, the term infant enters active rather than quiet sleep and spends more time in active sleep than does the adult.[32] Active sleep durations vary from 10 to 45 minutes, whereas quiet sleep lasts about 20 minutes.[32] The infant's sleep cycle is 50 to 60 minutes, as compared with the adult's 90 to 100-minute cycle.[6] On awakening from a sleep state, the newborn returns to that same state, but repeated awakenings result in prolonged wakefulness.[6] Infants exhibit a diurnal variation in the quality of their sleep—more quiet sleep occurs during afternoon naps.[106] As the infant matures, there is a decrease in active and an increase in quiet sleep.[32]

Babies have their own clock for sleep-wake, hunger, and feeding/fussy times. These often do not coincide with the family's rhythms and may cause disruption and conflict. The infant's maturity at birth greatly affects his rhythms and development of normal circadian rhythm. A term newborn has innate rhythms and over a period of time (about 18 weeks) develops adult regularity.

In preterm infants, active and quiet sleep are more poorly organized and of shorter duration.[31] Active sleep is "lighter" than quiet sleep—there is more response to stimuli in active sleep.[31] Quiet sleep is a more controlled state and occurs more frequently in term infants than in premature infants. Hence, a third sleep state, transitional sleep, has been identified for the premature infant.[92] This state is characterized by quiet sleep with periods of closed eyes, regular or periodic respirations, no bodily movements, and no rapid eye movement (REM). As the preterm infant matures, he or she spends progressively less time in transitional sleep, has more quiet than active sleep, and has more awake, alert time. However, the preterm who is 40 weeks postconceptional age does not have as well organized sleep patterns as the term newborn.[92]

Sleep disruption may interfere with growth and development by altering neuronal maturation and growth hormone secretion.[90] Human growth hormone has a rhythmic pattern associated with sleep-wake cycles. The highest peaks of growth hormone in infants occur during REM (active) sleep. The fetus (29 to 32 weeks) spends 80% of the time in utero in REM sleep; the term newborn's sleep is 50% REM sleep.[31,32] Since growth hormone secretion is dependent on the regular recurrence of sleep, any disturbance of the sleep-wake cycle results in irregular spikes of growth hormone during a 24-hour period.

An infant whose cycles are discrepant from his family's may be perceived as "difficult." Since this behavior does not fit parental expectations of regular eating/sleeping/eliminating, the parent-child interaction is off to a rocky start. Gradually, through care giving, parents teach the infant synchronization with family rhythms. By 9 months of age the term infant has developed day/night fluctuations that are similar to adult patterns.[29]

TABLE 24-4

Newborn States and Considerations for Care Giving

NEWBORN STATE	COMMENTS

Sleep states
Deep sleep (non-REM sleep)
  Slow state changes
  Regular breathing
  Eyes closed; no eye movements
  No spontaneous activity except startles and
    jerky movements
  Startles with some delay and suppresses
    rapidly
	Baby is very difficult if not impossible to arouse. Baby will not breastfeed or bottle-feed in this state, even after vigorous stimulation. Baby is unable to respond to environment; frustrating for care givers.
	Term babies may exhibit a "slow" heart rate (80-90 beats/min), which may trigger heart rate alarms and result in unnecessary stimulation by NICU staff.
	At birth, preterm infants have altered states of consciousness:
	  No deep sleep or crying state.
	  Early dominant states are light sleep, quiet, and active alert.
	  As maturation occurs, there is an increase in quiet alert.

Light sleep (REM sleep)
  Low activity level
  Random movements and startles
  Respirations irregular and abdominal
  Intermittent sucking movements
  Eyes closed, rapid eye movement
	Full-term infants begin and end sleep in active sleep; preterm infants are more responsive (than term infants) to stimuli in active sleep.
	Babies may cry or fuss briefly in this state and be awakened to feed before they are truly awake and ready to eat.

Awake states
Drowsy or semidozing
  Eyelids fluttering
  Eyes open or closed (dazed)
  Mild startles (intermittent)
  Delayed response to sensory stimuli
  Smooth state change after stimulation
  Fussing may or may not be present
  Respirations—more rapid and shallow
	Baby may awaken further or return to sleep (if left alone). Quietly talking and looking at the baby, or offering a pacifier or an inanimate object to see and listen to may arouse the baby to the quiet alert state.

Modified from Brazelton TB: Neonatal behavioral assessment scale, Philadelphia, 1973, Spastics International Medical Publishers/JB Lippincott Co; and Blackburn S: JOGN Nurs (suppl), p 805, May/June 1983.

Sensory capabilities

At birth, the neonate's senses are fully developed. The newborn is able to communicate—react to and initiate a reaction from those in the environment. As the neonate takes in the sensory information, he begins to associate features of the environment that occur together (i.e., sound, smell, sight, touch of "mother" or "father").[98] Later, a cue (e.g., sound, smell) of the familiar person initiates the newborn's memory.

TACTILE/KINESTHETIC

Touch is the major method of communication for neonates and infants. In utero, fetal existence has been primarily one of movement—within the zero gravity of the amniotic fluid and rhythmic maternal movements. The sense of touch, temperature, and pressure are all well developed, and receptors lie in the newborn's skin. The sensitivity to touch is especially well developed in the face, around the lips (i.e., root reflex), and in the hands (i.e.,

TABLE 24-4—cont'd

Newborn States and Considerations for Care Giving

NEWBORN STATE	COMMENTS
Awake states—cont'd	
Quiet alert, with bright look	Immediately after birth, term newborns exhibit a period of quiet alert, their first opportunity to "take in" their parents and the extrauterine environment. Dimmed lights, quiet talking, and stroking optimize this time for parents.
Focuses attention on source of stimulation	
Impinging stimuli may break through; may have some delay in response	
Minimal motor activity	This is best state for learning to occur, since baby focuses all of attention on visual, auditory, tactile, and sucking stimuli. This is also best state for interaction with parents—baby is maximally able to attend and reciprocally respond to parents.
Active alert—eyes open	Baby has decreased threshold (increased sensitivity) to internal (hunger, fatigue) and external (wet, noise, handling) stimuli. Baby may quiet self, may escalate to crying, or with consolation by caretaker become quiet alert or go to sleep.
Considerable motor activity—thrusting movements of extremities; spontaneous startles	
Reacts to external stimuli with increase in movements and startles (discrete reactions difficult to differentiate because of general higher activity level)	Baby is unable to maximally attend to caretakers or environment because of increased motor activity and increased sensitivity to stimuli.
Respirations irregular	
May or may not be fussy	
Crying—intense and difficult to disrupt with external stimuli	Crying is infant's response to unpleasant internal and/or external stimulation—infant's tolerance limits have been reached (and exceeded). Baby may be able to quiet self with hand-to-mouth behaviors; talking may quiet a crying baby; holding, rocking, or putting baby upright on caretaker's shoulder may quiet infant.
Respirations rapid, shallow, and irregular	

grasp reflex). Since newborns are nonverbal, they pick up messages via the manner in which they are held and handled—by the adult's "body language." Babies are often barometers for adult feelings—if the adult is tired and irritable, the baby knows and may respond with irritability and crying.

Babies love to be held, rocked, and carried—note the soothing effects on the crying infant. Adults do *not* spoil babies by providing this important stimuli. Increased carrying of babies contributes to less crying at 6 weeks of age.[10] In response to being held, infants adjust their body posture to the body of the care giver. Adults describe babies as "cuddly" (comfortable, relaxed curl; snuggles to adult body and attempts to root and/or suck) or "noncuddly" (sprawls, tenses or stiffens, and "pushes away"). The most comforting position for a crying baby is upright on an adult's shoulder.[64] Responsiveness to tactile stimulation has been found to be greater in female than in male neonates.[64]

HEARING

The fetus in utero has heard the voices of mother, father, and siblings from the fifth month of intrauterine life (approximately 20 weeks). These voices are "familiar" to the newborn, so that they "know" their family and are able to differentiate them from the voices of strangers.[26] The ability to hear the outside world, particularly the spoken word, is a prerequisite to further language development.

Neonates with an intact CNS are able to orient and respond to the auditory environment. In response to a sound, the neonate will:

1. Change motor activity (eye blink; decrease in activity, limb movements; head turn)
2. Change heart rate and/or respirations—if the infant is quiet, the heart rate increases with stimuli; if the infant is crying, the heart rate decreases with stimuli
3. Smile
4. Startle or grimace
5. Alert or arouse
6. Cry or cease to cry
7. Stop sucking

The response to sound is dependent on the sound's quality. When frequency and pitch are low, the infant is soothed and distress is decreased; high frequency and pitch alert and distress the infant. Therefore monotonous low-frequency sounds are an auditory soother and pacifier.

Frequencies below 4000 Hz (the range of human speech) produce the most newborn response.[87] Infants are maximally reactive to the human voice in typical speech patterns (rather than disconnected syllables). Infants prefer the high-pitched (such as female) voice over the low-pitched (such as male) voice. Note how adults and children instinctively pitch their voices higher when talking to a baby. Presented with a female and a male voice, the infant always turns toward the female voice. Parents who talk with their babies elicit increasing eye contact with the baby.[9]

Stimuli presented for 5 to 15 seconds elicit the best reaction. Stimuli lasting longer than several minutes are less effective, because the infant habituates to the sound and ceases responding. The ability to habituate to sound is indicative of an intact CNS. Infants will exhibit startle behavior if the stimulus rapidly reaches maximal loudness. A slower time to reach maximal loudness is associated with infant alerting and searching for the stimulus. Infant state is important in evaluation of response to auditory stimuli—light sleep is the optimal state. Infants quiet and soothe in response to rhythmic sounds (rather than disrhythmic ones). Neonates move their bodies in rhythmic synchrony with the spoken word. This ability is called entrainment and is possessed by both children and adults.

VISION

The ability to fix, follow, and alert is indicative of an intact CNS.[79] At birth, babies are able to see an object within 8 to 10 inches of the face (visual acuity of $20/140$).[37] By 45 hours after birth, the neonate is able to distinguish his or her mother's face from that of a stranger.[42] The cradled-in-the-arms position of feeding is the exact distance from the adult's face that the newborn can see. In response to an interesting visual stimulus, neonates stop sucking to look, alert and attend to the object, horizontally scan the object, and fix and follow a moving object in a 90-degree arc. Infants prefer the human face as a visual stimulus, prefer a patterned over a nonpatterned stimulus, and attend longer to larger patterns with more complex patterns and angles.[37,42] Babies are probably able to discriminate color but prefer black and white because of the greater contrast and will focus on the outside of a figure, where the contrast is the greatest.[79,80] Newborns are sensitive to bright light and will tightly close their eyes in its presence. They prefer moderate, diffuse lighting. Presentation of visual stimuli enables development of the neural pattern for vision. During the baby's first year of life, visual investigation of the environment is a primary mode of learning.

SMELL/TASTE[69,102]

Olfaction is well developed at birth. At 5 days of age, the neonate is able to differentiate his or her mother's breast pad and demonstrates a preference for the smell over that of a "stranger." The infant's response to pleasant odors is to arouse and suck. After several presentations of the stimuli, the infant will habituate to the odor. Babies withdraw from unpleasant odors such as vinegar and ammonia. They are also able to differentiate tastes, preferring sweet solutions and refusing bitter, acid, and sour substances. Asphyxiated infants demonstrate a loss of olfaction that parallels the suppressing of brainstem reflexes and activities.

COMMUNICATION SKILLS

The neonate's ability to communicate is a naturally endowed survival skill. Crying is the infant's language to communicate needs. Crying may also be a response to the environment—noisy, cold, overstimulating, multiple caretaking, or lack of synchrony. Since the cry brings someone to meet the need, the infant soon learns that the caretaker gives attention and the world is a trustworthy place. The more responsive the caretaker is to the infant's crying, thus the infant's needs, the less crying behavior is necessary.[10] Learning occurs as the infant associates comfort with the caretaker. The temperament of the individual baby and his or her ability to habituate to disturbing stimuli influence the amount of crying behavior. Tension of the caretaker and/or the environment is communicated nonverbally to the infant and may potentiate or contribute to the infant's crying.

The amount and tone of the newborn's cry is influenced by birth weight, gestational age, and the events of birth. Types of cries include birth cry, hunger cry, pain cry, and pleasure cry. The newborn's cry physiologically affects the mother—her breasts change and prepare to nurse. Brazelton has shown that many infants exhibit crying cycles for as much as 1¾ to 2¾ hours a day by the second to sixth week of life.[17] Neonates possess a repertoire of self-quieting behaviors when in a fussy state: (1) hand-to-mouth efforts, (2) sucking on fist or tongue, and (3) use of visual and/or auditory stimuli from the environment.[18]

The neonatal cry may be diagnostic of existing conditions or trauma. CNS insult often results in a high-pitched, shrill cry. The pain cry of asphyxiated newborns differs significantly from that of healthy term infants.[78]

The smiling infant is a joy to the care giver. Smiling is a learned response to the presentation of the human face. The ability to smile appears by the age of 2 to 6 weeks of life.[35] A smile is most easily elicited by the stimulus of a moving, smiling human face. There is a direct relationship between gestational age and the age of smiling.[44] The ability to learn to smile may begin before 40 weeks in the preterm infant exposed to en face stimuli.[44] The social implications of the smile include positive feedback to the care giver that the baby is happy and contented, which results in parental feelings of adequacy and competence.

ENVIRONMENT
Prenatal environment

In utero, preonates are totally dependent on their mother's health and well-being for their own. It is through her that they receive the nurturance, housing, and stimulation to develop their body, their sensory organs, and the rudiments of their personality and temperament.

SENSORY CAPABILITIES AND MEMORY

In utero, human sensory organs are developed and used by preonates. Tactile stimulation in utero includes a continuous bath of amniotic fluid, the rhythmic movements of the mother, and the flexion of the fetal position. As the fetus grows, it is able to touch the uterine walls, expanding the tactile kinesthetic, and vestibular experience through additional stimuli. In the last trimester the fetus receives continuous tactile stimuli as its body fills the uterine cavity, it is in constant contact with the uterine walls, and it feels where its world starts and stops.

After 20 weeks gestation, the human cochlea has normal adult function. Within the uterus, the fetus is able to hear the maternal heart beat at the sound level of 72 to 85 dB (a noise level "too loud" for environmental noise).[87] Extrauterine sounds such as traffic, music, and family voices are heard and responded to in utero.

Eye development begins at 22 days after conception. The eyelids fuse at about 10 weeks and remain fused till about the twenty-sixth week of gestation. At birth, photoreceptors are developed, but maturation is not complete for several months. The fetus is able to distinguish light from dark and recoils from a bright light shone at the mother's abdomen.

The development and function of taste buds in utero have been documented. The fetus increases its amniotic fluid consumption when saccharine is added to the fluid and decreases consumption with the injection of distasteful substances.[16] Taste may be a way the fetus monitors the intrauterine environment.[16]

Studies have suggested that preonates exhibit memory.[26,27] Newborns who had been read a particular story while in utero responded to the story reread to them after birth with a recognition and attentiveness that was not exhibited in response to unfamiliar stories.[26,27] Prebirth consciousness and memory have appeared in hypnotic and psychotherapeutic regressive research.[23]

INTRAUTERINE COMMUNICATION AND INFLUENCES ON DEVELOPMENT

The development, organization, and function of the preonate's sensory systems are influenced by the mother's psychophysioemotional constitution and personality. The quantity and intensity of the environmental stressors a pregnant woman experiences impact directly on her preonate's intrauterine and postpartal health and well-being. Continuous interpersonal tension during pregnancy is associated with increased morbidity for the infant.[110]

Three developmental stages in the communication process between preonates and their mothers have been described: physiologic, behavioral, and sympathetic.[112] Physiologic communication occurs during the first trimester when organ systems are being developed. Under stress, neurohormonal substances such as catecholamines and adrenocorticotropic hormone (ACTH) are secreted. Via the placenta these substances transmit the mother's emotional responses and imprint them within the preonate's "memory."[118] Thus a stressful experience has the same effect on the preonate and will elicit the same emotional response within the preonate that it does on the mother.

The mother's neurohormonal secretions also influence the development of the preonate's hypothalamus, endocrine system, and autonomic nervous system. Stress hormones impact on the developing hypothalamus, which sends messages to the autonomic nervous system to deal with the stress. Prolonged exposure of the developing hypothalamus and autonomic system to chronic maternal stress alters and impairs their organization and functioning.[118] Postpartally, these impairments will manifest as gastrointestinal and emotional (severe depression or anxiety) disorders.

Behavioral communication occurs during the second trimester when the preonate is sufficiently developed that its movements are felt by the mother. Maternal emotional stress or a sudden, loud noise will elicit a kicking (behavioral) response. Mothers often initiate communication with their preonates by rubbing and talking to their abdomen.

Sympathetic communication occurs during the last trimester, includes the two previous levels of communication, and adds an emotional/intuitive level. An interactional process occurring on a feeling level without the use of rational processes, sympathetic communication enables mothers and preonates to be sensitive to each other on a deep, subtle level. This emotional/intuitive type of communication has been described as the "meta" level of communication, a transmission of actual intention, feelings, and reality of situation and people (i.e., the meaning behind the words).[53] The message is transmitted through body language, voice tones, and the emotional affect of those communicating.

As a result of these intrauterine interactions, a reciprocal relationship of bonding is established. The quality of the relationship is dependent on the nature of the dynamics between mother and preonate. If the interaction has been good (i.e., the mother desires the baby throughout the stressors of pregnancy), then the bonding will be good. If the interaction has been negative (i.e., mother does not want/rejects the baby or is chronically inundated with major stressors), the bonding will not be good, resulting in some degree of postpartal behavioral, psychologic, or physiologic problems.[110]

Intrapartal environment

Birth is a major transition from physiologic dependence to physiologic independence. At term, the neonate's physiologic systems are developed, sensory organs function, and the rudiments of personality and temperament are established. Since they do not have defense mechanisms to deal with the bombardment of stimuli at birth, neonates are more open, receptive, and vulnerable.[48] Birth is disorienting and disruptive. The amount of disruption depends on the degree of trauma incurred during the labor and birth process. This experience is analogous to foreign travel in which an adult is confused and disoriented in a strange land and attempts to discover the familiar as a frame of reference.[48]

The physiologic changes of labor produce stress in the mother that is communicated (via neurohormonal secretions) to the fetus.[12,58,118] Not having a support system compounds the stress, often escalating it beyond the mother's tolerance and coping skills. Anxious and fearful women have longer labors and more delivery complications than women who are confident about themselves and their infants.[67] The recent shift toward family-centered birth enables mothers to receive support from their families, to be an active participant in the birth process, and to have immediate contact with their newborns.

Family-centered trends are both psychologically and physiologically sound for mothers and their babies. Physiologic adjustment to extrauterine life may be facilitated by maternal caretaking—rocking, cuddling, visual and verbal interaction, and nonnutritive suckling.[60,98,118] Likewise, the neonate contributes to the physiologic stability of the new mother by oxytocin and prolactin release with breastfeeding. Psychologically,

parental reactions and attitudes regarding the birth influence their interactions with the infant. Children with behavior disorders more often have a history of obstetric complications and prematurity. Parental feelings toward the infant have also been correlated with (1) the severity of the infant's illness at birth, (2) the mode of delivery, and (3) the interval between birth and parental first contact with the infant.[28]

Oxytocin stimulates labor contractions and induces neonatal amnesia (for the traumatic intensity of the process).[11,118] An uncomplicated delivery in which the mother is alert and minimally stressed (i.e., feels in charge of her delivery, is able to work with the contractions, is receiving emotional support) provides a birth passage with minimum neonatal trauma. When a mother feels afraid, alone, anxious, and unsupported, she produces the stress hormone ACTH, which stimulates memory.[58] ACTH overrides the amnesiac effect of oxytocin, causing the intense sensations of the birthing process to be physioemotionally imprinted within the neonate.[58,118] Thus one's birth experience influences "the foundations of human personality."[118]

The neonate is also influenced by medications and the events of labor and birth (see Chapter 2). Maternal medications for analgesia and anesthesia affect neonatal behaviors, resulting in decreased sucking ability, lethargy, and decreased habituation. Medicated babies are less able to evoke caretaker behaviors such as smiling, touching, and vocalization. They also give less feedback to their parents than unmedicated babies. The parents may feel rejected, tend to stimulate the infant less, and thus begin a pattern of aberrant interaction.

At birth the neonate no longer experiences the world as closeness and security, but as endless space. Note the naked newborn startle and Moro in the "freedom" of space—the newborn no longer knows where his or her world starts and stops. The force of gravity, cold, bright lights, unfamiliar voices/sounds, and antiseptic smells are diametrically opposed to the sensations within the uterus. Children birthed in a nonstressed, warm, dimly lit environment with immediate skin-to-skin contact and slow adjustment to the extrauterine environment have been found to be happy, alert, curious, more self-sufficient and relaxed, and quicker learners.[60,98,118]

Postnatal environment

Home and family are the primary medium through which newborns (1) reestablish their biorhythmic balance, (2) stabilize themselves in the extrauterine world, (3) develop a sense of self and mastery in the world, and (4) become socialized as human beings. Socialization teaches the adaptive psychosocial skills necessary for survival and functioning in society. Cultural and family values, behavioral expression, and ways of meeting social-emotional needs are learned within the family. Thus home/family environment is considered to be a "normalized" environment for human development.

CARETAKER FACTORS

A dyadic relationship exists between the caretaker and the infant—the behavior of one reinforces the behavior of the other. The infant's physical and emotional needs are satisfied by caretakers. Depending on their ability to perceive and receive ministrations, infants respond to their caretakers, who receive emotional satisfaction. Parental expectations have a major impact on their perceptions and their behavior, and ultimately affect the child's development. Parents must work out the discrepancy between the wished-for and the actual child, especially if the baby is preterm, ill, or anomalied. How attached the parents are to the baby influences their relationship to and ability to care for their infant (see Chapter 22). If the pregnancy has failed to produce a normal, healthy baby, the parents must grieve the loss of their expectations. Parents are unable to attach and caretake for the baby until they have completed their grief work (see Chapter 23).

A caretaker and infant have a reciprocal interaction when their cycles and signals are synchronized with each other. The biorhythmic cycle of the newborn has been in synchrony with one person (mother) while in utero, and the infant is accustomed to her cycles and rhythms for developing adaptive behavior. Mothers are more sensitive to the cues of their newborns and are more easily able to meet their needs than other care providers (including fathers and siblings).[39] Consistent maternal caretaking enables newborns to regulate their rhythms to the mother's and begin adapting to the postnatal environment. From her, they expand their adaptation to the family, and to the larger world of society.[39]

Experience in relating to infants does influence the caretaker's efficiency in interpretation and sensitivity to infant cues. Multiparous women have more sensitivity to infant cues than do primiparous mothers. Mothers with little or no experience exhibit more difficulty in quieting a crying baby. Maternal responses to infant cues include[19]:

1. Adjustment of her rhythm to the infant's cues for attention and withdrawal; adding her cues when the infant is receptive. This approach increases the amount of time the infant engages in eye contact with the mother.

2. Failure to decrease her stimulation although the infant's rhythm has changed or the infant has withdrawn. This approach increases the time the infant looks away and decreases the infant's attention to her cues when the baby does look at her.

3. Attempting to establish her own rhythm with that of the infant—there is an increase/decrease in stimuli that is out of phase with the infant. This approach may result in shortened, unsatisfying patterns of interaction.

Consistency in maternal responses is especially important as the infant learns the accepted patterns of cues from the caretaker. Cared for by one or two people, the infant is able to develop synchrony with and expectations of the parents. Single caretaking improves establishment of biorhythms for sleep-wake cycles, feeding, and visual attentiveness.[28,111] Consistent cues soon elicit a consistency of response from the infant. Consistency and promptness of maternal response result in less infant crying during the first year of life.[11] A predictable and responsive environment enables the infant to progress to varied types of communication (not just crying). Care by parents provides for mutual cuing and mastery of the environment through interaction. Inconsistent cues distress and confuse the infant. Multiple caretaking confuses the infant, increases distress with feeding, causes irritability, and upsets visual attention.[28,111] Consistency, communication, and interaction during care providing significantly affect the nature, quality, and normality/abnormality of infant development.

Regardless of how stable or unstable, consistent or inconsistent it is, family life has a rhythm, synchronicity, and predictability of its own. Through interaction with parents and siblings, infants develop their ability to form relationships. From these primary relationships, the foundation and format for other relationships are established. The quality of subsequent relationships is dependent on the quality of the relationship experienced within the primary family from birth throughout infancy.[50]

NEONATAL FACTORS

The neonate is not a passive recipient of the environment of the family, but is an active participant in shaping that environment. Infants send cues about their ability and readiness for interpersonal interactions. As described by Brazelton,[19] infants interact differently with persons than with inanimate objects (Figure 24-1). The excitement generated by interpersonal interaction is seen in the infant's arm and leg movements, bodily movement toward the other person, smiling, vocalizing, and increased visual attention. Because of the infant's immaturity, he or she is unable to maintain a continuous interaction. The infant attends for short periods and then turns away to decrease excitement and protect himself or herself from bombardment by overwhelming stimuli. Mater-

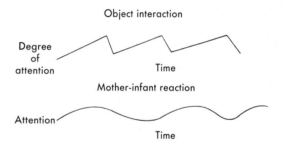

Figure 24-1. Interaction pattern with object and with mother. Object interaction is characterized by abrupt attention, excitement phases followed by sudden and abrupt looking away. Interaction with person is cyclical and involves initiation of interaction, orientation to person, acceleration of excitement, peak of excitement, deceleration of excitement, and withdrawal or turning away. (From Brazelton TB, Koslowski B, and Main M: The origins of reciprocity: the early mother-infant interaction. In Lewis M and Rosenblum LA, editors: The effect of the infant on its caregiver, New York, 1974, John Wiley & Sons, Inc.)

nal/care provider sensitivity to the attention-withdrawal cycle of interaction enables the adult to modulate her behavior in synchrony with the infant's cues. Successful interaction with an infant includes reading the baby's cues, responding appropriately, and not overwhelming the baby with too much stimulation (thus overstepping the baby's tolerance for interaction). Overwhelming the infant results in his or her withdrawal for progressively longer periods of time in order to protect himself or herself from overstimulating and insensitive others.[19]

Just as the parent has expectations, the infant also has expectations of the relationship. The infant expects relief or protection from painful experiences, maintenance of comfort, and homeostasis. Relief from the discomforts of hunger, cold, sleeplessness, and boredom enable the infant to respond positively to the care provider.

Care-eliciting behaviors are those neonatal cues used to signal the caretaker that attention is needed. Crying, visual following, and smiling are care eliciting. Newborn responses to care include

TABLE 24-5

Stages and Characteristics of Behavioral Organization in Preterm Infants

ALS ET AL*	GORSKI†
Physiologic homeostasis—stabilizing and integrating temperature control, cardiorespiratory function, digestion, and elimination. Characteristics: becomes pale, dusky, cyanotic, heart and respiratory rates change—all symptoms of disorganization of autonomic nervous system.	"In turning"—physiologic stage of mere survival characterized by autonomic nervous system responses to stimuli (rapid color changes due to swings in heart and respiratory rates); no or limited direct response; inability to arouse self spontaneously; jerky movements; asleep (and protecting the CNS from sensory overload) 97% of the time. Preterms (<32 weeks) are easily physiologically overwhelmed by stimuli.
Motor development may infringe on physiologic homeostasis, resulting in defensive strategies (vomiting, color change, apnea, and bradycardia). State development becomes less diffuse and encompasses full range: sleep, awake, crying. States and state changes may impact on physiologic/motor stability.	"Coming out"—first active response to environment may be seen as early as 34-35 weeks (provided some physiologic stability has been achieved). Characteristics: remains pink with stimuli; has directed response for short periods; arouses spontaneously and maintains arousal after stimuli ceases; if interaction begins in alert state: maintains quiet alert for 5-10 min, tracks animate/inanimate stimuli; spends 10%-15% of time in alert state with predictable interaction patterns.
Alert state is well differentiated from other states; may interfere with physiologic/motor stability.	"Reciprocity"—active interaction and reciprocity with environment from 36-40 weeks. Characteristics: directs response; arouses and consoles self; maintains alertness and interacts with both animate and inanimate objects; copes with external stress.

*Modified from Als H et al: Am Acad Child Psychiatry 2D:239, 1981.
†Modified from Gorski PA: Semin Perinatol 3:61, 1979.

quieting, suckling, clinging and cuddling, looking, smiling, and vocalizing. These social interactions positively reward the care provider and encourage and promote continued care. Infant characteristics that modify maternal attitudes include (1) a healthy or sickly infant; (2) an attractive, pretty baby or infant with obvious congenital anomaly; (3) a premature infant; (4) a calm and contented or fussy, irritable infant; (5) an infant responsive to or rejecting of maternal care. A maternal/care provider's ability to soothe the infant reinforces a feeling of success (or failure) in her feelings of competence.

The infant's sex also affects the cues and the care giver's response. Male infants exhibit more startles, more muscle activity, and more physical strength. In response, they receive more holding from care givers as a means of soothing.[64] Females exhibit more tactile and oral sensitivity, more smiling, and more responsivity to sweet taste. As a result, girls are more often soothed by talking, eye-to-eye contact, and a pacifier.[64]

The infant's level of neurophysiologic development influences the appropriateness of maternal/caretaking behaviors. The neurologically mature term baby who has already mastered autonomic, motoric, and state regulation is able to actively elicit and respond to caretaking behaviors.[3,39] Because of the immaturity of the CNS, the preterm infant lags behind the term baby in care eliciting and responsivity to the care provider. Als and Brazelton[3,20] have proposed a hierarchy of levels of organization in the developing infant. Gorski et al[50] have proposed stages of behavioral organization that describe the responses of preterm infants to their environment (both stimuli and caretakers) (Table 24-5). Since the young preterm infant's priority is mere survival, interaction with the environment and care providers is at the expense of physiologic stability. Since the preterm infant sends different cues than the term baby, knowledge of these stages enables caretakers to modulate their behavior and the environment. Whereas overwhelming the term baby results in withdrawal from interaction, overwhelming the preterm infant first results in a real threat to physiologic survival, then to withdrawal from interaction.

Since preterm infants are not as neurologically mature as term infants, the Brazelton Neonatal Behavioral Assessment Scale has little value with this population. Therefore Als and Brazelton[2] have devised a behavioral assessment scale for preterm infants, Assessment of Preterm Infant's Behavior (APIB), which assesses five developmental lines: autonomic, motor, state, attentional-interactive, and self-regulatory. This examination delineates the quality and duration of the preterm infant's response, the difficulty in eliciting the response, and the effort and cost to the preterm infant of achieving and maintaining a response. Since it, too, is an interactive test, the nature and amount of organization provided by the care provider is an indication of the preterm infant's lack of integrative skill. As the preterm infant matures and advances in development of organization, he or she is more able to interact with the environment (animate and inanimate). However, it must be remembered that this maturation process is "uneven"—as the preterm infant advances in one area of development, he or she may become, at least temporarily, more vulnerable (i.e., experience difficulties) in other areas such as physiologic stability.[50]

INTERVENTIONS

Life in a special care nursery is characterized by sensory deprivation of normal stimuli that the preterm infant would have experienced in the womb and that term babies would experience at home with their families. However, the NICU is also an environment of sensory bombardment—constant noise, light, and tactile stimulation; intrusive, invasive procedures; upset of sleep-wake cycles; multiple caretakers; etc. The impact of this environment is the focus of speculation, controversy, and recent research.[51]

Focus has changed from applying blanket infant stimulation to assessing the individual infant and deciding what types of interventions to facilitate development are needed.[25,116] Rather than too much or too little stimulation, infants in the NICU receive an inappropriate pattern of stimulation[40]—noncontingent, nonreciprocal, painful (rather than pleasant), multiple stimuli, etc. Since the immature CNS of the premature infant is unable to tolerate these stimuli, the easily overstimulated preterm infant protects himself or herself by physiologic and interactional defensive maneuvers that threaten survival and social ability and may lead to lifelong maladaptations.[31] Recent research has shown medical and developmental benefits to very low birth weight (VLBW) (<1250 g, <28 weeks gestation; <1800 g) infants from individualized behavioral and environmental care in the NICU.[5,97]

Preterm infants are not the only infants at risk from the stress of overstimulation in the NICU. Sick or anomalied term infants and chronically ill infants with prolonged hospitalization also experience stress.[52] The term infant with persistent pulmonary hypertension (see Chapter 17) is particularly vulnerable to repeated handling, procedures, and interventions that decrease PaO_2. Thus these infants are managed on a minimal intervention regimen—care is organized, coordinated, and individualized to decrease noxious stimuli and physical manipulations. The chronically ill infant with bronchopulmonary dysplasia (BPD) has been shown to improve when behavioral/environmental changes were initiated.[5,79,83] The term small-for-gestational-age (SGA) infant is sleepy and not alert in the first few weeks of life, which may result in the infant's being left alone or overstimulated to awaken for interaction.[4] After a few weeks, these infants become very irritable, fussy, and disorganized in spontaneous and social behaviors. Anticipatory guidance, reassurance that the disorganization is in the baby rather than a result of parental care, and practical intervention strategies enable the parents to shape the environment and the baby's response.[4,50]

The ultimate goal of intervention strategies in the NICU is to facilitate and promote infant growth and development and thus task mastery. Establishing biorhythmic balance and physiologic homeostasis is necessary for survival and is enhanced by a sensitive, responsive NICU environment. An unresponsive environment may so stress the preterm infant that apnea, bradycardia, and other physiologic instabilities severely compromise and prolong recovery.[3,49,50,52] For the hospitalized infant, development of the sense of self and trust is undermined by noncontingent stimulation that prevents a sense of competence and control of the environment from being established.[51] When the ventilated baby experiences hunger or is wet, he or she is unable to signal the care provider with a cry because of the tube. Thus the infant experiences a need, but is unable to signal and bring care and relief. The baby soon learns that he or she is not in control of the situation. Another intubated infant may be quietly asleep and not experiencing a need; yet it is "care time," so the nurse moves, wakes, changes, and generally disturbs the baby. This baby also soon learns about not being in control of the situation.

Hospitalized infants, especially those with prolonged stays, may exhibit the classic signs of institutionalized infants and/or infants suffering from maternal deprivation[46,107] (Table 24-6). It is the goal of "environmental neonatology"[51] to prevent this maladaptive behavior by altering the NICU to be more developmentally appropriate

TABLE 24-6

Classic Signs of "Hospitalitis"

Asocial affect
Gaze aversion—fleeting glances at caretaker with inability to maintain eye contact
Flat affect—social unresponsiveness (little fixing and following; smiling) to caretaker
Little/no quiet alert state—baby abruptly changes state and often is described as "either asleep or awake and crying" (crying is only "awake" state); out-of-control crying

Touch aversion*
Becomes hypotonic or hypertonic with caretaking or attempts at socialization
Fights, flails, and resists being cared for or held
Aversive responses (see Table 24-8) to caretaking or holding persist

Feeding difficulties
Have multiple origins, including delayed onset of oral feedings; touch aversion around mouth secondary to invasive procedures; multiple caretakers; feeding on schedule, rather than demand
Rumination syndrome—voluntary regurgitation, a form of self-comfort and gratification when environment is not nurturing or gratifying[104]

Failure to thrive
Poor or no weight gain despite adequate caloric intake
Develops mental delays (language, motor, social, emotional)

Data from Gardner LI: Sci Am 227(1):76, 1982; and Spitz R: Psychoanal Study Child 1:53, 1945.
*Baby associates human touch with pain.

for infants. Normalizing the environment begins with an assessment of the stimulation to which the individual baby is exposed. The type (i.e., noxious versus pleasant; contingent versus noncontingent), amount, and timing of stimulation should be noted. To decrease noxious stimuli, no infant should have "routine" care (e.g., all infants are suctioned every 2 hours; all infants have a Dextrostix test every 4 hours).[5,50] Care should be individualized by asking the questions: "Why are we doing this procedure?" and "Is this procedure necessary for *this* baby's care?" Overstimulation in the NICU occurs when procedures (81% to 94% of all contacts are medical/nursing procedures, an average of 40 to 132 times per day) are performed; it does *not* result from social interaction with parents.[51] Painful, invasive procedures that are not vital to the individual baby are stress-producing events that should be eliminated. Rest may be the most important environmental change.

The preonate in utero and the term baby at home relate to a minimum of caretakers and thus need to learn one or only a few sets of cues.[47,111] Multiple caretakers in the NICU confuse the infant by providing many care-related cues for the infant to learn—many techniques of handling and many emotional, nonverbal messages to decode. Primary nursing minimizes the number of care providers, since the primary nurse and one or two associates always (or as much as possible) care for the infant; assess, revise, and write the care plan; and coordinate care. Primary nursing also adds consistency and continuity for parents.

The infant's state or level of arousal provides an appropriate context for caretaking. Some babies exhibit a low threshold to stimuli—they are easily overwhelmed and fatigued. Others, with a higher threshold, are quieter, more difficult to arouse, initiate less, and thus receive less interaction.[11] Organizing care to be reciprocal to the baby's state reinforces the infant's competence in signaling a need (sense of self) and having it met (sense of trust). As the infant matures, feeding on demand rather than on a schedule not only teaches this valuable lesson, but also increases absorption and utilization of caloric intake.[31,50] If the baby is asleep, ask: "Do we need to do this now? Would another time be better?" In some centers physicians make an appointment with the nurse to examine the baby—at a time that is optimal for the baby.

Since preterm infants exhibit short duration of state cycles until around 38 weeks, they have decreased tolerance for stimuli. Some preterm infants tolerate all care done at once and long periods of rest; others do not and need care spread out to decrease overstimulation and decompensation. Even "premie growers" may be unable to tolerate more than one stimuli at a time—they feed best if visual, auditory, and social stimuli are not provided until *after* the feeding. As the baby matures and is able to tolerate integrated experience, multimodal stimuli are provided.

Alterations in the individual infant's daily schedule are made to accommodate a more flexible or structured schedule—whichever is better for the baby.[51] Assessing the infant before, during, and after an interaction/intervention guides the care provider in adapting care and the environment to the individual baby (Table 24-7). Table 24-8 outlines physiologic and behavioral cues indicative of readiness to interact (approach) and avoidance behaviors indicative of sensory overload. An intubated preterm infant cared for in an NICU with a strict suction "routine" every 2 hours responds with profound cyanosis, lowered $TcPO_2$/lowered pulse oximetry, and bradycardia, and requires bagging after every suction (with no secretions obtained)—an obviously unnecessary and stressful intervention. In a less rigid, more individualized care setting, that same infant may signal the need for suction by becoming restless, by a decrease in oxygenation, and/or by heart rate changes (tachycardia or bradycardia). Suctioning improves the infant's condition—the baby lies quietly, has improved oxygenation, and the heart pattern stabilizes. This infant has signaled his or her need, and the care providers have read the cues and responded with a stabilizing intervention—the baby has *not* been stressed by an unnecessary procedure.

Knowledgeable professionals are able to role model for and teach parents how to relate to their premature infant. Parents are taught to recognize and use infant states to maximize interaction. The drowsy premature infant may be unable to engage in eye-to-eye contact with the parents or be able to sustain it for too short (for the parents) a period of time. Waiting until the baby is more awake to initiate eye contact will be more rewarding to the

TABLE 24-7

Parameters for Assessing Interaction/Intervention with Neonates

Before

Gather baseline data *before* touching the baby
  Gestational age and postconceptional age
  Diagnosis
  Level of physiologic homeostasis
    Previous vital signs
    Oxygenation state—(continuous pulse oximetry
      or transcutaneous monitor)
  Neonatal state
    Sleep—deep, light, drowsy
    Awake—quiet alert, active alert, crying
    Approach behaviors ⎫
    Avoidance behaviors ⎭ see Table 24-8

During

Gently and as nonintrusively as possible assess
  physiologic and behavioral signs *during* intervention
  Level of (current) physiologic homeostasis: vital
    signs and changes
    Observation (without touching baby)—color,
      posture, general appearance, respiratory rate,
      temperature (skin, incubator), blood pressure

(transducer), oxygenation (from continuous
  monitor)
  Quiet (with minimal disturbance)—ausculate
    heart, lungs, and abdomen; axillary tempera-
    ture, blood pressure (cuff); head-to-toe
    assessment; oxygenation (saturation decreases
    with stressful, disturbing stimuli)
Neonatal state change
  Sleep—deep, light, drowsy
  Awake—quiet alert, active alert, crying
  Approach behaviors ⎫
  Avoidance behaviors ⎭ see Table 24-8

After

Assess physiologic and behavioral signs *after*
  intervention
  Level of physiologic homeostasis
    Vital signs—returned to baseline values? More/
      less stable than baseline values?
  Neonatal state change—return to baseline state?
    To a higher state? Unable to be consoled? More
    consolable left alone?

---

parent and less stressful to the baby. Role model for parents that this baby is an individual and, even though premature, is able to signal for more or less stimuli (Table 24-8).

The preterm infant who is lightly touched may startle, jerk, or withdraw from parental touch. In response, the parent suddenly and sadly pulls his or her hand away and is reticent to touch the baby again. Intervention includes helping parents read cues and learn appropriate responses to their baby. The baby may be interpreted to the parents: "Jamie likes firm touch . . . like this." Teach parents how to recognize a stressed baby and how to intervene. The prime rule of relating to infants is: the baby leads; the adult follows.

Feeding the premature infant may be difficult, since the baby "goes to sleep" or "gets lazy" during feedings. The usual parental ministrations of talk-ing to the baby, soothing with touch, or holding upright on the shoulder may not work with a fussy, irritable preterm infant. The preterm infant's be-havior may be so disorganized, unpredictable, or misunderstood by the parents that an appropriate response is not possible.[2,50] Thus parents often become exhausted, bewildered, and frustrated in their encounters with their preterm infants. Par-ents may define the preterm infant's behavioral response to their care as rejecting and unloving: "My baby doesn't like me."[39,60] Teach parents that their baby's disorganization with stimuli is due to prematurity (i.e., an immature CNS) and *not* to parent ministrations. Reassure them that as the premature infant grows and evidences matura-tional changes, he or she will be able to tolerate more stimulation and will be more responsive to their care.

TABLE 24-8

Approach versus Avoidance Behaviors

APPROACH BEHAVIORS	AVOIDANCE BEHAVIORS
Physiologic	
Cardiorespiratory changes: decrease in heart and/or respiration rate; regular, slow respirations	Cardiorespiratory changes: increase or decrease in respiratory rate; irregular respirations; apnea; increased blood pressure; sneezing, hiccoughs, coughing, sighing
	Color changes: cyanosis—central or generalized mottling or duskiness; pallor or plethora
	Gastrointestinal changes: abdominal distention; spitting up, vomiting; gagging; stooling
Behavioral	
Quieting of body movement	State changes
Self-quieting behaviors: hand to mouth, hand clasping, finger folding, sucking; decrease in extremity movement	Facial—wide-eyed "help me" look; frowning, grimacing; hypotonia; yawning; startles; averted gaze; tongue thrusting
Attentive behaviors: alert gaze, fixing and following visual stimuli, ceasing to suck/slowing of sucking rate, turning toward auditory stimuli	Neuromuscular—arching and flailing movements; hypertonia; tremors, jerkiness; startles; finger splaying—"stop sign"
Imitation: mouth opening; tongue extension; vocalizing, cooing, babbling	

Modified from Als H et al: J Am Acad Child Psychiatry 20:239, 1981.

Just as parent-infant interaction is responsible for normal development of the term baby, parent-infant interaction is crucial in the development of at-risk infants. Many parents of premature infants have been observed making heroic efforts, over long periods of time, to interact with their less alert, active, and responsive babies.[49,50] "Setting parents up to succeed" involves placing parents in situations where they will experience positive feedback from their infants. Suggesting and role-modeling intervention strategies show parents what and how to play and interact with their babies. Parent participation in intervention/stimulation strategies is assured by stressing how important it is to infant development, that professionals are too busy to provide all the stimulation necessary, and that they are in a unique position to provide developmental care in the hospital and at home after discharge. Parents (with help from professionals) are the ideal planners and providers of developmentally appropriate intervention strategies.

Rooming-in of parents and their at-risk newborns is the best environment for cues to be learned and care given according to these cues. Unlimited and unrestricted contact of parents and newborns should be the policy in every normal, medium, and high-risk nursery. Providing a "family room," "bonding room," or "apartment" where parents and their soon-to-be-discharged newborn can room in helps the transition from hospital to home care.

Intervention strategies

Since infants experience their environment through sensory capabilities, intervention strategies are based on tactile/kinesthetic, auditory, visual, olfactory/gustatory, and communication skills. Interventions must be individualized according to the infant's state, sensory threshold, physiologic homeostasis, and approach/avoidance cues.

CIRCADIAN RHYTHMS

In utero, the states of the fetus are regulated by the sleep-wake cycles of the mother. In the NICU multiple intrusions disrupt regulation; how this impacts on the infant is not fully known, although limited energy may be drained and the infant subjected to further stress.[2,51,52] To minimize interruptions and excessive handling, babies should not be awakened when asleep; if they must be awakened for care, it should be during active sleep.[31] Appointments for examinations should be made before feeding to decrease unnecessary disturbance of sleep but with enough rest time (if needed) before actual feeding.

Adequate numbers of caretaking encounters—physical assessment, vital signs, diaper/linen change, procedures—must be balanced against constant manipulations.[5,50] Since essentially all NICU (level II and III) babies are continuously monitored, "laying on of hands" every 1 to 2 hours is often unnecessary. Thorough physical assessment and vital sign recording every 4 hours is easily alternated with recordings from the monitors every 4 hours—thus the baby is evaluated every 2 hours but *not* disturbed that often. An acutely ill baby may need closer observation, but alternating "hands on" with monitor readings accomplishes the goal without overwhelming a baby with few reserves.

Day/night cycles are facilitated by afternoon nap time and nighttime in which the dimming of lights or covering of incubators and cribs with blankets and quieting of NICU noise enables babies to sleep. Deep, quiet sleep is facilitated by quiet and dark, soft (classical) music, gentle stroking of the head, and self-regulated task (self-sought proximity of infant to breathing bear).[112] Maintaining daily nap time and nighttime hours helps babies reset their diurnal rhythms and become accustomed to sleeping in dim light and a quiet environment (something that babies discharged from the hospital for even short stays have difficulty doing).

TACTILE/KINESTHETIC INTERVENTION

Since the sense of touch is highly developed in utero, even the very immature preterm has acute tactile sensitivity. For the newborn, human touch is the most important tactile stimulation. Tactile sensation both arouses and quiets—gentle but firm handling quiets babies, since they feel more secure; light, uncertain touch often results in agitation and withdrawal.

In the NICU babies who are repeatedly subjected to painful, intrusive procedures develop touch aversion—the association of human touch with pain. These infants cry uncontrollably, squirm away, flail arms and legs, and recoil when touched—knowing that pain will soon follow. The infant who was ventilated may have touch aversion around the mouth—the infant is averse to facial stroking and rooting, has a hypersensitive gag reflex, and refuses to nipple feed. Painful procedures should be minimized to those absolutely (medically) indicated—*no* baby should be subjected to "routine" painful procedures. During those necessary procedures, providing body containment, comfort measures (like a pacifier), and adequate pain relief (see Chapter 21) is essential.

Noncaretaking touch (i.e., social contact) should be provided by parents and professionals when the preterm infant is able to tolerate it.[41] Nonpainful touch such as stroking (the head, trunk, or hands) during care calms, soothes, and helps prevent touch aversion. If the preterm becomes more agitated with stroking, a hand firmly placed on the head or trunk often quiets. Additional stroking of stable preterm infants has been associated with increased activity, a faster regaining of birth weight, less crying, and better social scores.[64-66,98] As the preterm infant matures, head-to-toe massage (with lotion or vitamin E oil) at the rate of 12 to 16 strokes/min (for respiratory

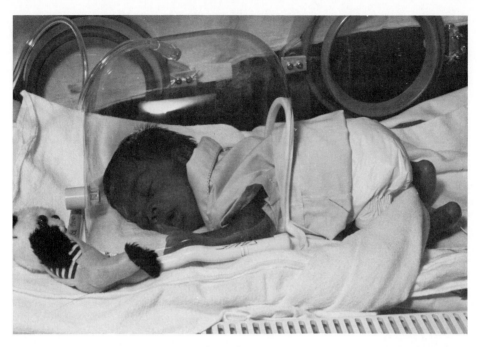

Figure 24-2. Preterm infant in oxygen hood that is large enough to accommodate upper body—to facilitate hand-to-mouth behavior. Note sling that helps maintain flexion without frog leg position.

homeostasis)[59] soothes, provides for tension release, and stimulates respiration, circulation, and gastrointestinal function. Confidence in parenting skills and tactile communication between parent and infant are encouraged when parents massage their baby. Parents may also tub bathe the premature grower, which provides a relaxing, tension-relieving experience of multiple textures (water, water temperature, soap, washcloth).

Varying sensation and touch pattern keeps the baby interested in stroking and massaging. As the preterm infant matures and is able to tolerate variety, he should be introduced to different textures (e.g., lambskins, stuffed toys, cotton, satin). Baby clothes provide various textures, make the baby more attractive ("He looks like a real baby!" "She looks like a girl, since her shaved head is covered.") and decrease heat loss (especially hats).

Hand-to-midline behaviors are encouraged by cradling the baby for feedings (for both bottle and gavage feedings if the baby tolerates it) with both arms in the midline. If the premature infant needs an oxygen hood, using one large enough so that the baby's whole upper body will fit inside encourages hand-to-mouth quieting (Figure 24-2). Use arm restraints only when necessary and immobilize the extremity in a physiologic position. Release and exercise the restrained extremity with each care-giving encounter. Avoid restraining both arms so that one is free for hand-to-mouth behaviors. If both must be restrained (e.g., the infant pulls out the orogastric tube), give the baby a pacifier.

POSITIONING. Preterm infants display different motor development than term infants. A continuous assessment of muscle tone, response to posi-

TABLE 24-9

Development of Tone*

GESTATIONAL AGE	DEVELOPMENT
28 weeks	Completely hypotonic and lacks all physiologic flexion
32 weeks	Hips and knees begin to show some flexion while arms remain extended
34 weeks	Flexor tone apparent in legs
36 weeks	Loose flexion of arms and legs evident and grasp reflex present
40 weeks (term)	Develops tone in utero and develops flexed position in intrauterine space; after birth, reflex activity and CNS maturity help term infant to unfold and extend; term infant holds all four limbs in flexed position

Data from Anderson J and Auster-Liebhaber J: Phys Occup Ther Pediatr 4(1):89, 1984; Dubowitz L et al: J Pediatr 77:1, 1970; and Palisano R and Short M: Phys Occup Ther Pediatr 4(4):43, 1984.
*Muscle tone develops in caudocephalic direction and interacts with simultaneous cephalocaudal development of movement to help affect posture.

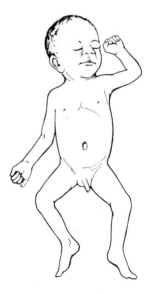

Figure 24-3. Premature infant resting posture exhibiting shoulder retraction and abduction, and frog leg position—hips abducted and externally rotated, and ankle and feet eversion. (From Pelletier JM and Palmeri A: High-risk infants. In Clark PN and Allen AS, editors: Occupational therapy for children, St Louis, 1985, The CV Mosby Co.)

tioning and handling, oral-motor function, and response to sensory stimuli provides data for individualizing intervention.[43,100,105] The goal of intervention is to provide opportunities for normal development and organization of the sensory systems, detect early developmental problems, and educate parents about stimulation, handling, and positioning.

Preterm infants usually have less developed physiologic flexion in the limbs, trunk, and pelvis than term newborns[7,33,91] (Table 24-9). For preterm infants long periods of immobilization without a positioning device, on a firm mattress with the influences of gravity, result in a number of abnormal characteristics: (1) increased neck extension with a right-sided head preference, (2) shoulder retraction and abduction (reduces forward rotation and ability to reach midline), (3) increased trunk extension with "arching" of the neck and back, (4) frog leg position—hips abducted and externally rotated, and (5) ankle and feet eversion[116] (Figure 24-3). Table 24-10 lists the reasons for proper positioning in the NICU.[93]

To prevent overstretching of the joints and to facilitate development of flexor tone, the infant should be provided with a variety of positions. Side lying (Figure 24-4) is used to improve visual awareness of hands, to encourage hands-to-midline movement, and to discourage the frog leg position. In this position the baby is able to bring hands to mouth for sucking and self-comforting.

Acutely ill preterms are often positioned supine with the head to the side or in the midline to accommodate their ventilators, umbilical catheters, and other devices. Supine positioning does not promote flexion and may be stressful to acutely ill infants.[1] Placed supine, babies experience more startle behaviors and sleep disturbance

TABLE 24-10

Reasons for Proper Positioning

1. Inhibits or shortens dystonic phase while baby remains in fetal position during postnatal period
2. Facilitates hand-to-midline and midline orientation
3. Stimulates visual exploration of environment (through head to midline)
4. Facilitates development of head control (making feeding easier and helping respiratory problems)
5. Helps balance flexors and extensors to facilitate symmetric posture
6. Helps develop antigravity movement
7. Enhances comfort and decreases stress
8. Has an organizing effect that facilitates development of flexor tone
9. Promotes normal and prevents abnormal development
10. Helps enhance development of motoric skills, reflexes, and postural tone

Data from Pelletier JM and Palmeri A: High-risk infants. In Clark PN and Allen AS, editors: Occupational therapy for children, St Louis, 1985, The CV Mosby Co.

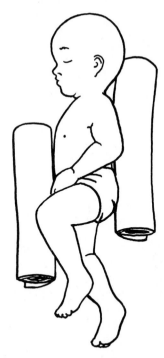

Figure 24-4. Side lying is obtained by using rolled blanket behind infant's head and trunk; additional support is added by placing another roll in front of infant's chest and abdomen with top leg over it. Placing blanket over infant and tucking it under mattress helps hold this position.

from environmental stimuli. Prolonged supine positioning is associated with the hypertonic "arched" position (hyperextension of head, neck, and shoulder girdle) of many chronically ventilated babies.[7] Supine positioning should promote as much flexion as possible (Figure 24-5). A positioning device of foam with the middle cut out sloping under the scapulae is another method of obtaining supine flexion. Pillows filled with polystyrene beads (i.e., premie bean bags) require skill for optimal positioning but are useful in providing positioning for very small premature infants (1000 to 1500 g).

Body containment increases the baby's feeling of security, promotes quieting and self-control, and enables stress to be better endured. Many premature infants "travel" (no matter how many times they are moved) to the sides or bottom of their incubator. Just as premature infants are able to seek proximity to a breathing bear,[112] they are able to seek out security. Parents and professionals are inclined to move the uncomfortable-looking baby back to the middle of a "boundary-less" world. Leave babies where they feel safe and comfortable—if they become uncomfortable they will let you know. Providing boundaries (i.e., blanket rolls) often stops this migration.

Small, acutely ill premature infants who are positioned supine are often extremely agitated, thrashing arms and legs, tachycardic, and expending precious energy and calories. Instead of medications, these babies are often calmed by providing a "nest" of blankets on either side and at the head and feet. The baby's limbs are then flexed

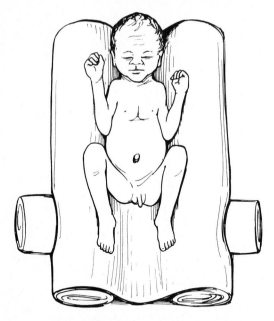

Figure 24-5. Supine positioning with rolled blankets or pads on either side of baby and under knees to provide secure boundaries and promote flexion. CAUTION: Supine positioning should be used with caution. Preterm infants who have not developed gag reflex (<36 weeks gestation) are at particularly high risk for aspiration. Supine positioning should not be used until majority of feeding has been absorbed (at least 1 to 1½ hours after feeding). (From Pelletier JM and Palmeri A: High-risk infants. In Clark PN and Allen AS, editors: Occupational therapy for children, St Louis, 1985, The CV Mosby Co.)

inside the "artificial womb" and the infant quietly rests (Figure 24-6). If agitation recurs, a limb (usually a leg) has extended outside the infant's secure boundary—flexing and returning it to the "womb" quiets the baby.[1,117]

Body containment maneuvers such as swaddling, holding onto a finger or hand, and crossing the baby's arms in the midline and holding them securely help with self-regulation during feeding, procedures, or other stressful manipulations. Picking the preterm infant up from a supine posi-

tion produces startles and head hyperextension.[38] A better technique is to roll the baby prone, which flexes the head, and then flex the limbs onto the trunk and pick the baby up.[117]

Prone positioning encourages the baby to work on using neck extension and promotes flexion of the extremities. This position does not require the use of any device—it merely encourages knee and arm flexion; a small roll or sling (see Figure 24-2) assists in maintaining flexion.[38] Prone (versus supine) positioning has numerous benefits and is the position of choice for many NICU babies (Table 24-11). Use of a sheep/lambskin helps to further facilitate flexion and prevents skin abrasion, especially on the knees.

A combination of vestibular and tactile stimulation increases quieting behaviors, decreases apneic and bradycardic episodes, increases visual and auditory fixation, and increases brain growth.[64-66,98] Waterbeds provide contingent stimuli, since they move in response to the infant's movement; oscillating waterbeds provide rhythmic motion. Kinesthetic stimulation is provided by rocking chairs, hammocks, baby swings, and baby carriers.[54] Carrying quiets the infant, provides sensory communication with the caretaker, changes the infant's environment, and provides visual and auditory as well as tactile stimuli. A nasal cannula (see Chapter 17) and portable tank enable mobility for the infant receiving oxygen.

AUDITORY INTERVENTION

The NICU is a noisy environment that has no diurnal rhythm—it is as noisy at night as in the daytime[51,81] (Table 24-12). The NICU infant is exposed to an onslaught of noise 24 hours a day for days, weeks, or months. At follow-up, preterm infants exhibit a lower threshold for sound.[55,84] Neonatal illnesses, drug therapies, and possibly acoustic insult account for the increased risk for sensorineural hearing loss in NICU babies (regardless of gestational age).

The first goal in auditory intervention is to assess the current level of noise in the NICU and to

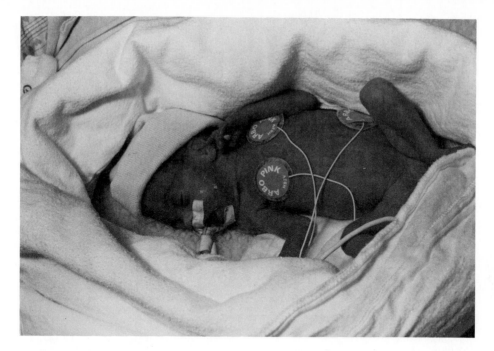

Figure 24-6. Very small premature infant resting quietly in a "nest" of pads and blankets.

TABLE 24-11

Effects of Prone Positioning

1. Improves oxygenation by 15% to 25%[74,119]
   a. Increased $TcPo_2$ values
   b. Increased Pao_2 values
2. Improves lung mechanics and lung volumes[119]
   a. Increased lung compliance
   b. Increased tidal volume
3. Decreases energy expenditure[75]
   a. Increased quiet sleep
   b. Decreased awake time
   c. Decreased caloric expenditure (median difference supine versus prone: +3.1 kcal/kg/day)
   d. (?) Decreased heat loss
4. Decrease in gastric reflux in prone position with head of bed elevated 30 degrees[88]

decrease the noise decibels wherever possible. Increased environmental noise levels are a stressor to all NICU babies—the preterm, as well as the ill term baby (e.g., persistent pulmonary hypertension of the newborn [PPHN]; drug withdrawal)—and cause increased startles, fussiness, apneic and bradycardic episodes, hypoxemia, and sleep disturbance.[49,50,70] The sudden high-pitched shrill, dysrhythmic noise of equipment alarms alerts the care provider, but it also results in infants manifesting an extreme hypersensitivity to sound (as a learned conditioned response).[55,84]

Strategies to minimize external auditory stimuli include quieting alarms with suction (and remembering to reset them); not taking a shift report

TABLE 24-12

Noise Levels in the NICU

LEVEL (dB)	COMMENTS
50-60	Normal speaking voice
50-60*†	Incubator (motor) noise
45-85‡	Noise in NICU (talking, equipment alarms, telephones, radio)
65-80†	Life support equipment (ventilator, IV pumps)
85	Noise level at which hearing damage is possible for adult; (?) neonatal effects
90§	Adult exposure for 8 hours requires protective device and hearing conservation program
92.8†	Opening incubator porthole
96-117†	Placing bottle of formula on top of incubator
110-116†	Closing one or both cabinet doors
114-124†	Closing one or both portholes
130-140†	Banging incubator to stimulate apneic premature infant
160-165	Recommendations for peak, single noise level not to exceed to prevent (adult) hearing loss; (?) neonatal effects

Modified from Mitchell SA: Semin Hear 5(1):17, 1984.
*American Academy of Pediatrics recommends incubator noise not to exceed 58 dB.
†Measures from inside the incubator.
‡Noise levels do not vary from morning to night.
§Occupational Safety and Health Administration (OSHA) standard.

over, or allowing medical rounds near, the baby's incubator; having noisy equipment repaired immediately; emptying sloshing water in ventilator/nebulizer tubing; and maintaining cardiac monitors in a quiet state with alarms on. Nursery design changes include smaller cubicles rather than one large room, soundproofing materials, lights for phones and alarm systems, and minimizing equipment noise. Placing a blanket on top of the incubator muffles the noise of equipment placement; gentle, considerate (to the baby) placement of equipment on or in the incubator muffles sound; and closing portholes and drawers gently decreases the structural noises of care giving. Pro-

hibiting placement of equipment (e.g., clipboards, stethoscopes, formula bottles) on top of the incubator prevents such noises.

No tapping (by parents or siblings) or banging (by medical, nursing, or ancillary personnel) on the incubator Plexiglas should ever be permitted. This (along with a brisk startle reflex from the baby) is an opportunity to teach about the noise levels generated by such activity. Babies should be kept in incubators as long as necessary to maintain heat balance. The incubator does *not* protect the infant from noise—a well-managed NICU environment may be much quieter than the continuous noise of an incubator. Prolonged stays in an incubator *do* expose the infant to repeated caregiving noises, as well as to a dearth of kinesthetic stimulation (e.g., carrying, holding, rocking, swinging, and sitting upright in an infant seat).

Radios have been banned in many NICUs. If music is played, it should be on a low volume (below the dB range of normal speech), should *not* be rock music, and preferably should be classical (babies prefer Brahms, Bach, and Beethoven). Day-night cycles (nap time; nighttime) when auditory stimulation is decreased should be established in the NICU. On discharge, NICU babies often will not sleep in a quiet room—softly playing a radio facilitates sleep, and the infant is gradually weaned from it. Signs such as: "Quiet . . . baby sleeping" or "Do not disturb— I'm asleep (talk to my nurse)" ensure undisturbed sleep—provided they are heeded.

The "in tuning" premature infant (see Table 24-5) of less than 34 weeks gestation probably receives enough auditory input from the NICU— auditory enhancement at this stage is probably overstimulation. Just as high-frequency sounds arouse, low-frequency ones—like the heart beat, respiratory sounds, and vacuums—quiet.[31] Music boxes with a repetitive lullaby and tape recordings of mother's/father's/siblings' voices (reading stories, poems, or singing) soothe the infant. Watch for the infant's reaction and use if the baby is soothed. If the baby becomes restless, turning the volume lower and/or placing the device on the outside, rather than inside, of the incubator may be more relaxing. Rattles, bells, and squeeze toys alert and ready the baby for interaction.

The human voice is the most preferred sound. Teach parents the neonatal preference for high-pitched voices, speaking in typical speech patterns (not baby talk). Role model and teach parents to gently talk to the infant while touching and giving care. Teach parents to talk to their infant while presenting their faces in the infant's range of vision. Watch for infant tolerance and increase or decrease talk time to avoid overload. Imitate the baby's coos and babbles—this reinforces and encourages vocalizations.

For the neonate, hearing may initially be more important than vision for attachment and bonding to the parents. By 45 hours after birth newborns are able to discriminate and prefer their mother's face—they have connected her familiar voice with her unfamiliar face.[42] A high index of suspicion regarding hearing loss is warranted if caretakers do not observe normal responses to sound stimulation. All newborns, especially those with a history of familial hearing loss, hyperbilirubinemia (>15 mg in preterm infant; >20 mg in term infant), congenital viral infections, defects of the ear, nose, and throat, small preterm infants (<1500 g), and those receiving ototoxic drugs, should have a hearing screening before discharge.

VISUAL INTERVENTION

The NICU is lit with bright cool-white fluorescent lights 24 hours a day to enable immediate and ongoing visibility of all infants. Although there is no neonatal research on the hazards of this type of lighting, there is abundant animal, child, and adult research documenting negative biochemical and physical effects (change in endocrine function, increased hypocalcemia, cell transformations, immature gonadal development, and chromosome breakage).[51]

The first goal in visual intervention is to assess the current level of light and decrease it wherever possible. The very immature preterm infant is accustomed to the muted light of the uterus—light filtered through the abdominal and uterine walls—and has fused (if <26 weeks gestation) eyelids. Draping blankets on top of the incubator decreases the light at the infant's level but allows immediate maximal illumination when the blanket is pulled back. Since babies are continuously monitored, not all babies need to be maximally illuminated at all times.[51] Dimming the lights (to 65 to 75 foot candles), especially in day-night cycles, helps establish diurnal rhythms.[31] Another recommendation is to use indirect full-spectrum light (which may require color assessment adjustments) at each bedside, since it does not have the side effects of cool-white light and can be individually controlled.[51]

Visual attentiveness is correlated with birth weight and gestational age—the more mature the baby, the more the baby is able to fix and follow. The 28-week gestation infant fixes and follows but may become apneic as a result. Visual stimulation is very tiring and taxing (increases the heart rate) to the immature baby—those of more than 34 weeks gestation probably receive enough stimulation from the NICU environment. When these infants reach the "coming out stage" (see Table 24-5) they are ready for visually enhancing activities.

Babies receiving phototherapy are visually sensory deprived because of their protective eye pads. These should be removed during care and feeding and interaction with parents and professionals. Providing interesting visual stimuli includes inanimate (e.g., toys, black and white faces and patterns, pictures of family members, artwork from siblings, mobiles) and animate (faces of parents, siblings, and professionals) objects (Figure 24-7). Babies prefer the human face as a visual stimulus, especially the talking face, which stimulates both visual and auditory pathways. Parents often need to be encouraged that *their* faces, rather than all the baby's toys, are what their infant prefers to listen to and watch.

Teach parents the abilities of the infant and appropriate methods of visual stimulation:

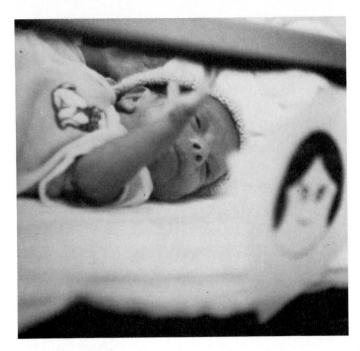

Figure 24-7. Premature infant fixing on black and white face.

1. Place mobiles, pictures, and faces within the visual range of the newborn—8 to 12 inches for term infants, a little closer for preterm infants.
2. Quiet alert is the best state for visual encounters—after feedings, if awake; swaddle infant to quiet or unwrap infant to arouse; hold infant upright.
3. Place infant on abdomen with objects of various sizes and shapes within visual range.
4. Change toys and visual stimuli—babies become bored with the same thing.
5. When the preterm infant tolerates multiple stimuli, hold infant in en face position (see Chapter 22) to feed, talk to, and rock. Whether the infant is nipple or gavage fed, alternate sides so the infant sees both sides of the care provider's face (especially important if the preterm infant exhibits the com-

mon preference for right-sided head turning).
6. Place infant at varied heights (in baby carrier, crib, swing, infant seat, on floor) so the infant sees the world from various angles.
7. Place infant so that he or she is able to bring hands to midline—and can see hands and fingers and eventually reach for toys.

Babies who exhibit gaze aversion should not be "pursued" by the face of the parent or professional, since this only potentiates the time "spent away" with their gaze to protect themselves from overload.[19] Gaze aversion, flat facial affect, and absence of a smile may cast doubt on the ability of these infants to see, since there is no eye language or caretaker feedback of preference, recognition, and delight. These infants *do* see, but they fix only fleetingly. Minimizing care providers is crucial so that the infant deals with as few caretaker cues, styles, and ways of being handled as possible.

SMELL/TASTE INTERVENTION

The neonate's well-developed sense of smell is not stimulated in the NICU with pleasant odors. The high-risk infant is stimulated by the smell of forgotten alcohol, skin prep, or povidone-iodine (Betadine) pads inside the incubator. Since the premature infant is unable to respond by crying or moving away, the infant responds to noxious smells by a decrease in respiratory rate, transient apnea, and/or an increase in heart rate. Removal of noxious odors from the incubator is as critical as removal of sharp instruments after a procedure.

Enhancing the olfactory environment includes having parents hold the infant or sit close if the infant cannot yet be held. The smell of the mother's breast milk is especially pleasant and may elicit a suckling reflex. Placing one drop on the baby's lips with a cotton ball or gauze sponge helps the baby to recognize the mother's smell and to associate that smell with food and feeding when the baby is able to nipple feed.

Nonnutritive suckling (during gavage and between feedings) is associated with better oxygenation, quieter, more restful behavior, increased readiness for nipple feedings, and better weight gain. Sucking on a pacifier satisfies the infant's sucking needs and may facilitate early learning that satiety and sucking are associated. However, nutritive and nonnutritive suckling are *not* alike (see Chapter 12); because the baby vigorously sucks on a pacifier does not mean the baby will be able to suckle nutritively, since the expressive and swallow phases have not been present in nonnutritive suckling. This is very confusing to most parents and many professionals.

High-risk infants often undergo prolonged periods of nothing by mouth (NPO), when their hunger cries and pains are not relieved. Although pacifiers are soothing, these babies may learn that sucking and satiety are not related. NICU babies also undergo many aversive stimuli around and within the mouth (i.e., oral intubation, oral and endotracheal tube suction; intermittent gavage) that result in touch aversion of the mouth and a hypersensitive gag reflex. Feeding difficulties may be the result of (1) neurologic damage (e.g., intravascular hemorrhage [IVH]); (2) structural abnormalities (e.g., cleft palate or submucous cleft, recessed chin); (3) prematurity—baby is too neurologically immature and tires easily with "work" of feeding; (4) aversive feeder (acquired or developmental sucking defect, psychologic—"hospitalitis," rumination); or (5) a combination of these types.

The goals of intervention include (1) a safe feeding (i.e., diminished risk of aspiration); (2) a functional feeding (i.e., adequate caloric intake with minimal energy expenditure); and (3) a pleasant, social interactive experience for infant and parents/care givers. Table 24-13 outlines intervention strategies to facilitate nipple feeding.

A feeding plan must be individualized for each infant and posted at the bedside. All care providers must adhere to the plan for consistency of stimuli and to promote infant learning.

Tommy was a 28-week preterm infant with severe idiopathic respiratory distress syndrome (IRDS), prolonged ventilation, and now BPD. He is now 38 weeks postconceptual age, receiving hood/nasal cannula oxygen, and trying to learn to nipple feed. In the morning report, the night nurse says that Tommy "has bradycardia with tube passage so that 24 hours ago he had a cardiorespiratory arrest that required bag/mask ventilation, cardiac massage, and epinephrine. He also has bradycardia and tachypnea with bottle feeding."

Tommy's nurse evaluated his initial attempts to bottle feed (after waiting for him to demand) and wrote the care plan (see boxed material on p. 661) after feeding him 45 ml in 20 minutes without tachypnea, cyanosis, or bradycardia.

CRYING/SMILING INTERVENTION

Crying is the infant's innate care-eliciting behavior—a signal that the infant needs attention. Immediate response decreases physiologic stress,

TABLE 24-13

Strategies to Facilitate Nipple Feeding

I. Minimize noxious stimuli to the mouth
   A. Suction *only* as needed (*not* routinely)
   B. Consider indwelling gastric tube rather than intermittent gavage (a baby fed every 2 hours would have gavage tube passed 12 times a day)
   C. Pass intermittent gavage tube
      1. Down mouth through hole in pacifier nipple
      2. If baby has hypersensitive gag, passing smaller tube down nose stimulates gag reflex less than passing tube down mouth
   D. Use *only* orthodontic nipples/pacifiers if mother wants to breastfeed—straight nipples promote tongue thrust and nipple confusion, an acquired sucking defect
   E. Perioral/intraoral stimulation techniques
      1. Are only *more aversive,* rather than therapeutic, on babies with touch aversion at mouth area
      2. When performing oral exercises, do so with care—do *not* stimulate aversive reflexes (e.g., gag reflex)
II. Enhance pleasant stimuli to the mouth
   A. Have baby smell/taste breast milk
   B. Provide nonnutritive suckling with tube feeding
   C. Facilitate hand-to-mouth behaviors
   D. Orthodontic pacifier—does not promote sucking defect; may be too hard/too big for premature infant
   E. Firm nipple—a too-soft nipple increases flow, stimulates anxiety and/or gag reflex, and causes bradycardia
   F. Perioral/intraoral stimulation—(?) facilitates development of normal sucking behaviors
   G. Use Lact-Aid nursing supplementer (see Chapter 12)
      1. Never frustrate baby with a dry breast
      2. Positive reinforcement for baby to nurse
      3. Calorically and energy efficient method
      4. Oral therapy—teaches baby proper nutritive suckle
III. Positioning—use proper position to facilitate swallow and improve suction
   A. Hold with feedings (even gavage) as much as possible
   B. Consistent caretakers—parents, primary nurses, foster grandparents
   C. Swaddle
      1. Decreases startles
      2. Infant may become too warm and sleepy
   D. Facilitate swallowing
      1. Position with chin tucked
      2. If breastfeeding, turn baby's whole body toward mother so head/trunk are in alignment (baby is not trying to swallow with head turned to one side)
      3. Upright position with neck, shoulders, and back supported—slows gravitational flow of formula from nipple (as when baby is in semireclined position)
      4. Cuddling, semireclined position—increases flow of formula by gravity—may be too fast, regardless of nipple chosen; results in increased gags, choking, and bradycardia
      5. Prone with neck extended (slightly)
         a. Keeps tongue forward and airway unobstructed
         b. Good for aversive feeder who chokes
      6. Gentle, upward pressure under chin or at base of tongue facilitates swallowing, since it mimics upward thrust of tongue with swallowing
   E. Improve formation of suction
      1. Semireclining (>45-degree angle) on lap of caretaker—frees both hands to work with baby on oral control
      2. Cupping both cheeks with fingers of free hand (i.e., hand not holding bottle) improves lip closure and suction formation
      3. Gentle tugging at nipple (as if to take it out of mouth) causes baby to begin/continue suckling

TABLE 24-13—cont'd _____

Strategies to Facilitate Nipple Feeding

IV. Timing
- A. Do not allow baby to cry to exhaustion before feeding—baby will be too tired to eat
- B. Keep external stimuli to a minimum in immature preterm infants (<34 weeks) for optimal intake and weight gain
- C. If satiated, baby will not suck
   1. Feed on demand/when alert[50]
   2. If feeding on schedule, note if baby is active, restless, and hungry before feeding
   3. If feeding on schedule, space time and see if baby "feels hungry and demands"
   4. First, nipple what baby is able to feed; then tube feed
- D. Try to nipple feed for no longer than 20 minutes (baby becomes too tired and uses up energy and calories to feed, instead of to grow)
- E. Infants of advanced age (around 6 months) may be unable to nipple if they have never had the opportunity; it may be more developmentally appropriate to cup or spoon-feed child

---

TOMMY'S FEEDING PLAN

1. *Sit upright.* This decreases the flow of formula from the bottle and thus decreases:
   a. His gag reflex, which causes the bradycardia
   b. His anxiety caused by a bolus of formula in his mouth
2. *Use a blue nipple.* This is the shortest nipple and decreases stimulation of his hypersensitive gag reflex, which causes his bradycardia. (All other nipples stimulated him to gag.)
3. *Gently push up under his chin when he gets a mouthful of formula.* This pushes his tongue upward against his palate, the same way the tongue moves during swallowing. (Reader, swallow and watch your tongue motion.) He becomes frightened (i.e., eyes wide open and fearful; increased respiratory rate; arching and struggling) when he has a mouthful of formula, since he is used to only sucking on a dry pacifier and having nothing to swallow. His fear raises his heart rate, his respiratory rate, and his gag reflex, which causes bradycardia.
4. *Talk to him.* Softly and gently, tell him he can swallow and praise him when he does.
5. *Nipple.* Have him do this as much as possible (he will only get better with practice) and supplement feeding with the *indwelling* NG tube (no more intermittent tube passage).

---

increases trust in the environment, and enhances the sense of self and of control over the world. The need to escalate to "out of control" crying is decreased with immediate response, so that babies are easier to soothe. Consoling the crying infant also helps the baby change states so he or she is able to attend and interact with the environment.

Term babies vocalize, cry, and look at their caretaker more than do preterm and ill infants.[51] NICU babies exhibit fewer care-eliciting behaviors (some preterm infants in one study never cried, vocalized, or looked at the caretaker).[51] Preterm infants are thus less responsive to the caretakers (both parents and professionals), who receive less positive feedback from the infant and hence are less rewarded. In one study those NICU babies who were able to cue the care provider (cry, look, vocalize) were contingently responded to 80% to 100% of the time.[51]

Intubated babies who are unable to produce an audible cry signal their needs by agitation, heart rate changes, and changes in oxygenation. Preterm infants (<32 weeks) may recover better from agitation when left alone, since active consolation is overstimulating.[50] How caretakers attempt to soothe a crying baby (while giving NICU care) include no response to cries (58.1% of the time), response by talking (29.2% of the time), response by social touching (5.5% of the time), and response by talk and social touching (7.2% of the time).[51]

Teach parents (and staff) to use graduated interventions in quieting a crying baby:

1. Soothe with gentle high-pitched talking (loud enough that the infant is able to hear it above his crying).
2. Place the palm of the hand across the infant's chest or hold arms on chest with the palm of the care provider's hand.
3. Swaddle with blankets to decrease self-upsetting startles.
4. Pick up infant, hold (upright is the most soothing position), and rock.
5. Offer a pacifier.

Most stimulation in the NICU is procedural. The lack of social stimulation in the NICU not only affects the infant, but also teaches parents that their baby is too weak, fragile, uninterested, or incapable of social interaction. Again, social stimulation must be paced according to the stage of development and stability of the infant (see Table 24-5). Enhancing the infant's social environment includes presenting the smiling, moving, talking care provider's face to the alert infant; touching and stroking; and soothing and consoling the distressed infant.

In many busy NICUs parents and a foster grandparent program provide this sensory integrated social experience. If the baby has been transported to a referral center, parents may live some distance away and be unable to visit daily. The chronically ill 4- to 5-month-old infant who begins to recognize the foster grandmother may smile, relax, and feed better for her and is often fussier and more irritable on her day off. A foster grandparent program benefits both infants and seniors—the infant receives love and socialization, and the senior "has a reason to get up in the morning."

If at all possible, parents should be encouraged to perform the "firsts" with their baby (e.g., first nipple feeding, first bath, first time out of the incubator). Since parents are not always present,

they will miss some important milestones for their baby (e.g., extubation). Many NICUs have developed baby diaries (or calendars) where the nurses, physicians, and foster grandparents write important information about the baby's day (as if the baby were the author). The text is accompanied by self-developing pictures with humorous captions (e.g., "Look at me—I've got my tube out!"). Staff are very creative in relating "what's been happening" so that the parents not only have a verbal report (that over time will be forgotten), but also a keepsake of NICU progress.

Long-term care in the NICU

Since smaller, more immature preterm infants are now surviving, some babies spend months in the NICU. To facilitate the development of these chronically hospitalized infants, parents and professionals must have realistic expectations of their developmental levels. A preterm infant who reaches 40 weeks postconceptual age is not as mature in sleep-wake cycles, attentiveness, or soothability as a 40-week term baby.[50] In evaluating the developmental performance of a preterm infant, one must correct for the weeks of prematurity. For example: Susie is chronologically 8 months old; she was 32 weeks gestation at birth, so her developmental age would be:

8 months − 8 weeks (2 months) preterm = 6 months

Susie will be developmentally appropriate in performance if she functions at a 6-month level; developmental delay would be functioning below the 6-month level.

Table 24-14 outlines developmental expectations for infants from birth to 1 year. Remember to correct for prematurity.

OUTCOME

Even though the survival rate of preterm, including VLBW preterm infants, has dramatically improved as a result of education of care providers, regionalization of care, and improved technology, there has not been a corresponding change in neonatal morbidity.[40,62,63] These infants are still at increased risk for physical and psychosocial emotional disabilities (Table 24-15) despite recent NICU advances.[24,62,63,108] Low birth weight and the need for assisted ventilation are the risk factors associated with the highest risk of sequelae—developmental delay of 25% in infants weighing 1500 g or less;[96] in infants with assisted ventilation, neurologic deficit and developmental delay is as high as 45%.[101] The risk of developmental delay is 0% to 45% for corrected age and up to 88% if postconceptual age is used[22,71] (i.e., correction is not made for prematurity).

There is an increased incidence of failure to thrive and child abuse and neglect in preterm infants.[61] Separation of infants and parents at birth is disruptive of parent-infant attachments and increases the risk of parenting disorders (see Chapters 22 and 23). In the first year of life, preterm infants are often more "difficult" and less "easy" to care for: are difficult to soothe, less adaptive, less able to habituate, state labile, negative in mood, and withdrawn.[76,120] Many families (40%) of VLBW infants experience feeding difficulties in the first year of the infant's life.[120] The parent who finds the preterm infant "too difficult" may become less responsive to and involved with the infant and thus escalate the infant's difficult behavior. By the second year of life the prematurely born is less difficult (although the child may still not be an "easy" toddler) and is at less risk developmentally.[103] Whereas an unsupportive environment may increase the difficult behavior, a supportive parent-infant interaction benefits the infant (i.e., the infant makes developmental gains).

The increased risk of cognitive impairment with decreasing birth weight may diminish with time and a supportive environment or may persist till school age.[22,71,76,85] Preterm infants are more likely to function below their genetic potential because of increased incidence of mental retardation, cerebral palsy, and learning disabilities.[57,86,113] Children who were preterm infants require more special education, repeat grades, and do less well on reading and math achievement tests than children who were born at term. Even when NICU graduates perform well on developmental tests, they may have neurosensory difficulties (i.e., problems with visual-motor integration, spatial relationships, and speech and language development) and passive, withdrawn behavior that negatively affects school accomplishment.[62] Early identification of cognitive/learning difficulties enables the infant/toddler/preschool years to be the optimal time for intervention.[57]

Graduate preterms are at increased risk for motor impairment, particularly gross motor skills (i.e., rolling over, sitting, crawling, standing, and walking). Rather than neurologic impairment, some of these deficits may be due to abnormal positioning and handling in the NICU.[38,76,103,105]

Just as the ability of parents to attach and caretake for their infant is disrupted by illness and hospitalization (see Chapters 22 and 23), the ability of the newborn to form a symbiotic attachment to the parents is disrupted by the NICU experience. The unattached child results when the infant internalizes the rage associated with unmet needs.[72,107] Because of a lack of contingent, reliable, and consistent caretaking, these infants do not develop a sense of trust in parents, self, or humankind. Unmet needs may be a result of (1) lack of parental attachment and caretaking; (2) asynchrony between caretakers and infant, so that the infant's cues are not interpreted and responded to appropriately; (3) neglect and abuse; or (4) multiple caretaking.

The emotional disruptions of the unattached child are the same as the psychologic outcomes of the battered child[72,94,99,107]:

1. The infant's ego development is derived primarily from sensations from the body surface.
2. When the body suffers pain, there is a decrease in the pleasure principle as a guide to development and an increase in violent, aggressive tendencies, since the caretaker, who should comfort, is inflicting pain.
3. The infant identifies with and incorporates

Text continued on p. 671.

TABLE 24-14

Neonatal and Infant Development (0-12 months)*

AGE	AUDITORY	LANGUAGE	VISUAL
0-1 month	Reacts to vocal sounds (recognizes and is soothed by mother's/caretaker's voice) Smiles when spoken to by mother Locates sound by turning head toward it Distinguishes volume and pitch; prefers high voice	Randomly produces crying/mewing sounds Communicates with body movements and cries Quiets when picked up	Sees within 8-10 inches from face—watches and recognizes mother's face Fixes—follows moving objects, lights; stops sucking to look Sense of location/direction established by 1 month
1-2 months	Vocally responds to and imitates sounds of mother/caretaker Babbling accompanied by motor activity (1-6 months) Quiets to voice	Imitates sounds of others Babbles/coos and repeats sounds with intention Deliberately cries for assistance	Binocular vision begins (6 weeks) Gives equal time and concentration to familiar or unfamiliar objects (6-8 weeks) Prefers linear patterns over curves; prefers people over objects Discriminates horizontal and vertical patterns Quiets to face
2-3 months	Sound has stimulus-response effect Stops sucking to listen; searches for sound with eyes	Refines intonation through interaction with caretaker Coos one syllable sounds—ooh, ah, ae; gurgles, chuckles Cries less Vocalizes when talked to	Prefers looking at new things Begins facial differentiating with focus on eyes (2 months) Color vision begins functioning Prefers curves to lines (2-6 months)
3-4 months	Distinguishes mother's/caretaker's voice from other female voices Turns head toward sound immediately	Organizes behaviors into expressive acts—coos are pitch-modulated and sustained for 15-20 minutes Makes sounds and recreates them to recapture experience	Discovers hands (3 months) Differentiates patterns and shapes (3 months) Color vision same as adult's Binocular vision well established; sees 15-inch distance

*This table represents a generalized/normative grouping of developmental ages in which an infant accomplishes these tasks. Since some infants develop faster and some slower, this table is to be used as a guideline and not a literal interpretation of the milestone age for accomplishing a developmental task.

TACTILE-MOTOR	COGNITIVE-MENTAL	SOCIAL-EMOTIONAL

Primitive reflexes
  Hands fisted—random grasp
    with intention
  Prone—tucked position
  Supine—tonic neck position
Pulled to sit: head lags—back is
  rounded with head rolled for-
  ward
Tactile contact aids in reestablish-
  ing biorhythmic balance and de-
  veloping sense of self and con-
  fidence
	Reflex reactions (i.e., grasp, Moro
	  root, suckle, etc.)
	Organizes incoming stimuli
	Internal and external world are not
	  differentiated—all are experi-
	  enced as a part of the self
	Actions done with little indication
	  of purpose or intention
		Task-development of trust versus
		  mistrust through constancy and
		  reliability of environment; re-
		  sponse to infant's cries is essen-
		  tial
		Spends two thirds of time sleeping
		  (7-8 short naps/day)
		Shuts out noxious stimuli

Rolls from supine to side-lying
  position
Hands open or loosely closed—
  manipulative play with hands
  and fingers (6 weeks)
Deliberate holding grasp when fin-
  ger placed in hand (8 weeks)
Raises head to vertical position
  (45-degree angle) when prone
Begins unfolding body, extending
  and kicking legs (6-12 weeks)
	Attracted to unfamiliar and novel
	  stimuli (0-6 months)
	Converting reflexes into intentional
	  responses through movement
	  (i.e., body exploration) (1-4
	  months)
	Developing rudimentary problem-
	  solving skills (begins 5th-12th
	  week and evolves throughout in-
	  fancy); expects feeding at certain
	  time; associates people with
	  behaviors (e.g., mother with
	  food)
		Accepts/tolerates substitute care
		  giver
		Begins formulating sense of mas-
		  tery through interaction with
		  environment
		Sleeps 2-4 long periods/day (6
		  weeks); awake 10 hours/day
		Responds positively to comfort
		  and care; negatively to pain and
		  need
		Smiles at familiar voice/face—
		  mother, father, and siblings
		Does not discriminate odd ele-
		  ments in a matrix
		Swipes at objects
		Tears when crying

Prone position favored—raises
  head 90 degrees and holds for
  several seconds; turns from
  prone to side-lying position
Supine—slight head lag when
  pulled to sit; sits supported with
  head erect and bobbing
Reciprocal kicking (precursor to
  crawling)
Discovers hands (3 months); grasp
  reflex decreasing (3 months);
  reaches for object with both
  hands
	Learning is sensory-kinetic (physi-
	  cal through movement)
	Engages in purposeful activity—
	  repeat actions; associates action
	  with result
	Distinguishes near from distant
	  objects
	Begins to exhibit memory
	Begins to become aware of self
		Gives different responses to emo-
		  tions expressed by others
		Duplicates mother in facial move-
		  ments and sometimes affect
		Is developing a sense of mastery
		Cries when mother leaves
		Attracts mother's attention

Hand-to-mouth relationship well
  established
Tonic neck and Moro reflex
  decreasing
Attempts to grasp from visual
  cues; transfers toy from one
  hand to the other
	Is refining perceptual abilities (e.g.,
	  awareness of facial features, in-
	  cluding differentiating unfamiliar
	  faces; aware of differences in
	  depth and distance; stares at
	  place from which object drops)
	Is aware of strange situations
		Regulation of patterns of eating,
		  sleeping, alert
		Takes several naps of couple hours
		  duration (in morning and after-
		  noon); sleeps 10 hours a night
		Laughs when socializing
		Shows anticipation

Continued.

TABLE 24-14—cont'd

Neonatal and Infant Development (0-12 months)*

AGE	AUDITORY	LANGUAGE	VISUAL
3-4 months— cont'd		Smiles, squeals, coos when talked to	Differentiates aberrant facial features Raises and moves hand toward object seen Smiles and vocalizes at mirror image
4-5 months	Locates sound to the side but cannot locate sound above or below (4-7 months) Turns head and looks for speaker Understands name	Utters vowel sounds and a few consonant sounds (d, b, l, m) Spontaneously vocalizes to self, toys Stops crying when talked to Protests if another tries to take toy	Sees but is unable to pick up small objects Visually directed movement (contacts object) Differentiates facial features (more refined)—focuses on mouth and oval head shapes Smiles and vocalizes to mirror image Makes face to imitate Looks for fallen objects
5-6 months	Discriminates p/t; b/g; i/a	Enjoys playing vocal games—attempts to repeat sounds Combines vowel and consonants—sounds contain intonation patterns Imitates and differentiates p/t; b/g; i/a	Distinguishes live, animated faces from no expression/ affect Responds to or ignores familiar objects and focuses on new/less familiar
6-7 months	Listens quietly to sounds— babbles when sounds stop in order to elicit further sounds Coos, hums, stops crying with music	Uses tone, pitch, and stress in voice to communicate Has more control of sounds Babbles and becomes active with exciting sounds and to female voices Vocalizes pleasure and displeasure	Discerns and enjoys uniqueness of individual faces Is visually alert 50% of daytime hours Inspects objects at length

TACTILE-MOTOR	COGNITIVE-MENTAL	SOCIAL-EMOTIONAL
On tummy may rock like an airplane, arching back and extending limbs Sits supported, head erect and steady, back firm	Is aware of self from others and objects Discriminates—may prefer one object/person over others	Responds to and enjoys handling; not content to lie alone in bed
Head and hand activities at midline—grasps bidextrously Voluntarily reaches for and bats objects; raises arms to be picked up Sits supported with upper back erect and head steady—no head lag when pulled to sit Prone—lifts head at 90-degree angle; lifts head and chest, supporting weight on forearms Prefers novel to known stimuli	Discovers actions have effect on environment Is developing intentional behavior (4-8 months)—objects exist only in relation to infant; they have no meaning or existence separately Indicates existence of memory	Solidifies attachment with mother/primary caretaker who is base from which to explore world Is becoming aware of others as separate beings and that needs are met by another Responds to differing emotions in people Smiles and vocalizes for social contact
Uses hands and mouth to learn about world Supine—holds head upright; reaches for objects; can hold bottle independently; shakes and pounds objects on surface and in air; releases object in one hand while grasping with the other ("mirror reflex"); sits supported with head steady and lower back erect; full head control in supine and prone positions Prone—supports weight on palms with arms extended; rolls from prone to supine to prone position (5-7 months)	Endows mental representations with meaning and attributes Organizes and develops schema of world Watches actions as a spectator and gestures to have act repeated Directs visual attention to unfamiliar objects Is surprised when encounter is unexpected	Eats pureed foods Distinguishes/discriminates mother/primary caretaker from others (i.e., unfamiliar from familiar)—is beginning to prefer the familiar and known; resents strangers
Sits unsupported with arms propped forward Transfers objects from hand to hand; wants to finger-feed self, holds own bottle Reaches for objects spontaneously, without apprehension or reticence Mobility becomes medium through which infant learns about self and world	Is aware of a person as a whole object Perceives existence of objects and their movements dependent on infant's actions (things do not exist when they are not seen) Senses relationship of hands to objects they touch Plays games—peek-a-boo, come and get me, go and fetch	"Separation/stranger anxiety" begins (6-12 months) First teeth—volitional biting; begins chewing solids; feeds self cracker Many sleep through the night Regulates behavior by emotional responses of others Smiles at mirror image Differentiates adults from children—reaches for child

Continued.

TABLE 24-14—cont'd

Neonatal and Infant Development (0-12 months)*

AGE	AUDITORY	LANGUAGE	VISUAL
7-8 months	Is aware of sound below, but cannot directly locate (7-9 months) Listens to own sounds and those of others Distinguishes friendly from angry voices	Makes different sounds for need demands and conversation responses	Has increased attention span and is interested in detail Distinguishes near and far objects and space Briefly looks for toy that disappears
8-9 months	Recognizes names of objects and body parts (8-10 months) Turns toward sounds and own name	Says primary words: "mama" and "dada" (8-10 months) Imitates an object in imitation of its sound Pushes away what he or she does not want Rejects confinement	Differentiates faces regarding features and identity Puts objects "in" and "out" of container Searches for object if hidden while he or she watches
9-10 months	Locates sounds below (9-13 months) Responds when called by name Responds to other words such as "no-no" Carries out simple commands	Utters first intentional "word"/sound (10-14 months) Repeats syllable or larger sequence of sounds	Is aware of vertical space—fears heights Recognizes large from small objects (uses both hands or finger and thumb) Uncovers object he or she has seen hidden
10-11 months	Listens to familiar words with interest Understands and obeys words and commands: "Give me your bottle"	Uses sounds to intentionally communicate Develops symbolic representations for sounds and/or objects—waves "bye-bye"; shakes head for "no" Incessantly repeats word, which becomes response for everything Says 1-2 words besides "mama" and "dada"	Reaches behind for an object (without seeing it) Looks inside container for an object Searches for object he sees hidden; will search in second place

TACTILE-MOTOR	COGNITIVE-MENTAL	SOCIAL-EMOTIONAL
Holds head upright when held supine and prone (6-8 months)	Expects repetition of event	Begins chewing
"Parachute reaction": puts down arms and legs to catch self when prone	Remembers parts of a situation; small series of actions in immediate past	Moves away from parent/primary caretaker in exploring the environment
Crawls backward on abdomen	Associates picture of baby to self and vocalizes to it	Shows humor; teases
Reaches for, grasps, mouths, shakes, and bangs objects	Is aware of and compares size differences of similar objects	Wishes to be included in social interaction
Requires independence in feeding		Resists doing what he or she does not want to do
		Plays with toys
Uses hands (without thumb grasp) to scoop object up	Has intentional behavior for problem solving—uses means to accomplish goal (e.g., removes object in the way of desired object) (8-12 months)	Bites cracker, chews and swallows
Sits erect without support and leans forward		Holds bottle without help
Moves from sitting to prone (8-10 months)		Manages finger foods
Crawls forward and backward on abdomen	Has rudimentary sense of self as separate being from others	Takes 2-3 naps/day
Stands while leaning against object; pulls to stand	Objects only exist in place where first appeared	Has longer time between wetting—occasional dryness when sleeping
	Anticipates events; solves simple problems	Cries when mother leaves; separation anxiety is more obvious
Begins thumb-finger grasp	Coordinates motor activity to midline	Controls mouth muscles—less drooling; vertical chewing begins
Picks up small objects; reaches for objects seen hidden	Has beginning awareness of objects existing when out of sight	Feeds self crackers
Pulls up onto feet with help; pulls to stand and sustains with support	Is easily bored with repetition	Plays games such as "so big," "peek-a-boo," and "patty cake"
Sits up with straight lower spine	Remembers experience from previous day	Recognizes mother from self
Sustains kneeling position and moves on knees	Anticipates reward, and return of person or object	Performs for audiences; repeats if applauded
Brings two objects together at midline and releases one for the other	Refuses to be distracted—is persistent	Protects self; is sensitive to crying child
Drops smaller object into larger one		Initiates play
Walks with help if not yet walking on own; cruises	Objects begin having symbolic representation (i.e., meaning/existence external to infant—they exist outside the self)	Establishes regular elimination pattern (10-12 months)
Probes with index finger		Begins sexual identity
Creeps on hands and knees	Imitates behaviors	Shows moods and feelings
Moves from prone to sitting position (10-12 months)	Prefers one hand to the other	Is sensitive to other children
Sits, rotates, pivots without losing balance (10-12 months)	Points to body parts	Prefers some toys; "loves" doll or animal
Releases objects from grasp (in air as well as on surfaces)		Helps dress self

Continued.

TABLE 24-14—cont'd

Neonatal and Infant Development (0-12 months)*

AGE	AUDITORY	LANGUAGE	VISUAL
11-12 months	Discriminates and responds to differences in vocabulary, tone, and person speaking	Applies language or labels to familiar objects and events in the environment May express thoughts and desires with single word Says "no" and knows what it means	Eye muscles are mature in movement Points at objects

TABLE 24-15

Sequelae Associated with Prematurity

Physical
1. Failure to thrive[46,95,107]
   a. Organic (i.e., physiologic cause)
   b. Nonorganic (i.e., attachment problems; neglect)
2. Child abuse and neglect[61,72,108]—psychologic sequelae ("the unattached child")
   a. Feelings of powerlessness—learned helplessness
   b. Poor ego development—low self-esteem, insecurity, oriented outside the self for cues and guidance
   c. Lack of trust in self and others
   d. Needy dependence
   e. Increasingly prone to depression
   f. Difficulty or inability in establishing and maintaining intimate relationships with others
   g. Increased irritability
3. Developmental delay in gross motor skills[76,103,105,114]
   a. Neurologic impairment (e.g., IVH, cerebral palsy)
   b. Nursery-acquired positioning malformations

Psychosocioemotional
1. Cognitive impairment—decrease in intelligence quotient (IQ) and developmental quotient (DQ)*
2. Learning disorders†
   a. Visual and/or auditory perceptual difficulties
   b. Visual and/or auditory motor incoordination
   c. Normal or delayed acquisition of speech/language
3. Difficult behavioral style[21,76,103]
   a. Difficult to soothe
   b. Less adaptive—difficulty with habituation; state lability; arrhythmicity
   c. Negative mood
   d. Withdrawn and/or highly active
4. Emotional sequelae—(the "unattached child")[72,94,99,108]
   a. Feelings of powerlessness—learned helplessness
   b. Poor ego development—low self esteem, insecurity, oriented outside the self for cues and guidance
   c. Lack of trust in self and others
   d. Needy dependence
   e. Prone to depression
   f. Difficulty or inability in establishing and maintaining intimate relationships with others
   g. Increased irritability
5. Social sequelae[72,94,99,108]
   a. Lack of social conscience: violent or aggressive behaviors toward self and others; no guilt or remorse for behavior
   b. Difficulty or inability in developing intimate relationships with others

*References 9, 22, 57, 71, 85, 86, 101, 109.
†References 21, 57, 62, 85, 86, 108.

TACTILE-MOTOR	COGNITIVE-MENTAL	SOCIAL-EMOTIONAL
Masters forefinger and thumb movements and grasp; hand dominance is evident Plays ball and pull toys; picks up objects and throws them down; brings one object above another Some are standing with support for a few minutes, whereas others are walking alone Moves from sitting to creeping to prone position and reverses process Restrains motor action with unexpected events	Displays conceptual awareness/manual orientation to spatial relationships Is aware of existence of unperceived objects Is aware of similarities in objects Imitates unfamiliar acts and attempts to copy adults Memory retrieval is available and used; shows guilt	Imitates other's behavior Knows body parts Begins rotary chewing Drinks from a cup Feeds self finger foods Cooperates (somewhat) in being dressed (extends arm/leg) Takes off clothes Obeys commands, yet is not always cooperative Parallel play Increasing negativism

the abusive caretaker into the infant's own ego development.

4. The caretaker's control in the relationship negates the needs, feelings, and states of the infant, who also learns to discount himself or herself and inhibits self-initiated activity—is passive with learned helplessness.

Unattached and battered children exhibit poor self-esteem, difficulty or inability in developing close, intimate relationships, lack of a social conscience, and a preoccupation with or increase in violent tendencies.[72,94,99,108]

NICU infants are at risk for being unattached because (1) they have multiple caretakers; (2) the parents are not always present and after a prolonged stay of the baby may be "strangers" to the baby; (3) the needs of the multiple caretakers and baby may be asynchronous (e.g., it is "care time," but the baby is asleep); and (4) lifesaving care in the NICU is intrusive, noxious, and painful. Rather than the soothing, pleasurable nurturing of family, the NICU baby is constantly bombarded with painful touch, handling, and stimuli. From the infant's perspective, the altruistic pain of lifesaving care is indistinguishable from the pain of child abuse.[108] The infant is cognitively unable to distinguish or be taught the difference—he or she merely subjectively experiences

the pain. As one mother stated, "To Joshua, cauterizing his gastrostomy site with a silver nitrate stick was no different than if I'd burned him with a cigarette. To him, his mother was causing him pain."[34]

Although some VLBW (<1500 g) infants may suffer CNS damage because of IVH,[97] it is unclear if developmental delays are due totally to organic insults, the impact of the NICU environment on an immature CNS, or a combination of insults. The environmental characteristics of the NICU, with their potentially adverse effects on the newborn, have been and are currently being researched. The effects of many developmental programs are unclear.[21] Recent studies indicate developmental (and physiologic) improvement from individualized management of the NICU environment.[5,97] Long-term effects of individualized developmental NICU care are not yet known.

The impact on the neonate's experience of hospitalization may be ameliorated or exacerbated by such variables as maturity at birth, severity of illness, length of hospital stay, primary nursing, genetic endowment, temperament, maternal education and caretaking, and postdischarge follow-up and interventions. Since keeping parents involved is so important to outcome, parents need anticipatory guidance about "taking their premie home." Instead of telling parents that preterm infants are "more difficult," a more positive "preterm infants need more help from parents in the first year of life" is warranted. Concrete techniques to soothe, feed, and interact with *their* baby and "rooming-in" practice help parents be more confident in caretaking. Absolving parental guilt (i.e., "What am I doing wrong?") by teaching parents that the *baby* has a problem, helps keep parents involved with the baby. Teaching appropriate play activities assists parents in enjoying their baby while providing the baby with vital sensory and social experience for development.[9]

Care of preterm infants began with a minimal handling policy. Research and knowledge of the unique anatomy and physiology of the neonate preceded the development of high-technology devices and high touch to manage both machines and newborns. Observation and research has documented the impact of the NICU environment on its vulnerable inhabitants. Individualized developmental interventions in the NICU and beyond have resulted in decreased developmental delay as well as medical benefits. Further observation and research will assist in creating a healthy, humane environment that promotes optimal infant development.

REFERENCES

1. Als H: Toward a synactive theory of development: promise for assessment and support of infant individuality, Infant Ment Health J 3(4):229, 1982.
2. Als H: Infant individuality: assessing patterns of very early development. In Call JD, Galenson MD, and Tyson R, editors: Frontiers of infant psychiatry, New York, 1983, Basic Books, Inc.
3. Als H and Brazelton TB: A new model of assessing the behavioral organization in preterm and full term infants, J Am Acad Child Psychiatry 20:239, 1981.
4. Als H et al: The behavior of the full-term yet underweight newborn infant, Dev Med Child Neurol 18:590, 1976.
5. Als H et al: Individualized behavioral and environmental care for the VLBW preterm infant at high risk for BPD: neonatal intensive care unit and developmental outcome, Pediatrics 78(6):1123, 1986.
6. Anders T: Maturation of sleep patterns in the newborn infant, Adv Sleep Res 2:43, 1975.
7. Anderson J and Auster-Liebhaber J: Developmental therapy in the NICU, Phys Occup Ther Pediatr 4(1):89, 1984.
8. Barnard K and Erickson M: Teaching children with developmental problems, ed 2, St Louis, 1976, The CV Mosby Co.
9. Beckwith L: The influences of caregiver-infant interaction on development. In Sell EJ: Follow up of the high-risk infant, Springfield, Ill, 1980, Charles C Thomas, Publisher.
10. Bell SM and Ainsworth MD: Infant crying and maternal responsiveness, Child Dev 43:1171, 1972.
11. Blackburn S: Fostering behavioral development in high risk infants, JOGN Nurs (suppl), p 805, May/June 1983.
12. Bohus B et al: Oxytocin, vasopressin and memory: opposite effects on consolidation and retrieval processes, Brain Res 157:414, 1978.
13. Bowlby J: Attachment, New York, 1973, Basic Books, Inc.
14. Bowlby J: Separation, New York, 1973, Basic Books, Inc.
15. Bowlby J: Loss, New York, 1980, Basic Books, Inc.
16. Bradley RM and Mistretta CM: Fetal sensory receptors, Physiol Rev 3:353, 1975.
17. Brazelton TB: Crying in infancy, Pediatrics 14:579, 1954.
18. Brazelton TB: Neonatal behavioral assessment scale, Philadelphia, 1973, Spastics International Medical Publishers/JB Lippincott Co.
19. Brazelton TB: The origins of reciprocity: the early maternal-infant interaction. In Lewis M and Rosenblum LA, editors: The effect of the infant on its caregiver, New York, 1974, John Wiley & Sons, Inc.
20. Brazelton TB and Als HA: Four early stages in the development of maternal-infant interaction, Psychoanal Study Child 34:349, 1979.
21. Campbell SK: Effects of developmental interventions in the special care nursery, Adv Dev Behav Pediatr 4:165, 1983.
22. Caputo DV et al: The development of prematurely born children through middle childhood. In Field T et al, editors: Infants born at risk, New York, 1978, Spectrum Books.
23. Chamberlain DB: Consciousness at birth: the range of empirical evidence. In Verny T, editor: Pre- and perinatal psychology, an introduction, New York, 1987, Human Sciences Press, Inc.
24. Cohen RS et al: Favorable results of neonatal intensive care for very low birth weight infants, Pediatrics, 69:621, 1982.
25. Cole JG: Infant stimulation reexamined: an environmental- and behavioral-based approach, Neonatal Network 3(5):24, 1985.
26. DeCasper AJ and Fifer WP: Of human bonding: new-

borns prefer their mother's voices, Science 208:1175, 1980.

27. DeCasper AJ and Spence MJ: Prenatal maternal speech influences newborn's perception of speech sounds, Infant Behav Dev 9:133, 1986.

28. deChateau P: The importance of the neonatal period for the development of synchrony in the maternal-infant dyad—a review, Birth Fam J 4(1):10, 1977.

29. Deters GE: Circadian rhythm phenomenon, MCN 5: 249, 1980.

30. Dobbing J and Sands J: Quantitative growth and development of the human brain, Arch Dis Child 48:757, 1973.

31. Dreyfus-Brisac C: Organization of sleep in preterms: implications for caretaking. In Lewis M and Rosenblum LA, editors: The effect of the infant on its caregiver, New York, 1974, John Wiley & Sons, Inc.

32. Dreyfus-Brisac C: Ontogenesis of brain bioelectric activity and sleep organization in neonates and infants. In Faulkner F and Tanner JM, editors: Human growth, vol 3, New York, 1979, Plenum Publishing Corp.

33. Dubowitz L et al: Clinical assessment of gestational age in the newborn infant, J Pediatr 77:1, 1970.

34. Eickner S: Personal communication, 1987.

35. Emde RN and Harmon RJ: Endogenous and exogenous smiling systems in early infancy, J Am Acad Child Psychiatry 11:177, 1972.

36. Erickson E: Childhood and society, New York, 1950, WW Norton & Co.

37. Fantz RL, Fagan JF, and Miranda SB: Early visual selectivity as a function of pattern variables, previous exposure, age from birth and conception and expected cognitive deficit. In Cohen L and Salaptic P, editors: Infant perception, vol 1, New York, 1975, Academic Press, Inc.

38. Fay MJ: The positive effects of positioning, Neonatal Network 6(5):23, 1988.

39. Field TM: Interaction patterns of preterm and term infants. In Field TM, editor: Infants born at risk, New York, 1979, Spectrum Books.

40. Field TM: Infants born at risk. In Friedman S and Sigman M, editors: Preterm birth and psychological development, New York, 1980, Academic Press, Inc.

41. Field TM: Supplemental stimulation of preterm neonates, Early Hum Dev 4(3):301, 1980.

42. Field TM et al: Mother-stranger face discrimination by the newborn, Infant Behav Dev 7:19, 1984.

43. Field TM et al: Tactile/kinesthetic stimulation effects on preterm neonates, Pediatrics 77(5):654, 1986.

44. Foley H: When do preterms and light for dates babies smile? Dev Med Child Neurol 19:757, 1977.

45. Freedman DG: Ethnic differences in babies, Hum Nature 2(1):36, 1979.

46. Gardner LI: Deprivation dwarfism, Sci Am 227(1):76, 1982.

47. Gardner SL: Mothering: the unconscious conflict between nurses and new mothers, Keeping Abreast: J Hum Nurt 3:192, 1978.

48. Garland KR: Newborns are people, too! Keeping Abreast: J Hum Nurt 3:206, 1978.

49. Gorski PA: Premature infant behavioral and physiological responses to caregiving interventions in the intensive care nursery. In Call JD, Galenson E, and Tyson RL, editors: Frontiers in infant psychiatry, New York, 1983, Basic Books, Inc.

50. Gorski PA, Davison MF, and Brazelton TB: Stages of behavioral organization in the high risk neonate: theoretical and clinical considerations, Semin Perinatol 3:61, 1979.

51. Gottfried AW and Gaiter JL: Infant stress under intensive care: environmental neonatology, Baltimore, 1985, University Park Press.

52. Gunderson LP and Kenner C: Neonatal stress: physiologic adaptation and nursing implications, Neonatal Network 6(1):37, 1987.

53. Haley J: Strategies in psychotherapy, New York, 1969, Grune & Stratton, Inc.

54. Harbin RE: Is there a place for a rocking chair in your newborn nursery: a review of studies on the effect of rocking the newborn, Pediatr Nurs, p 16, July/Aug 1975.

55. Hyde BB and McCown DE: Classical conditioning in neonatal intensive care nurseries, Pediatr Nurs 12(1):11, 1986.

56. Illingworth RS: The development of the infant and young child, ed 5, Edinburgh, 1972, Churchill Livingstone.

57. Jacob S et al: Cognitive, perceptual and personal-social development of prematurely born preschoolers, Percept Mot Skills 58:551, 1984.

58. Kastin J et al: The effects of MSH and MIF on the brain. In Stumpf WE and Grant LD, editors: Anatomical neuroendocrinology, New York, 1975, S Karger.

59. Katlwinkel J et al: Apnea of prematurity, J Pediatr 86: 588, 1975.

60. Klaus M and Kennell J: Parent-infant bonding, St Louis, 1982, The CV Mosby Co.

61. Klein M and Stern L: Low birth weight and the battered child syndrome, Am J Dis Child 22:15, 1971.

62. Klein N et al: School performance of normal intelligence VLBW children, Pediatr Res 17:98A, 1983.

63. Knoblock H et al: Considerations in evaluating changes in outcome for infants weighing less than 1,501 gms., Pediatrics 69:285, 1982.

64. Korner AF: The effect of the infant's state, level of arousal, sex and ontogenetic stage on the caregiver. In Lewis M and Rosenblum LA, editors: The effect of the

infant on its caregiver, New York, 1974, John Wiley & Sons, Inc.

65. Korner AF and Thoman EB: The relative efficacy of contact and vestibular-proprioceptive stimulation in soothing neonates, Child Dev 2:443, 1972.

66. Korner AF et al: Effects of waterbed flotation on premature infants: a pilot study, Pediatrics 56:361, 1975.

67. Lederman RP et al: The relationship of maternal anxiety, plasma catecholamines, and plasma cortisol to progress in labor, AJOB Nurs 11:495, 1970.

68. Lewis M and Michalson L: The socialization of emotional pathology, Infant Ment Health J 3:125, 1984.

69. Lipsitt LP: The study of sensation and learning processes of the newborn, Clin Perinatol 4(1):163, 1977.

70. Long JG et al: Noise and hypoxemia in the intensive care nursery, Pediatrics 65:143, 1981.

71. Lubchenco LO et al: Long term follow up studies of prematurely born infants. I. Relationship of handicaps to nursery routines, J Pediatr 80(3):501, 1972.

72. Magid K and McKelvey CA: High risk: children without a conscience, Colorado, 1987, Mand M Publishing.

73. Mahler M et al: The psychological birth of the human infant, New York, 1975, Basic Books, Inc.

74. Martin RJ et al: Effect of supine and prone positions on arterial oxygen tension in the preterm infant, Pediatrics, 63:528, 1979.

75. Masterson J et al: Prone and supine positioning effects on energy expenditure and behavior of low birth weight neonates, Pediatrics 80:689, 1987.

76. Medoff-Cooper B and Schraeder BD: Developmental trends and behavioral styles in VLBW infants, Nurs Res 31(2):68, 1982.

77. Meltzoff AN and Moore MK: Imitation of facial and manual gestures by human neonates, Science 198(4312): 74, 1977.

78. Michelson K, Sirvio P, and Wasz-Hockert O: Pain cry in full term asphyxiated newborn infant correlated with late finding, Acta Paediatr Scand 66(5):611, 1977.

79. Miranda SB and Fantz RL: Visual abilities and pattern preference of preterm infants and full term neonates, J Exp Child Psychiatry 10:189, 1970.

80. Miranda SB and Fantz RL: Distribution of visual attention of newborn infants among patterns varying in size and number of details, Proceedings of the American Psychologic Association, Washington, DC, 1971.

81. Mitchell SA: Noise pollution in the neonatal intensive care nursery, Semin Hear 5(1):17, 1984.

82. Montague A: Prenatal influences, Springfield, Ill, 1962, Charles C Thomas, Publisher.

83. Montague A: Touching, New York, 1971, Harper & Row, Publishers, Inc.

84. Murphy TF, Nichter CA, and Liden CB: Developmental outcomes of the high-risk infant: a review of methodological issues, Semin Perinatol 6:353, 1982.

85. Nichol R et al: School performance of children with birth weight of 1000 grams or less, Am J Dis Child 136:105, 1982.

86. Noble-Jamieson CM et al: Low birth weight children at school age: neurological, psychological and pulmonary function, Semin Perinatol 6:266, 1982.

87. Northern J and Downs MA: Hearing in children, Baltimore, 1974, Williams & Wilkins.

88. Orenstein SR and Whitington PF: Positioning for prevention of gastroesophageal reflux, J Pediatr 103(4):534, 1983.

89. Osofsky JD and Danzger B: Relationships between neonatal characteristics and mother-infant interaction, Dev Psychol 1:124, 1974.

90. Oswald J: Human brain protein, drugs and dreams, Nature 233:893, 1969.

91. Palisano R and Short M: Methods for assessing muscle tone and motor function in the neonate: a review, Phys Occup Ther Pediatr 4(4):43, 1984.

92. Pamalee AH: Sleep states in premature infants, Dev Med Child Neurol 9:70, 1967.

93. Pelletier JM and Palmeri A: Infants at risk. In Clark PN and Allen AS, editors: Occupational therapy for children, St Louis, 1985, The CV Mosby Co.

94. Prescott J: Body pleasure and the origins of violence, Futurist 2:64, 1975.

95. Provence S and Lipton RC: Infants in institutions, New York, 1962, International Universities Press.

96. Regional Perinatal Intensive Care Centers Program Annual Report FY 1983-84, Tallahassee, Fla, DHRS, 1984.

97. Resnick MB et al: Developmental intervention for low birth weight infants: improved early developmental outcome, Pediatrics 80(1):1987.

98. Rice R: Maternal-infant bonding: the profound long-term benefits of immediate, continuous skin and eye contact at birth. In Stewart D and Stewart L, editors: 21st century obstetrics, now! Chapel Hill, NC, 1977, NAPSAC, Inc.

99. Rice R: Infant stress and the relationship to violent behavior, Neonatal Network 5:39, 1985.

100. Ross E: Review and critique of research on the use of tactile and kinesthetic stimulation with premature infants, Phys Occup Ther Pediatr 4(1):35, 1984.

101. Ruiz MPD et al: Early development of infants of birth weight less than 1,000 grams with reference to mechanical ventilation in the newborn period, Pediatrics 68:330, 1981.

102. Sarnat HB: Olfactory reflexes in newborn infants, J Pediatr 92(4):624, 1978.

103. Schraeder BD and Medoff-Cooper B: Development and temperament in very low birth weight infants—the second year, Nurs Res 32(6):331, 1983.

104. Sheagren TG et al: Rumination—a new complication of neonatal intensive care, Pediatrics 66(4):551, 1980.

105. Siegel LS: Reproductive, perinatal and environmental variables as predictors of development of preterm (<1501 gm) and full term children at 5 years, Semin Perinatol 6:274, 1982.

106. Sostek AM, Anders TF, and Sostek AJ: Diurnal rhythms in two to eight week old infants: sleep-wake state organization as a factor of age and stress, Psychosom Med 38(4):250, 1976.

107. Spitz R: Hospitalism, Psychoanal Study Child 1:53, 1945.

108. Steele BF: The effect of abuse and neglect on psychological development. In Call JD, Galenson E, and Tyson RL, editors: Frontiers of infant psychiatry, New York, 1983, Basic Books, Inc.

109. Stewart AL et al: Outcome for infants of very low birth weights: survey of world literature, Lancet 1:1038, 1981.

110. Stott DH: Follow up study from birth of the effects of prenatal stresses, Dev Med Child Neurol 15:770, 1973.

111. Sugarman M: Perinatal influences on maternal-infant attachment, Am J Orthopsychiatry 47:407, 1977.

112. Thoman EB and Graham SE: Self-regulation of stimulation by premature infants, Pediatrics 78(5):855, 1986.

113. Thomas A, Chess S, and Birch HG: The origins of personality, Sci Am 223:102, 1970.

114. Towbin A: Cerebral dysfunction related to perinatal organic damage: clinical neuropathologic correlations, J Abnorm Psychol 87:617, 1978.

115. Tudor M: Child development, New York, 1981, McGraw Hill Book Co.

116. Updike C et al: Positional support for premature infants, Am J Occup Ther 40(10):712, 1986.

117. Vandenberg KA: Revising the traditional model: an individualized approach to developmental interventions, Neonatal Network 3(5):32, 1985.

118. Verny T and Kelly J: The secret life of the unborn child, New York, 1981, Dell Publishing Co, Inc.

119. Wagaman MJ et al: Improved oxygenation and lung compliance with prone positioning of neonates, J Pediatr 94:787, 1979.

120. Wingert WA et al: Pediatric nurse practitioners in follow up care of high risk infants, Am J Nurs 80:1485, 1980.

CHAPTER 25

Ethics in neonatal intensive care

JULIE SANDLING · BRIAN CARTER · CLAUDIA MOORE · JOHN W. SPARKS

Clinical decision making is influenced by the values of the individuals involved. In the neonatal intensive care unit (NICU), these include the preservation of life, decreasing morbidity, and relieving pain and suffering. Many health care professionals agree that the art of clinical medicine, combined with societal and personal values, can result in sound clinical decisions.

Recent technologic advances in medicine have benefited many patients. We are better able to prolong life; at the same time, we are more often in a position to make deliberate decisions about when and how death will occur. Concomitantly, it has become necessary for society to reassess whether the value of prolonging life conflicts with other values, such as relieving pain and suffering, and reducing morbidity. In such cases values of society, the family, and the health care professional necessarily enter into and influence the decision-making process.

Ethical reasoning insists that we understand the role of values as well as medical data in making decisions.

HISTORY

Ethical questions in clinical practice are not new (Table 25-1), but in recent years the questions of appropriate treatment of handicapped and seriously ill newborns have become a matter of increasing public concern. This interest has been influenced by a number of dramatic cases, such as Baby Doe or the Quinlan case,[42] in which con-

cern has focused on the withholding and withdrawing of treatment and allowing patients to die.

The majority of newborns treated in NICUs grow up to lead active, productive lives. But not all seriously ill newborns fare well with even the most aggressive of treatments.[34] Recognizing the risks and benefits of technology, Eisenberg[13] stated, "At long last, we are beginning to ask, not *can* it be done, but *should* it be done."

Discussion of treatment of seriously ill newborns was stimulated by the 1973 publication of Duff and Campbell.[12] Their seminal article described the selective nontreatment or withdrawal of treatment for 43 seriously ill newborns at Yale–New Haven Hospital (between 1970 and 1972) whose "prognosis for meaningful life was extremely poor or hopeless." They recognized that survivors of neonatal intensive care are often healthy; they also recognized that some infants remain severely disabled by congenital malformations that, until recently, would have resulted in premature death. Duff and Campbell were legitimately concerned about the quality of life for these severely impaired survivors and their families.

Before this report, ethical and legal concerns in neonatal medicine focused on the risks and benefits of available technology. Such issues included oxygen therapy, with the offsetting dilemma that treatment could possibly cause blindness whereas nontreatment might result in cerebral palsy

TABLE 25-1

Selected Issues in Perinatal/Neonatal History of Ethical Import

TIME	FETAL DIAGNOSIS	FETAL THERAPY	NEONATAL THERAPY
1900s (early)			Temperature regulation, nutrition; limited survival in LBW and anomalied infants
			Recognition of congenital rubella syndrome
			Cardiovascular surgery in the newborn period
			Modern incubator developed
			Oxygen therapy for respiratory distress
1950s		Tocolysis (ETOH)	EBF (Rh) incompatibility recognized
			Oxygen toxicity recognized: RLF/blindness in treated infants; CP and mortality in those untreated
			Other iatrogenic diseases
			Antibiotic usage broadens
1960s	Placentocentesis	Intraperitoneal blood transfusion for EBF	"Birth" of NICUs
	Early ultrasound		Field of teratology develops following thalidomide disaster
	FHR monitoring		Improved outcome for infants <2500 g
	Fetal scalp pH assessment		Surgical management of meningomyelocele becomes an issue
	Amniocentesis		
	Chromosomal analysis		
1970s	Fetoscopy	Intravascular blood transfusion for EBF	CPAP, modern neonatal ventilator
	Real-time ultrasound		Improved outcome for infants <1500 g
	Improved structural, chromosomal, and metabolic diagnostics	Beta-adrenergic agonists for tocolysis	BPD recognized
		Corticosteroids for lung maturation	Problems of the VLBW infant: IVH, BPD, NEC
			TPN/HAL becomes available
		Legalization of abortion	Improved pediatric surgery
1980s	Chorionic villous sampling	Fetal surgery for hydrocephalus	Newborn metabolic screening
	Cordocentesis	Prophylactic penicillin for group B streptococcus infection	High-frequency ventilation
	Doppler flow studies of placenta and umbilical vessels		Prophylactic phenobarbital
			Surfactant replacement therapy
	New reproductive technology		Improved survival in infants <1000 g
	AFP monitoring		Prophylactic antibiotics

(1950s), and the results of treating newborns with congenital anomalies such as meningomyelocele (1960s). Treatment of premature infants and infants with birth defects, especially meningomyelocele, became technically possible in the 1950s and has progressed steadily since then (Table 25-1). The controversy since the early 1960s has been over how vigorously to treat newborns.

Zachary[59] and Shurtleff[48] advocated aggressive management, which increased survival rates but offered questionable quality of life for those more severely affected. Lorber[29,30] was less optimistic about the effects of aggressive management of infants with meningomyelocele and is noted for his selective nontreatment of some of these infants. According to Duff and Campbell[12]:

Both treatment and nontreatment constitute unsatisfactory dilemmas for everyone. . . . When maximum treatment was viewed as unacceptable by families and physicians in our unit, there was a growing tendency to seek early death as a management option, to avoid that cruel choice of gradual, often slow, but progressive deterioration of the child.

Most recently, the unnamed Johns Hopkins baby (1970s) and "Baby Doe" (1980s) have become the focus of this controversy over the issue of withholding treatment and nutrition from handicapped infants.[5,22,38,54] Both were born with Down's syndrome and intestinal atresia. Both were denied relatively uncomplicated surgical repair of the atresia, and both died of starvation. In the Bloomington Baby Doe case, the court upheld the parents' decision to deny treatment. The federal government later responded to this case with regulations monitoring and intervening in the medical care of handicapped newborns (1980s).

Throughout this short, though focused, "history" of ethical issues in neonatal care, it has become increasingly apparent that there are numerous individuals involved in the decision-making process. More people become involved as technologic advances increase treatment options. Parents have always been presumed to be the best decision makers on their child's behalf. Health care providers have also been committed to providing what is in the best interests of their patients. Historically, decisions were made privately between parents and their physician. In the modern NICU, decisions are made in the context of a health care team composed of professionals from various moral communities who offer specialized input into the care of the neonate and the family. Children have also been protected against decisions that are detrimental to their best interests by statutes on child abuse and neglect. Respect for clinical decision making, preferably made by parents and clinicians together, and protection of children against harm are concerns constantly being balanced, both ethically and legally.

DEFINITION OF BIOETHICS

Ethics is the study of rational processes for determining the most morally desirable course of action in view of conflicting value choices. Ethics is a branch of philosophy that considers competing values in order to obtain the best possible outcome to a given situation. The most morally desirable course of action is determined by whether, and how, that action adheres to certain ethical principles held by those involved in making decisions. Conflicts arise when competing values and/or principles cannot be satisfied; thus an ethical dilemma exists.

In order for an ethical dilemma to exist, a real choice between possible courses of action must exist. Further, different values must be held for possible courses of action by parties involved in the process.

An ethical statement considers what is right or wrong, better or worse, and implies by its "ought" that it applies to all people in relevantly similar situations. Universalizability may be inherent in ethical statements. It does not mean that moral principles apply universally to everyone regardless of their moral positions, but that any moral choice must, for those accepting it, apply universally in relevantly similar circumstances.[7]

Bioethics seeks to determine the most morally desirable course of action in health care given the conflicting values inherent in varying treatment options.[4] Most often, when a conflict of values does not exist, moral conflict does not exist. That is, when the health care providers and parents all agree that it is most beneficial to an infant not to treat the infant aggressively and to allow the infant to die, no dilemma or conflict between them exists. Of course, that they agree does not mean that conflict does not exist with moral views of outside parties or principles. Regardless, the goal is to determine the most morally desirable course of action under a given set of circumstances.

THEORIES OF ETHICS

We base clinical-ethical judgments on fundamental theories and principles. There are a variety of theoretical approaches, of which two concern us here.

Utilitarian approach

The utilitarian, or consequentialist, approach is based on the principle of utility—what is most desirable is to maximize the good, or intrinsic positive value of an outcome, for the greatest number of individuals affected. The utilitarian gauges the worth of actions by their outcomes. Thus in determining what is morally right and wrong behavior, the utilitarian looks for the better or best outcomes or consequences. Restated, the utilitarian promotes the greatest balance of value over disvalue. No action in and of itself is generally considered right or wrong.

Utilitarians may disagree about what a "good" outcome is. Is it happiness? Love? Pleasure? Elimination of suffering? The act utilitarian calculates the desirable outcome from different possible courses of action and chooses that action that promotes the greatest "good." The rule utilitarian believes that some principles (beneficence, justice) promote ethical behavior. The principles that yield the greatest utility for each situation are chosen and enforced.

Deontological approach

The deontological, or formalist, position asserts that some acts are intrinsically right or wrong independent of their consequences. The goodness of an act is inherent in the act itself. For instance, formalists may claim that lying is wrong because intentional deception is morally unacceptable, even if the deception is intended to be, or is, benevolent. Formalists do not ignore the consequences of their actions; however, unlike utilitarians, they base their decisions on certain principles that they follow absolutely in all decisions. Thus the obligation to uphold these principles takes ethical precedence over the consequences of individual acts.

Principles of autonomy, beneficence, nonmaleficence, and justice are frequently deontologically based. The foundation of other deonto-

logic approaches may be belief in the sanctity of life, fidelity, or honesty. Adherence to these principles, based on religious or other sets of rules, is of primary importance. A good or right decision can then be derived and a course of action taken. These principles may conflict. The formalist must prioritize them to determine which principle takes precedence.

Formalists disagree about which principles are right or wrong, inviolable or not, just as utilitarians disagree about what constitutes the greatest "good" as a moral goal. Most people agree that certain principles such as beneficence and justice are positive principles and should be upheld. The formalist gauges the worth of actions by adherence to certain held principles and the values they are based on, not by their outcomes.

These moral theories and their variants are operative in decisions regarding neonates, as in other areas of health care. The utilitarian and the formalist may arrive at the same, or opposite, conclusions that are nonetheless each ethically justifiable. Either approach may be used to establish the most morally acceptable actions and outcomes possible.

These theoretical schools of thought are systematic approaches to ethics that are undergirded by moral principles, rules, and judgments. Judgments are conclusions about certain actions; rules raise those conclusions to a level of "ought." Rules state that actions ought or ought not to be done because they are right or wrong. Principles are more broad and serve as the basis and justification of rules. Ethical principles, in their broad scope, are inclusive of judgments and rules, and form the foundation of ethical theories.

PRINCIPLES OF ETHICS

Bioethical principles are at the heart of decision making in the NICU. These principles aid individual decision makers in determining what their moral obligations and duties are in times of moral dilemma. Each principle is based on specific values, moral rules, and responsibilities. Whether one is a deontologist or a utilitarian determines which and how these principles are considered.

The major principles are autonomy, beneficence and nonmaleficence, and justice. Although each principle can be theoretically defined, in the clinical setting they have a multitude of interpretations and applications. Each principle carries with it a significant interrelationship with the others, and at times may create emotional tension and conflict between persons. Often health care professionals find themselves in situations where following one principle violates another. Or, one professional's ethics may be strictly deontologic whereas another team member's or the parent's ethics may be strongly utilitarian. Deciding which ethical theory and which moral duties should prevail is at the center of bioethics. Each decision maker brings with him or her a personal ethical theory and perhaps a professional ethical theory. It is *how* individuals apply these theories and principles that creates the basis for decision making in the NICU.

Principle of autonomy

The principle of autonomy is based on the right to self-determination. This principle cannot be applied directly to the neonate, because he or she is not competent and never has been. The neonate has no known values, morals, or beliefs to bring to the decision-making process. Decisions must always be made for this patient by third parties. These third parties extend from the parents to the health care team, ethics committees, and possibly to the court system. Each member of the decision-making process brings with him or her an idea of what type of care is in the best interest of the patient. Considerations of "best interest" can be as opposite as black and white—life and death. Each consideration carries with it personal values and morals demanding that certain duties and obligations be met. And each consideration must be based on adequate information being understood and applied to the particular situation.

In the NICU autonomy applies to the right of the parent(s) or designated guardian to make a decision about the patient's care. Autonomy has prima facie (all things being equal) value here, even for the rule deontologist. For example, though the parents of a seriously anomalous infant want "everything possible done," this is usually weighed against the harm inflicted, the risks to be taken, and, at times, what resources or possible treatments are available to implement and/or continue care. Because the patient is not competent, the decisions are made by proxies with an expected standard of "reasonableness." Even the rule deontologist, who values autonomy as an absolute, must consider whose best-interest standard takes precedence.

As with all of the bioethical principles, autonomy can be interpreted in many ways within the NICU setting. For example, some believe that the autonomy of the parents is conditional and that it must be so because of the stress inherent in having a sick or dying newborn. Others believe to the contrary; they trust that parents can and should make these difficult decisions because they will eventually live with the results. Still others believe that parents can never understand the problems involved in the decision-making process and that difficult decisions should therefore be made by the physician and the health care team; this is called a paternalistic outlook. When conflict arises, whose values take precedence? Shelp[47] suggests that the parents' view of best interest should take precedence, within reason. He lists "instances in which parental refusal of treatment would be reasonable . . . (1) where there is no proven procedure or where there is conflicting medical advice, e.g., trisomy 13 and bleeding in the brain . . . (2) where there is less than a high probability that the result of treatment will be a normal or near normal life . . . (3) where intervention would be futile . . . (4) where treatment would impose a grave burden on the infant or others." Shelp's "standard of reasonableness limits the discretion of parents without stipulating what the decision should be."[47] He is a consequentialist. Ramsey,[43] a deontologist, stipulates "best interest" to always lean toward life-sustaining treatments (except when the patient is already dying).

PATERNALISM

Paternalism views the best-interest standard from the perspective that one individual, usually the physician, knows best. The Hippocratic image of physicians and their authority over patients was not only accepted, but expected, by society over the last 2500 years. Only recently has our society's increasing emphasis on self-knowledge and self-determinism led us to a position where the traditional physician is no longer considered purely autonomous in patient care discussions.

Paternalism is formally defined as "(1) the intentional limitation of the autonomy of one person by another, (2) where the person who limits autonomy appeals exclusively to grounds of beneficence for the person whose autonomy is limited.... The essence of paternalism, then, is an overriding of the principle of respect for autonomy on grounds of the principle of beneficence."[8]

Paternalistic interventions restrict the patient's autonomy and freedom. However, in terms of giving autonomy to a neonatal patient, it is obvious that the neonate's state of incompetence creates a unique situation. In this case the freedom of the patient's family to be self-determining is at issue. When another's substituted judgment (i.e., usually the parent's) must prevail, there remain many questions about the propriety of their decisions. Engelhardt[16] upholds the need for some paternalism. However, he, like others, acknowledges the inherent and continuing problem with deciding whose paternalistic judgment should prevail. Whose substituted judgment brings the best outcome for the patient? Although the physician's knowledge and authority is still of utmost importance in decision making, it is now being considered with much more care and discretion by the family members, the health care team, and by society as a whole.[36]

Sometimes situations exist where paternalism is justified in the NICU. For example, if a family is obviously too stressed to give an informed consent in an emergency situation, the health care team must do what is in the best interest of the patient first. Often emergency care is required for a period of time before long-term treatment plans can be made. Time is frequently a critical factor with sick neonates, requiring instantaneous decisions by the ever-present health care team. Without such paternalistic interventions the neonate may die. The best-interest standard in the NICU continues to side with life until there is information available to the contrary.

In the past the physician usually belonged to the same moral community as the patient and his or her family. Values were generally similar and options generally limited. Today's high-tech NICUs and mobile society inhibit the simple best-interest standards of the past. Consequently, it is imperative to construct avenues for consideration of the varied and divergent moral communities present today. However, resolving the dilemma of who should decide does not solve the problem of what ought to be done. The principle of beneficence works to answer this question.

PROXY DECISION MAKERS: BEST INTEREST AND SUBSTITUTED JUDGMENT

In perinatal cases it is self-evident that fetuses or newborns are not competent to act autonomously in making their own decisions. As discussed earlier, in the never-competent patient, beneficence and nonmaleficence become the dominant principles. This incompetence raises subsidiary questions of who decides what is best for the patient, and how the decision is made.

One standard of proxy action seeks to determine the patient's best interest. The best-interest standard "requires a surrogate to do what, from an objective standpoint, appears to promote a patient's good, without reference to the patient's actual or supposed preferences." Thus only the "best interest" of the patient is considered, and the course of action is chosen on the basis of what seems best for that patient, regardless of the patient's wishes. Since newborns have not expressed their wishes, this standard is frequently preferred for newborns.

Another standard of proxy action is "substituted judgment." In this case the responsibility of the proxy moral agent is to make the decision the incompetent person would have made if competent. This in essence grants the incompetent patient respect as a moral agent deserving of autonomy. The distinction between "best interest" and "substituted judgment" is subtle in the context of the neonate. The parents or other proxy decision makers in the first instance decide what is in the best interest of the child. The child is the decision maker in the second instance, with parents or other proxies expressing a belief concerning what the child would have chosen. The distinction becomes practical when the child's beliefs may or may not be assumed to coincide with the beliefs of the parent. For instance, as in the case of blood transfusions for children of Jehovah's Witness parents, the child's undetermined beliefs cannot be assumed to coincide with the parents' beliefs. Therefore transfusions are generally permitted.

Of course, substituted judgment is difficult in neonates because they have not expressed any values or decisions for themselves. The necessity for some surrogate process of decision making, whether by best-interest standard or substituted judgment, is clear in perinatal cases. The appearance of "wrongful life" suits in the legal setting parallels the ethical dilemma of decision making for incompetent minor patients. In such cases children mature to express disagreement with parental decisions previously made in their behalf.

Principles of beneficence and nonmaleficence

Beneficence is broadly defined as "active goodness, kindness, charity."[7] This principle summons moral agents to do "good" for another. This "good" is impossible to pin down in our pluralistic society. Many individuals demand that their personal interpretation take precedence.[47] So where does that leave us? It is a dynamic situation—one where moral agents are exposed to an increasingly diverse perception of what one's moral duties and responsibilities entail. Where once beneficence meant preserving life at all cost, it now includes consideration of when to stop preserving life—when to withdraw or withhold life-sustaining treatment. In some situations death may be seen as a "good." This would be a utilitarian perspective. The deontologist, however, would see the "good" as preserving life regardless of its quality. Whereas the utilitarian views life as a relative good, the deontologist usually views life as an absolute good. Therefore withdrawing or withholding available technology from a sick or anomalous newborn would be unacceptable to the deontologist unless the newborn were already dying. Withdrawal or withholding of treatment could be an option for the utilitarian even if the neonate were only experiencing prolonged, irreversible pain and suffering.

The Hippocratic Oath expresses a duty of beneficence: "I will use treatment to help the sick according to my ability and judgment, but I will never use it to injure or wrong them." While one's duty is to do "good" (i.e., help the sick—beneficence), it is also expected that one will do no "harm" (i.e., never injure or wrong them—nonmaleficence).

Nonmaleficence is primarily associated with the maxim "primum non nocere—above all, or first, do no harm." Although the exact origin of this maxim is unknown, its importance is not questioned. Often in conflict situations, "we can expect nonmaleficence to be overriding" the principle of beneficence.[7] Whereas the principle of beneficence requires positive acts such as preventing or removing evil and doing or promoting good, the principle of nonmaleficence requires avoidance of certain acts that inflict harm or injury to the patient. Beauchamp and Childress[7] have constructed a model that shows today's clinical interpretation of the "goods" and "harms":

Goods	Harms
Health	Illness
Prevention, elimination, or control of disease and injury	Disease (morbidity and injury)
Relief from unnecessary pain and suffering	Unnecessary pain and suffering
Amelioration of handicapping conditions	Handicapping conditions
Prolonged life	Premature death

Where withdrawing or withholding treatment from a very anomalous infant would be viewed as inflicting harm and morally wrong by some deontologists, it could also be viewed by utilitarians as harmful *not* to withdraw or withhold treatment so as not to prolong pain and suffering or continue a life too tragic to exist. Finding an answer frequently entails weighing the "goods" against the "harms."

The principles of beneficence and nonmaleficence and the moral rules and obligations they require are not absolute. They are at best prima facie principles. For example, it is acceptable to inflict some pain and suffering in order to achieve a cure or to prevent a worse harm (i.e., death). However, any time harm is inflicted, there is a need for moral justification.[7]

Engelhardt[16] and Shelp[47] agree that the difficulty with the principle of beneficence lies in the fact that it is not able to reach across varied communities. Shelp[47] considers this possible scenario in the NICU:

The parents may be Southern Baptist, the nurse a Reform Jew, the neonatologist an atheist, and the social worker a Roman Catholic. It is possible, even probable, that each party could reach a different reasonable decision, given their individual moral commitments, about what interventions ought to occur.

When confronted with such a diversity of perspectives and values, one no doubt wonders how to proceed. There is no absolute answer at this point. Some ethicists believe that the parents as decision makers are motivated by beneficence and can best determine what is the "greatest good" for their child. But since no one can know what the patient would consider "good," surrogates must effect beneficence and nonmaleficence in deciding what is reasonable treatment in each situation.

There is a very fine line between doing "good" for the patient and doing "harm." What would sometimes be considered an immoral practice could be accepted as a moral act. For example, killing is an immoral practice; however, letting a patient die could be a moral act. "Many beliefs about principles and consequences are applied to practices or rules rather than directly to acts."[7] So in some individual cases exceptions can be justified morally (i.e., letting an anencephalic newborn or a newborn with trisomy 18 die without giving extraordinary care). However, this does not mean that most acts can be justified this way. There are situations where specific acts, though they may seem morally right, must be prohibited so as to maintain the trust necessary for an effective professional-patient relationship.[7] "Mercy killing" is often considered in this light. While we are both morally and legally bound not to kill, this is still a prima facie principle.

In the best situation, all relevant decision makers agree on what is good. This is rare today, especially since our federal government has impacted on the decision-making process. Its opinion of "good" must also be taken into account. The Baby Doe regulations reflect the moral atmosphere of the 1980s (i.e., aggressive treatment of sick and anomalous newborns). This moral atmosphere considers all treatment, extraordinary and ordinary, to be a given right to all newborns, no matter what their potential quality of life. Many physicians and other health care providers feel this presence in the nursery. This expectation of aggressive treatment exemplifies how one moral community and its moral rules can succeed in influencing society as a whole.

Society does, however, maintain a pluralistic interpretation of what is good versus what is harmful. There is a necessary balance between these two. For example, how much pain can be inflicted on a patient, and for how long, before the harm outweighs the "good"? How long does one wait for a "good" outcome? These would be questions from a utilitarian. The deontologist might ask: "Is there any new technology available to give the patient another chance?" Or, "Have we done all that we can for the patient?" These are not just medical questions. Their basis lies in assumed moral duties and obligations.

Beauchamp and Childress[7] state that the duty of nonmaleficence includes not only actual harms, but also risks of harm. The greater the risk of harm, the greater the need for solid moral reasoning as justification. This is a standard of care maintained by all health care professionals. This standard does not give blanket promises for cures in all cases. Instead, it reduces the probability of errors in diagnosis and treatment by requiring that moral agents act thoughtfully, carefully, and reasonably. Harms are not always intentional; in fact, it is possible to violate the principle of nonmaleficence by accident. Concern for the patient's "greatest good" inherently examines what risks or actual harms could be involved in treatment or nontreatment—too little technologic support or too much. Since uncertainty is common in the NICU, each team member should consider the balance between these two principles on a daily basis. Each parent with a sick or anomalous newborn comes in contact with the realities of treatment more and more the longer their infant is in the NICU. The decision-making dilemma can find solutions by beginning with mutual respect for varied moral viewpoints and acceptance that no moral agent need violate his or her own moral stance. Then the decision-making process can proceed. The next step is to examine the decisions in terms of the principle of justice. Moral decision making in the NICU does not exist in a vacuum. Indeed, as our world changes, so too does the distribution of its goods and services—its benefits and burdens.

Principle of justice

The concept of justice dates back to the Greek philosophers. Aristotle has been credited with one of the most basic premises of justice: equals ought to be treated equally and unequals may be treated unequally. This principle of formal justice does not give specific prescriptions for interpreting equals or unequals. In the NICU each neonate is potentially equal to all other humans. His or her potential, however, is not only immeasurable at the time of treatment; it is also one with varied interpretations (i.e., potential for what?). For example, can we compare the potential life of a 480 g, 24-week infant with a teenage "suicidal" mother with that of a term infant with Down's syndrome who has two loving parents? Some would say yes, and some would say emphatically no. Or, is there a difference between having a seriously premature infant as one's first versus one's third or fourth child? Having a preexisting family may create different considerations for many people. Family resources—financial, emotional, physical, and spiritual—are not bottomless. Controversy over what is "due" each neonate often hinges on one's interpretation of "personhood" and consequent rights.

The concept of justice entails "giving to each his right or due."[7] Although our society generally believes all individuals are of equal worth, disparities of allocation still exist. The material principles of justice help to identify alternative bases on which to balance the distribution or allocation of benefits and burdens[7]:

1. To each person an equal share
2. To each person according to individual need
3. To each person according to individual effort
4. To each person according to societal contribution
5. To each person according to merit

It is likely that when one basis for justice is used, an alternative basis for justice is negated or at least neglected. These material principles specify only prima facie duties. They must be weighed with other bioethical principles in particular situations. The acceptability of each material principle of justice rests on its moral justification. For example, critically ill neonates use health care dollars at an unequal rate compared with those newborns who do not need extraordinary high-tech help. Is it morally "just" to use $175,000 to produce one 700 g survivor when the money could be used to feed, counsel, and educate dozens of socially deprived children instead? Since resources are limited, trying to do everything for everyone leaves "fewer resources to meet the needs of those who are unserved or underserved."[31]

How might we properly allocate our health care dollars? How can we help families to make the best decision for their neonate considering their own personal resources? These questions must be considered. Some advise that a basic health care minimum be provided for all individuals. Others suggest that health care dollars would be better spent on preventive care for many rather than intensive care for a few. Many infants and their families could avoid the trauma of a premature birth if research and education were given higher priority in resource allocation.

Just distribution of resources to meet an acceptable standard of health care is particularly problematic as resources become increasingly scarce. On a societal or macroeconomic scale, we question how to best distribute our scarce resources. These are issues of distributive justice. On an individual or microeconomic scale, we consider the competing claims for resources between affected individuals. It can be considerably problematic to balance macroeconomic theories with microeconomic claims. For example, if a hospital's ability to stay open depends on the majority of the patients paying their bills, then one must critically consider the consequences of frequently giving free care. On a microlevel, it is morally wrong to allow finances to enter into the allocation of health care. However, on a macroscale, finances can determine whether a hospital stays open. Do we provide health care to all no matter what the consequences? Do we provide all that is

available to each individual, or do we allocate our scarce resources by setting standards and limits to care? Macroallocation and microallocation policies are not mutually exclusive. They influence each other in the determination of goods and services available.

The fundamental needs of individuals are met because our society feels a moral obligation to us—rich or poor. Some consider equal access to a respectable minimum of health care to be the right of all members of society, whereas others consider health care to be a superogatory (not obligatory) duty of society. The problem with supplying all of society with minimum health care comes both in setting limits so that there is enough to go around and in specifying standards so that all get equal treatment. Inherent in this problem is who should set these limits and standards. Should it be the government? The hospital corporation? Ethics committees? Physicians? The moral community? These are moral questions underlying the principle of distributive justice.

Medical technology is moving ahead faster than economics. "Health care now devours nearly 11% of the country's gross national product."[21] Lamm calls health care a "fiscal black hole" (cited in Greene[21]). Specifically with neonatal care, there has been a revolution in technologic advances over the past 15 to 20 years. "The cost of intensive care for tiny babies of less than 800 gram birth weight is of the same order as that of heart transplants, liver transplants and bone-marrow transplants ($100,000-$200,000)."[37] Whereas transplants remain relatively rare, delivery of neonates weighing less than 800 g is relatively frequent. Consequently, the resources needed to maintain this population constitute a significant part of our limited health care resources. Priority setting becomes increasingly necessary as technology expands treatment options. New technologies do not promise certain cures; however, they do promise new controversies over resource allocation. Although the concept of rationed medical care concerns many, it has until now been a part of our social policy. A technologic imperative does not necessarily optimize health care. Health care can evolve and improve on a balanced scale with our available resources if we set humane and compassionate goals.

ETHICAL ISSUES OF PARTICULAR IMPORTANCE IN THE NICU
Personhood

Decision making in the NICU often revolves around the concept of "personhood." Determining what this means depends on which moral community is consulted. Designation of personhood is morally significant because it determines if and what duties and obligations are owed to a particular newborn.

Some communities believe personhood is present at the moment of conception; they equate "human" with "person." Shelp[47] refers to this as the "genetic theory of personhood." Others believe personhood depends on the presence or absence of certain basic human qualities. Shelp calls this moral theory "property based." Although with the latter theory there is agreement that the concept of personhood is nongenetic, there are differences regarding which qualities qualify for "person" status.

Fletcher[19] and Engelhardt[14] support this stance. They believe that there are human lives that are "subpersonal." They say that "it is not what is natural but what is personal which has the first-order value in ethics."[19] They believe that neocortical function is required for personhood. Engelhardt[14] relates qualities such as self-consciousness, rationality, and self-determination to personhood. He distinguishes between persons in a moral sense and persons in a social sense. Infants are deemed persons only in a social sense, not a strict sense where societal rights are obligatory. The rights of the infant, according to Engelhardt, are held in trust by his or her parents; therefore "decision(s) about treatment . . . belong properly to the parents because the child belongs to them in a sense that it does not belong to anyone else, even to itself."[14] In this sense, then, infanticide does carry moral significance. All such decisions must be properly justified. Engelhardt does consider that financial, emotional, and spiritual costs can be morally valid reasons to justify infanticide.

Tooley[51] suggests "that the ability to see oneself as existing over time is a necessary condition for the possession of a right to life."[26] If Tooley's reasoning is correct, then no infant has a right to life, at least not for some time. Whereas the "prolife" moral community assigns person status to all with potential life, Tooley denies that potential has anything to do with a right to life. Advocates of quality-of-life standards for personhood give a qualified endorsement to infanticide. When a life is full of intractable pain and suffering, death is seen as a morally acceptable option. In fact, it is sometimes considered a relatively better outcome than continuing life.

Ramsey,[43] Robertson,[45] and the Catholic church hold a contrasting view. For them, death is never better than life; quality-of-life assessments are not part of their moral reasoning. Life is considered sacred—an absolute good. Both the fetus and newborn are considered a person with a right to live. Therefore "death must always be imposed nonhumanly by God or nature or some other cosmic arbiter."[19] This "prolife" position supports the moral right of deformed fetuses and deformed newborns to whatever care would be given a normal infant, implying that abortion and infanticide are morally reprehensible. If antibiotics would be given to a normal infant, then they must also be administered to a newborn infant with trisomy 18.

If one is deemed a "person," then society owes one certain obligations and expects certain duties. If one is not deemed a "person," then it is morally reasonable for societal benefits to be withheld or withdrawn. Whatever justification is needed for a particular moral dilemma in the NICU extends from this beginning. There is no final answer, no final definition of personhood.

Patienthood

A primary problem confronting the perinatal clinician is the fundamental question: Who is the patient? The adult patient is generally competent and worthy of respect as a moral agent. However, in the case of a newborn, the newborn, the family, and, in some circumstances, society have been variously considered the "patient." The accordance of rights to the newborn as an independent agent is a relatively recent occurrence. Neonatal cases are inextricably bound in the context of complicated family and societal situations. Nonetheless, decisions need to be made in perinatal cases, often in the face of societal disagreement and indecision, perhaps unduly posing special burdens on perinatal clinicians. The fundamental question remains: To whom is the moral duty owed?

Professional-patient relationship

The importance of the professional-patient relationship cannot be underestimated, since this is the human context in which decision making occurs. With neonates, this includes a relationship between parents as surrogates and the health care team.

When the four major principles—autonomy, beneficence, nonmaleficence, and justice—are applied to health care relationships, several moral rules can be derived. These moral rules include fidelity, truth telling, and confidentiality. The professional-patient relationship is considerably impacted on by the meaning and extent of these rules.

Fidelity, or promise keeping, may be derived from the principle of autonomy. The duty to keep promises may promote the greatest good (utilitarian) or be seen as an obligation (formalist). Many relationships between professionals and patients (or surrogates) involve promises or contracts, whether implicitly or explicitly made. For example, once professionals have established a relationship with a patient, their duty of fidelity includes not abandoning or neglecting that pa-

tient. An obvious problem in dealing with surrogates may be conflicting duties to the parents and the patient. Promises made by professionals are binding except when they are superseded by stronger obligations.

Truth telling, like fidelity, can be derived from the principle of autonomy or respect for persons. It implies an implicit contract between parties that the truth will be told. At the heart of truth telling is trust, which gives professional-patient relationships their integrity. Lying violates implicit contracts, respect for persons, and trust. It also impedes informed consent.

Utilitarians and formalists may agree on the duty to tell the truth, though they may disagree on the duty not to deceive. Cases have been made for "benevolent deception," when intentional deception is morally justifiable if its primary intent is for the benefit of the patient. In such cases telling the truth may be a violation of beneficence and nonmaleficence. Others argue that deception, benevolent or not, is morally wrong because it violates respect for persons and trust. Ultimately, the professional-patient relationship erodes. Respect for persons involves acknowledging patient autonomy to know, or not to know, the truth of his or her particular situation.

It is generally agreed that confidentiality should prevail in professional-patient relationships. With minors, confidentiality extends to the parents or legal guardians. Part of the implied contract is that information gained by both parties will be kept confidential. From the earliest days of medicine, protecting the patient's privacy has been a fundamental tenet of clinical practice. There are, of course, instances where confidentiality is justifiably breached. It is at this point that many ethical dilemmas arise.

Breach of confidentiality may be morally and legally justified in order to protect the life of a patient or the lives of others who may be endangered. The value of human life overrides the relationship, but the professional should be able to demonstrate clear danger before violating a patient's privacy. This may also be seen as a violation of autonomy. "The health care professional's breach of confidentiality thus cannot be justified unless it is necessary to meet a strong conflicting duty."[7]

Obviously, health care professionals can be torn between conflicting moral obligations, such as between the patient and society. Such instances where a breach may be justified include child abuse and neglect, and certain communicable diseases. But there is strong justification among both utilitarians and formalists for maintaining the privacy and confidentiality of patient information. Most important, the genuine integrity of the professional-patient relationship will be enhanced and preserved when confidentiality, like fidelity and truth telling, is respected and upheld. This integrity of relationship then becomes the basis of the decision-making process.

Nursing ethics

Nurses play a central role in health care. Their knowledge and abilities have taken quantum leaps in the twentieth century. Nurses are expected, as are physicians, to maintain their expertise in a rapidly changing world of high technology. Whereas in the past nurses have been primarily responsible for the "caring" aspects of medical care, they are now involved with the "curing," too. With this expanded role nurses find themselves in the middle of ethical dilemmas on a daily basis. Ethical dilemmas involve suffering and deep personal conflicts. Nurses in the NICU are especially vulnerable to controversial situations. Not only are they dealing with helpless, incompetent patients whose potentials are uncertain, but, often decisions regarding treatment have very long term effects. Decisions made in an emergency situation may result in serious handicaps for the patient and excessive burdens for the family, or they may turn the infant around to a renewed quality of life.

Nurses are on the front line of neonatal care. They are with the patient for 8- to 12-hour stretches. They closely monitor the subtle changes, the rapid changes, the intricate responses inherent in neonatal care. They form close relationships with the families of their patients, and they integrate the support services needed by the patient and/or family (e.g., social services, physical therapy, Aid to Families with Dependent Children [AFDC], Visiting Nurse Service [VNS], support groups, etc.). Whereas the physician sees the patient and/or family for a relatively short period, the nurse provides the continuity of care that families in stressful situations yearn for. Parents ask questions; they seek certainty, reassurance, and compassion. They want their fears allayed, their anxieties lessened, and their problems solved. Nurses are captive audiences for "stressed out" parents.

Often the frustrations of the parents are shed on the nurses. Intimidated by physicians, families turn to nurses to explain what is happening to their baby, what it means, and what will be the outcome. Although nurses are patient advocates along with the families of sick newborns, they are not always active in decision making about their patients. Sometimes the decisions made about their patients contradict their own moral viewpoint. Sometimes the information given by the physician is too general and the family members want more but are afraid to ask, or they do not understand the information. Sometimes physicians are overwhelmed by the severity of a case and fail to take responsibility for making crucial decisions. And sometimes families want inappropriate treatment for their newborn—either too much or too little. What is the nurse's role in such situations?

There is a need for teamwork and consensus decision making. "Conducted well, staff meetings on decisions in the NICU make it possible to share responsibility for difficult decisions and, it is to be hoped, produce decisions ethically more sound than those made by individuals without consultation."[24] When life and death decisions are needed, those professionals carrying out such treatments require support, emotional and spiritual. By sharing the burden, everyone benefits.

Nurses are involved in a significant relationship with physicians. Ethical dilemmas may arise out of this. Nurses are caught, at times, between two competing obligations—one, to carry out the physician's orders and, the other, to ensure that the patient's rights and best interests come first. The nurse's assessment of the patient may differ from the physician's. Frequently, the nurse, who is "at the bedside," is able to notice subtle changes that the physician misses in rounds or during a brief examination. It is not unlikely that the nurse's knowledge of the patient and his or her family would suggest a different treatment plan from that of the physician.

It is always the nurse's obligation to make sure the patient's best interests are being met. If the physician does make an unsound medical judgment, it is the nurse's obligation to clarify the intention and correct the situation if necessary. Tensions can exist when the parents want different treatment for their child than the physician does, when the parents feel intimidated by the physician and complacently say that all is fine, or when parents consent to certain treatments without being fully informed of the risks and benefits. What are the obligations of the nurse in such situations? Should the nurse arbitrate between the family and the physician? Should the nurse reinforce the physician's information or persuade the family to speak with the physician directly? Finally, should the nurse allow a treatment to proceed without adequate informed consent from the family?

Mappes and Kroeger[32] suggest that such situations are not really moral dilemmas but instead manifest "a tension between doing what is morally right and what is least difficult practically. . . . The problem is not that the nurse's obligation is unclear, but that in actual situations fulfilling this moral obligation is extremely difficult."

Moral dilemmas do enfold nurses at times if their moral values conflict with the physician's or the parents'. Nurses are often caught in very stressful situations. Their professional obligations may conflict with those of their chosen moral

community. Important decisions must be made by nurses during conflicts of this sort. No one on the health care team is required to ignore his or her personal values if deep conflict exists. A nurse, as well as any other health care professional, may withdraw from a case. Conflicting values are inherent in the NICU; consequently nurses must first understand their own values and then create a plan for dealing with moral dilemmas. Although the patient's "best interest" is paramount for the nurse professional, there may be times when the nurse's "best interest" requires separation from the patient, physically and/or emotionally.

It is time that nurses become equal members of the health care team. Not only will this aid in achieving the patient's best interest, but it will also help the entire health care team in times of intense moral dilemmas.

Informed consent

The issue of valid informed consent has been raised repeatedly in the environment of the NICU. Information given to parents may be poorly understood for many reasons, including the complex nature of the information; the emotional or physical state of the parents following the birth of a sick, premature, or anomalous infant; physical separation of the parents from their newborn; or feelings of bewilderment and intimidation leading to uncontested paternalism. Indeed, there are indications that valid informed consent is an ideal toward which we work but one that, within the realities of practice, may rarely be obtained. Consent should be sought, however, and open lines of communication and parental education established in order to facilitate some level of understanding and enable more than token participation in decision making by the parents.

One standard that has been put forth in an effort to accomplish informed consent is the "reasonable person standard," which consists of the following considerations:

1. All relevant material information for a decision must be given.

2. All known risks of significant bodily harm or death must be given.
3. The "reasonable person" reflects an ideal composite of what a reasonable person in society is—the individual person in the case at hand is not in question unless he or she is extraordinary in some aspect (e.g., family values, etc.).
4. The standards of disclosure in medicine are the same as in other professions in which relationships are built on trust.

There are several ways in which the reasonable person standard might be enacted in the NICU, thus ensuring that more valid informed consent is obtained. First, early contact should be made with the parents or family regarding the expected course of problems and special management needs of the newborn. This consultation may even be initiated before delivery. Second, information should be provided by the clinical staff in a factual, compassionate manner. Parents may need continued orientation or reorientation to the NICU environment. This may be especially necessary for parents who are geographically separated from their child. Third, phone calls and photographs are important means for parents to maintain emotional involvement with their child. Fourth, social workers, clergy, or other support structures should be contacted and utilized early in order to manage emotional distress and to facilitate communication. Fifth, regular patient care conferences with the parents should be scheduled. This will keep parents apprised of the newborn's status and will keep the staff informed about the parents' level of understanding, perspectives, and values. Additional efforts to communicate must be made at the time of special procedures, tests, or therapies to enhance everybody's understanding and the informed consent process.

An integral part of the informed consent process and one that directly affects decision making is the principle of fidelity—commonly referred to as truth telling. Issues of what to tell, how and when to tell, and whom to tell become a daily part of the staff's interaction with each other and the families of affected newborns. A high level of respect for patient and family confidentiality needs to be maintained, and members of the staff need to be cautious about discussing cases and exchanging information given in confidence. Once again, however, open lines of communication and exchange of relevant information regularly will facilitate smooth operation in the NICU.

In practice, the issue of truth telling is considered an essential component of the physician-family relationship, thus allowing for ethical decision making and generally not conflicting with other competing values such as nonmaleficence, beneficence, autonomy, or justice. Information should be shared among staff members and presented to the family truthfully, compassionately, and without bias.

Double effect

The principle of "double effect" asserts that an action may be considered good if the intent of the action is a positive value, even if the secondary effects of the action might be considered harmful if undertaken as the primary goal; further, the good effect should be commensurate with the harm. Thus even the most conservative foe of abortion might defend abortion undertaken to save the life of the mother, an overriding positive value. Similarly, while less dramatic, an emergency cesarean section for fetal indications may be ethically defensible: while the mother does not "need" an operative delivery and may indeed suffer increased resultant morbidity, the positive value of preserving the life and health of the fetus/newborn may be found to dominate over the smaller risk of potential harm to the mother. With advances in antenatal diagnosis, such conflicts between mother and fetal needs are becoming increasingly common. Double effect is used frequently in the NICU, although it is rarely explicitly identified. An example is the use of narcotics in a dying newborn: the positive goal is reduction of suffering, even at the expense of shortening life.

DECISION MAKING IN THE NICU

In the NICU decisions of serious proportion are encountered regularly, based on medical facts and nonmedical values. From the moment of birth, and in some cases even earlier, a foremost issue is that of determining the appropriate level of treatment (or nontreatment) of sick or anomalous newborns. While entire texts have been devoted to this issue,[26,56] some of the primary concerns are outlined here regarding decisions of when to treat, when to limit treatment or not treat at all, and who should be involved in the decision-making process.

A frequently encountered treatment problem requiring attention, other than the much publicized anomalous infant, is the extremely premature or very low birth weight (VLBW) infant whose course is marked by slow or absent progress despite appropriate and seemingly heroic intervention. The development of complications from disease is of further concern. In concert, these may portend a guarded or very poor prognosis.

These cases may prompt "quality of life" and "ordinary versus extraordinary treatment" discussions. However, such terms, while commonly used, are vague and value laden. The President's Commission[39] noted that "there is no basis for holding that whether a treatment is common or unusual, or whether it is simple or complex, is in itself significant to a moral analysis of whether treatment is warranted or obligatory"—a view that had been previously voiced by moral philosophers. Further, while "quality of life" may seem to be a straightforward phrase, its interpretation depends on one's moral perspective and value system. We would do better to facilitate the best decision for each case.

Steps in ethical decision making

The approach to any of the varied "hard cases" encountered in the newborn nursery should follow a method that clearly demonstrates the practice of applied clinical ethics. As stated by Pellegrino,[35] the goal of applied ethics is making right and good moral decisions for and with a particular patient. Such a decision requires first, however, that the decision maker, whether that be a parent, health care provider, or other, understand his or her own (1) philosophy of relationship to the patient (or family), (2) interpretation of ethical principles and values, (3) theoretical basis of ethics used (utilitarian, deontologic, etc.), and (4) source from which morality is derived. An ethical "workup" is then undertaken (see below), in which substantive issues are identified and worked through, resulting in a decision.[50] Implementing decisions requires determining who shall decide, by what criteria they shall be allowed to do so, and subsequently how the decisions or actions are to be implemented in an acceptable fashion that does not override the values of others.

The essential steps to decision making in neonatal cases where a dilemma exists include the following[9,20] (Table 25-2):

1. Consider who is involved in making and implementing the decision.
2. Determine who shall make the decision. Is this an easily resolved issue for the parents/family, physician, and other health care team members, or is referral to an ethics committee or even a judicial body in order? This is often not clear initially, but it may become more evident as the following steps are undertaken.
3. Establish and evaluate all of the medical "facts": alternatives to treatment that are positive, reasons and indications for medical intervention, and expected consequences of any intervention or lack of intervention.
4. Understand the significant human factors and values in the case. These should be determined for the patient, family, and health care team.
5. Identify all major theoretic and value conflicts in the case. Realize which ethical principles or duties are at odds (e.g., truth telling, beneficence, autonomy, nonmaleficence, and justice). Determine which values

have priority in the case. This should prove to be consistent with the values of the patient/family when possible and may not reflect the values of the health care team. The use of a committee to examine and reflect on such prioritization and facilitate subsequent decision making has been helpful in a number of institutions, though such a process may take place without convening a committee.

TABLE 25-2

Approach to Ethical Dilemmas in Neonatology

1. Consider who is involved in making and implementing the decision (family, guardians, clinicians, society).
2. Decide who will make the final decision.
3. Clarify all of the medical facts within the case—consider indications, alternatives, and consequences of each action or inaction.
4. Understand significant human factors and values.
5. Identify the ethical dilemma or conflict.

	DEONATOLOGIC (FORMALIST) POSITION	*UTILITARIAN (CONSEQUENCE-ORIENTED) POSITION*
6. List options.	a. List rules/principles (Ten Commandments, Kant's categorical imperative, social contract, etc.). b. List all options as solutions to problem.	a. Identify all options as solutions to problem. b. List positive and negative consequences for each option. c. Quantify these positive and negative consequences.
7. Weigh/prioritize values.	Compare principles with options; eliminate those that are unacceptable: (1) Only one option is ethically consistent with your rules. *or* (2) Two or more options are consistent; choose one. *or* (3) An option may be in harmony with one principle but violates another; appeal to higher or more general principle.	a. List values you would consider in sorting out the options open to you. b. Assign weights; quantify the importance of your values or selection criteria.
8. Make a decision.	a. The conflict is resolved by using a higher principle. *or* b. No resolution; dilemma remains and proper action is still not evident.	a. Select and implement the option that has the most harmony with your values and results in the greatest positive and least negative consequence score. b. If you cannot carry out any of the above steps, the decision is stymied until you can work around the difficulty.

9. Check for moral and rational defensibility.

Modified from Francoeur RT: From then to now. In Harris CC and Snowden F, editors: Bioethical frontiers in perinatal intensive care, Natchitoches, La, 1985, Northwestern State University Press; and Brody H: Ethical decisions in medicine, Boston, 1981, Little, Brown & Co, Inc.

6. Make a decision.
7. Review each step to determine the moral and rational defensibility of the action taken.

This process need not always be invoked in full. Often, when the case is carefully dissected and medical facts, treatment alternatives, and expected prognoses are revealed, issues that at first seemed in question are clarified, and it becomes apparent that no real dilemma exists.

Good ethics, then, start with good facts and effective communication. Clinicians should be aware of all relevant facts, be they medical, social, human value, or legal in nature. Decisions should not be based on personal opinion or insufficient data. The value placed on one's medical well-being may differ between the health care team and the patient/family, and discrepancy may lead to a perceived problem. This serves to remind us of the need for a formal approach to problem solving in hard cases.

A viable patient-professional relationship that facilitates the clarification of facts, human values and feelings, and the interests of all relevant parties is essential to ethical decision making. Decisions made should ideally reflect a moral choice that is good for the patient involved and is morally and rationally defensible. We should all work toward achieving a position that is both morally congruent with the values deemed of greatest worth in an individual case and applicable within the moral community as a whole. In the NICU the values most often dealt with are expressed in the principles described earlier.

Certain problems may arise that can seemingly impair this process (Table 25-3). Often there is

TABLE 25-3

Problems that Impair Ethical Decision Making

1. Inadequate time
2. Inadequate information
3. Limitations in current knowledge
4. Uncertain prognoses
5. Limitations of human wisdom

inadequate information or time, but decisions must be made, even at odd hours and with limited reflection on process. Limited foresight is available in prognosticating, especially in the individual case, and often very difficult value-laden predictors are required. Some have gone so far as to say that imagination is at least as important as facts in making decisions. But this is not unique to ethical decision making. As Brody[9] states, "We must always take action on the basis of some degree of uncertainty. The goal is to reduce that uncertainty to manageable proportions, and to insure that we have at least considered all the major consequences that we are able to predict with our current level of understanding of the world."

While it may be arguable whether the patient is the neonate, the nuclear family, the extended family, or another societal group, it would appear prudent to develop a consensus wherever possible and thus minimize conflict among the interested parties. Early involvement of the parents in the care of their child, along with sensitive and thorough presentation of clinical information to the parents, helps minimize the stresses on the parents and prepares them to participate in decision making regarding the care of their child. In our nurseries at the University of Colorado, we have created the position of family care coordinator, whose role is to work with families and to determine both what was said and what was heard in order to facilitate communication and care of the family. This position has been held by an NICU nurse (without other direct patient care responsibility) with considerable insight into family dynamics, and this person has been invaluable in facilitating communication and support in times of great stress. With careful attention to the needs of patients, families, and staff, many conflicts can be resolved at an early stage before positions are hardened and emotional investment is high, resulting in a development of consensus and minimization of conflict.

In a minority of cases, conflict is unavoidable. In some cases medical care raises issues that are highly controversial either within the group of clinicians providing care or in the broader context of societal problems. In many cases the family is far from homogeneous in its expression of wishes. Many parents are young and in the process of achieving independent adulthood with well-developed values. Single-parent families are not uncommon. The birth of a critically ill infant may serve as a focus to crystallize disagreements between spouses or may aggravate conflicts between the parent(s) and the extended family. In such cases a more formal process, such as a formal conference between clinicians and the family, appeal to an ethics committee, or even involvement of the legal system, may help to resolve or minimize conflicts of values.

PROBLEMS OF UNCERTAINTY

A major difficulty in ethical considerations is the medical uncertainty on which they are based. It is difficult to determine what may be in the best interest of the child when the prognosis remains unclear. And even when the prognosis seems clear, there are always those children who confound science, whose outcomes are far from expected.

Some of the most frequent problems in working with perinatal cases arise as a result of this uncertainty. Parents always ask, "Will my baby be okay when he (or she) grows up?" and are often answered with a variety of unsatisfying or incomprehensible replies. In most cases with premature infants, "truth telling" may compel an answer that when reduced to its simplest form says, "I don't know." A statistical approach to answer the question may be: "Most babies like yours grow up to be normal." Or, "Some babies like yours have serious problems." These answers are often followed by a litany of statistical probabilities of each morbidity. Neither approach answers the mother's question of what *her particular* baby will be like. Such approaches serve to complicate the clinician's relationship with parents over issues such as expertise, veracity, and disclosure. The statistical approach may answer the NICU's question of quality of care, but few parents understand such statistics or are willing to apply them to a loved one. Nonetheless, uncertainty is a way of life in many perinatal cases, and this observation significantly compromises the resolution of ethical problems in the NICU.

In considering medical uncertainty, however, it is important to recognize two general classes of perinatal cases. NICU patients can be generally classified as either (1) premature infants without known anomalies or (2) near-term infants with major anomalies, either syndromic or nonsyndromic. For infants with known syndromes or major anomalies, prognoses from the literature are describable with reasonable accuracy. Thus the prognosis for an infant with trisomy 18 can be given with a fairly high degree of accuracy, permitting reasonable application of these processes.

"Extreme prematurity, on the other hand, is characterized by enormous uncertainty. . . . In these cases predictions of outcome at birth are probabilistic at best."[44] While a detailed review of neonatal outcome is beyond the scope of this chapter, several conclusions appear justified. First, infant mortality has declined rapidly since the establishment of NICUs, and the major mortality groups are in lower weight and younger gestational age groups. Examination of the mortality curves from the University of Colorado over successive time periods reveals an impressive increase in survival of younger and smaller babies.[25] National data, while less available, parallel these findings.[34] Second, coincident with the decline in mortality have come major improvements in neonatal morbidity. Summarizing the reported major morbidity from the literature, a government case study[34] noted a decline in major morbidity from nearly 50% in the pre-NICU era to current figures in the range of 15% from many institutions. Third, the absolute number of normal premature survivors has increased dramatically, and the absolute number of moderately and severely affected survivors appears to have increased as well.[34] Similar conclusions may be reached for individual morbidities, such as retinopathy of prematurity (retrolental fibroplasia).

Such data are helpful from a public health standpoint but do little to assure a concerned parent. The statistical message is necessarily ambivalent: "Today your child has a much improved chance of surviving to be a normal child, but you have a slightly greater chance of having a surviving child with a major handicap than if your child had been born 20 years ago."

If one's values deny the admissibility of quality-of-life considerations in clinical decisions, then such considerations are moot. However, for those perinatal clinicians who consider quality of life a major consideration, it remains an exceedingly difficult practical problem to predict which particular child will be significantly handicapped. The predictive value of nursery evaluations in estimating long-term handicap is low.

The morbidities in premature survivors are variable in nature, but central nervous system (CNS) morbidities generally include visual impairment and blindness, speech and hearing impairment, neuromuscular impairment, and serious retardation. Few premature survivors require long-term institutional care.[34] The combined risk for one or more of these handicaps is in the range of 15% to 20%. Most would agree that these are indeed serious handicaps, with major impact on the patient and family. However, in using such morbidities to withhold or withdraw care, one must ask whether such morbidities meet the criterion of universalizability: would (or should) such morbidities be sufficient individually or in combination to withdraw or withhold treatment from other patients with similar conditions?

The intent of raising these questions is to underscore the complexity of ethical discussions as particularly applied to problems in the modern NICU. This in no way reduces the enormity of such problems for the patient, the family, health care providers, or society. Technologic advances may resolve old uncertainties but often seem to carry new uncertainties that are equally perplexing.

Strategies for dealing with factual uncertainty in ethical discussions

Rhoden[44] has summarized several strategies for dealing with uncertainty in perinatal cases: (1) the "wait until certainty" approach, (2) the statistical prognosis approach, and (3) the individualized prognostic strategy.

In the first approach aggressive care is continued until the clinical situation becomes more medically certain. Then ethical principles may be applied to evaluate the clinical situation. Such an approach "errs on the side of life." It supports the value of preserving life and may have other positive values for the patient, clinician, and society, while at the same time it has the major potential drawbacks of interfering with the autonomy of the patient (best interest), or parents (substituted judgment), increasing suffering (nonmaleficence), and perhaps increasing morbidity.

In the second approach statistical prognosis is accepted as the basis for withholding or withdrawing care, with the positive goal of minimizing the number of infants who suffer long drawn-out deaths or who live with serious handicaps. According to Rhoden[44]:

Since statistical data about categories of infants are seldom as good as information about a particular infant gained during a trial period of treatment, the statistical approach undoubtedly loses more salvageable survivors than is necessary or justifiable. . . . A pure statistical strategy brings with it the dual dangers of rigidity and minimization of the ethical component.

The individualized prognostic strategy involves starting treatment and then reevaluating it based on response. Thus initial treatment is a diagnostic as well as therapeutic trial, and the initial decision to treat is not irrevocable. Ethically speaking, there is no difference between withholding and withdrawing treatment. The advantages of such an approach are that it preserves the chance of life in borderline cases while at the same time it permits withdrawal of support based on individualized information. This strategy permits a wide variation in care within a statistical group and leads to potential confusion and errors in execution. It also supports the role of parents and other surrogate agents in ethical decision making. "When medical uncertainty leads to moral uncertainty, it seems preferable, albeit harder, to confront these dual ambiguities than to bury them under statistical criteria or unrelenting moral certitude."[44] Clearly, such an approach leads to practical difficulties. As noted above, the process of prognostication is usually far from precise, and judgments may frequently be made that later prove to be incorrect at a time when the withdrawal or withholding of support may no longer be an issue.

Proxy decision makers

In dealing with newborns who are, by their very nature, incompetent and cannot make decisions for themselves, value conflicts must be resolved with the input of a proxy or surrogate decision maker acting on the infant's behalf. This may be the parents, a family member, friend, guardian ad litem, or the physician. To be considered a valid surrogate, the person should be competent, knowledgeable of integral values of the patient or family, free from conflicting interests, and without serious emotional conflicts in dealing with the case.

Society has for many reasons allocated to the parents the primary authoritative role in collaborating with health care providers in making decisions about their newborn's care. In most instances the parents are best suited for such matters and have the infant's best interests in mind. They are usually present when possible, are concerned for their infant's well-being, and are willing to hear the facts of their infant's condition, as well as learn of needed therapies. Of all people, they also know best the values of the family culture or environment in which the infant will be raised. At the same time, however, parents are rarely free of conflicting interests or without serious emotional conflicts in considering treatment options.

Parents may be less than dispassionate decision makers. They are understandably overwhelmed at times, both physically and emotionally exhausted, and baffled or intimidated by the hi-tech environment of the NICU and the complexities of their infant's care. Amidst feelings of grief, fear, anxiety, and wonderment over their premature or anomalous infant, they may be uncertain of their proper role and responsibilities as parents. Health care providers need to give daily updates on the infant's condition and anticipated course. Parents' needs for emotional support and avenues to both vent their frustrations and explore their concerns over economic, marital, family/sibling, and career effects of their predicament make resources such as nurses, social workers, and chaplains essential in providing assistance to allow them to participate in difficult decision making. Occasionally it will be necessary to assess the level of parental competency in assuming the role of surrogate, recognizing when additional help or support for them is needed in fulfilling this role.

Physicians as decision makers, an oft-cited traditional paternalistic role, are yet another option. They know and understand the complexities of the medical condition and treatment more than do parents, and should promote the patient's best interests in advocating treatment. They may be more objective about individual cases and are not emotionally overwhelmed, as the parents might be. Also, based on experience, they offer a perspective of effectiveness of treatments and can be consistent in treating similar cases.

However, physicians may also encounter problems when they act as the principal decision makers. While their knowledge of medical facts is the most complete of all persons, it is at the same time, unfortunately, incomplete. Accurate diagnoses and certainty in prognoses are at times elusive. Medical knowledge does have limitations. While statistics are helpful for groups of similarly affected and treated patients, individual outcomes are difficult to predict. Further, while having the degree of specialized information and knowledge they do, physicians do not necessarily possess any more moral expertise than do parents or others.

Treatment versus nontreatment decisions are ultimately moral, not simply medical, decisions. Great care must be taken to consider the values brought into the decision-making process by all involved parties.

Physicians do not work in isolation from the health care team when making decisions about patients. Nurses, social workers, and chaplains are vital members of the decision-making team. A potential problem with each of these clinicians as surrogates is that there may exist a conflict of interest between them and the patients they are deciding for. Members of the health care team may be biased toward the prolongation of life, have preconceived and strong biases about euthanasia, or be influenced by issues unrelated to the patient, including advancement of care, financial issues, or societal issues. Hence they may not fully take into account the best interests of the patient or the values of the involved family. There may also be a lack of consistency in their application of principles to similar cases, and they may give in to strong pressures (real or perceived) exerted by the law or very assertive parents. In contrast to parents, it has been argued that physicians are not present years later to see the end results of their actions and decisions—be they good or bad.

Various factors should contribute to minimizing the potential problems in parents and health care professionals reaching morally defensible decisions in the best interest of the premature or anomalous infant. The professionalism of health care team members who are committed to serving the health and interests of their patients is a foremost consideration that serves this purpose. A sense of duty leads these professionals to assist families in achieving their life goals, through facilitating open communication and discussion of their varied concerns. A great sense of personal and professional satisfaction may be derived by helping families accept and deal with their emotions, questions, and concerns for their infant and their own circumstances. Professionals may benefit from the support afforded by each other and

certainly will avoid problems if efforts are made to communicate well with each other.

In recent years hospital ethics committees have been given an increasing role in facilitating ethical decision making for sick neonates and have, in rare instances, actually functioned as proxy decision makers. As more institutions are establishing committees, their roles are more focused on education, policy interpretation, and advisory functions as opposed to decision making. Decision making by committees might be problematic in that it may threaten the traditional physician–patient/family relationship and usurp both the physician's authority and the parents' autonomy. Siegler[49] recently noted a number of ways in which a committee "can constrain and modify physician-patient decisions," including the imposition of administrative and regulatory burdens. The mechanics of the committee process, time, and distant relationship to the family and case have also been raised as problems in utilizing committees.

Weir[56] notes that a committee, especially an infant bioethics committee, may have the potential of meeting all of the criteria for a proxy decision maker. Ethics committees are multidisciplinary in composition and have the goals of emotional stability, objectivity, impartiality, and consistency. Ideally they may facilitate the resolution of conflicts between parents and physicians in matters of treatment and be more capable of both addressing and working through the ethical or moral aspects of cases than parents, health care professionals, or other individuals. In reality, their most useful role seems to be one of improving effective communication between staff and families. Finally, they may prove to be a safeguard for infants where parents and professionals are working toward an end that may be perceived as contrary to the infant's best interests.

Surely, much reflective thinking should be invested in our decisions, as individuals, parents, or members of a committee. However, a small number of cases will proceed beyond institutional review to a court. While many attorneys might advocate this process, there are strengths and weaknesses to consider. Courts may present many of the criteria for being good proxies—they are disinterested parties, free of emotional involvement, and mostly consistent in reasoning from case to case. They can ensure that all relevant facts are presented and considered, and judges are capable of exercising unmatched control of data collection, investigation, questioning of experts, and seeking of alternative solutions. A judge can also appoint a guardian ad litem to be the patient's advocate when necessary.

Yet, there are at least a few weaknesses in courts as proxies. They are removed from the NICU and have no contact with the case, patient, staff, or family whose problem they are deciding—as such they are more remote than other possible proxy decision makers. Time may be consumed in working through cases, which may result in additional problems, changes in pertinent facts, or prolongation of suffering. Decisions rendered by judges may also reflect some bias based on personal considerations of the judge rather than consistent judicial decisions across lines of legal jurisdiction. Also, some would argue that courts are by design adversarial, using force to resolve conflict rather than promoting cooperation.

Standard of best interest

The best-interest standard has been advocated by the President's Commission and others seeking to accomplish valid moral decision making in difficult neonatal cases.[39,55,56] We are obliged "to try to evaluate benefits and burdens from the infant's own perspective."[39] This standard is accepted in the case of newborns over the autonomy-promoting "substituted judgment," since substituted judgment can only be applied hypothetically to a never-competent newborn. This standard is accepted as the best method available to "reasonable" adults who have to make decisions for neonates. The Commission also urges us to consider "not whether a normal adult would rather die than suffer from severe mental and physical impairments, but rather whether this child, who has never known the satisfactions and aspirations of the normal world, would prefer nothing to what he or she has."[39] In other words, it is difficult if not impossible for a "normal" adult to judge how an impaired person would feel about his or her limited condition. Certainly, normal adults would view a severe mental or physical handicap as a serious loss. But an impaired newborn would never have the privilege of such a comparison and would not feel the pain of this loss.

The potential for self-seeking by the decision maker is easy to understand and has been recognized. The interests of parents, siblings, physicians, hospital staff or administration, and society may all seem to compete with those of the newborn. But the interests of others—be they emotional, economic, or otherwise problematic—cannot justifiably override those of the patient[6] based on the actual or potential personhood of the critically ill neonate. Individual or societal problems or perceived burdens are generally not viewed on the same moral plane as a person's claim to life. Perhaps by promoting the critically ill neonate's interests despite the protests of others, society will be called to recognize its failure to accept, provide for, and integrate its "handicapped" members. In an effort to minimize such conflicts of interest and promote the best possible insight into determining the newborn's best interests, infant bioethics committees have been formed and put to work.

Certainly there will be cases that stretch the best-interest standard to its limits. Cases of protracted treatment with uncertain prognoses beg the question of quality of existence (in which nonmaleficence is the principle of concern) and will require consideration of more than mere suffering and pain. Indeed, in the words of Arras,[6] "sometimes circumstances may be so extreme and the consequences so dreadful that the priority of justice can no longer be maintained." In this sense, we need to find the best balance of beneficence, nonmaleficence, and justice.

We must also consider other morally relevant

concerns of sick neonates who may be doomed to brief lives with less than recognizably "human" existence. Human capacities (ability to think, be aware of self, and relate to other people) may be different from biologic human life. The preservation of biologic human life bereft of the benefit of distinctly human capacities is controversial and has been challenged in quality-of-life decisions.[6,12,26,29,56] Arras[6] suggests the "relational potential standard" (Does this child have the ability, or potential, to relate to physical space and time and to communicate with others?) as a means to address these concerns more aptly than the "misapplied best interest standard," calling on society itself to give inquiry "into the conditions of valuable human life."

Priority should be given to attempts at effecting a cure in these ill infants; when a cure cannot be achieved, patient comfort should be sought. Some maintain that life itself may not always be an absolute good; thus it may be morally justifiable to withhold or withdraw futile treatment associated with inhumane risks or harms that would prolong dying. Mitchell,[33] a member of the American Nurses Association Committee on Ethics, has stated:

Some infants are so premature and underweight, so profoundly impaired, so hopelessly diseased, or so severely asphyxiated that their foreshortened lives are full of misery for them and those around them. For infants who are so impaired that medical therapies are futile or . . . would only prolong suffering, invasive medical procedures and surgery are morally as well as medically inappropriate.

She calls on nurses to shift their focus in such cases to "seek primarily to provide comfort, relieve suffering and help a grieving family."

Killing versus letting die

A controversial area in treatment and nontreatment decisions is that of the moral (or, as some perceive, strictly procedural) decision of killing versus letting die. Many believe that philosophically and morally there is no difference between these two actions (i.e., allowing someone to die is the same as killing that person). Others claim that such a distinction clearly points to regard for the intrinsic value of human life. Ramsey[43] argues that in the context of neonatal medicine, "letting die" actually connotes "benign neglect." No moral distinction can be made between this neglect—presumably taken as an act of beneficence—and euthanasia. He states that the "benign neglect of defective infants—who are not dying, who cannot themselves refuse treatment, who are most in need of human help—is the same as directly dispatching them: involuntary euthanasia," a course he clearly rejects.

This argument is changed dramatically, however, when the neonate is determined to be dying and decisions to withhold further treatment have been made. In such an instance, taking the step of active euthanasia (i.e., actively doing something to effect the neonate's death) is considered by some to be more beneficent and nonmaleficent than purporting to enact passive euthanasia, or letting the neonate die. Such advocates claim that by "letting nature take its course" one simply avoids the difficult decision-making process for convenience, yet does not ensure imminent death—and may even prolong suffering.[26,56]

Another model in which this dichotomy can be seen is that of the technical, and sometimes moral, imperative to intervene within the NICU. Some individuals, as well as certain religious groups, believe that it is imperative to implement any means to treat patients. They call on technical, religious, and ethical arguments to support the prolongation of life.

In contrast, many individuals favor the rejection of the technical or moral imperative to preserve life at all costs. Vaux[52] reflects this view by calling for the withdrawal of our dependence on perceived technical, legal, and economic necessities and accepting an ethic that "honors the intrinsic value of newborns, the crucial capacities and needs of the family and community, and the finality of God."

Either of the above models may lead one to

consider the distinctions between what is termed the "sanctity of life" (holding life and its preservation in all circumstances as the preeminent condition or rule), and the "quality of life" (realizing or assigning value to life based on the conditions in which it will exist or by its possessing certain, characteristically human, attributes). Either line of reasoning can lead to acceptance or rejection of the idea of withholding or withdrawing treatment or life support. And either will conclude that society can or cannot apply certain standards that would justify actively seeking to bring about a dying newborn's death.

Some would advocate selective euthanasia for suffering neonates in whom treatment has been withheld or withdrawn, although this is certainly not the normal process in this country. It is also entangled with legal considerations, uncertain consequences, and slippery moral slopes. Further discussion in this area is sure to come in the next decade.

ETHICS COMMITTEES AND INFANT BIOETHICS COMMITTEES

When disputes over treatment decisions arise, it is preferable to keep the decision-making responsibility within the professional-patient relationship. In the vast majority of cases, members of the health care team and the parents do have the infant's best interests in mind. Yet, in view of the vast dimensions and difficulties of some of these decisions, many people may consult with an Infant Bioethics Committee (IBC). Where there is agreement about a treatment plan, the committee might be consulted for confirmation of that plan; where there is a dispute about a proposed course of treatment, the committee might be consulted for clarification of ethical principles, values, and various treatment options that would be consistent with ethical and legal standards.

The stimulus to the establishment of IBCs in the United States was the controversy over and death of Baby Doe in Bloomington, Indiana, when society (and government) became acutely aware of the moral issues surrounding what many

perceived to be wrongful nontreatment. This incident provided strong moral justification for committee review of infant cases, particularly when treatment is being withheld or withdrawn to effect the termination of life. The government, in response, proposed a series of regulations to monitor the medical treatment of handicapped newborns.* The most recent regulation is the Child Abuse Prevention and Treatment Act amendment[2] to protect disabled infants with life-threatening conditions from medical neglect. These guidelines, along with the recommendations of the American Academy of Pediatrics, encourage hospitals to create IBCs or to have access to one for consultation. "The Academy believes the creation of infant bioethical review committees constitutes a direct, effective and appropriate means of addressing the existing education and information gaps."[3] Members are necessarily from various disciplines and areas of expertise: physicians, nurses, lawyers, clergy, social workers, ethicists, administrators, and community representatives. It is intended that such an interdisciplinary group will represent both the practical knowledge that is crucial to total case management and the various values that enter into treatment decisions. Their purpose is to promote quality decisions regarding treatment of ill newborns.

Most decisions within hospitals carry ethical implications but are resolved through other channels (Table 25-4). Although IBCs and ethics committees are relatively new resources within hospitals, established to help resolve ethical conflicts within patient care decisions,[46] many hospitals now have them. The President's Commission concluded[39]:

When the benefits of therapy are less clear, an "ethics committee" or similar body might be designated to review the decision making process. This approach would ensure that an individual or group whose function is to promote good decision making reviews the

---

*The original statute stated that no handicapped individual could be discriminated against solely on the basis of handicap.[41] See also articles by Angell[5] and Victoroff.[54]

TABLE 25-4

Clinical Problems with Ethical Implications

PROBLEM	EXAMPLE
Quality assurance	Quality assurance committees
Prognosis determination	Quinlin case
Regulatory review	Baby Doe regulations
Clinical research	Human subjects committees
Legal review	Hospital counsel, risk management
Ethical consultation	Ethics committees and/or
Ethical education	infant bioethics
Hospital policies	committees

most difficult cases. Cases included in this category should certainly encompass those in which a decision to forego life-sustaining therapy has been proposed because of a physical or mental handicap, as well as cases where a dispute has arisen among caregivers and surrogates over the proper course of treatment.

IBCs are a resource for consultation and advice. They are not a decision-making body, although some groups are moving toward a consensus model. Different committees have different procedures.[18,27] Committee functions and responsibilities may include (1) offering counsel and ethical review in cases involving disabled infants, (2) educating hospital personnel and families of disabled infants with life-threatening conditions, (3) reviewing prospectively the components of federal and state guidelines regarding care and management of such infants, (4) reviewing retrospectively case management and any deviations from federal and state guidelines as they exist, and (5) developing any policy statements for the institution as they are appropriate or necessary. Typically, anyone involved in a particular case may request a consultation from the IBC.

The legal status of ethics committees and IBCs remains unclear. Much of the time an ethical solution is legal, and vice versa, though exceptions do exist. The legal liability of an ethics committee

was pronounced in a recent court case.[57] Since committee records can be used as evidence in litigation, some committees are keeping detailed records of case involvement, whereas others are not keeping any at all. Legal responsibility of all participants in case management and decision making is consistent with that of any surrogate. Although members of an ethics committee may not be making medical or legal decisions, they may be indicted on ethical advice they offer that significantly influences a patient's outcome.

"BABY DOE" REGULATIONS

The Child Abuse Prevention and Treatment Act amendment (1984),[2] more commonly known as the "Baby Doe" guidelines, considers medical neglect as a form of child abuse. Invoking these regulations requires that parents be accused of denying appropriate care for their child—a poor start for dialogue and problem solving.

The guidelines purport that "it is ethically and legally justified to withhold medical or surgical procedures which are clearly futile and will only prolong the act of dying."[41] They also require that everything reasonable be done to protect the disabled infant's life. There are three exceptions to the requirement that treatment, other than "appropriate nutrition, hydration and medication,"[41] must be provided to disabled infants. Exceptions, as determined by medical judgment, are[41]:

1. The infant is irreversibly comatose.
2. The provision of such treatment would merely prolong dying and would be futile in terms of the infant's survival.
3. The provision of such treatment would be virtually futile in terms of the infant's survival, and the treatment itself would be inhumane.

Federal guidelines deliberately specify that "quality of life" may not be considered in determining an exception.

In modern practice, until an accurate diagnosis and prognosis is determined, liveborn infants who might survive are resuscitated. In most instances it is deemed better to "err on the side of life" until appropriate evaluation is completed. If the infant can be stabilized, further decisions based on "reasonable medical judgment" are made. Ethically, legally, and practically speaking, treatment begun can be withdrawn.

Treatment should be attempted if it is clearly beneficial, possibly beneficial with minimal burden to the infant, or remotely beneficial but prognosis is fatal without it and it is in accordance with the parents' wishes. Treatment may be foregone if the infant is permanently comatose, treatment is clearly futile, or treatment is virtually futile and is unacceptably burdensome for the infant.

Perhaps most important, these guidelines advise hospitals to establish IBCs to offer counsel in those cases involving disabled infants with life-threatening conditions. If, after consultation with an IBC, treatment dispute persists, the state child protection professionals may need to be consulted. They may, if necessary, obtain temporary guardianship to seek court-ordered treatment of a disabled infant to ensure what the court determines to be humane and ethical treatment of that child.

SOCIAL ETHICS

Moral judgments made in the hospital setting do not occur in isolation from the larger social context of which institutions and individuals are a part. Such judgments can be considerably impacted on by prevailing social values and perspectives. Further, while decisions in the nursery generally are interpersonal in nature, they may also have significant impact on the larger community. Technologic advancements have enabled some severely disabled infants to survive and grow, albeit with mental and physical handicaps. These persons often require numerous hospitalizations and costly rehabilitation. Society frequently bears the financial, physical, and social costs of these individuals.

Social ethics reflects on the sociocultural aspects of human life. It considers how individuals as moral agents are accountable for their behavior in social structures and public policy issues. It can also refer to shared patterns of moral judgment. Moreover, it focuses on how social contexts influence individual moral behavior and what the range of moral responsibility is.

In a pluralistic society such as ours, there is no one social ethic. Some believe in rugged individualism, others in equality of opportunity, worth, and treatment; others believe that we bear mutual responsibility for one another. An underlying concern of most socioethical systems is concern for both the individual and the common good.

In NICUs bioethics and social ethics converge. Treatment decisions have social implications; societal values influence treatment decisions. Yet, rarely is a paradox of values so apparent as in the treatment of disabled infants. No matter how poor an infant's prognosis is at birth, our society seems determined to treat virtually every newborn with whatever technology is available at whatever cost (emotional, physical, or financial). While federal guidelines advocate the use of "reasonable medical judgment" in treating these infants, these regulations may be interpreted as increasing the obligation to treat. Through the government, society expresses the determination to treat; yet, societal commitment to long-term care of these patients and families is wholly insufficient. Public funds for such care have typically been reduced, while urgency for treatment of these patients has increased. The values inherent in our public policy decisions regarding initial and long-term treatment are curiously disparate.

After comparing the health care and social policies of the United States with the seemingly more equitable policies of Great Britain and Sweden, Young[58] concludes, "We need to strive for a better balance between aggressive treatment in the neonatal intensive care units initially, and the resources currently allocated for the long-term care of the disabled." Such a balance might include being more selective about aggressive treatment, as well as learning more about prematurity and trying to prevent it. "To the extent that society fails to ensure that seriously ill newborns have the opportunity for an adequate level of continuing care, its moral authority to intervene on behalf of a newborn whose life is in jeopardy is compromised."[58]

PSYCHOLOGIC IMPACT OF ETHICAL DECISION MAKING

The psychologic impact of ethical decision making must not be neglected or negated, since in any given clinical situation human life is at stake. Philosophical constructs, when applied, must take into consideration human realities and capacities to tolerate and integrate the awesome responsibilities concerning life and death issues. What parents would not be overwhelmed by their severely disabled infant? The prospect of lifetime rehabilitation? The reality or prospect of suffering? The prospect of death of their newborn?

Parents play a vital role in the decision-making process because they, along with the infant, are the most affected. No matter what their religious or sociocultural background, almost all parents experience shock and grief over their disabled infant, or even over the need for intensive care. They deal with this in better and worse ways. For many parents the ability to participate in ethical decision making is impaired while they are in such an acute stage of shock. Usually, prenatal diagnosis of anomalies gives parents time to adjust to their child's condition before birth and/or before decisions have to be made. This adjustment time can be most valuable. To participate in ethical decision making, particularly decisions about withholding or withdrawing treatment, parents must have achieved some degree of emotional reorganization and acceptance. Staff assistance in helping them move from emotional disorganization to reorganization is crucial to further decisions that need to be made. At this point, parents may be better able to absorb medical data, ethical values, and principles. While there may not be a theoretical difference between withholding and withdrawing treatment, there is a large emotional difference. The sound clinician, as well as the ethicist, must be sensitive to both.

As noted in Chapters 22 and 23, there is a wide range of parental reactions to premature and seriously ill newborns. The grief stages have been identified.[11,28] Where parents are in their adaptation will affect their decision-making capacities. For instance, a mother's desire to treat even the most severely disabled child may evidence her denial (or misunderstanding) of her child's condition, rather than a sanctity-of-life ethic. The already grief-stricken parents are faced with an overlay of agonizing decisions about letting their child die.

Choices about treatment and nontreatment do affect the grieving process. Questions such as "Am I just prolonging suffering by keeping her alive?" are countered by, "Am I not giving her a chance and playing God by allowing her to die?" Duff and Campbell[12] report families experiencing "a normal mourning for their losses" after allowing their seriously ill infants to die. What remains for many parents are doubts that their choice was correct. For some, decisions based on certain religious principles or other value criteria offer moral justification of behavior that assists in the mourning process. For others, the justification may be logically, but not emotionally, clear. In these instances grieving can become more complex and difficult.

A valuable role of an IBC may be to offer input into, if not confirmation of, the parents' decision in a way that helps to allay guilt that can interrupt normal grieving. Ethics, while at once highly theoretical and intellectual, must consider that the situations with which it most intimately deals are highly emotional. For parents, the psychologic trauma will impact on their ethical considerations, and ethical decisions will have further psychologic impact.

A real value of an interdisciplinary health care team is the particular attention paid to the many complex aspects of a patient's living and dying. Many treatment decisions have major individual and social ramifications. When parents are facing the death of their child, the entire team may be involved in assisting them. Nurses and physicians, social workers, clergy, and psychologists may all be intimately involved with monitoring the patient's comfort level and deteriorating course, and with comforting grieving parents. Baptisms (when appropriate) and, especially, funerals are important ritualistic ways of organizing the meaning of the traumatic event. The entire staff should encourage parents to offer all that they can to their dying child. They should provide maximum comfort for the patient and maximum support to the family. Helping patients and families cope with death is a privilege. It can be personally and professionally satisfying, and ultimately immeasurably helpful to everyone involved, to enter emotionally into this process. Often care of the living means care of the dying.

Psychologic trauma and impact should also be recognized among the health care team, since their concern and involvement with the infant is usually significant. Helping someone through the dying process can be a traumatic, though rewarding, experience. In such instances professionals may agree with the decision (hopefully the par-

ents') to withhold or withdraw treatment. Professionals may also disagree with the decision but may place a higher value on the parents' autonomy to decide than on the decision itself. Respecting this, they may abide by the parents' wishes for their child. No one should be forced to compromise personal or professional integrity, however, and in such cases where one's ethical integrity is being violated, the case may be transferred. Preferably, professionals can learn about the range of ethically defensible options and can support the parents in choices different from their own.

IMPACT OF NEW TECHNOLOGIES IN PERINATAL-NEONATAL MEDICINE

There are a number of technologies and methodologies in reproductive medicine, perinatology, and neonatology that are currently in use, under study, or being developed that may pose questions of ethical import. The issues in Table 25-5 are offered in an effort to raise the level of awareness among health care providers and to stimulate in-

---

TABLE 25-5

Advances in Perinatal Care and Moral/Ethical Implications

Fetal cell implants

What, if any, research and experimentation of fetuses/abortuses is acceptable?

Do we have moral obligations to the fetus? The mother? The recipient of fetal tissues?

Is proxy consent necessary? From the mother? From whom?

Is it problematic that abortion is used to meet this end?

What abusive potentials exist for obtaining fetal tissues in this manner?

Anencephalic infants as transplantation donors

Are such infants brain dead? Born dying?

Should the definition of brain death be changed for these infants?

Are such infants "persons?" If personhood is denied, what does this say about the value of the pregnancy (or subsequent pregnancies)?

Does such an infant have any "rights" to health care for its brief life?

Is prolonging such an infant's life or arranging for transplantation simply "using" the infant, leading us to do what ordinarily would not be done in order to attain a "justifiable" end?

What abusive potentials exist for such a practice?

Surfactant replacement therapy for respiratory distress syndrome

Which infants should receive this therapy? Will it be accessible to all such infants?

What should such a therapy cost, considering the potential for decreasing lengths and costs of hospitalization?

High-frequency ventilation and extracorporeal membrane oxygenation

Which infants should receive these therapies?

How should these scarce resources be equitably allocated and utilized? Should infants suffering multiorgan system dysfunction and having questionable or grim prognoses receive such therapy to prolong life?

quiry into the moral and ethical appropriateness of these advances and their consequences for individuals and our society. Should parents be told of these advances? Should parents be offered these advances regardless of their experimental nature? Because we have these new technologies and methodologies, are we obligated to use them?

We can attempt to answer these and countless other questions by understanding what ethical principles they address or involve and by looking at what individual as well as social values are at stake. In doing so, we can apply the ethical work-up in an effort to come up with rationally defensible solutions to these continually vexing issues.

CONCLUSION

The intent of the present chapter has been to provide a basic overview of bioethics within the context of the NICU. It is important for neonatal clinicians to develop an understanding of their own values and a sensitivity to the values of others. NICUs function in the real world, with real patients and real problems, and despite the best efforts and intentions, conflicts of values are inevitable. It is therefore essential to develop and maintain effective processes for resolving ethical conflict.

The history of neonatal care has been, and continues to be, one of rapid technologic development, imposing new confrontations in values. We believe that professional development of ethical as well as clinical skills will help to meet these ongoing challenges.

GLOSSARY

Best interest A standard used to determine the validity of proxy consent in decision making. Treatment decisions are based on what most "reasonable persons" would assess as the burdens and benefits that would likely accompany the child's life. This standard leads clinicians to seek treatment, resulting in a "net benefit" to the child.

Deontology (formalism) A theory of ethics that holds that the moral rightness of an act must be decided totally independent of the consequences of that act. Duty is independent of consequential good,

and certain moral commands (rules) operative under fundamental principles must be obeyed under all circumstances.

Dilemma A situation that exists when more than one possible course of action exists and differing values are held for each possible course of action by the parties involved. Moral dilemmas arise when an appeal to moral considerations can be made for opposing courses of action; when it is apparent that an act can be considered both morally right *and* morally wrong and that on moral grounds there is a sense of "ought" *and* "ought not" to perform the act.

Double effect A principle, often viewed within the larger context of nonmaleficence, that claims that an act having a harmful effect is not always morally prohibited. Any harmful effect of an act is viewed as indirect, unintended, or simply as a foreseen effect but not as the direct and intended effect (e.g., if an act, as in treatment, brings about death, it is not always to be prohibited). Four conditions are often given to clarify this principle for specific acts:
1. The action itself must be "good" or at least morally indifferent.
2. The agent must intend only the good effect and not the evil effect.
3. The evil effect cannot be a means to the good effect.
4. There should be a favorable balance between the good and evil effects of the action.

Ethics The study of moral conduct, systems, and ideas.

Moral rules Rules that are founded or justified by principles and state that actions of a certain kind ought (or ought not) to be done because they are right (or wrong).

Morals The conduct and codes of conduct of individuals and groups. Three popular uses exist: (1) in contrast to immoral (right versus wrong), (2) in contrast to nonmoral (actions that have no bearing or question of right and wrong), and (3) "morals"—the behavior pattern of an individual or group.

Paternalism The principle and practice of ruling like a "father." This typically presupposes benevolence and making decisions for others—overriding of a person's wishes or actions (autonomy) for beneficent reasons.

Personhood A characteristic that may be used in decision making that is based on the idea that possession of certain capabilities (typically higher brain functions such as consciousness, rationality, perception of space and time, and the ability to communicate) constitute personhood; and that only "persons" have any moral claim to life, treatment, etc.

Prima facie   A term that qualifies a "right," "wrong," "duty," or "obligation," indicating a first appearance or self-evident/apparent condition of facts. Prima facie duties, for example, are those that are binding in all circumstances except when they are in conflict with equal or stronger duties.

"Proxy" decision maker (surrogate)   A designated person who will act on behalf of an individual who is incapable of making decisions.

Reasonable person standard   A standard by which the validity of informed consent is measured. Information to be disclosed is determined by referring to a hypothetical "reasonable person" and determining whether such a person would see any significance in the information in assessing risk and deciding whether to submit to a treatment or procedure.

Rights   Those things to which people have a just claim; a claim to a condition to which the individual is entitled.

Substituted judgment   A standard used to determine the validity of proxy consent in decision making. Treatment decisions are based on what has been determined to be that choice an incompetent person would make in a given situation (if that person were actually competent). This standard attempts to uphold patient autonomy even in the incompetent.

Utilitarianism (consequentialism)   A theory in ethics that holds that an act is right when it brings about a good outcome for the greatest number of people, upholds the greatest balance of "good" over "evil," and seeks to effect "utility" or the most useful outcome. "The end justifies the means." This may be developed into rules that are adhered to in order to maximize benefits and minimize harms (rule utilitarian) or simply appealed to in individual actions (act utilitarian).

Values   Those things that have worth or are desirable to an individual or group.

Virtues   A habit, disposition, or trait that a person may possess or aspire to possess; specifically, a moral virtue upholds what is morally right or praiseworthy.

Wrongful birth   A legal action (a tort suit) sought by the parents of a handicapped child in which the claim is made that such handicaps are the result of the defendant's negligence.

Wrongful life   A legal action (typically a tort suit) sought by a handicapped child in which the claim is made that birth (and the ensuing life) resulted from the defendant's negligence.

REFERENCES

1. Aiken HD: Reason and conduct, New York, 1978, Alfred A Knopf, Inc.
2. Amendments to the Child Abuse Prevention and Treatment Act, 98 Stat 1749, 1984; 45 CFR PART 1340, April 15, 1985.
3. American Academy of Pediatrics: Components of the American Academy of Pediatrics on proposed rule regarding nondiscrimination on the basis of handicap relating to health care for handicapped infants, Undated manuscript.
4. American Hospital Association: Report of the Special Committee on Biomedical Ethics: Values in conflict: resolving ethical issues in hospital care, Chicago, 1985, American Hospital Publishing, Inc.
5. Angell M: The Baby Doe rules, N Engl J Med 314:642, 1986 (editorial).
6. Arras JD: Toward an ethic of ambiguity, Hastings Cent Rep 14:25, 1984.
7. Beauchamp T and Childress J: Principles of biomedical ethics, ed 2, New York, 1983, Oxford University Press.
8. Beauchamp T and McCulloch L: Medical ethics: the moral responsibility of physicians, Englewood Cliffs, NJ, 1984, Prentice-Hall, Inc.
9. Brody H: Ethical decisions in medicine, Boston, 1981, Little, Brown & Co, Inc.
10. Caplan AL and Murray TH, editors: Which babies shall live? Humanistic dimensions of the care of imperiled newborns, Clifton, NJ, 1985, Humana Press.
11. Cohen M: Ethical issues in neonatal intensive care: familial concerns. In Jonsen A and Garland M, editors: Ethics of newborn intensive care, San Francisco, 1976, University of California.
12. Duff R and Campbell AGM: Moral and ethical dilemmas in the special care nursery, N Engl J Med 289:890, 1973.
13. Eisenberg L: The human nature of human nature, Science 176:123, 1972.
14. Engelhardt HT Jr: Viability and use of the fetus. In Bondeson WB et al, editors: Abortion and the status of the fetus, Dordrecht, Netherlands, 1983, D Reidel Publishing Co.
15. Engelhardt HT Jr: Ethical issues in aiding the death of young children. In Mappes TA and Zembaty JS, editors: Biomedical ethics, ed 2, New York, 1986, McGraw-Hill Book Co.
16. Engelhardt HT Jr: The foundations of bioethics, New York, 1986, Oxford University Press.
17. Firth R: Ethical absolutism and the ideal observer, Philosophy Phenomenol Res 12:317, 1952.

18. Fleischman A and Murray T: Ethics committees for infants Doe? Hastings Cent Rep 13:5, 1983.

19. Fletcher J: Humanhood: essays in biomedical ethics, Buffalo, NY, 1979, Prometheus Books.

20. Francoeur RT: From then to now. In Harris CC and Snowden F, editors: Bioethical frontiers in perinatal intensive care, Natchitoches, La, 1985, Northwestern State University Press.

21. Greene R: What price life? Forbes 140(5):42, 1987.

22. Gustafson JM: Mongolism, parental desires, and the right to life, Perspect Biol Med 19:247, 1976.

23. Hart HLA: Law, liberty and morality, Stanford, Calif, 1963, Stanford University Press.

24. Jameton A: Nursing practice—the ethical issues, Englewood Cliffs, NJ, 1984, Prentice-Hall, Inc.

25. Koops BL, Morgan LJ, and Battaglia FC: Neonatal mortality risk in relation to birth weight and gestational age: update, J Pediatr 101:969, 1982.

26. Kuhse H and Singer P: Should the baby live? New York, 1985, Oxford University Press.

27. Leiken S: Children's hospital ethics committees, Am J Dis Child 141:954, 1987.

28. Lindemann E: Symptomatology and management of acute grief, Am J Psychiatry 101:141, 1944.

29. Lorber J: Results of treatment of myelomeningocele, Dev Med Child Neurol 13:279, 1971.

30. Lorber J: Early results of selective treatment of spina bifida cystica, Br Med J 4:201, 1973.

31. Lyon J: Playing god in the nursery, New York, 1985, WW Norton & Co, Inc.

32. Mappes E and Kroeger J: Ethical dilemmas for nurses: physician's orders versus patient's rights. In Mappes TA and Zembaty JS, editors: Biomedical ethics, ed 2, New York, 1986, McGraw-Hill Book Co.

33. Mitchell C: Care of severely impaired infant raises ethical issues, Am Nurse 16:9, 1984.

34. Neonatal intensive care for low birth weight infants: costs and effectiveness, December 1987, Health Technology Case Study 38, Congress of the United States, Office of Technology Assessment, Washington, DC, US Government Printing Office.

35. Pellegrino ED: The anatomy of clinical ethical judgments in perinatology, Semin Perinatol 11:202, 1987.

36. Pellegrino ED and Thomasma DC: A philosophical basis of medical practice: toward a philosophical ethic of healing professions, New York, 1981, Oxford University Press.

37. Pemberton PJ: The tiniest babies—can we afford them? Med J Aust 146:63, 1987.

38. Pless JE: The story of Baby Doe, N Engl J Med 309:663, 1983.

39. President's Commission for the Study of Ethical Problems in Medicine and Biomedical and Behavioral Research: Deciding to forego life-sustaining treatment, Washington, DC, 1983.

40. The price of life: ethics and economics, Report of the Task Force on the Affordability of New Technology and Highly Specialized Care: Life at any price? Minneapolis, Minnesota, Coalition on Health Care Costs 7:41, 1984.

41. Proposed Rule 45 CFR Part 84: Nondiscrimination on the basis of handicap relating to health care for handicapped infants, Fed Register 48(129), July 5, 1983. Repealed 1986.

42. *In re* Quinlan, 70 NJ 10, 355 A 2d 647, cost devised, 429 US 922, 1976.

43. Ramsey P: Ethics at the edges of life, New Haven, Conn, 1978, Yale University Press.

44. Rhoden NK: Treating Baby Doe: the ethics of uncertainty, Hastings Cent Rep 16:34, 1986.

45. Robertson JA: Involuntary euthanasia of defective newborns. In Mappes TA and Zembaty JS, editors: Biomedical ethics, ed 2, New York, 1986, McGraw-Hill Book Co.

46. Ross JW: Handbook for hospital ethics committees, Chicago, 1986, American Hospital Publishing, Inc.

47. Shelp EE: Born to die? Deciding the fate of critically ill newborns, New York, 1986, The Free Press.

48. Shurtleff D: Care of the myelodysplastic patient. In Green M and Haggerty R, editors: Ambulatory pediatrics, Philadelphia, 1986, WB Saunders Co.

49. Siegler M: Ethics committees: decisions by bureaucracy, Hastings Cent Rep 16:22, 1986.

50. Thomasma DC: Training in medical ethics: an ethical workup, Forum Med •:33, 1978.

51. Tooley M: Abortion and infanticide, New York, 1983, Oxford University Press.

52. Vaux KL: Ethical issues in caring for tiny infants, Clin Perinatol 13:477, 1986.

53. Veatch RM: Emphasis on values prompting a change in medical practice, Kennedy Inst Ethics Newsletter 1:1, 1987.

54. Victoroff M: The ballad of Baby Doe: parental discretion or medical neglect? Prim Care 13:271, 1986.

55. Weil WB: Issues associated with treatment and nontreatment decisions, Am J Dis Child 138:519, 1984.

56. Weir RF: Selective nontreatment of handicapped newborns, New York, 1984, Oxford University Press.

57. Wolf S: Ethics committees in the courts, Hastings Cent Rep 16:9, 1986.

58. Young EWD: Caring for disabled infants, Hastings Cent Rep 13:15, 1983.

59. Zachary R: Ethical and social aspects of treatment of spina bifida, Lancet 2:274, 1968.

Index